# Lecture Notes in Artificial Intelligence        8265

## Subseries of Lecture Notes in Computer Science

### LNAI Series Editors

Randy Goebel
  *University of Alberta, Edmonton, Cana.*
Yuzuru Tanaka
  *Hokkaido University, Sapporo, Japan*
Wolfgang Wahlster
  *DFKI and Saarland University, Saarbrück    ...uny*

### LNAI Founding Series Editor

Joerg Siekmann
  *DFKI and Saarland University, Saarbrücken, Germany*

Félix Castro   Alexander Gelbukh
Miguel González (Eds.)

# Advances in Artificial Intelligence and Its Applications

12th Mexican International Conference
on Artificial Intelligence, MICAI 2013
Mexico City, Mexico, November 24-30, 2013
Proceedings, Part I

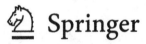 Springer

Volume Editors

Félix Castro
Universidad Autónoma del Estado de Hidalgo
Hidalgo, Mexico
E-mail: fcastro@uaeh.reduaeh.mx

Alexander Gelbukh
Centro de Investigación en Computación
Instituto Politécnico Nacional
Mexico City, Mexico
E-mail: gelbukh@gelbukh.com

Miguel González
Tecnológico de Monterrey
Estado de México, Mexico
E-mail: mgonza@itesm.mx

ISSN 0302-9743                          e-ISSN 1611-3349
ISBN 978-3-642-45113-3                  e-ISBN 978-3-642-45114-0
DOI 10.1007/978-3-642-45114-0
Springer Heidelberg New York Dordrecht London

Library of Congress Control Number: 2013953891

CR Subject Classification (1998): I.2.1, I.2.3-11, I.4, I.5.1-4, J.3, H.4.1-3, F.2.2, H.3.3-5, H.5.3

LNCS Sublibrary: SL 7 – Artificial Intelligence

*Typesetting:* Camera-ready by author, data conversion by Scientific Publishing Services, Chennai, India

Printed on acid-free paper

Springer is part of Springer Science+Business Media (www.springer.com)

# Preface

The Mexican International Conference on Artificial Intelligence (MICAI) is a yearly international conference series organized by the Mexican Society of Artificial Intelligence (SMIA) since 2000. MICAI is a major international AI forum and the main event in the academic life of the country's growing AI community.

MICAI conferences publish high-quality papers in all areas of AI and its applications. The proceedings of the previous MICAI events have been published by Springer in its *Lecture Notes in Artificial Intelligence* (LNAI) series, vols. 1793, 2313, 2972, 3789, 4293, 4827, 5317, 5845, 6437, 6438, 7094, 7095, 7629, and 7630. Since its foundation in 2000, the conference has been growing in popularity and improving in quality.

The proceedings of MICAI 2013 are published in two volumes. The first volume, *Advances in Artificial Intelligence and Its Applications*, contains 45 papers structured into five sections:

- Logic and Reasoning
- Knowledge-Based Systems and Multi-Agent Systems
- Natural Language Processing
- Machine Translation
- Bioinformatics and Medical Applications

The second volume, *Advances in Soft Computing and Its Applications*, contains 45 papers structured into eight sections:

- Evolutionary and Nature-Inspired Metaheuristic Algorithms
- Neural Networks and Hybrid Intelligent Systems
- Fuzzy Systems
- Machine Learning and Pattern Recognition
- Data Mining
- Computer Vision and Image Processing
- Robotics, Planning and Scheduling
- Emotion Detection, Sentiment Analysis, and Opinion Mining

The books will be of interest for researchers in all areas of AI, students specializing.in related topics, and for the general public interested in recent developments in AI.

The conference received 284 submissions by 678 authors from 45 countries: Algeria, Argentina, Australia, Austria, Bangladesh, Belgium, Brazil, Bulgaria, Canada, Chile, China, Colombia, Cuba, Czech Republic, Egypt, Finland, France, Germany, Hungary, India, Iran, Ireland, Italy, Japan, Mauritius, Mexico, Morocco, Pakistan, Peru, Poland, Portugal, Russia, Singapore, South Africa, South Korea, Spain, Sweden, Switzerland, Thailand, Tunisia, Turkey, UK, Ukraine,

Uruguay, and USA. Of these submissions, 85 papers were selected for publication in these two volumes after a peer-reviewing process carried out by the international Program Committee. In particular, the acceptance rate was 29.9%.

MICAI 2013 was honored by the presence of such renowned experts as Ildar Batyrshin of the IMP, Mexico; Erik Cambria of the National University of Singapore; Amir Hussain, University of Stirling, UK; Newton Howard, Massachusetts Institute of Technology, USA; and Maria Vargas-Vera, Universidad Adolfo Ibáñez, Chile, who gave excellent keynote lectures. The technical program of the conference also featured tutorials presented by Roman Barták (Czech Republic), Ildar Batyrshin (Mexico), Erik Cambria (Singapore), Alexander Garcia Castro (Germany), Alexander Gelbukh (Mexico), Newton Howard (USA), Ted Pedersen (USA), Obdulia Pichardo and Grigori Sidorov (Mexico), Nelishia Pillay (South Africa), and Maria Vargas-Vera (Chile). Four workshops were held jointly with the conference: the First Workshop on Hispanic Opinion Mining and Sentiment Analysis, the 6th Workshop on Hybrid Intelligent Systems, the 6th Workshop on Intelligent Learning Environments, and the First International Workshop on Semantic Web Technologies for PLM.

In particular, in addition to regular papers, the volumes contain five invited papers by keynote speakers and their collaborators:

- "Association Measures and Aggregation Functions," by Ildar Batyrshin
- "An Introduction to Concept-Level Sentiment Analysis," by Erik Cambria
- "The Twin Hypotheses. Brain Code and the Fundamental Code Unit: Towards Understanding the Computational Primitive Elements of Cortical Computing," by Newton Howard
- "Towards Reduced EEG Based Brain-Computer Interfacing for Mobile Robot Navigation," by Mufti Mahmud and Amir Hussain
- "Challenges in Ontology Alignment and Solution to the Contradictory Evidence Problem," by Maria Vargas-Vera and Miklos Nagy

The authors of the following papers received the Best Paper Award on the basis of the paper's overall quality, significance, and originality of the reported results:

| | |
|---|---|
| 1st place: | "A Bayesian and Minimum Variance Technique for Arterial Lumen Segmentation in Ultrasound Imaging," by Sergio Rogelio Tinoco-Martínez, Felix Calderon, Carlos Lara-Alvarez, and Jaime Carranza-Madrigal (Mexico) |
| 2nd place: | "The Best Genetic Algorithm I. A Comparative Study of Structurally Different Genetic Algorithms," by Angel Kuri-Morales and Edwin Aldana-Bobadilla (Mexico) |
| | "The Best Genetic Algorithm II. A Comparative Study of Structurally Different Genetic Algorithms," by Angel Kuri-Morales, Edwin Aldana-Bobadilla, and Ignacio López-Peña (Mexico) |

3$^{rd}$ place:    "A POS Tagger for Social Media Texts Trained on Web Comments," by Melanie Neunerdt, Michael Reyer, and Rudolf Mathar (Germany)[1]

The authors of the following paper selected among all papers of which the first author was a full-time student, excluding the papers listed above, received the Best Student Paper Award:

1$^{st}$ place:    "A Massive Parallel Cellular GPU Implementation of Neural Network to Large Scale Euclidean TSP," by Hongjian Wang, Naiyu Zhang, and Jean-Charles Créput (France)

We want to thank all the people involved in the organization of this conference. In the first place, the authors of the papers published in this book: It is their research work that gives value to the book and to the work of the organizers. We thank the track chairs for their hard work, and the Program Committee members and additional reviewers for their great effort spent on reviewing the submissions.

We are grateful to Dr. Salvador Vega y León, the Rector General of the Universidad Autónoma Metropolitana (UAM), Dr. Romualdo López Zárate, the Rector of the UAM Azcapotzalco, Dr. Luis Enrique Noreña Franco, Director of the Fundamental Science and Engineering Division, M.Sc. Rafaela Blanca Silva López, Head of the Systems Department, M.Sc. Roberto Alcántara Ramírez, Head of the Electronics Department, and Dr. David Elizarraraz Martínez, Head of the Fundamental Science Department, for their invaluable support of MICAI and for providing the infrastructure for the keynote talks, tutorials and workshops. We are also grateful to the personnel of UAM Azcapotzalco for their warm hospitality and hard work, as well as for their active participation in the organization of this conference. We greatly appreciate the generous sponsorship provided by the Mexican Government via the Museo Nacional de Antropología, Instituto Nacional de Antropología e Historia (INAH).

We are deeply grateful to the conference staff and to all members of the local Organizing Committee headed by Dr. Oscar Herrera Alcántara. We gratefully acknowledge the support received from the following projects: WIQ-EI (Web Information Quality Evaluation Initiative, European project 269180), PICCO10-120 (ICYT, Mexico City Government), and CONACYT-DST (India) project "Answer Validation through Textual Entailment." The entire submission, reviewing, and selection process, as well as preparation of the proceedings, was supported for free by the EasyChair system (www.easychair.org). Last but not least, we are grateful to the staff at Springer for their patience and help in the preparation of this volume.

October 2013                                          Félix Castro
                                               Alexander Gelbukh
                                          Miguel González Mendoza

---

[1] This paper is published in a special issue of the journal *Polibits* and not in this set of books.

# Conference Organization

MICAI 2013 was organized by the Mexican Society of Artificial Intelligence (SMIA, Sociedad Mexicana de Inteligencia Artificial) in collaboration with the Universidad Autónoma Metropolitana Azcapotzalco (UAM Azcapotzalco), Universidad Autónoma del Estado de Hidalgo (UAEH), Centro de Investigación en Computación del Instituto Politécnico Nacional (CIC-IPN), and Tecnológico de Monterrey (ITESM).

The MICAI series website is at: www.MICAI.org. The website of the Mexican Society of Artificial Intelligence, SMIA, is at: www.SMIA.org.mx. Contact options and additional information can be found on these websites.

## Conference Committee

| | |
|---|---|
| General Chairs: | Alexander Gelbukh, Grigori Sidorov, and Raúl Monroy |
| Program Chairs: | Félix Castro, Alexander Gelbukh, and Miguel González Mendoza |
| Workshop Chair: | Alexander Gelbukh |
| Tutorials Chair: | Félix Castro |
| Doctoral Consortium Chairs: | Miguel Gonzalez Mendoza and Antonio Marín Hernandez |
| Keynote Talks Chair: | Jesus A. Gonzalez |
| Publication Chair: | Ildar Batyrshin |
| Financial Chair: | Grigori Sidorov |
| Grant Chairs: | Grigori Sidorov and Miguel González Mendoza |
| Organizing Committee Chair: | Oscar Herrera Alcántara |

## Track Chairs

| | |
|---|---|
| Natural Language Processing | Sofia N. Galicia-Haro |
| Machine Learning and Pattern Recognition | Alexander Gelbukh |
| Data Mining | Félix Castro |
| Intelligent Tutoring Systems | Alexander Gelbukh |
| Evolutionary and Nature-Inspired Metaheuristic Algorithms | Oliver Schütze, Jaime Mora Vargas |
| Computer Vision and Image Processing | Oscar Herrera Alcántara |
| Robotics, Planning and Scheduling | Fernando Martin Montes-Gonzalez |
| Neural Networks and Hybrid Applications Intelligent Systems | Sergio Ledesma-Orozco |

Logic, Knowledge-Based Systems,
 Multi-Agent Systems and               Mauricio Osorio, Jose Raymundo
 Distributed AI                         Marcial Romero
Fuzzy Systems and Probabilistic
 Models in Decision Making             Ildar Batyrshin
Bioinformatics and Medical             Jesus A. Gonzalez, Felipe
 Applications                           Orihuela-Espina

## Program Committee

Ashraf Abdelraouf              Félix Castro
Juan-Carlos Acosta             Martine Ceberio
Teresa Alarcón                 Michele Ceccarelli
Alfonso Alba                   Gustavo Cerda Villafana
Fernando Aldana                Niladri Chatterjee
Rafik Aliev                    Edgar Chavez
Javad Alirezaie                Zhe Chen
Oscar Alonso Ramírez           David Claudio Gonzalez
Leopoldo Altamirano            Maria Guadalupe Cortina Januchs
Jose Amparo Andrade Lucio      Stefania Costantini
Jesus Angulo                   Nicandro Cruz-Ramirez
Annalisa Appice                Heriberto Cuayahuitl
Alfredo Arias-Montaño          Erik Cuevas
García Gamboa Ariel Lucien     Iria Da Cunha
Jose Arrazola                  Oscar Dalmau
Gustavo Arroyo                 Justin Dauwels
Serge Autexier                 Enrique De La Rosa
Gideon Avigad                  Maria De Marsico
Juan Gabriel Aviña Cervantes   Beatrice Duval
Victor Ayala Ramirez           Asif Ekbal
Sivaji Bandyopadhyay           Michael Emmerich
Maria Lucia Barrón-Estrada     Hugo Jair Escalante
Ildar Batyrshin                Ponciano Jorge Escamilla-Ambrosio
Albert Bifet                   Vlad Estivill-Castro
Bert Bredeweg                  Gibran Etcheverry
Ivo Buzon                      Eugene Ezin
Eduardo Cabal                  Denis Filatov
Felix Calderon                 Juan J. Flores
Hiram Calvo                    Pedro Flores
Nicoletta Calzolari            Andrea Formisano
Oscar Camacho Nieto            Anilu Franco
Sergio Daniel Cano Ortiz       Claude Frasson
Jose Luis Carballido           Juan Frausto-Solis
Mario Castelán                 Alfredo Gabaldon
Oscar Castillo                 Ruslan Gabbasov

Sofia N. Galicia-Haro
Ana Gabriela Gallardo-Hernández
Carlos Hugo Garcia Capulin
Ma. de Guadalupe Garcia Hernandez
Arturo Garcia Perez
Alexander Gelbukh
Onofrio Gigliotta
Pilar Gomez-Gil
Eduardo Gomez-Ramirez
Arturo Gonzalez
Jesus A. Gonzalez
Miguel Gonzalez
José Joel González Barbosa
Miguel Gonzalez Mendoza
Felix F. Gonzalez-Navarro
Efren Gorrostieta
Carlos Gracios
Monique Grandbastien
Christian Grimme
De Ita Luna Guillermo
Joaquin Gutierrez
D. Gutiérrez
Rafael Guzman Cabrera
Hartmut Haehnel
Dongfeng Han
Jin-Kao Hao
Yasunari Harada
Antonio Hernandez
Donato Hernandez Fusilier
Eva Hernandez Gress
J.A. Hernandez Servin
Oscar Herrera
Dieter Hutter
Pablo H. Ibarguengoytia
Mario Alberto Ibarra Manzano
Oscar Gerardo Ibarra Manzano
Rodolfo Ibarra-Orozco
Berend Jan Van Der Zwaag
Héctor Jiménez Salazar
W. Lewis Johnson
Laetitia Jourdan
Pinar Karagoz
Timoleon Kipouros
Olga Kolesnikova
Konstantinos Koutroumbas

Vladik Kreinovich
Angel Kuri-Morales
James Lam
Ricardo Landa
Dario Landa-Silva
Reinhard Langmann
Adriana Lara
Bruno Lara
Yulia Ledeneva
Sergio Ledesma Orozco
Yoel Ledo
Juan Carlos Leyva Lopez
Derong Liu
Rocio Alfonsina Lizarraga Morales
Aurelio Lopez
Omar Lopez
Virgilio Lopez
Juan Manuel Lopez Hernandez
Gladys Maestre
Tanja Magoc
Claudia Manfredi
Stephane Marchand-Maillet
Jose Raymundo Marcial Romero
Antonio Marin Hernandez
Luis Martí
Ricardo Martinez
Rene Alfredo Martinez Celorio
Francisco Martínez-Álvarez
José Fco. Martínez-Trinidad
Jerzy Martyna
Ruth Ivonne Mata Chavez
María Auxilio Medina Nieto
R. Carolina Medina-Ramirez
Jorn Mehnen
Patricia Melin
Ivan Vladimir Meza Ruiz
Efren Mezura
Mikhail Mikhailov
Vicente Milanés
Sabino Miranda-Jiménez
Dieter Mitsche
Joseph Modayil
Luís Moniz Pereira
Raul Monroy
Fernando Montes

Héctor A. Montes
Fernando Martin Montes-Gonzalez
Manuel Montes-y-Gómez
Carlos Rubín Montoro Sanjose
Jaime Mora Vargas
Marco Antonio Morales Aguirre
Guillermo Morales-Luna
Masaki Murata
Michele Nappi
Juan Antonio Navarro Perez
Jesús Emeterio Navarro-Barrientos
Juan Carlos Nieves
Juan Arturo Nolazco Flores
Leszek Nowak
C. Alberto Ochoa-Zezatti
Ivan Olmos
Felipe Orihuela-Espina
Eber Enrique Orozco Guillén
Magdalena Ortiz
Mauricio Osorio
Helen Pain
Rodrigo Edgar Palacios Leyva
Vicente Parra
Mario Pavone
Ted Pedersen
Hayde Peregrina-Barreto
Héctor Pérez-Urbina
Alexey Petrovsky
Obdulia Pichardo-Lagunas
David Pinto
Carlos Adolfo Piña-García
Natalia Ponomareva
Volodymyr Ponomaryov
Joel Quintanilla Dominguez
Marco Antonio Ramos Corchado
Risto Rangel-Kuoppa
Luis Lorenzo Rascon Perez
Carolina Reta
Alberto Reyes
Orion Fausto Reyes-Galaviz
Carlos A. Reyes-Garcia
Bernardete Ribeiro
Alessandro Ricci
François Rioult
Erik Rodner

Arles Rodriguez
Horacio Rodriguez
Katia Rodriguez
Eduardo Rodriguez-Tello
Leandro Fermín Rojas Peña
Alejandro Rosales
Paolo Rosso
Horacio Rostro Gonzalez
Samuel Rota Bulò
Imre Rudas
Salvador Ruiz Correa
Marta Ruiz Costa-Jussa
Jose Ruiz Pinales
Leszek Rutkowski
Klempous Ryszard
Andriy Sadovnychyy
Abraham Sánchez López
Raul Enrique Sanchez Yañez
Guillermo Sanchez-Diaz
Antonio-José Sánchez-Salmerón
Jose Santos
Paul Scheunders
Oliver Schütze
Friedhelm Schwenker
J.C. Seck-Tuoh
Nikolay Semenov
Shahnaz Shahbazova
Oleksiy Shulika
Patrick Siarry
Grigori Sidorov
Gerardo Sierra
Bogdan Smolka
Jorge Solís
Elliot Soloway
Peter Sosnin
Humberto Sossa Azuela
Mu-Chun Su
Luis Enrique Sucar
Shiliang Sun
Salvatore Tabbone
Atsuhiro Takasu
Hugo Terashima
Miguel Torres Cisneros
Luz Abril Torres-Méndez
Genny Tortora

Gregorio Toscano-Pulido
Leonardo Trujillo
Fevrier Valdez
Edgar Vallejo
Antonio Vega Corona
Josue Velazquez
Francois Vialatte
Javier Vigueras
Manuel Vilares Ferro
Jordi Vitrià

Panagiotis Vlamos
Zhanshan Wang
Qinglai Wei
Cornelio Yáñez-Márquez
Iryna Yevseyeva
Alla Zaboleeva-Zotova
Ramon Zatarain
Zhigang Zeng
Claudia Zepeda Cortes

## Additional Reviewers

Roberto Alonso
Miguel Ballesteros
Somnath Banerjee
Jared Bernstein
Veronica Borja
Ulises Castro Peñaloza
Ning Chen
Santiago E. Conant-Pablos
Joana Costa
Victor Darriba
Agostino Dovier
Milagros Fernández Gavilanes
Santiago Fernández Lanza
Samuel González López
Braja Gopal Patra
Esteban Guerrero
Daniela Inclezan
Yusuf Kavurucu
Anup Kolya
Kow Kuroda
Pintu Lohar
Maricarmen Martinez

Alfonso Medina Urrea
Alev Mutlu
Fernando Orduña Cabrera
Santanu Pal
Yan Pengfei
Soujanya Poria
Gerardo Presbitero
Francisco Rangel
Juan Carlo Rivera Dueñas
Edgar Rodriguez
Mark Rosenstein
Nayat Sanchez-Pi
Alejandro Santoyo
Yasushi Tsubota
Nestor Velasco
Darnes Vilariño
Esaú Villatoro-Tello
Francisco Viveros Jiménez
Shiping Wen
Xiong Yang
Daisuke Yokomori

## Organizing Committee

Local Chair:                           Oscar Herrera Alcántara
Local Arrangements Chair:              R. Blanca Silva López
Finance Chair:                         Elena Cruz M.
Logistics Chair:                       Iris Iddaly Méndez Gurrola
Student Chair:                         Eric Rincón
International Liaison Chair:            Dr. Antonin Sebastien P.

# Table of Contents – Part I

## Logic and Reasoning

## Knowledge-Based Systems and Multi-Agent Systems

## Natural Language Processing

*Invited Paper:*

## Machine Translation

# Bioinformatics and Medical Applications

*Invited Paper:*

*Best Paper Award, First Place:*

# Table of Contents – Part II

## Evolutionary and Nature-Inspired Metaheuristic Algorithms

## Neural Networks and Hybrid Intelligent Systems

### Best Student Paper Award:

## Fuzzy Systems

### Invited Paper:

## Machine Learning and Pattern Recognition

## Data Mining

## Computer Vision and Image Processing

## Robotics, Planning and Scheduling

*Invited Paper:*

## Emotion Detection, Sentiment Analysis, and Opinion Mining

*Invited Paper:*

# Some Properties of Logic N-GLukG

Mauricio Osorio[1], José Luis Carballido[2], and Claudia Zepeda[2]

[1] Universidad de las Américas,
Sta. Catarina Mártir, Cholula, Puebla, México
osoriomauri@gmail.com
[2] Benemérita Universidad Autónoma de Puebla,
Facultad de Ciencias de la Computación, Puebla, México
{jlcarballido7,czepedac}@gmail.com

**Abstract.** We present an extension of GLukG, a logic that was introduced in [8] as a three-valued logic under the name of $G'_3$. GLukG is a paraconsistent logic defined in terms of 15 axioms, which serves as the formalism to define the p-stable semantics of logic programming. We introduce a new axiomatic system, N-GLukG, a paraconsistent logic that possesses strong negation. We use the 5-valued logic $N'_5$, which is a conservative extension of GLukG, to help us to prove that N-GLukG is an extension of GLukG. N-GLukG can be used as the formalism to define the p-stable semantics as well as the stable semantics.

**Keywords:** paraconsistent, knowledge representation semantics, logic programming semantics.

## 1 Introduction

The present work is a theoretical contribution to the study of logics. There are two main ways of defining logics, and different logics have different properties, which characterize the logics as members of certain important group. Classical logic has been the framework most mathematicians use when building their theories, as it counts among its theorems results that conform to our common sense, like the law of the excluded middle $a \lor \neg a$, the explosion principle $a \land \neg a \to b$, and the double negation equivalence $a \leftrightarrow \neg\neg a$ . Some other logics follow the more radical point of view advocated by Brouwer, who refuses to accept the universality of the law of the excluded middle: it is not valid to conclude that there exists an object $x$ such that not $P(x)$ from the negation of the proposition for all $x, P(x)$. From the point of view of these theories one must construct such an object. More recently, the development of computer sciences and the increasing need to automate human-like behavior have boosted the study of logics and semantics useful to model knowledge representation, in particular non-monotonic reasoning. Due to these trends the study of paraconsistent logics has become more relevant. Briefly speaking, following Béziau [1], a logic is paraconsistent if it has a unary connective $\neg$, which is paraconsistent in the sense that $a, \neg a \nvdash b$, and at the same time has enough strong properties to be called a negation.

F. Castro, A. Gelbukh, and M. González (Eds.): MICAI 2013, Part I, LNAI 8265, pp. 1–11, 2013.

There is no paraconsistent logic that is unanimously recognised as a good paraconsistent logic [1], and as result, there are different proposals for a definition of what a paraconsistent logic should be [2].

In this work we study a new paraconsistent logic called N-GLukG. N-GLukG has a strong negation besides having the native paraconsistent negation, and it is capable of expressing both, the p-stable and the stable semantics, these semantics have helped in the modeling of knowledge representation. With the help of the 5-valued logic $N_5'$ [5], we prove that N-GLukG is an extension of GLukG. Furthermore, N-GLukG can be used as the formalism to extend the p-stable semantics to a version that includes strong negation in a similar way as the stable semantics has been extended to include such a negation [7]. We prove that N-GLukG is sound with respect to $N_5'$, namely, every theorem in N-GLukG is a tautology in $N_5'$. We also show that not every tautology in $N_5'$ is a theorem in N-GLukG. We present a substitution theorem for N-GLukG and translate some other results from $N_5'$ to N-GLukG. We prove one of the main results, it is related to the theory of knowledge representation, and states that N-GLukG can express both the stable and the p-stable semantics. We explore the relation between N-GLukG and GLukG. This paper extends [9] by adding new theorems and presenting new proofs. In fact [5,9]and the current paper present the theory of new logics that extend Nelson logic N5 that have potential applications in Logic Programming and Non-Monotonic Resaoning.

Our paper is structured as follows. In section 2, we summarize some definitions and logics necessary to understand this paper. In section 3, we introduce a new logic that is an extension of a known logic, this new logic satisfies a substitution theorem, and can express the stable semantics as well as the p-stable semantics. Finally, in section 4, we present some conclusions.

## 2   Background

We present several logics that are useful to define and study the logic N-GLukG. We assume that the reader has some familiarity with basic logic such as chapter one in [6].

### 2.1   Syntax of Formulas

We consider a formal (propositional) language built from: an enumerable set $\mathcal{L}$ of elements called *atoms* (denoted $a$, $b$, $c$, ...); the binary connectives $\wedge$ (*conjunction*), $\vee$ (*disjunction*) and $\rightarrow$ (*implication*); and the unary connective $\neg$ (*negation*). Formulas (denoted $\alpha$, $\beta$, $\gamma$, ...) are constructed as usual by combining these basic connectives together with the help of parentheses.

We also use $\alpha \leftrightarrow \beta$ to abbreviate $(\alpha \rightarrow \beta) \wedge (\beta \rightarrow \alpha)$. It is useful to agree on some conventions to avoid the use of so many parentheses in writing formulas. This will make the reading of complicated expressions easier. First, we may omit the outer pair of parentheses of a formula. Second, the connectives are ordered as follows: $\neg$, $\wedge$, $\vee$, $\rightarrow$, and $\leftrightarrow$, and parentheses are eliminated according to the rule that, first, $\neg$ applies to the smallest formula following it, then $\wedge$ is to connect the smallest formulas surrounding it, and so on.

A *theory* is just a set of formulas and, in this paper, we only consider finite theories. Moreover, if $T$ is a theory, we use the notation $\mathcal{L}_T$ to stand for the set of atoms that occur in the theory $T$. A literal $l$ is either an atom or the negation of an atom.

## 2.2    Hilbert Style Proof Systems

One way of defining a logic is by means of a set of axioms together with the inference rule of Modus Ponens.

As examples we offer two important logics defined in terms of axioms, which are related to the logics we study later.

$C_\omega$ logic [3] is defined by the following set of axioms:

| | |
|---|---|
| **Pos1** | $a \to (b \to a)$ |
| **Pos2** | $(a \to (b \to c)) \to ((a \to b) \to (a \to c))$ |
| **Pos3** | $a \wedge b \to a$ |
| **Pos4** | $a \wedge b \to b$ |
| **Pos5** | $a \to (b \to (a \wedge b))$ |
| **Pos6** | $a \to (a \vee b)$ |
| **Pos7** | $b \to (a \vee b)$ |
| **Pos8** | $(a \to c) \to ((b \to c) \to (a \vee b \to c))$ |
| $C_\omega 1$ | $a \vee \neg a$ |
| $C_\omega 2$ | $\neg\neg a \to a$ |

The first eight axioms of the list define positive logic. Note that these axioms somewhat constraint the meaning of the $\to$, $\wedge$ and $\vee$ connectives to match our usual intuition. It is a well known result that in any logic satisfying axioms **Pos1** and **Pos2**, and with *modus ponens* as its unique inference rule, the *Deduction Theorem* holds [6].

## 2.3    Axiomatic Definition of GLukG

We present a Hilbert-style axiomatization of $G'_3$ that is a slight (equivalent) variant of the one presented in [8]. We present this logic, since it will be extended to a new logic called N-GLukG, which possesses a strong negation and is the main contribution of this work.

GLukG logic has four primitive logical connectives, namely $\mathcal{GL} := \{\to, \wedge, \vee, \neg\}$. *GLukG*-formulas are formulas built from these connectives in the standard form. We also have two defined connectives:

$-\alpha := \alpha \to (\neg\alpha \wedge \neg\neg\alpha).$
$\alpha \leftrightarrow \beta := (\alpha \to \beta) \wedge (\beta \to \alpha).$

GLukG Logic has all the axioms of $C_\omega$ logic plus the following:

**E1**  $(\neg\alpha \to \neg\beta) \leftrightarrow (\neg\neg\beta \to \neg\neg\alpha)$
**E2**  $\neg\neg(\alpha \to \beta) \leftrightarrow ((\alpha \to \beta) \wedge (\neg\neg\alpha \to \neg\neg\beta))$
**E3**  $\neg\neg(\alpha \wedge \beta) \leftrightarrow (\neg\neg\alpha \wedge \neg\neg\beta)$
**E4**  $(\beta \wedge \neg\beta) \to (--\alpha \to \alpha)$
**E5**  $\neg\neg(\alpha \vee \beta) \leftrightarrow (\neg\neg\alpha \vee \neg\neg\beta)$

Note that Classical logic is obtained from GLukG by adding to the list of axioms any of the following formulas: $\alpha \to \neg\neg\alpha$, $\alpha \to (\neg\alpha \to \beta)$, $(\neg\beta \to \neg\alpha) \to (\alpha \to \beta)$. On the other hand, $-\alpha \to \neg\alpha$ is a theorem in GLukG, that is why we call the "$-$" connective a strong negation.

In this paper we consider the *standard* substitution, here represented with the usual notation: $\varphi[\alpha/p]$ will denote the formula that results from substituting the formula $\alpha$ in place of the atom $p$, wherever it occurs in $\varphi$. Recall the recursive definition: if $\varphi$ is atomic, then $\varphi[\alpha/p]$ is $\alpha$ when $\varphi$ equals $p$, and $\varphi$ otherwise. Inductively, if $\varphi$ is a formula $\varphi_1 \# \varphi_2$, for any binary connective $\#$. Then $\varphi[\alpha/p]$ will be $\varphi_1[\alpha/p] \# \varphi_2[\alpha/p]$. Finally, if $\varphi$ is a formula of the form $\neg\varphi_1$, then $\varphi[\alpha/p]$ is $\neg\varphi_1[\alpha/p]$.

## 2.4   GLukG as a Multi-valued Logic

It is very important for the purposes of this work to note that GLukG can also be presented as a multi-valued logic. Such presentation is given in [4], where GLukG is called $G'_3$. In this form it is defined through a 3-valued logic with truth values in the domain $\mathcal{D} = \{0, 1, 2\}$ where 2 is the designated value. The evaluation functions of the logic connectives are then defined as follows: $x \wedge y = \min(x, y)$; $x \vee y = \max(x, y)$; and the $\neg$ and $\to$ connectives are defined according to the truth tables given in Table 1. We write $\models \alpha$ to denote that the formula $\alpha$ is a tautology, namely that $\alpha$ evaluates to 2 (the designated value) for every valuation.

In this paper we keep the notation $G'_3$ to refer to the multi-valued logic just defined, and we use the notation GLukG to refer to the Hilbert system defined at the beginning of this section.

There is a small difference between the definitions of $G'_3$ and Gödel logic $G_3$: the truth value assigned to $\neg 1$ is 0 in $G_3$. $G_3$ accepts an axiomatization that includes all of the axioms of intuitionistic logic. In particular, the formula $(a \wedge \neg a) \to b$ is a theorem, therefore $G_3$ is not paraconsistent.

**Table 1.** Truth tables of connectives in $G'_3$

| $x$ | $\neg x$ |
|---|---|
| 0 | 2 |
| 1 | 2 |
| 2 | 0 |

| $\to$ | 0 | 1 | 2 |
|---|---|---|---|
| 0 | 2 | 2 | 2 |
| 1 | 0 | 2 | 2 |
| 2 | 0 | 1 | 2 |

The next couple of results are facts we already know about the logic $G'_3$

**Theorem 1.** *[8] For every formula $\alpha$, $\alpha$ is a tautology in $G'_3$ iff $\alpha$ is a theorem in GLukG.*

**Theorem 2 (Substitution theorem for $G'_3$-logic).** *[8]Let $\alpha$, $\beta$ and $\psi$ be GLukG-formulas and let $p$ be an atom. If $\alpha \leftrightarrow \beta$ is a tautology in $G'_3$ then $\psi[\alpha/p] \leftrightarrow \psi[\beta/p]$ is a tautology in $G'_3$.*

**Corollary 1.** *[8]Let $\alpha$, $\beta$ and $\psi$ be GLukG-formulas and let $p$ be an atom. If $\alpha \leftrightarrow \beta$ is a theorem in GLukG then $\psi[\alpha/p] \leftrightarrow \psi[\beta/p]$ is a theorem in GLukG.*

## 2.5   The Multi-valued Logic $N'_5$

Now we present $N'_5$, a 5-valued logic defined in [5]. We will use the set of values $\{-2, -1, 0, 1, 2\}$. Valid formulas evaluate to 2, the chosen designated value. The connectives $\wedge$ and $\vee$ correspond to the *min* and *max* functions in the usual way. For the other connectives, the associated truth tables are in table 2.

**Table 2.** Truth tables of connectives in $N'_5$

| $\rightarrow$ | -2 | -1 | 0 | 1 | 2 |
|---|---|---|---|---|---|
| -2 | 2 | 2 | 2 | 2 | 2 |
| -1 | 2 | 2 | 2 | 2 | 2 |
| 0 | 2 | 2 | 2 | 2 | 2 |
| 1 | -1 | -1 | 0 | 2 | 2 |
| 2 | -2 | -1 | 0 | 1 | 2 |

| $\neg$ | |
|---|---|
| -2 | 2 |
| -1 | 2 |
| 0 | 2 |
| 1 | 2 |
| 2 | -2 |

| $\sim$ | |
|---|---|
| -2 | 2 |
| -1 | 1 |
| 0 | 0 |
| 1 | -1 |
| 2 | -2 |

| $\leftrightarrow$ | -2 | -1 | 0 | 1 | 2 |
|---|---|---|---|---|---|
| -2 | 2 | 2 | 2 | -1 | -2 |
| -1 | 2 | 2 | 2 | -1 | -1 |
| 0 | 2 | 2 | 2 | 0 | 0 |
| 1 | -1 | -1 | 0 | 2 | 1 |
| 2 | -2 | -1 | 0 | 1 | 2 |

A very important result is that $N'_5$ logic is a conservative extension of $G'_3$ logic, as the following theorem shows.

**Theorem 3.** *[5] For every GLukG-formula $\alpha$, $\alpha$ is a tautology in $N'_5$ iff $\alpha$ is a tautology in $G'_3$.*

## 3   The Logic N-GLukG

In this section we introduce a new logic we will call N-GLukG. We prove that N-GLukG is an extension of GLukG (Theorem 5), that it satisfies a substitution theorem (Theorem 6), and that it can express the stable semantics as well as the p-stable semantics. N-GLukG is defined in terms of an axiomatic system. The axioms are chosen in such a way that N-GLukG is sound with respect to $N'_5$, i.e. every theorem of N-GLukG is a tautology in $N'_5$. The only inference rule is modus ponens. Here is our list of 19 axioms:

$\mathbf{C_\omega 2}$    $\neg\neg a \rightarrow a$

**NPos1**   $\neg\neg(a \rightarrow (b \rightarrow a))$

**NPos2**   $\neg\neg((a \rightarrow (b \rightarrow c)) \rightarrow ((a \rightarrow b) \rightarrow (a \rightarrow c)))$

**NPos3**     $\neg\neg(a \wedge b \rightarrow a)$
**NPos4**     $\neg\neg(a \wedge b \rightarrow b)$
**NPos5**     $\neg\neg(a \rightarrow (b \rightarrow (a \wedge b)))$
**NPos6**     $\neg\neg(a \rightarrow (a \vee b))$
**NPos7**     $\neg\neg(b \rightarrow (a \vee b))$
**NPos8**     $\neg\neg((a \rightarrow c) \rightarrow ((b \rightarrow c) \rightarrow (a \vee b \rightarrow c)))$
**NC$_\omega$1**     $\neg\neg(a \vee \neg a)$
**NC$_\omega$2**     $\neg\neg(\neg\neg a \rightarrow a)$
**NE1**     $\neg\neg((\neg a \rightarrow \neg b) \leftrightarrow (\neg\neg b \rightarrow \neg\neg a))$
**NE2**     $\neg\neg(\neg\neg(a \rightarrow b) \rightarrow ((a \rightarrow b) \wedge (\neg\neg a \rightarrow \neg\neg b)))$
**NN1**     $\neg\neg(\sim (a \rightarrow b) \leftrightarrow a \wedge \sim b)$
**NN2**     $\neg\neg(\sim (a \wedge b) \leftrightarrow \sim a \vee \sim b)$
**NN3**     $\neg\neg(\sim (a \vee b) \leftrightarrow \sim a \wedge \sim b)$
**NN4**     $\neg\neg(a \leftrightarrow \sim\sim a)$
**NN5**     $\neg\neg(\sim \neg a \leftrightarrow \neg\neg a)$
**NN6**     $\neg\neg(\sim a \rightarrow \neg a)$

We have a defined connective: $\alpha \leftrightarrow \beta := (\alpha \rightarrow \beta) \wedge (\beta \rightarrow \alpha)$. Also we note that the connective $\vee$ is not an abbreviation.

Observe that the inclusion of axiom C$_\omega$2 assures that each of the other 16 axioms becomes a theorem in N-GLukG when dropping the double negation in front of them, this way we recover as theorems the axioms that define the positive logic as well as some of those that define GLukG. The convenience of having double negation in front of all these axioms is key in the proof of the substitution property (Theorem 6) presented at the end of this section. In particular the deduction theorem is valid in N-GLukG: $\alpha \vdash \beta$ if and only if $\vdash \alpha \rightarrow \beta$.

Next we present some of the first results about N-GLukG:

**Theorem 4.** N-GLukG *logic is sound with respect to* $N_5'$ *logic.*

*Proof.* It is easy to check that each axiom of N-GLukG is a tautology in $N_5'$. Also, according to the truth table for the implication of $N_5'$, modus ponens preserves tautologies, i.e. if $\alpha \rightarrow \beta$ and $\alpha$ are tautologies then $\beta$ is a tautology. Then it follows that every theorem in N-GLukG is a tautology in $N_5'$.     □

From this result we conclude that the logic N-GLukG is paraconsistent, since the formula $(\neg a \wedge a) \rightarrow b$ is not a theorem.

The converse of Theorem 4 does not hold. In order to prove this we need to look at the next logic along with some facts.

Let us define a 4-valued logic called $P - four$ in terms of the truth tables in Table 3.

**Definition 1.** *Let the logic* $P - four$ *be defined by the connectives according to the following tables, and where 3 is the only designated value.*

It is straightforward to check that each of the axioms that define N-GLukG is a tautology in $P - four$ and that given two tautologies of the form $\alpha$ and $\alpha \rightarrow \beta$ in $P - four$ then $\beta$ must be a tautology, i.e. Modus Ponens preserves tautologies in $P - four$.

From this, we have the following proposition.

**Table 3.** Truth tables of connectives in $P - four$

| $A$ | $\neg A$ | $A$ | $\sim A$ | $\to$ | 0 1 2 3 | $\wedge$ | 0 1 2 3 | $\vee$ | 0 1 2 3 |
|---|---|---|---|---|---|---|---|---|---|
| 0 | 3 | 0 | 3 | 0 | 3 3 3 3 | 0 | 0 0 0 0 | 0 | 0 1 2 3 |
| 1 | 3 | 1 | 2 | 1 | 2 3 2 3 | 1 | 0 1 0 1 | 1 | 1 1 3 3 |
| 2 | 3 | 2 | 1 | 2 | 1 1 3 3 | 2 | 0 0 2 2 | 2 | 2 3 2 3 |
| 3 | 0 | 3 | 0 | 3 | 0 1 2 3 | 3 | 0 1 2 3 | 3 | 3 3 3 3 |

**Proposition 1.** N-GLukG *is sound with respect to* $P - four$.

As a consequence, we can prove now that $N_5'$ is not complete with respect to N-GLukG.

**Proposition 2.** *Not every tautology in* $N_5'$ *is a theorem in* N-GLukG.

*Proof.* The formula $\neg\neg(\alpha \vee \beta) \to (\neg\neg\alpha \vee \neg\neg\beta)$ is a tautology in $N_5'$, but it is not a tautology in $P - four$ as we can see by taking a valuation $\nu$ such that $\nu(\alpha) = 1, \nu(\beta) = 2$ since it evaluates to zero.

We conclude then that the formula is not a theorem in N-GLukG according to proposition 1. □

The reader may wonder whether any tautology in $P - four$ is a theorem in N-GLukG. This is not the case, as the formula known as Pierce axiom: $((\alpha \to \beta) \to \alpha) \to \alpha$ shows. This formula is a tautology in $P - four$ but not in $N_5'$ as it is shown by assigning the values 1 and 0 to $\alpha, \beta$ respectively. Then according to Theorem 4, it can not be a theorem in N-GLukG.

Now we continue looking at some properties of N-GLukG. In particular we have that the connective $\sim$ of N-GLukG is not a paraconsistent negation as the following proposition shows.

**Proposition 3.** *The formula* $(a\wedge \sim a) \to b$ *is a theorem in* N-GLukG.

*Proof.* The formula $\neg\neg((a \to ((b \to a) \to a)) \to ((a \to (b \to a)) \to (a \to a)))$ is an instance of axiom NPos2, we apply NE2 to conclude that $\neg\neg((a \to (b \to a)) \to (a \to a))$ is a theorem. Repeating the same argument to this last formula, but now using NPos1 and NE2 we conclude that $\neg\neg(a \to a)$ is a theorem.

Now from $a, \sim a$ let us prove $b$. Given $a\wedge \sim a$ we use NN1 and $C_\omega 2$ to obtain $\sim (a \to a)$, and then by applying NN6 and $C_\omega 2$ we obtain $\neg(a \to a)$. From this and the formula $\neg\neg(a \to a)$ we conclude $b$, since $(\neg\alpha \wedge \neg\neg\alpha) \to \beta$ is a theorem in GLukG [8]. □

We also have the following result as a consequence of Theorem 4.

**Theorem 5.** *Every theorem in* N-GLukG *that can be expressed in the language of* GLukG, *is a theorem in* GLukG.

*Proof.* If $\vdash_{\text{N-GLukG}} \alpha$, then by theorem 4 $\models_{N5'} \alpha$. Then according to Theorem 3 $\models_{G_3'} \alpha$, and then by Theorem 1 it follows that $\vdash_{\text{GLukG}} \alpha$. □

Now we present a substitution theorem for N-GLukG logic. The next lemma is interesting on its own and plays a role in the proof of the theorem.

**Lemma 1.** *If $\Psi$ is a theorem in N-GLukG, then $\neg\neg\Psi$ is also a theorem in N-GLukG.*

*Proof.* Let us prove this fact by induction on the size of the proof of $\Psi$. First we check that $\neg\neg\Psi$ is a theorem whenever $\Psi$ is an axiom of N-GLukG. Observe that, from axiom $C_\omega 2$, the formula $\neg\neg\neg\alpha \to \neg\alpha$ is a theorem, and applying $E1$, it follows that the formula $\neg\neg\alpha \leftrightarrow \neg\neg\neg\neg\alpha$ is a theorem in N-GLukG for any formula $\alpha$. If $\Psi$ is an axiom of N-GLukG and $\Psi$ has the form $\neg\neg\alpha$ then $\neg\neg\Psi$ is a theorem by the fact just mentioned and modus ponens. If $\Psi = \neg\neg\alpha \to \alpha$ then $\neg\neg\Psi$ is axiom $NC_\omega 2$ and therefore a theorem. Next, let us assume that the result is true for any theorem whose proof in N-GLukG consists of less than $n$ steps and let $\Psi$ be a theorem whose proof consists of $n$ steps where the last step is an application of modus ponens to two previous steps, say $\alpha$ and $\alpha \to \Psi$. Then by hypothesis $\neg\neg\alpha$ and $\neg\neg(\alpha \to \Psi)$ are theorems, and by using $E2$, $\neg\neg\alpha \to \neg\neg\Psi$ is a theorem. We reach the conclusion by an application of Modus Ponens.  □

For the next result, we introduce the notation $\alpha \Leftrightarrow \beta$ as equivalent to the formula $(\alpha \leftrightarrow \beta) \wedge (\sim\alpha \leftrightarrow \sim\beta)$.

**Theorem 6.** *Let $\alpha$, $\beta$ and $\psi$ be $N_5'$-formulas and let $p$ be any atom. If $\alpha \Leftrightarrow \beta$ is a theorem in N-GLukG then $\psi[\alpha/p] \Leftrightarrow \psi[\beta/p]$ is a theorem in N-GLukG.*

Let us prove the Theorem. First, we observe that we will use some basic consequences from the axioms of positive logic, specifically:

*Remark 1.* $A \leftrightarrow B, C \leftrightarrow D \vdash (A \to C) \leftrightarrow (B \to D)$, also $A \leftrightarrow B, C \leftrightarrow D \vdash (A \wedge C) \leftrightarrow (B \wedge D)$ and $A \leftrightarrow B, C \leftrightarrow D \vdash (A \vee C) \leftrightarrow (B \vee D)$

*Proof.* Induction on the size of $\psi$.

Base case:

If $\psi = q$, $q$ an atom, we have:

$$\psi[\alpha/p] \Leftrightarrow \psi[\beta/p] = \begin{cases} q \Leftrightarrow q \text{ if } p \neq q \\ \alpha \Leftrightarrow \beta \text{ if } p = q, \end{cases}$$

$q \Leftrightarrow q$ is a theorem since $\eta \to \eta$ is a theorem for any formula $\eta$. $\alpha \Leftrightarrow \beta$ is a theorem by hypothesis.

Now we assume the statement true for the formulas $\phi, \phi_1, \phi_2$.

Case 1) $\psi = \neg\phi$.

We want to prove that $\neg\phi[\alpha/p] \leftrightarrow \neg\phi[\beta/p]$ and $\sim\neg\phi[\alpha/p] \leftrightarrow \sim\neg\phi[\beta/p]$ are theorems.

Since by hypothesis $\phi[\alpha/p] \Leftrightarrow \phi[\beta/p]$ is a theorem, then $\phi[\alpha/p] \leftrightarrow \phi[\beta/p]$ is a theorem and $\sim\phi[\alpha/p] \leftrightarrow \sim\phi[\beta/p]$ is also a theorem. By the previous lemma $\neg\neg(\phi[\alpha/p] \leftrightarrow \phi[\beta/p])$ is a theorem, and by using $E2$ we conclude that $\neg\neg(\phi[\alpha/p]) \leftrightarrow \neg\neg(\phi[\beta/p])$ is a theorem. Now according to $E1$, $\neg(\phi[\beta/p]) \leftrightarrow \neg(\phi[\alpha/p])$ is a theorem. According to $NN5$ and the first part of remark 1, $\sim\neg\phi[\alpha/p] \leftrightarrow \sim\neg\phi[\beta/p]$ is also a theorem.

Case 2) $\psi = \sim\phi$.

We want to prove that $\sim\phi[\alpha/p] \leftrightarrow \sim\phi[\beta/p]$ and $\sim\sim\phi[\alpha/p] \leftrightarrow \sim\sim\phi[\beta/p]$ are theorems. The first formula follows from the induction hypothesis. The second formula follows from the fact that $\eta \leftrightarrow \sim\sim\eta$ is a theorem ($NN4$) for any formula $\eta$, from remark 1, and from inductive hypothesis.

Case 3) $\psi = \phi_1 \rightarrow \phi_2$.

We assume that $(\phi_i[\alpha/p] \Leftrightarrow \phi_i[\beta/p])$ is a theorem for $i \in \{1, 2\}$. We need to prove that the two following formulas are theorems: $(\phi_1[\alpha/p] \rightarrow \phi_2[\alpha/p]) \leftrightarrow (\phi_1[\beta/p] \rightarrow \phi_2[\beta/p])$ and $\sim(\phi_1[\alpha/p] \rightarrow \phi_2[\alpha/p]) \leftrightarrow \sim(\phi_1[\beta/p] \rightarrow \phi_2[\beta/p])$. The first statement follows from the remark above. For the second one we use the theorem: $\sim(\theta \rightarrow \eta) \leftrightarrow (\theta \wedge \sim\eta)$, which is consequence of $NN1$. According to this, it is enough to show that $(\phi_1[\alpha/p] \wedge \sim\phi_2[\alpha/p]) \leftrightarrow (\phi_1[\beta/p] \wedge \sim\phi_2[\beta/p])$ is a theorem, but this follows from the hypothesis and the remark above.

Case 4) $\psi = \phi_1 \wedge \phi_2$.

Assume $(\phi_i[\alpha/p] \Leftrightarrow \phi_i[\beta/p])$ is a theorem for $i \in \{1, 2\}$. From the last remark it follows that $(\phi_1[\alpha/p] \wedge \phi_2[\alpha/p]) \leftrightarrow (\phi_1[\beta/p] \wedge \phi_2[\beta/p])$ is a theorem. As for $\sim(\phi_1[\alpha/p] \wedge \phi_2[\alpha/p]) \leftrightarrow \sim(\phi_1[\beta/p] \wedge \phi_2[\beta/p])$, we use the De Morgan law which is $N2$ after dropping the double negation, to transform the biconditional into $(\sim\phi_1 \vee \sim\phi_2)[\alpha/p] \leftrightarrow (\sim\phi_1 \vee \sim\phi_2)[\beta/p]$, which is a theorem according to the inductive hypothesis and the remark above.

Case 5) $\psi = \phi_1 \vee \phi_2$.

Assume $(\phi_i[\alpha/p] \Leftrightarrow \phi_i[\beta/p])$ is a theorem for $i \in \{1, 2\}$. From the last remark it follows that $(\phi_1[\alpha/p] \vee \phi_2[\alpha/p]) \leftrightarrow (\phi_1[\beta/p] \vee \phi_2[\beta/p])$ is a theorem. As for $\sim(\phi_1[\alpha/p] \vee \phi_2[\alpha/p]) \leftrightarrow \sim(\phi_1[\beta/p] \vee \phi_2[\beta/p])$, we use the De Morgan law which is $NN3$ after droping the double negation to transform the biconditional into $(\sim\phi_1 \wedge \sim\phi_2)[\alpha/p] \leftrightarrow (\sim\phi_1 \wedge \sim\phi_2)[\beta/p]$ which is a theorem according to the inductive hypothesis and the remark above.    □

So far we have looked at some properties of logics N-GLukG and $N'_5$. Now we would like to point out the theoretical value of these logics in the context of logic programming and knowledge representation.

**Lemma 2.** *In* N-GLukG *the weak explosion principle is valid: For any formulas $\alpha, \beta$, the formula $\neg\alpha \wedge \neg\neg\alpha \rightarrow \beta$, is a theorem.*

*Proof.* From $\neg\alpha$ as premise, we prove $\neg\neg\alpha \rightarrow \beta$. By $Pos1$ we have $\neg\alpha \rightarrow (\neg\beta \rightarrow \neg\alpha)$. Using the premise and Modus Ponens we obtain $\neg\beta \rightarrow \neg\alpha$. Next we use $E1$ and Modus Ponens to obtain $\neg\neg\alpha \rightarrow \neg\neg\beta$. Using $Cw2$ it follows that $\neg\neg\alpha \rightarrow \beta$.    □

According to this, we can define a bottom particle in N-GLukG.

**Definition 2.** *For any fixed formula $\alpha$ let us define the bottom particle $\bot$ as $\neg\alpha \wedge \neg\neg\alpha$.*

**Lemma 3.** *The fragment of* N-GLukG *defined by the symbols $\wedge, \vee, \rightarrow, \bot$ contains all theorems of intuitionism.*

*Proof.* By defining a new negation $\backsim A : A \to \bot$, it is not difficult to prove with the use of the explosion principle and the deduction theorem the following two formulas: $(A \to B) \to ((A \to \backsim B) \to \backsim A)$ and $\backsim A \to (A \to B)$.

These two formulas along with the axioms that define positive logic define intuitionism.                                                                    □

As indicated in the introduction, logic GLukG(as some other paraconsistent logics) can be used as the formalism to define the p-stable semantics in the same way as intuitionism (as some other constructive logics) serves as the mathematical formalism of the theory of answer set programming (stable semantics) [10]. Accordingly we can state the next result.

**Theorem 7.** N-GLukG *can express the stable semantics as well as the p-stable semantics.*

*Proof.* It follows from the previous lemma and theorem 5.                      □

## 4 Conclusions and Future Work

We presented, by means of a family of axioms, the N-GLukG logic, also with two negations, and having the property that any of its theorems is a tautology in $N_5'$. The N-GLukG logic contains as axioms most of the axioms that define the GLukG logic. In fact we proved that any theorem in N-GLukG that can be expressed in the language of GLukG is also a theorem in GLukG. We also presented a substitution theorem for N-GLukG. We also proved that with logic N-GLukG we can express the stable and p-stable logic programming semantics. Finally, as mentioned in the introduction, we are interested in exploring possible ways of extending the p-stable semantics to a more expressive semantics by using a logic with strong negation. $N_5'$ and GLukG seem to be suitable candidates for the formalization of such a semantics.

**Funding.** This work was supported by the Consejo Nacional de Ciencia y Tecnología [CB-2008-01 No.101581].

## References

1. Béziau, J.-Y.: The paraconsistent logic z a possible solution to jaśkowski's problem. Logic and Logical Philosophy 15(2), 99–111 (2006)
2. Carnielli, W., Coniglio, M.E., Marcos, J.: Logics of formal inconsistency. In: Handbook of Philosophical Logic, pp. 1–93. Springer (2007)
3. Da Costa, N.C.A.: On the theory of inconsistent formal systems. Notre Dame Journal of Formal Logic 15(4), 497–510 (1974)
4. Galindo, M.O., Pérez, J.A.N., Ramírez, J.A.R., Macías, V.B.: Logics with common weak completions. Journal of Logic and Computation 16(6), 867–890 (2006)
5. Carballido, J.L., Osorio, M., Zepeda, C., et al.: Mathematical Models. Section 2: N'5 as an extension of G'3. In: Mathematical Models and ITC: Theory and Applications. Benemérita Universidad Autónoma de Puebla Press

6. Elliot Mendelson. Introduction to mathematical logic. CRC Press (1997)
7. Ortiz, M., Osorio, M.: Strong negation and equivalence in the safe belief semantics. Journal of Logic and Computation 17(3), 499–515 (2007)
8. Galindo, M.O., Carranza, J.L.C.: Brief study of g'3 logic. Journal of Applied Non-Classical Logics 18(4), 475–499 (2008)
9. Galindo, M.O., Carranza, J.L.C., Cortes, C.Z.: $N_5^t$ and some of its properties. To appear in Electronic Proceedings of 7th Alberto Mendelzon International Workshop on Foundations of Data Management (AMW 2013). CEUR Workshop Proceedings, ceur-ws.org (2013), http://ceur-ws.org/
10. Pearce, D.: Stable inference as intuitionistic validity. The Journal of Logic Programming 38(1), 79–91 (1999)

# The Inverse Method for Many-Valued Logics*

Laura Kovács[1], Andrei Mantsivoda[2], and Andrei Voronkov[3]

[1] Chalmers University of Technology
[2] Irkutsk State University
[3] The University of Manchester

**Abstract.** We define an automatic proof procedure for finitely many-valued logics given by truth tables. The proof procedure is based on the inverse method. To define this procedure, we introduce so-called *introduction-based sequent calculi*. By studying proof-theoretic properties of these calculi we derive efficient validity- and satisfiability-checking procedures based on the inverse method. We also show how to translate the validity problem for a formula to unsatisfiability checking of a set of propositional clauses.

## 1   Introduction

The inverse method of theorem proving was developed in the 1960s [12, 17–19], see [10] for an overview. The method is essentially orthogonal to the tableau method and is based on the bottom-up proof-search in sequent calculi. The inverse method is based on the idea of specialising a sequent calculus by a given goal, using the subformula property of sequent calculi. The inverse method was successfully applied to a number of non-classical logics, including intuitionistic logic and some modal logics [32, 34, 22].

The inverse method can be efficiently implemented for classical logic [31] and some non-classical logics [33]. In this paper we give a presentation of the inverse method for finite many-valued logics. We show how to apply the inverse method to obtain a proof procedure for many-valued logics. Nearly all known methods of automated reasoning have been extended to many-valued logic in [8, 9, 24, 25, 2, 27, 5, 14, 26, 15, 3], but to the best of our knowledge it is the first ever presentation of the inverse method.

This paper is organised as follows. In Section 2 we define many-valued logics, their syntax and semantics. Section 3 defines so-called introduction-based sequent calculi and proves results about their soundness and completeness. The main results of this section are that soundness and completeness are "local" properties, which can easily be checked. We also discuss minimal calculi (which result in more efficient proof procedures) and prove admissibility of the cut rule. In Section 4 we introduce a key definition of *signed subformula*. It is interesting that this definition depends not only on the semantics of a logic, but also on a sequent calculus we choose.

* We acknowledge funding from the Austrian FWF grant S11410-N23 and the Austrian WWTF grant ICT C-050.

F. Castro, A. Gelbukh, and M. González (Eds.): MICAI 2013, Part I, LNAI 8265, pp. 12–23, 2013.
© Springer-Verlag Berlin Heidelberg 2013

Section 5 presents the main technique used by the inverse method: the specialisation of a sequent calculus to prove a particular goal, using the subformula property. In Section 6 we show that the inverse method can be efficiently implemented by translation to propositional satisfiability. Finally, in Section 7 we discuss some related work and future research directions. Detailed proofs of theorems are not included in this paper but can be found in its longer version[1].

## 2   Many-Valued Logics

This section contains all basic definitions. Many of them are quite standard and included mostly for the sake of unambiguity. Results of this section are not original. We only consider many-valued logics with a finite set of truth values.

**Definition 1.** *A finite many-valued logic $\mathcal{L}$ is a triple $(V, Con, arity, val)$ where*

1. *$V$ is a finite non-empty set of* truth values;
2. *Con is a finite non-empty set of* connectives;
3. *arity is a mapping from Con to the set of non-negative integers, called the* arity mapping;
4. *val is a function from Con to the set of functions on $V$, called the* valuation *function, such that the arity of $val(c)$ is $arity(c)$, for all $c \in Con$.*

*If $arity(c) = m$, then we call $c$ an $m$-ary connective. The logic $\mathcal{L}$ is called a $k$-valued logic if $k$ is the number of elements in $V$.*

For the rest of this paper we assume an arbitrary, but fixed $k$-valued logic $\mathcal{L} = (V, Con, arity, val)$. We also assume to have a countably infinite set *Atom* of *propositional variables*.

**Definition 2.** *The set of* formulas *of logic $\mathcal{L}$ is defined as follows:*

1. *Every propositional variable $A \in Atom$ is a formula;*
2. *If $c \in Con_m$ and $F_1, \ldots, F_m$ are formulas, then $c(F_1, \ldots, F_m)$ is a formula.*

In many-valued logics we prove that a formula always has a given truth value or a given set of truth values. We will introduce a notation for expressing that a formula $F$ has a truth value $t$.

**Definition 3.** *A* signed formula *is a pair $(F, t)$, denoted $F^t$, where $F$ is a formula and $t \in V$. A* sequent *is a finite set $\{F_1^{t_1}, \ldots, F_m^{t_m}\}$ of signed formulas. For simplicity, we will write such a sequent as a sequence $F_1^{t_1}, \ldots, F_m^{t_m}$.*

In [14, 26] signed formulas are signed with *sets of* truth values. For simplicity, we only consider single truth values as signs. However, we can generalize our results to sets of signs as well.

---

[1] Available upon request, due to authors' anonymity.

The intuitive meaning of the signed formula $F^t$ is that the formula $F$ has the truth value $t$. Sequents are needed to define the semantics and the proof theory of many-valued logics. The intuitive meaning of a sequent $F_1^{t_1}, \ldots, F_m^{t_m}$ is that at least one of the $F_i$'s has the truth value $t_i$.

For sequents $S_1, S_2$, we will write $S_1 \cup S_2$ as simply $S_1, S_2$. Likewise, for a sequent $S$ and formula $F^t$, we will write $S \cup \{F^t\}$ simply as $S, F^t$, and similarly for multiple sequents and formulas.

The semantics of many-valued logics is defined via the notion of an truth assignment.

**Definition 4.** *A* truth assignment *is any mapping* $\alpha : Atom \to V$. *The truth value* $\alpha(A)$ *is the value of the variable* $A$ *under the truth assignment* $\alpha$.

*Truth assignments can be extended to arbitrary formulas* $F$ *of logic* $\mathcal{L}$ *in the following way. For any* $c \in Con$ *of arity* $m$, *let*

$$\alpha(c(F_1, \ldots, F_m)) \overset{\text{def}}{=} val(c)(\alpha(F_1), \ldots, \alpha(F_m))$$

We shall also extend evaluations to signed formulas and sequents. Each signed formula and sequent will be either true or false. More precisely, we extend the mapping $\alpha$ to a mapping from signed formulas and sequents to the set of boolean values $\{true, false\}$ as follows:

$$\alpha(F^t) \overset{\text{def}}{=} \begin{cases} true, \text{ if } \alpha(F) = t \\ false, \text{ otherwise} \end{cases}$$

$$\alpha(F_1^{t_1}, \ldots, F_n^{t_n}) \overset{\text{def}}{=} \begin{cases} true, \text{ if } \alpha(F_i^{t_i}) = true \text{ for some } i = 1, \ldots, n \\ false, \text{ otherwise} \end{cases}$$

**Definition 5.** *A sequent* $S$ *is called* valid *in a logic* $\mathcal{L}$ *if for all truth assignments* $\alpha$ *we have* $\alpha(S) = true$.

The semantics of connectives in finitely-valued logics can conveniently be represented via *truth tables*. A truth table for a connective $c$ is a table whose rows are all tuples of the graph of $val(c)$. For example, in a two-valued logic with truth values $\{t, f\}$ the ternary connective $c$ such that $val(c)(t_1, t_2, t_3) = t$ iff $t_1 = t_2 = t$ or $(t_1 = t_3 = t \text{ and } t_2 = f)$ can be represented by the following truth table:

| $A_1$ | $A_2$ | $A_3$ | $c(A_1, A_2, A_3)$ |
|---|---|---|---|
| $t$ | $t$ | $t$ | $t$ |
| $t$ | $t$ | $f$ | $t$ |
| $t$ | $f$ | $t$ | $t$ |
| $t$ | $f$ | $f$ | $f$ |
| $f$ | $t$ | $t$ | $f$ |
| $f$ | $t$ | $f$ | $f$ |
| $f$ | $f$ | $t$ | $f$ |
| $f$ | $f$ | $f$ | $f$ |

# 3   Sequent Calculi

The main goal of proof systems for many-valued logics is to prove validity of sequents. There is a technique allowing a sound and complete sequent calculus to be constructed from a given many-valued logic [30, 4]. In this section we define *introduction-based sequent calculi*. A naive way of constructing a sound and complete sequent calculus creates however many redundancies. We try to avoid this by using a *minimal* sequent calculi.

When presenting sequent calculi, we will use the terminology of [6, 10]. Namely, an *inference* has the form

$$\frac{\{S_1, \cdots, S_n\}}{S} \ ,$$

where $n \geq 0$, an *inference rule* is a collection of inferences and a *calculus* is a collection of inference rules. In the inference above, the sequent $S$ is called the *conclusion*, and $S_1, \ldots, S_n$ the *premises* of this inference. For simplicity, we will write such inferences as

$$\frac{S_1 \quad \cdots \quad S_n}{S} \ .$$

As in [6, 10], a *derivation* in a calculus is any tree built from inferences in this calculus. A sequent is *derivable* if it has a derivation.

**Definition 6.** *A calculus $G$ of sequents is called* introduction-based *if*

1. *$G$ contains the inferences rule*

$$\overline{A^{t_1}, \ldots, A^{t_k}} \tag{1}$$

   *where $A$ is an arbitrary propositional variable and $t_1, \ldots, t_k$ are all truth values of the logic.*
2. *$G$ contains some inference rules of the form*

$$\frac{\{S_j, F_j^{t_j} \mid j \in J\}}{\bigcup_{j \in J} S_j, c(F_1, \ldots, F_n)^t} \tag{2}$$

   *where $J$ is a fixed subset of $\{1, \ldots, n\}$, the $F_j$'s are arbitrary formulas and the $t_j$'s and $t$ are fixed truth values. Such an inference rule will be called an introduction rule* for c.
3. *$G$ contains no other rules.*

Note that in this definition the set of indices $J$ may form a proper subset of $\{1, \ldots, n\}$ and the truth values $t_j$'s should not necessarily be pairwise different. An introduction rule represents an infinite set of inferences, obtained by varying formulas $F_1, \ldots, F_n$.

To illustrate this definition and any other material in this paper we will use the standard two-valued logic $\mathcal{L}_2$ with truth values *true* and *false*, the standard connectives like the conjunction and a ternary connective *ite* (if-then-else). The valuation function of $\mathcal{L}_2$ for all connectives is considered as standard.

The following are familiar introduction rules for the conjunction $\wedge$:

$$\frac{S, F_1^{false}}{S, (F_1 \wedge F_2)^{false}} \qquad \frac{S, F_2^{false}}{S, (F_1 \wedge F_2)^{false}} \qquad \frac{S_1, F_1^{true} \quad S_2, F_2^{true}}{S_1, S_2, (F_1 \wedge F_2)^{true}}$$

The following is an introduction rule for *ite*:

$$\frac{S_1, F_1^{true} \quad S_2, F_2^{true}}{S_1, S_2, ite(F_1, F_2, F_3)^{true}}$$

In the sequel a calculus means an introduction-based calculus, unless otherwise is clear from the context.

**Definition 7.** *An introduction rule (2) is called* sound *if for every inference of this rule, whenever all premises of the rule are true, the conclusion is also true. A calculus is called* locally sound *if every rule of this calculus is sound. A calculus is called* sound *if every derivable sequent is true.*

**Theorem 8.** *A calculus is sound if and only if it is locally sound. Every locally sound calculus is sound, i.e. every sequent provable in a calculus locally sound for $\mathcal{L}$, is valid in $\mathcal{L}$.*

**Definition 9.** *A calculus $G$ is called* subset-complete *if for every valid sequent $S$ there exists a derivable sequent $S'$ such that $S' \subseteq S$. A calculus $G$ is called* locally complete *if for every n-ary connective $c$ and truth values $t_1, \ldots, t_n, t$ such that $t = val(c)(t_1, \ldots, t_n)$, there exist a set $J \subseteq \{1, \ldots, n\}$ such that rule (2) belongs to $G$.*

Note the non-standard formulation of completeness caused by the absence of the weakening rule in the calculus. Consider, for example, the logic $\mathcal{L}_2$. The sequent $A^{true}, A^{false}, B^{true}$, where $A$ and $B$ are propositional variables, is valid, but not derivable in *any* introduction-based calculus, since it does not have the form (1) and contains no connectives. However, its proper subset $A^{true}, A^{false}$ is derivable in *every* such calculus, since it is an instance of (1). It is not hard to argue that the following theorem holds.

**Theorem 10.** *A calculus $G$ is subset-complete if and only if it is locally complete.*

From Theorems 8 and 10 we obtain the following result.

**Theorem 11.** *An introduction-based calculus is sound and subset-complete if and only if it is both locally sound and locally complete.*

Let us introduce the *weakening rule*, or simply *weakening*:

$$\frac{S}{S, F^t} .$$

Obviously, weakening preserves validity. We call an *introduction-based calculus with weakening,* or simply *calculus with weakening,* any calculus obtained from an introduction-based calculus by adding the weakening rule.

**Definition 12.** *A calculus is called* complete *if every valid sequent is derivable in this calculus.*

**Theorem 13.** *A calculus with weakening is sound and complete if and only if it is both locally sound and locally complete.*

**Definition 14.** *Let* $\{t_1, \ldots, t_n\}$ *be all truth values of a logic* $\mathcal{L}$. *The* cut rule *for this logic is defined as follows*

$$\frac{S_1, F^{t_1} \quad \cdots \quad S_n, F^{t_n}}{S_1, \ldots, S_n}$$

**Theorem 15.** *The cut rule is admissible in any calculus with weakening which is both locally sound and locally complete, that is, every sequent derivable in this calculus with the use of the cut rule, is also derivable without the cut rule.*

*Proof.* It is enough to note that the cut rule is sound and apply Theorem 13.

It is not hard to find a locally sound and locally complete calculus. Consider the calculus defined by all inference rules of the form

$$\frac{S_1, F_1^{t_1} \quad \cdots \quad S_n, F_n^{t_n}}{S_1, \ldots, S_n, c(F_1, \ldots, F_n)^t}$$

where $val(c)(t_1, \ldots, t_n) = t$. It is straightforward to show that this calculus is both locally sound and locally complete.

Let us introduce a partial order $\leq$ on inference rules of introduction-based calculi as the smallest order such that

$$\frac{S, F_r^{t_r} \quad \cdots \quad S, F_s^{t_s}}{S, c(F_1, \ldots, F_n)^t} \quad \leq \quad \frac{S, F_p^{t_p} \quad \cdots \quad S, F_q^{t_q}}{S, c(F_1, \ldots, F_n)^t}$$

whenever $\{r, \ldots, s\} \subseteq \{p, \ldots, q\}$.

**Example 16.** *Consider the following three rules for the classical disjunction:*

$$\frac{S, F_2^{true}}{S, (F_1 \vee F_2)^{true}} \tag{3}$$

$$\frac{S, F_1^{false} \quad S, F_2^{true}}{S, (F_1 \vee F_2)^{true}} \tag{4}$$

$$\frac{S_1, F_1^{true} \quad S_2, F_2^{true}}{S_1, S_2, (F_1 \vee F_2)^{true}} \tag{5}$$

*Then* (3) $\leq$ (4) *and* (3) $\leq$ (5), *but rules* (4) *and* (5) *are incompatible w.r.t.* $\leq$.

The relation $\leq$ can be generalised to a partial order $\preceq$ on introduction-based calculi by comparing their sets of rules using the finite multiset extension of $\leq$, see [11] for a precise definition. We are interested in calculi minimal w.r.t. $\preceq$ since smaller calculi have a more compact presentation of inference rules. Consider, for example, introduction rules for *ite* in $\mathcal{L}_2$. It is not hard to argue that the following are all such inference rules minimal w.r.t. $\leq$:

$$\frac{S_1, F_1^{true} \quad S_2, F_2^{true}}{S_1, S_2, ite(F_1, F_2, F_3)^{true}}$$
$$\frac{S_1, F_1^{false} \quad S_3, F_3^{true}}{S_1, S_3, ite(F_1, F_2, F_3)^{true}}$$
$$\frac{S_2, F_2^{true} \quad S_3, F_3^{true}}{S_2, S_3, ite(F_1, F_2, F_3)^{true}}$$

$$\frac{S_1, F_1^{true} \quad S_2, F_2^{false}}{S_1, S_2, ite(F_1, F_2, F_3)^{false}}$$
$$\frac{S_1, F_1^{false} \quad S_3, F_3^{false}}{S_1, S_3, ite(F_1, F_2, F_3)^{false}}$$
$$\frac{S_2, F_2^{false} \quad S_3, F_3^{false}}{S_2, S_3, ite(F_1, F_2, F_3)^{false}}$$

It has the least locally sound and locally complete calculus consisting of the first four of the above rules. This example shows that finding minimal calculi may be non-trivial, since the last two inference rules are minimal, but not occur in the least calculus.

One can also show that, in general, the least calculus may not exist.

## 4   The Subformula Property

The theorem proving problem for a many-valued logic consist of determining the validity of a sequent. If the formula is valid, one may also want to have a derivation of this formula in some calculus. If it is not valid, one generally requires to find a truth assignment that makes the formula false. To design a proof-search algorithm based on the inverse method, we will use a subformula property. Interestingly, our definition of (signed) subformula will not be given in terms of the logic itself: it will be based on a locally sound and locally complete calculus. In the sequel we assume that such a calculus $G$ is fixed.

**Definition 17.** *Let $G$ contain an inference rule (2). Then we say that each signed formula $F_j^{t_j}$ is the* immediate signed subformula *of $c(F_1, \ldots, F_n)^t$. The notion of a* signed subformula *is the reflexive and transitive closure of the notion of immediate signed subformula. A* signed subformula *of a sequent $S$ is any signed subformula of a signed formula in $S$.*

Suppose that for two calculi $G_1$ and $G_2$ we have $G_1 \preceq G_2$. It is interesting that, if a signed formula $s_1$ is a signed subformula of a signed formula $s_2$ with respect to $G_1$, then $s_1$ is also a signed subformula of $s_2$ with respect to $G_2$. This means that smaller calculi give smaller "signed subformula" relations.

Our main interest in the subformula property can be explained by the following theorem.

**Axioms** Axioms of $G_\gamma$ are all sequents of the form

$$A^1, \ldots, A^k$$

such that each $A^i$ is a signed subformula of a signed formula in $\gamma$.

**Introduction rules** These are all rules of $G_\gamma$ are all rules of the form (2) restricted to signed subformulas of $\gamma$.

**Fig. 1.** The sequent calculus $G_\gamma$

**Theorem 18.** *Let $\Pi$ be a derivation of a sequent $S$. Then all signed formulas occurring in $\Pi$ are signed subformulas of signed formulas in $S$.*

*Proof.* Straightforward by induction on the depth of $\Pi$.

## 5 The Inverse Method

The inverse method tries to construct derivations from axioms to the goal, using the subformula property. Paper [10] contains a detailed explanation on how one can design the inverse proof search based on sequent calculi having a suitable subformula property. This can be done in two steps: first, given a sequent $\gamma$ to be proved, build a specialised sequent calculus intended to only prove $\gamma$ and second, organise proof-search in this specialised calculus. For some modal and other non-classical logics the second step can be highly non-trivial, as, e.g., in [34]. In this paper we show that, for many-valued logics, the second step can be delegated to a propositional SAT solver.

For the rest of this section we assume that $\gamma$ is a fixed sequent whose validity is to be established. Also, for simplicity of notation, we assume that the set of truth values is the set of integers $\{1, \ldots, k\}$. The specialised calculus $G_\gamma$ is shown on Figure 1.

It is not hard to argue that $G_\gamma$ has the following properties:

**Proposition 19.** *The following statements are true about $G_\gamma$:*

1. *Every sequent derivable in $G_\gamma$ consists of signed subformulas of $\gamma$.*
2. *The set of sequents used in $G_\gamma$ is finite.*

Further, we also have the following property.

**Theorem 20 (Soundness and completeness of $G_\gamma$).** *The sequent $\gamma$ is valid if and only if it is provable in $G_\gamma$.*

This theorem serves as a foundation of a proof procedure for many-valued logics. In the next section we show how one can use SAT solvers to search for derivations.

## 6   Inverse Method and Resolution

In this section we generalize to many-valued logics a well-known translation of sequent derivations into hyperresolution derivations. For classical logic it was described in different forms in [18, 16, 23, 10]. In this section we will use the standard terminology in propositional resolution, including (positive and negative) literals and clauses. We will consider a clause both as a set and a disjunction of literals.

Consider the set $S_\gamma$ of all signed subformulas of $\gamma$. We will now treat each signed formula in $S_\gamma$ as a propositional variable. These propositional variables should not be confused with the propositional variables in *Atom*.

Consider any introduction rule $R$ in $G_\gamma$:

$$\frac{\{S_j, F_j^{t_j} \mid j \in J\}}{\bigcup_{j \in J} S_j, c(F_1, \ldots, F_n)^t} \ . \tag{6}$$

Denote by $C_R$ the following propositional clause using variables in $S_\gamma$:

$$\bigvee_{j \in J} \neg F_j^{t_j} \vee c(F_1, \ldots, F_n)^t.$$

We recall that positive (propositional) hyperresolution is the following inference rule on propositional clauses:

$$\frac{C_1 \vee p_1 \quad \cdots \quad C_n \vee p_n \quad \neg p_1 \vee \ldots \vee \neg p_n \vee C}{C_1 \vee \ldots \vee C_n \vee C} \ , \tag{7}$$

where $p_1, \ldots, p_n$ are propositional variables and $C_1, \ldots, C_n, C$ are clauses consisting only of positive literals. The conclusion of this rule is called a *hyperresolvent of the clauses* $C_1 \vee p_1, \ldots, C_n \vee p_n$ *against the clause* $\neg p_1 \vee \ldots \vee \neg p_n \vee C$.

The following proposition is straightforward:

**Proposition 21.** *For every instance of (6), the conclusion of this inference is a hyperresolvent of the premises against $C(R)$. Vice versa, every inference of the form (7) against $C(R)$, where all clauses $C_i \vee p_i$ consist of variables in $S_\gamma$, is an instance of $R$.*

Suppose that $\gamma = s_1, \ldots, s_m$. Define the set $C(\gamma)$ of clauses consisting of clauses of three kinds:

1. All clauses $A^1 \vee \ldots \vee A^k$, such that $A^1, \ldots, A^k$ are signed subformulas of $\gamma$;
2. All clauses $C(R)$, such that $R$ is a rule of $G_\gamma$;
3. The (unary) clauses $\neg s_1, \ldots, \neg s_m$.

Using Proposition 21 one can prove the following theorem:

**Theorem 1.** *The sequent $\gamma$ is valid if and only if the set $C(\gamma)$ is unsatisfiable.*

One can use this theorem not only for establishing validity, but also for finding sequent derivations of (subsets of) $\gamma$. To this end, one should find an arbitrary resolution refutation of $C(\gamma)$ and transform it into a hyperresolution refutation. The details are included in a longer version of this paper.

Likewise, for any sequent that is not valid one can find a countermodel, as follows. Take any model $M$ of $C(\gamma)$, for example, found by a SAT solver. We have to find a truth assignment $\alpha$ that makes $\gamma$ false. Suppose that $A \in Atom$. If all $A^1, \ldots, A^k$ are signed subformulas of $\gamma$, then $A^1 \vee \ldots \vee A^k$ is a clause in $C(\gamma)$, hence for at least one $j$ we have $M \models A^j$. In this case we pick any such truth value $j$ and define $\alpha(A) \overset{\text{def}}{=} j$. If some of $A^1, \ldots, A^k$ is not a signed subformulas of $\gamma$, we pick such $A_j$ and define $\alpha(A) \overset{\text{def}}{=} j$.

Note that there is an interesting variation of our translation, where we add clauses $\neg A^i \vee \neg A^j$ for all $i \neq j$. It requires experiments on large and hard formulas to understand whether it improves validity checking. On the one hand, we obtain a large set of clauses. On the other hand, we obtain many binary clauses, which may result in better performance because of improved unit propagation.

# 7    Conclusion and Related Work

By proof-theoretic investigation of sequent calculi for many-valued logics, we show how to design an inverse method calculus for a given sequent $\gamma$. Further, we show that validity checking for $\gamma$ can be done by a SAT solver by building a set of propositional clauses $C(\gamma)$ such that $C(\gamma)$ is unsatisfiable if and only if $\gamma$ is valid.

Theorem proving for many-valued logics is an area that attracted attention of many researchers. Some papers were already cited above, let us now mention papers most relevant to this paper. Papers [2, 3] build a resolution calculus for many-valued logics. Our calculus uses the inverse method and our hyper-resolution simulation is different since the result of our translation is the set of ordinary propositional clauses. There are several papers providing translation from many-valued clausal logic into SAT, including [1, 7]. On the contrary, we focus on non-clausal formulas. Paper [15] discusses translation of formulas in many-valued logics to short normal forms, however these normal forms are many-valued too. Contrary to all these papers, we design an optimised translation by studying proof-theoretic properties of sequent calculi. For example, our notion of signed subformula is proof-theoretic and in general gives smaller sets of signed subformulas than in other approaches. The proof-theoretic investigation in this paper uses many ideas from [10]. However, [10] does not discuss many-valued logics and the translation to propositional resolution.

In future our results may benefit from results and ideas in the above mentioned papers. For example, using sets of signs instead of single signs is an interesting avenue to exploit. We are also interested in handling quantifiers.

# References

1. Ansótegui, C., Bonet, M.L., Levy, J., Manyà, F.: Mapping CSP into Many-Valued SAT. In: Marques-Silva, J., Sakallah, K.A. (eds.) SAT 2007. LNCS, vol. 4501, pp. 10–15. Springer, Heidelberg (2007)
2. Baaz, M., Fermüller, C.G.: Resolution for many-valued logics. In: Voronkov, A. (ed.) LPAR 1992. LNCS, vol. 624, pp. 107–118. Springer, Heidelberg (1992)
3. Baaz, M., Fermüller, C.G.: Resolution-based theorem proving for many-valued logics. Journal of Symbolic Computations 19, 353–391 (1995)
4. Baaz, M., Fermüller, C.G., Ovrutcki, A., Zach, R.: MULTLOG: a system for axiomatizing many-valued logics. In: Voronkov, A. (ed.) LPAR 1993. LNCS, vol. 698, pp. 345–347. Springer, Heidelberg (1993)
5. Baaz, M., Fermüller, C.G., Zach, R.: Systematic construction of natural deduction systems for many-valued logics. In: Proc. 23rd International Symposium on Multiple-Valued Logics, Los Gatos, CA, pp. 208–213. IEEE Computer Society Press (1993)
6. Bachmair, L., Ganzinger, H.: Resolution theorem proving. In: Robinson, A., Voronkov, A. (eds.) Handbook of Automated Reasoning, ch. 2, vol. I, pp. 19–99. Elsevier Science (2001)
7. Beckert, B., Hähnle, R., Manyà, F.: Transformations between signed and classical clause logic. In: ISMVL, pp. 248–255 (1999)
8. Carnielli, W.A.: Systematization of finite many-valued logics through the method of tableaux. Journal of Symbolic Logic 52(2), 473–493 (1987)
9. Carnielli, W.A.: On sequents and tableaux for many-valued logics. Journal of Non-Classical Logics 8(1), 59–76 (1991)
10. Degtyarev, A., Voronkov, A.: The inverse method. In: Robinson, A., Voronkov, A. (eds.) Handbook of Automated Reasoning, ch. 4, vol. I, pp. 179–272. Elsevier Science (2001)
11. Dershowitz, N., Plaisted, D.A.: Rewriting. In: Robinson, A., Voronkov, A. (eds.) Handbook of Automated Reasoning, ch. 9, vol. I, pp. 535–610. Elsevier Science (2001)
12. Gentzen, G.: Untersuchungen über das logische Schließen. Mathematical Zeitschrift 39, 176–210, 405–431 (1934); Translated as [13]
13. Gentzen, G.: Investigations into logical deduction. In: Szabo, M.E. (ed.) The Collected Papers of Gerhard Gentzen, pp. 68–131. North Holland, Amsterdam (1969); reprinted from [12]
14. Hähnle, R.: Automated Deduction in Multiple-Valued Logics. Clarendon Press, Oxford (1993)
15. Hähnle, R.: Short conjunctive normal forms in finitely valued logics. Journal of Logic and Computation 4(6), 905–927 (1994)
16. Lifschitz, V.: What is the inverse method? Journal of Automated Reasoning 5(1), 1–23 (1989)
17. Yu, S.: Maslov. An inverse method for establishing deducibility of nonprenex formulas of the predicate calculus. Soviet Mathematical Doklady 172(1), 22–25 (1983); reprinted as [20]
18. Maslov, S.Y.: Relationship between tactics of the inverse method and the resolution method. Zapiski Nauchnyh Seminarov LOMI 16 (1969) (in Russian); Reprinted as [21]
19. Maslov, S.Y.: Proof-search strategies for methods of the resolution type. In: Meltzer, B., Michie, D. (eds.) Machine Intelligence, vol. 6, pp. 77–90. American Elsevier (1971)

20. Maslov, S.Y.: An inverse method for establishing deducibility of nonprenex formulas of the predicate calculus. In: Siekmann, J., Wrightson, G. (eds.) Automation of Reasoning (Classical papers on Computational Logic), vol. 2, pp. 48–54. Springer (1983); reprinted from [17]

21. Yu Maslov, S.: Relationship between tactics of the inverse method and the resolution method. In: Siekmann, J., Wrightson, G. (eds.) Automation of Reasoning (Classical papers on Computational Logic), vol. 2, pp. 264–272. Springer (1983); Reprinted from [18]

22. McLaughlin, S., Pfenning, F.: Efficient intuitionistic theorem proving with the polarized inverse method. In: Schmidt, R.A. (ed.) CADE-22. LNCS, vol. 5663, pp. 230–244. Springer, Heidelberg (2009)

23. Mints, G.: Gentzen-type systems and resolution rules. Part I. Propositional logic. In: Martin-Löf, P., Mints, G. (eds.) COLOG 1988. LNCS, vol. 417, pp. 198–231. Springer, Heidelberg (1990)

24. Murray, N.V., Rosenthal, E.: Improving tableau deductions in multiple-valued logics. In: Proceedings of the 21st International Symposium on Multiple-Valued logics, Los Alamitos, pp. 230–237. IEEE Computer Society Press (1991)

25. Murray, N.V., Rosenthal, E.: Resolution and path dissolution in multiple-valued logics. In: Proceedings International Symposium on Methodologies for Intelligent Systems, Charlotte (1991)

26. Murray, N.V., Rosenthal, E.: Signed formulas: a liftable meta-logic for multiple-valued logics. In: Komorowski, J., Raś, Z.W. (eds.) ISMIS 1993. LNCS, vol. 689, pp. 230–237. Springer, Heidelberg (1993)

27. O'Hearn, P., Stachniak, Z.: A resolution framework for finitely-valued first-order logics. Journal of Symbolic Computations 13, 235–254 (1992)

28. Robinson, J.A.: Robinson. Automatic deduction with hyper-resolution. International Journal of Computer Mathematics 1, 227–234 (1965); Reprinted as [29]

29. Robinson, J.A.: Automatic deduction with hyperresolution. In: Siekmann, J., Wrightson, G. (eds.) Automation of Reasoning. Classical Papers on Computational Logic, vol. 1, pp. 416–423. Springer (1983); Originally appeared as [28]

30. Rousseau, G.: Sequents in many-valued logic 1. Fundamenta Mathematikae, LX, 23–33 (1967)

31. Voronkov, A.: LISS — the logic inference search system. In: Stickel, M.E. (ed.) CADE 1990. LNCS, vol. 449, pp. 677–678. Springer, Heidelberg (1990)

32. Voronkov, A.: Theorem proving in non-standard logics based on the inverse method. In: Kapur, D. (ed.) CADE 1992. LNCS, vol. 607, pp. 648–662. Springer, Heidelberg (1992)

33. Voronkov, A.: Deciding $K$ using $kk$. In: Cohn, A.G., Giunchiglia, F., Selman, B. (eds.) Principles of Knowledge Representation and Reasoning (KR 2000), pp. 198–209 (2000)

34. Voronkov, A.: How to optimize proof-search in modal logics: new methods of proving redundancy criteria for sequent calculi. ACM Transactions on Computational Logic 2(2), 182–215 (2001)

# A Parametric Interpolation Framework for First-Order Theories

Laura Kovács[1], Simone Fulvio Rollini[2], and Natasha Sharygina[2]

[1] Chalmers University of Technology
[2] USI

**Abstract.** Craig interpolation is successfully used in both hardware and software model checking. Generating good interpolants, and hence automatically determining the quality of interpolants is however a very hard problem, requiring non-trivial reasoning in first-order theories. An important class of state-of-the-art interpolation algorithms is based on recursive procedures that generate interpolants from refutations of unsatisfiable conjunctions of formulas. We analyze this type of algorithms and develop a theoretical framework, called a parametric interpolation framework, for arbitrary first-order theories and inference systems. As interpolation-based verification approaches depend on the quality of interpolants, our method can be used to derive interpolants of different structure and strength, with or without quantifiers, from the same proof. We show that some well-known interpolation algorithms are instantiations of our framework.

## 1 Introduction

Craig interpolation [3] provides powerful heuristics for verifying software and hardware. In particular, interpolants extracted from proofs of various properties are used in invariant generation and bounded model checking, see e.g. [5, 9, 14].

There exist various methods to compute interpolants from proofs. The work of [12] introduces an interpolation algorithm for propositional logic, and is generalized in [13] to generate interpolants in the combined theory of uninterpreted functions and linear arithmetic. The approaches of [7, 11, 15] propose another interpolation algorithm for propositional logic which is later extended in [17] to address a class of first-order theories. More recently, [4] introduces a framework that generalizes [12, 15], by analyzing the logical strength of interpolants. The work of [4] has been extended in [16] to interpolation in the hyper-resolution system. The methods described in [6, 10] give a general interpolation algorithm that can be used with arbitrary first-order calculi and inference systems. This algorithm is, however, restricted to local proofs [10] or split proofs [9].

While interpolation-based verification techniques crucially depend onto which extent "good" interpolants can be generated, there is no general criterion for defining the notion of "good". Finding a good interpolant is a hard problem, whose solution justifies spurious program paths or helps proving correctness of

F. Castro, A. Gelbukh, and M. González (Eds.): MICAI 2013, Part I, LNAI 8265, pp. 24–40, 2013.

program properties. Given a computer program to be verified, a natural question to ask is therefore "what makes some interpolants better than others?", or "what are the essential program properties for which a good interpolant can be derived"? If the program is small or manipulates only a restricted class of data structures, one can expect a programmer to identify possible program errors and hence characterize the set of interpolants justifying these errors. For example, if a program implements linear arithmetic operations over integers, a good interpolant might be a conjunction of linear integer inequalities over program properties [2]. The works of [4,8] remark that interpolants of different strength can be beneficial in different verification frameworks. When dealing with properties over quantifier-free linear arithmetic and uninterpreted functions, [8] emphasizes the need for logically strong interpolants in model checking and predicate abstraction; however, when restricting interpolation to propositional logic, [4] suggests instead that logically weaker interpolants are more useful in verification.

While [2,4,8] answer our question of what a good interpolant can be, these methods are restricted to specific logic fragments and the qualitative measure of their interpolants cannot be easily extended to more general logics. For example, when a program implements also array operations, like array initializations, a good interpolant should summarize that all array elements have been initialized. This interpolant is a first-order property and can be expressed in first-order logic with quantifiers and array symbols. Computing and describing the quality of first-order interpolants is however a non-trivial problem. One could come up with various syntactic measures of quality, e.g. a small amount of quantifiers, as discussed in [6]; nevertheless, such a syntactic approach is limited, since it cannot be used to characterize semantic features like logical strength.

In this paper we introduce a new theoretical framework, called *parametric interpolation framework*, for arbitrary theories and inference systems. We show that the aforementioned interpolation procedures can be considered elements of a class of algorithms characterized by specific structural properties. Our method supports the generation of multiple interpolants of different strength and structure. For example, our approach can generate quantifier-free interpolants on examples where current methods are only able to compute quantified interpolants. Our approach also provides flexibility in adjusting the logical expressiveness of the computed interpolants, and hence can yield interpolants, even quantifier-free ones, that are stronger/weaker than the ones generated by current methods. We therefore believe that our contribution helps to answer the fundamental AI problem delineated above: by comparing structure and strength of interpolants in first-order theories we propose a theoretical framework to explore "good" interpolants. Investigating the impact of our approach on concrete verification problems is a very interesting task which needs extensive experimentation, and we leave it as future work.

**Contributions.** The main contribution of this paper comes with the *theoretical formalization of a new parametric interpolation framework* (§4). We show that this framework generalizes existing interpolation algorithms for first-order theories and, as a consequence, also for propositional logic (§5). We illustrate the kind of interpolants we produce (§3) and show how the interpolation algorithms of [4, 10, 16] can be regarded as special cases of our method in the context of first-order and hyper-resolution inference systems.

When compared to [10], the differences and benefits of our approach can be summarized as follows. We derive an algorithm for arbitrary first-order theories and inference systems, which extracts interpolants as boolean combinations of formulas from a refutation proof. Our algorithm can be applied to a class of proofs strictly larger than the class of local proofs in [10]; it can also produce a family of interpolants which contains the interpolants of [10]. Within this family, we relate and compare the interpolants by their logical strength. The results of [10] about the existence of local proofs in the superposition calculus and turning non-local proofs into local ones in the style of [6] can be naturally extended to our framework. Remarkably, our method allows to compute *quantifier-free interpolants* for problems on which [10] can only derive quantified interpolants.

Referring to [4, 16], our approach is different in the following aspects. We integrate the hyper-resolution system into our first-order interpolation algorithm, and discuss the applicability of the family of interpolants proposed there. We then extend the class of proofs from first-order theories to arbitrary hyper-resolution refutations, and show how the structure of the formulas and inference rules allows to obtain additional interpolants, containing those generated by [16]. Finally, we also compare the produced interpolants by their logical strength.

## 2    Preliminaries

This section fixes our notation and recalls some required terminology by adapting the material of [10] to our setting.

We consider the language of standard first-order logic with equality. We assume that the language contains boolean connectives and quantifiers, as well as the logical constants $\top$ and $\bot$ respectively denoting the *always true* and *always false* formulas. For a formula $A$ we write $\overline{A}$ to mean $\neg A$, that is the negation of $A$. We write $A_1, \ldots, A_n \vdash A$ to denote that $A_1 \land \cdots \land A_n \to A$ is valid.

We call a *symbol* a predicate symbol, a function symbol or a constant. Individual (logical) variables are thus not symbols. We use capital letters $A, B, C, D, I, R$, possibly with indices, to denote formulas. Terms are denoted by $s, t$, variables by $x, y, z$, constants by $a, b, c$, and functions by $f, g$, all possibly with indices. A *signature* $\Sigma$ is a finite set of symbols. The signature of a formula $A$, denoted by $\Sigma_A$, is the set of all symbols occurring in $A$. For example, the signature of $g(a, x)$ is $\{g, a\}$. The language of a formula $A$, denoted by $\mathcal{L}_A$, is the set of all formulas built from $\Sigma_A$.

Consider a formula $A$ whose free variables are $x_1, \ldots, x_m$. Then $\forall A$ denotes the formula $(\forall x_1, \ldots, x_m)A$; similarly, $\exists A$ is the formula $(\exists x_1, \ldots, x_m)A$.

**Inference Systems and Derivations.** An *inference rule*, or simply *inference*, is an $n + 1$-ary relation on formulas, where $n \geq 0$. It is usually written as: $\frac{A_1 \quad \cdots \quad A_n}{A}$ where $A_1, \ldots, A_n$ are the *premises* and $A$ the *conclusion*. An *inference system* is a set of inference rules. An *axiom* is the conclusion of an inference with 0 premises. An inference with 0 premises and conclusion $A$ will be written without the bar line as $A$. A *derivation*, or a *proof*, of a formula $A$ is a finite tree built from inferences in the inference system, such that the root of the tree is $A$ and all leaves are axioms; nodes correspond to formulas. A node $A$ with parents $A_1, \ldots, A_n$ represents the conclusion $A$ of an inference with premises $A_1, \ldots, A_n$. A derivation of $A$ is *from assumptions* $A_1, \ldots, A_n$ if every leaf is either an axiom or one of the formulas $A_1, \ldots, A_n$. A *refutation* is a derivation of $\perp$. A sub-tree of a derivation is called a *sub-derivation*.

**Colored Symbols and Formulas.** Let us now fix two sentences $R$ and $B$ and give all definitions relative to them. We define $\Sigma_{RB} = \Sigma_R \cap \Sigma_B$ as the set of symbols occurring both in $R$ and $B$ and take $\mathcal{L}_{RB} = \mathcal{L}_R \cap \mathcal{L}_B$. The signature symbols from $\Sigma_{RB}$ are called *grey* symbols. Signature symbols occurring only in $\Sigma_R \setminus \Sigma_{RB}$ will be called *red*, and symbols occurring only in $\Sigma_B \setminus \Sigma_{RB}$ are *blue*. A symbol that is not *grey* is also called *colored*. A formula $A$ is called *grey* if it contains only grey symbols. Grey formulas are thus in $\mathcal{L}_{RB}$. A formula $A$ that is not grey is called *colored*. A formula $A$ is called *red* if it contains only red and grey symbols, but at least one red symbol. Similarly, $A$ is said to be *blue* if it only contains blue and grey symbols, but at least one blue symbol. Red formulas will be denoted by $R$ and blue formulas by $B$, possibly with indices.

An *RB-derivation* is any derivation $\Pi$ satisfying the following conditions:

(RB1) for every leaf $C$, we have: $\vdash \forall C$ and $C \in \mathcal{L}_R$ or $B \vdash \forall C$ and $C \in \mathcal{L}_B$;

(RB2) for every inference $\dfrac{C_1 \quad \cdots \quad C_n}{C}$ of $\Pi$, we have: $\forall C_1, \ldots, \forall C_n \vdash \forall C$.

We call *RB-refutation* an *RB-derivation* of $\perp$.

**Craig Interpolation.** Given two formulas $R$ and $B$ such that their conjunction is unsatisfiable, that is $R \wedge B \vdash \perp$, an *(Craig) interpolant* of $R$ and $B$ is any grey formula $I$ such that $A \vdash I$ and $B \wedge I \vdash \perp$. Hence, $I \in \mathcal{L}_{RB}$. Note that we are interested in interpolants $I$ of red $R$ and blue $B$ formulas. For simplicity, in this paper we assume that neither $R$ or $B$ are trivially unsatisfiable, that is $R \nvdash \perp$ and $B \nvdash \perp$. As proved in [10], Craig interpolation can also be defined modulo theories. Symbols occurring in a theory are called *interpreted*, while all other symbols are *uninterpreted*.

## 3   Example

We start with an example showing what kind of interpolants we can compute.

*Example 1.* Let us take $\forall z (z = c) \wedge a = c \wedge g(b) = g(h)$ as $R$, and $f(a) \neq f(h) \wedge h = b$ as $B$. Then, $c, g$ are red symbols, $a, b, h$ are grey, and $f$ is blue. Clearly, $R \wedge B$ is unsatisfiable. A refutation $\Pi$ of $R \wedge B$ is given in Fig. 1. A possible interpolant of $R$ and $B$ is the quantified formula $\forall z (z = a)$, which would be computed, for example, by the interpolation algorithm of [10].

However, when applying our method on Fig. 1, besides $\forall z (z = a)$ we are able to compute $a = b$ and $h \neq b \vee (a = b \wedge h = b)$ as interpolants of $R$ and $B$.

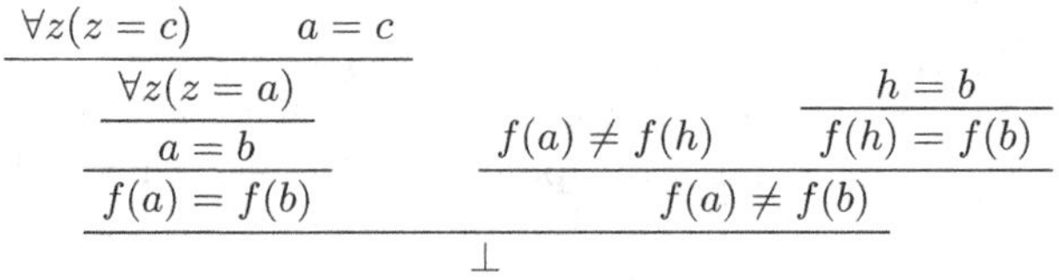

$$\dfrac{\dfrac{\dfrac{\forall z(z = c) \qquad a = c}{\forall z(z = a)}}{\dfrac{a = b}{f(a) = f(b)}} \qquad \dfrac{f(a) \neq f(h) \quad \dfrac{h = b}{f(h) = f(b)}}{f(a) \neq f(b)}}{\bot}$$

**Fig. 1.** Local refutation $\Pi$ of $R \wedge B$

Note that these two additional interpolants are quantifier-free, and of different strength. Our method thus offers the possibility of computing *quantifier-free interpolants* for problems on which [10] could only derive quantified interpolants. When applying our method to quantifier-free inference systems, for example to the propositional hyper-resolution system, our approach also generates a range of quantifier-free interpolants, including those coming from [16]. The main advantage of our approach hence comes with the flexibility of *choosing between more than one "good" interpolant* and *generating interpolants of different boolean structure and strength, with or without quantifiers, from the same proof.*

## 4    A Parametric Interpolation Framework

We now present a new interpolation framework that describes a class of recursive interpolation procedures computing so-called *partial interpolants* from refutation proofs. These procedures start by deriving partial interpolants for the leaves; then, they derive partial interpolants for (some of) the inner nodes, by relying on the previously computed partial interpolants. In what follows, we first define the notion of partial interpolants. Then our *parametric interpolation algorithm* is given (Alg. 1), and the soundness of our approach is discussed. The algorithm will be later instantiated into a specific interpolation algorithm in first-order, as well as propositional systems. (§5).

Let $\Pi$ be an RB-refutation, corresponding to the unsatisfiability proof of $R \wedge B$. Following [10], we generate an interpolant $I$ of $R$ and $B$ such that $I$ is a boolean combination of formulas of $\Pi$. Recall that $R \vdash I$, $B \vdash \overline{I}$ and $I \in \mathcal{L}_{RB}$. Our framework is parametric in a chosen *partition* of $\Pi$, i.e. a set of derivations $\mathcal{P} = \{\Pi'_i\}$ such that (i) each $\Pi'_i$ is a sub-derivation of $\Pi$, (ii) a leaf of a sub-derivation $\Pi'_i$ represents the root of another sub-derivation $\Pi'_j$ or a leaf of $\Pi$, (iii) each inference of $\Pi$ belongs to some $\Pi'_i \in \mathcal{P}$. We call the leaves of a sub-derivation $\Pi'_i \in \mathcal{P}$ *sub-leaves* of $\Pi'_i$; note that a sub-leaf might also be a leaf of $\Pi$. Similarly, the root of a sub-derivation $\Pi'_i$ is called a *sub-root* of $\Pi'_i$. The aim of our algorithm is to build an interpolant from $\Pi$, by using the partition $\mathcal{P}$ of $\Pi$. To this end, we first define the notion of a *partial interpolant* of a formula $C$.

**Definition 1.** *[Partial Interpolant] Let $C$ be a formula, and let $f$ and $g$ denote functions over formulas such that $f(\bot) = g(\bot) = \bot$. A formula $I_C$ is called a* partial interpolant of $C$ with respect to $R$ and $B$ if it satisfies:

$$R \vdash I_C \vee f(C), \quad B \vdash \overline{I_C} \vee g(C), \quad I_C \in \mathcal{L}_{RB}. \tag{1}$$

When $C$ is $\perp$, a partial interpolant $I_C$ is an interpolant of $R$ and $B$, since we have $R \vdash I_C$ and $B \vdash \overline{I_C}$. Note also that Def. 1 generalizes the notion of C-interpolants from [10]. Namely, by taking $f(C) = C$ and $g(C) = C$ a partial interpolant $I_C$ is just a C-interpolant in the sense of [10], when $C$ is grey.

Let us emphasize that in Def. 1 we are not restricted to a particular choice of $f$ and $g$, which can be arbitrary functions over formulas. For example, the value of $f(C)$ and $g(C)$ might not even depend on $C$, or $f$ and $g$ can be defined using $\mathcal{P}$; the only restriction we impose is that eq. (1) holds. Such a generality allows us to build various (partial) interpolants, as presented later in §5.

Using partial interpolants, our framework is summarized as follows. Given a partition $\mathcal{P}$ of $\Pi$, we first compute partial interpolants of the leaves of $\Pi$. Next, for each sub-derivation $\Pi'_i \in \mathcal{P}$ with root $C$ and leaves $C_1, \ldots, C_n$, we build a partial interpolant $I_C$ of $C$, proceeding inductively. We use the sub-leaves $C_1, \ldots, C_n$, and respectively compute their partial interpolants $I_{C_1}, \ldots, I_{C_n}$. $I_C$ is then obtained as a boolean combination of (some of) $C$, $C_1, \ldots, C_n$, and $I_{C_1}, \ldots, I_{C_n}$. As a consequence, a partial interpolant of the root $\perp$ of $\Pi$ is an interpolant $I$ of $R$ and $B$.

When computing partial interpolants of a formula $C$, we make a case distinction whether $C$ is a leaf (base case) or a sub-root of $\Pi$ (induction step). We now address each case separately and formulate requirements over a formula to be a partial interpolant of $C$ (see eq. (2) and (5)).

**Partial Interpolants of Leaves.** Let $C$ be a leaf of $\Pi$. Then, by the property (RB1) of $RB$-derivations, we need to distinguish between $R \vdash C$ and $B \vdash C$. The following *conditions over a partial interpolant $I_C$ of $C$* are therefore imposed in order to satisfy (1):

$$R \vdash C \wedge \overline{f(C)} \rightarrow I_C, \qquad B \vdash I_C \rightarrow g(C), \quad I_C \in \mathcal{L}_{RB}, \qquad \text{if } R \vdash C;$$
$$R \vdash \overline{f(C)} \rightarrow I_C, \qquad B \vdash I_C \rightarrow \overline{C} \vee g(C), \quad I_C \in \mathcal{L}_{RB}, \qquad \text{if } B \vdash C. \quad (2)$$

**Partial Interpolants of Sub-roots.** Let $C$ be the root of a sub-derivation $\Pi'$ of $\Pi$. We assume that $\Pi'$ consists of more than one formula (otherwise, we are in Case 1) and that the leaves of $\Pi'$ are $C_1, \ldots, C_n$. By the property (RB2), we conclude $\bigwedge C_i \vdash C$. By the induction hypothesis over $C_1, \ldots, C_n$, we assume that the partial interpolants $I_{C_1}, \ldots, I_{C_n}$ of the sub-leaves $C_i$ are already computed. Using eq. (1), we have:

$$R \vdash I_{C_i} \vee f(C_i), \quad B \vdash \overline{I_{C_i}} \vee g(C_i), \quad I_{C_i} \in \mathcal{L}_{RB}. \quad (3)$$

From a simple combination of $\bigwedge C_i \vdash C$ and eq. (3), we have:

$$R \vdash \bigwedge (I_{C_i} \vee f(C_i)) \wedge (\bigvee \overline{C_i} \vee C), \quad B \vdash \bigwedge (\overline{I_{C_i}} \vee g(C_i)) \wedge (\bigvee \overline{C_i} \vee C). \quad (4)$$

Using (1) in conjunction with (4), we derive the *following constraints over a partial interpolant $I_C$ of $C$*:

$$R \vdash \bigwedge(I_{C_i} \vee f(C_i)) \wedge (\bigvee \overline{C_i} \vee C) \wedge \overline{f(C)} \rightarrow I_C, \qquad\qquad I_C \in \mathcal{L}_{RB},$$

$$B \vdash I_C \rightarrow \bigvee(I_{C_i} \wedge \overline{g(C_i)}) \vee (\bigwedge C_i \wedge \overline{C}) \vee g(C). \qquad\qquad (5)$$

**Parametric Interpolation Algorithm.** Our interpolation algorithm is given in Alg. 1. It takes as input an $RB$-derivation $\Pi$, a partition $\mathcal{P}$ of $\Pi$, and the functions $f$ and $g$. In addition, Alg. 1 depends on a *construct* function which builds partial interpolants of leaves and sub-roots of $\Pi$, by using $f$ and $g$. That is, for a formula $C$, *construct* returns a *set $\Phi$ of partial interpolants $I_C$* by making a case distinction whether $C$ is a leaf or a sub-root of $\Pi$. Hence, setting $f_C = f(C), g_C = g(C), f_i = f(C_i), g_i = g(C_i), I_i = I(C_i)$, *construct* is defined as:

$$construct(C, C_i, I_i, f_C, g_C, f_i, g_i) = \begin{cases} \Phi_1, & \text{if } C \text{ is a leaf} \\ \Phi_2, & \text{if } C \text{ is a sub-root} \end{cases} \qquad (6)$$

where each $I_C \in \Phi_1$ satisfies (2) and each $I_C \in \Phi_2$ satisfies (5). Note that the arguments $C_i, I_{C_i}, f(C_i), g(C_i)$ of *construct* become trivially empty whenever $C$ is a leaf. For simplicity of notation, *we therefore write construct$(C, f(C), g(C))$ whenever $C$ is a leaf.* The behavior of *construct*, in particular the choice of $\Phi_1$ and $\Phi_2$, is specific to the inference system in which $\Pi$ was produced. We will address one choice of $\Phi_1$ and $\Phi_2$ in §5.

Assuming *construct*, $f, g$ are fixed, Alg. 1 returns an interpolant $I$ of $R$ and $B$. First, the leaves of $\Pi$ are identified (line 2). For each leaf $C$ of $\Pi$, a set $\Phi_1$ of partial interpolants satisfying (2) is constructed. Then, the partial interpolant of $C$ is selected from $\Phi_1$ (line 5). Next, partial interpolants of the sub-roots $C$ of $\Pi$ are recursively computed (lines 9-18). To this end, each sub-derivation $\Pi' \in \mathcal{P}$ with root $C$ and leaves $C_1, \dots, C_n$ is analyzed. A set $\Phi_2$ of partial interpolants of $C$ is built by using the partial interpolants of $C_1, \dots, C_n$ (line 13). The partial interpolant of $C$ is selected from $\Phi_2$ (line 14). Finally, the partial interpolant of $\bot$ is returned as the interpolant of $R$ and $B$ (line 19).

**Algorithm 1.** *Parametric Interpolation Algorithm*
**Input:**    *Formulas $R$ and $B$ such that $R \wedge B \rightarrow \bot$, an $RB$-refutation $\Pi$ of $R \wedge B$, a partition $\mathcal{P}$ of $\Pi$, and functions $f, g, construct$.*
**Output:**    *Interpolant $I$ of $R$ and $B$*
**Assumption:**    *$f$ and $g$ satisfy (1), construct produces grey formulas*

  1   **begin**
      *Compute Partial Interpolants of Leaves*
  2   $L := leaves(\Pi)$;
  3   **for**   *each formula $C$ in $L$* **do**
  4      $\Phi_1 := construct(C, f(C), g(C))$;
  5      $I_C := select(\Phi_1)$;
  6   **endfor** ;
      *Compute Partial Interpolants of Sub-Roots*
  7   $\mathcal{I} := \bigcup_{C \in L} I_C$, *where $\mathcal{I}[C] := I_C$*;
  8   $\mathcal{P}_* = \{\}$;

```
9  repeat
10    for  each Π' in P such that leaves(Π') ⊆ L do
11       C := root(Π');
12       for  each Cᵢ in leaves(Π')  do  I_{Cᵢ} := I[Cᵢ]  endfor ;
13       Φ₂ := construct(C, Cᵢ, I_{Cᵢ}, f(C), g(C), f(Cᵢ), g(Cᵢ));
14       I_C := select(Φ₂);
15       I := I ∪ {I_C};   L := L ∪ {C};
16    endfor ;
17    P* := P* ∪ {Π'};
18  until P* = P;
      Compute Interpolant
19  return I[⊥]
```

Alg. 1 depends on the choice of $f, g$, and *construct*, as well as of the partition $\mathcal{P}$; *select* denotes a function that picks and returns a formula from a set of formulas. A *parametric interpolation framework* is thus implicitly defined by $f, g, construct$, and $\mathcal{P}$, yielding different interpolation algorithms based on Alg. 1.

In the sequel we present a concrete choice of $f, g$ and *construct*, together with $\mathcal{P}$, yielding an interpolation procedure for arbitrary first-order inference systems. It is then not hard to argue that our method also yields an interpolation procedure in the propositional hyper-resolution system. Further, we show that Alg. 1 generalizes the interpolation algorithms of [10, 16].

## 5    Interpolation in First-Order Systems

We present an interpolation procedure for arbitrary first-order inference systems, by fixing the definition of $f, g, construct$ and $\mathcal{P}$ in Alg. 1 as follows.

**Definition of $f$ and $g$.** We take $f$ and $g$ such that $f(C) = g(C) = C$, for every formula $C$. Clearly, the condition $f(\bot) = g(\bot) = \bot$ from Def. 1 is satisfied.

**Definition of $\mathcal{P}$.** We are interested in a special kind of partition, which we call *RB-partition* and define below.

**Definition 2.** *[RB-partition] Let $\Pi$ be an RB-derivation and consider a partition $\mathcal{P} = \{\Pi'_j\}$ of $\Pi$ into a set of sub-derivations $\Pi'_j$. The partition $\mathcal{P}$ of $\Pi$ is called an RB-partition if the following conditions hold:*

*– the sub-root $C$ of each $\Pi'_j$ is grey;*
*– the sub-leaves $C_i$ of each $\Pi'_j$ satisfy one of the following conditions: (a) every $C_i$ is grey, or (b) if some of the $C_i$ are colored, then the colored sub-leaves $C_j$ are also leaves of $\Pi$ and $C_j$ are either all red or all blue. Hence, a colored sub-leaf $C_j$ cannot contain both red and blue symbols.*

In this section we fix $\mathcal{P}$ to be an *RB-partition*. We are now left with defining the input function *construct* of Alg. 1. We make a case distinction on the sub-roots of the proof, and define the sets $\Phi_1$ and $\Phi_2$ of partial interpolants as follows.

**Definition of** *construct* **for Partial Interpolants of Leaves.** Let $C$ be a leaf of $\Pi$. Since $f(C) = g(C) = C$, eq. (2) yields the following constraints over $I_C$:

$$R \vdash \bot \to I_C, \qquad B \vdash I_C \to C, \qquad I_C \in \mathcal{L}_{RB}, \qquad \text{if } R \vdash C;$$
$$R \vdash \overline{C} \to I_C, \qquad B \vdash I_C \to \top, \qquad I_B \in \mathcal{L}_{RB}, \qquad \text{if } B \vdash C.$$

In principle, any formula $I_C \in \mathcal{L}_{RB}$ such that $\overline{C} \to \overline{I_C}$ if $R \vdash C$, and $\overline{C} \to I_C$ if $B \vdash C$ can be chosen as partial interpolant. Depending on whether $C$ is grey or not, we define the set $\Phi_1$ of partial interpolants as follows:

- If $C$ is grey, we take:      $\Phi_1 = \{C, \bot\}$, if $R \vdash C$;    $\{\overline{C}, \top\}$, if $B \vdash C$.
- If $C$ is colored, we take: $\Phi_1 = \{\bot\}$, if $R \vdash C$;    $\{\top\}$, if $B \vdash C$.

**Definition of** *construct* **for Partial Interpolants of Sub-roots.** Let $C$ be the root of a sub-derivation $\Pi' \in \mathcal{P}$, and let $C_1, \ldots, C_n$ denote the sub-leaves of $\Pi'$. As $f(C) = g(C) = C$ and $f(C_i) = g(C_i) = C_i$, eq. (5) yields the following constraints over $I_C \in \mathcal{L}_{RB}$:

$$R \vdash \bigwedge (I_{C_i} \vee C_i) \wedge (\bigvee \overline{C_i} \vee C) \wedge \overline{C} \to I_C,$$
$$B \vdash I_C \to \bigvee (I_{C_i} \wedge \overline{C_i}) \vee (\bigwedge C_i \wedge \overline{C}) \vee C. \tag{7}$$

Any formula $I_C \in \Phi_2$ needs to satisfy eq. (7). A potential set $\Phi_2$ of partial interpolants consists of the following ten formulas (annotated from (a) to (j)):

(a) $\bigwedge (I_{C_i} \vee C_i) \wedge (\bigvee \overline{C_i} \vee C) \wedge \overline{C}$    (f) $\bigvee (I_{C_i} \wedge \overline{C_i})$

(b) $\bigwedge (I_{C_i} \vee C_i) \wedge (\bigvee \overline{C_i})$    (g) $\bigvee (I_{C_i} \wedge \overline{C_i}) \vee C$

(c) $\bigwedge (I_{C_i} \vee C_i) \wedge (\bigvee \overline{C_i} \vee C)$    (h) $\bigvee (I_{C_i} \wedge \overline{C_i}) \vee (\bigwedge C_i \wedge \overline{C})$    (8)

(d) $\bigwedge (I_{C_i} \vee C_i) \wedge \overline{C}$    (i) $\bigvee (I_{C_i} \wedge \overline{C_i}) \vee (\bigwedge C_i)$

(e) $\bigwedge (I_{C_i} \vee C_i)$    (j) $\bigvee (I_{C_i} \wedge \overline{C_i}) \vee (\bigwedge C_i \wedge \overline{C}) \vee C$

It is not hard to argue that every formula from (8) satisfies eq. (7). However, not any formula from (8) could be used as a partial interpolant $I_C$, as partial interpolants need to be grey. Note however that $\mathcal{P}$ is an $RB$-partition; this means that the root of $\Pi'$ is grey, yielding that $f(C) = g(C) = C$ are grey formulas. Hence, whether a formula from (8) is grey depends only on whether the leaves of $\Pi'$ are also grey. To define the set $\Phi_2$ of partial interpolants, we therefore exploit the definition of RB-partitions and adjust (8) to the following three cases. In the sequel we refer by (a), ..., (j) to the formulas denoted by (a), ..., (j) in (8). *Case (i).* All leaves $C_i$ of $\Pi'$ are grey. Any formula from (8) is a partial interpolant and:

$$\Phi_2 = \{(a), (b), (c), (d), (e), (f), (g), (h), (i), (j)\}.$$

*Case (ii). Some leaves of $\Pi'$ are red.* Let us write $\{C_i\} = \{D_k\} \cup \{C_j\}$, where $C_j$ are the grey leaves and $D_k$ denote the red leaves of $\Pi'$. Using the definition of $RB$-partitions, $D_k$ are also leaves of $\Pi$. From property (RB1), we conclude $R \vdash \bigwedge D_k$ and take $I_{D_k} = \bot$ as the partial interpolants of $D_k$. From (RB2), we have $\vdash \bigvee \overline{C_i} \vee C$. Then from $R \vdash \bigwedge D_k$ and $\vdash \bigvee \overline{C_i} \vee C$, we derive $R \vdash \bigvee \overline{C_j} \vee C$.

Thus, restricting ourselves to the grey leaves $C_j$, the constraints (5) become:

$$R \vdash \bigwedge (I_{C_j} \vee C_j) \wedge (\bigvee \overline{C_j} \vee C) \wedge \overline{C} \rightarrow I_C, \qquad B \vdash I_C \rightarrow \bigvee (I_{C_j} \wedge \overline{C_j}) \vee C.$$

Let (a′),(b′),(c′),(f′),(g′) denote the formulas obtained from (a),(b),(c),(f),(g), by replacing $C_i$ with $C_j$. It is not difficult to prove that any formula (a′),(b′),(c′),(f′), (g′) can be taken as a partial interpolant $I_C$ of $C$. Hence:

$$\Phi_2 = \{(a'), (b'), (c'), (f'), (g')\}.$$

*Case (iii). Some leaves of $\Pi'$ are blue.* Using the notation of Case (ii), eq. (5) imposes the following constraints over $I_C$:

$$R \vdash \bigwedge (I_{C_j} \vee C_j) \wedge \overline{C} \rightarrow I_C, \qquad B \vdash I_{C_j} \rightarrow \bigvee (I_{C_j} \wedge \overline{C_j}) \vee (\bigwedge C_j \wedge \overline{C}) \vee C.$$

Let (d′),(e′),(h′),(i′),(j′) denote the formulas obtained from (d),(e),(h),(i),(j), by replacing $C_i$ with $C_j$. Then, (d′),(e′),(h′),(i′),(j′) are partial interpolant $I_C$ of $C$. Hence:

$$\Phi_2 = \{(d'), (e'), (h'), (i'), (j')\}.$$

**Interpolation Algorithm for First-Order Inference Systems.** Alg. 1 yields *a new interpolation procedure for arbitrary first-order inference systems,* as follows. It takes as input an $RB$-refutation $\Pi$ and an $RB$-partition $\mathcal{P}$ of $\Pi$. The input functions $f, g$ of Alg. 1 satisfy the condition $f(C) = g(C) = C$, for every $C$, whereas the *construct* function is defined by using the above given sets $\Phi_1$ and $\Phi_2$ in (6). With these considerations on its inputs, Alg. 1 returns an interpolant $I$ of $R$ and $B$ by recursively computing the partial interpolants of leaves and sub-roots of $\Pi$. The (partial) interpolants derived by Alg. 1 are of different strength and are computed from the same proof. We next discuss the strength of our partial interpolants, and relate them to other methods, in particular to the local derivation framework of [10].

**Logical Relations among Partial Interpolants.** Fig. 2 shows the relationship among the formulas from (8) in terms of logical strength. An arrow is drawn between two formulas denoted by (x) and (y) if (x)→(y). All implications in Fig. 2 are valid, which can be shown by simply applying resolution on (x)∧(y). The logical relations of Fig. 2 correspond to Case (i) above; the relations corresponding to Cases (ii) and (iii) are special cases of Fig. 2.

Based on the partial interpolants of (8), we believe that we are now ready to answer the questions raised in §1 about interpolants quality. As illustrated in Fig. 2, *our partial interpolants differ in their logical strength.* Different choices of partial interpolants yield weaker or stronger interpolants in Alg. 1. While previous methods, e.g. [4,8,16], also address logical strength, they are restricted to quantifier-free interpolants. Our approach instead characterizes interpolants strength in full first-order logic, and can be used to derive interpolants in arbitrary first-order theories. The quality of interpolants clearly depends on their

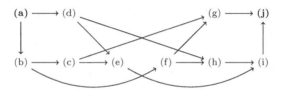

**Fig. 2.** Implication graph of partial interpolants in first-order inference systems

application to program verification, and weaker/stronger interpolants might yield better scalability of interpolation-based verification approaches.

**The Local Derivations Framework.** The interpolation algorithm of [10] extracts interpolants from so-called *local derivations*, also called *split derivations* in [9]. An inference in a local derivation cannot use both red and blue symbols; inferences of local derivations are called local inferences. It is easy to see that local proofs are special cases of $RB$-derivations.

Given a local $RB$-derivation $\Pi$, by making use of our notation, the algorithm of [10] can be summarized as follows. A partition $\mathcal{P}$ of $\Pi$ is first created such that each sub-derivation $\Pi'$ of $\Pi$ is a maximal red or a maximal blue sub-derivation. Next, partial interpolants are constructed as given below:

- If $C$ is a grey sub-leaf of $\Pi$, then: $\Phi_1 = \{C\}$, if $R \vdash C$;   $\{\overline{C}\}$, if $B \vdash C$.

- If $C$ is a grey sub-root of a sub-derivation $\Pi'$ with leaves $C_1, \ldots, C_n$, then $C_1, \ldots, C_n \vdash C$. Let $\{C_j\}$ denote the set of grey leaves of $\Pi'$. Hence, $\{C_j\} \subseteq \{C_1, \ldots, C_n\}$ and:

$$\Phi_2 = \begin{cases} \{\bigwedge_j (C_j \vee I_{C_j}) \wedge \bigvee_j \overline{C_j}\}, & \text{if } \Pi' \text{ is a red sub-derivation;} \\ \{\bigwedge_j (C_j \vee I_{C_j})\}, & \text{if } \Pi' \text{ is a blue sub-derivation.} \end{cases}$$

It is therefore not hard to argue that the algorithm of [10] is a special case of Alg. 1. The partial interpolants generated by [10] are a subset of the partial interpolants we compute. In particular, if $\Pi'$ is a red (respectively, blue) sub-derivation, then the partial interpolant of the sub-root $C$ of $\Pi'$ in [10] corresponds to our formula (b') (respectively, (e')) defined before.

Note that the sets $\Phi_1$ and $\Phi_2$ computed by [10] contain exactly one formula, giving thus exactly one interpolant, while the cardinality of $\Phi_1$ and $\Phi_2$ in our method can be greater than 1 (lines 4 and 13 of Alg. 1). Moreover, some of our interpolants cannot be obtained by other methods – see Example 1.

*Example 2.* We illustrate our first-order interpolation procedure by using the formulas $R$ and $B$ of Example 1. Consider the $RB$-refutation $\Pi$ given in Fig. 1 and take the $RB$-partition $\mathcal{P} = \{\Pi', \Pi''\}$, where $\Pi'$ and $\Pi''$ are respectively given in Fig. 3 and Fig. 4.

By applying Alg. 1, we first visit the sub-derivation $\Pi''$ and compute $I_{a=b}$. Since $\Pi''$ has red leaves, the set of partial interpolants corresponding to the root

$a = b$ of $\Pi''$ is: $\{(a'), (b'), (c'), (f'), (g')\}$. Since all the sub-leaves of $\Pi''$ are colored leaves, $(a'),(b'),(c'),(f'),(g')$ respectively reduce to $a = b \wedge a \neq b$, $\bot$, $a = b$, $\bot$, $a = b$. The set of partial interpolants $I_{a=b}$ is thus given by: $\{a = b, \bot\}$. Next, we

$$\frac{\dfrac{a = b}{f(a) = f(b)} \qquad \dfrac{f(a) \neq f(h) \qquad \dfrac{h = b}{f(h) = f(b)}}{f(a) \neq f(b)}}{\bot}$$

Fig. 3. Sub-derivation $\Pi'$

$$\frac{\dfrac{\forall z(z = c) \qquad a = c}{\forall z(z = a)}}{a = b}$$

Fig. 4. Sub-derivation $\Pi''$

visit the sub-derivation $\Pi'$. As $\Pi'$ has blue leaves, the set of partial interpolants corresponding to the root $\bot$ of $\Pi'$ is $\{(d'), (e'), (h'), (i'), (j')\}$. Since $\Pi'$ has two grey sub-leaves, namely $a = b$ and $h = b$, the formulas $(d'),(e'),(h'),(i'),(j')$ are simplified, yielding the following set of partial interpolants $I_\bot$: $\{(I_{a=b} \vee a = b) \wedge (I_{h=b} \vee h = b), (I_{a=b} \wedge a \neq b) \vee (I_{h=b} \wedge h \neq b) \vee (a = b \wedge h = b)\}$. To derive the partial interpolant $I_{h=b}$, note that $h = b$ is the only grey leaf of $B$. Therefore, the set of partial interpolants $I_{h=b}$ is given by $\{\top, h \neq b\}$. Using these results, the set of (partial) interpolants $I_\bot$ finally given by $\{a = b, h \neq b \vee (a = b \wedge h = b)\}$.

The $RB$-partition we used here is different from the one used in [10]. The flexibility in choosing $RB$-partitions in Alg. 1 allows us to derive *quantifier-free interpolants* from Fig. 1.

Summarizing, Fig. 2 characterizes the logical strength of the interpolants derived by our method, and hence offers a theoretical approach in finding a good interpolant when one is interested in deriving a logically strong/weak interpolant. A natural question to be further studied is whether a given refutation admits an $RB$-partition $\mathcal{P}$. It is even more interesting to understand which inference systems yield always an $RB$-partition of an $RB$-refutation. To some extent, the works of [6,10] answer these questions by considering *local derivations*. In [6], it is shown that non-local derivations in some cases can be translated into local ones, by existentially quantifying away colored uninterpreted constants; such a transformation comes thus at the price of introducing quantifiers. Further, [10] proves that an extension of the quantifier-free superposition calculus with quantifier-free linear rational arithmetic always guarantees local derivations. Since local derivations are special cases of $RB$-derivations, the results of [6, 10] also apply to our framework. Deriving sufficient and/or necessary conditions over $RB$-partitions of $RB$-derivations is an interesting task to be further investigated.

## 5.1 Interpolation in the Labeled Hyper-Resolution Framework

Alg. 1 yields a new interpolation procedure for arbitrary first-order inference systems and generalizes existing first-order interpolation methods [6,10]. It is not hard to prove that, by appropriately choosing $f, g, construct$ and $\mathcal{P}$ in Alg. 1, our approach also yields a new interpolation procedure for the propositional hyper-resolution inference system. Moreover, when adjusting Fig. 2 to that system, our method is able to generate the interpolants produced by the labeled hyper-resolution framework of [16], as well as additional interpolants that are logically weaker/stronger. In the following, we briefly sketch how Alg. 1 can be instantiated in the hyper-resolution system; for a detailed presentation we refer the reader to [1].

The *hyper-resolution (HR) system* is an inference system that uses a single inference rule, called the *hyper-resolution rule*:

$$\frac{\overline{p_1} \vee \cdots \vee \overline{p_{n-1}} \vee E \qquad D_1 \vee p_1 \qquad \ldots \qquad D_{n-1} \vee p_{n-1}}{\bigvee D_i \vee E}$$

where $p_1, \ldots, p_n$ are literals, called *pivots*, and $D_1, \ldots, D_n, E$ are clauses.

Let $\Sigma$ be a signature. We introduce a *restriction operator* $|_\Sigma$ over clauses $C$: $C|_\Sigma$ is the disjunction of the literals $l_j$ of $C$ such that $l_j$ are in $\Sigma$. We denote $C|_R = C|_{\Sigma_R \setminus \Sigma_{RB}}$, $C|_B = C|_{\Sigma_B \setminus \Sigma_{RB}}$, $C|_{RB} = C|_{\Sigma_{RB}}$ and say that $C$ is respectively restricted to its red, blue, grey symbols. For each clause $C$ and inference in $\Pi$, we define two arbitrary subsets $\Delta_R^C, \Delta_B^C \subseteq \Sigma_{RB}$ of grey symbols, where $\Delta_R^C \cup \Delta_B^C = \Sigma_{RB}$, and write $C|_{R\Delta_R^C} = C|_R \vee C|_{\Delta_R^C}$, $C|_{B\Delta_B^C} = C|_B \vee C|_{\Delta_B^C}$. $\Delta_R^C, \Delta_B^C$ need not to be the same for the inferences where $C$ is involved: for example, a grey symbol of $C$ can be treated as red in the inference where $C$ is the conclusion, and as blue in an inference where $C$ is a premise. We now define $f, g, \mathcal{P}, construct$ of Alg. 1, by adapting the notation of §5 to the HR system.

**Definition of $f$ and $g$.** We take $f$ and $g$ such that, for every $C$:

$$f(C) = C|_{R\Delta_R^C}, \quad g(C) = C|_{B\Delta_B^C}. \tag{9}$$

**Definition of $\mathcal{P}$.** We fix the partition $\mathcal{P}$ of an $RB$-derivation to a so-called *HR-partition*, so that for each sub-derivation with root $C$ and leaves $C_0, \ldots, C_{n-1}$, the inference $\frac{C_0 \ \cdots \ C_{n-1}}{C}$ is an application of the hyper-resolution rule.

**Definition of $construct$ for Partial Interpolants of Leaves.** The constraints of (2) over the partial interpolants $I_C \in \mathcal{L}_{RB}$, for a leaf $C$, reduce to:

$$R \vdash C \wedge \overline{C|_{R\Delta_R^C}} \to I_C, \qquad\qquad B \vdash I_C \to C|_{\Delta_B^C}, \qquad \text{if } R \vdash C;$$

$$R \vdash \overline{C|_{\Delta_R^C}} \to I_C, \qquad\qquad B \vdash I_B \to \overline{C} \vee C|_{B\Delta_B^C}, \qquad \text{if } B \vdash C.$$

A set $\Phi_1$ of partial interpolants is defined as:

$$\Phi_1 = \{C|_{\Delta_B^C}\}, \text{ if } R \vdash C; \quad \{\overline{C|_{\Delta_R^C}}\}, \text{ if } B \vdash C.$$

**Definition of $construct$ for Partial Interpolants of Sub-roots.** Let $C$ be the root of a sub-derivation $\Pi' \in \mathcal{P}$, and let $C_0, \ldots, C_{n-1}$ denote the leaves of

$\Pi'$. Further, denote by $\Delta_R^i = \Delta_R^{C_i}$ and $\Delta_B^i = \Delta_B^{C_i}$. The constraints of eq. (5) over the partial interpolants $I_C \in \mathcal{L}_{RB}$ are simplified to:

$$R \vdash \bigwedge(I_{C_i} \vee C_i|_{R\Delta_R^i}) \wedge (\bigvee \overline{C_i} \vee C) \wedge \overline{C|_{R\Delta_R^C}} \rightarrow I_C,$$

$$B \vdash I_C \rightarrow \bigvee(I_{C_i} \wedge \overline{C_i|_{B\Delta_B^i}}) \vee (\bigwedge C_i \wedge \overline{C}) \vee C|_{B\Delta_B^C} \qquad (10)$$

Any formula $I_C \in \Phi_2$ thus satisfies eq. (10). A potential set $\Phi_2$ of partial interpolants can be built as in eq. (8), with the logical relationship among them similar to Fig. 2. For brevity, we only mention here:

(d)   $(I_{C_0} \vee (E \vee \bigvee \overline{p_i})|_{R\Delta_R^0}) \wedge \bigwedge(I_{C_i} \vee (D_i \vee p_i)|_{R\Delta_R^i}) \wedge (\overline{\bigvee D_i \vee E})|_{R\Delta_R^C};$

(g)   $(I_{C_0} \wedge \overline{(E \vee \bigvee \overline{p_i})}|_{B\Delta_B^0}) \vee \bigvee(I_{C_i} \wedge \overline{(D_i \vee p_i)}|_{B\Delta_B^i}) \vee (\bigvee D_i \vee E)|_{B\Delta_B^C}.$

where (d)$\rightarrow$ (g). Similarly to §5, we conclude that our parametric interpolation framework derives various interpolants in the HR system. The logical relations among these interpolants allow one to explore the strength and structure of interpolants, deriving hence interpolants which are good in the sense of their logical expressiveness.

**The Labeled Hyper-Resolution Framework.** We now relate our method to the labeled hyper-resolution framework of [16].

The algorithm of [16] relies on a *labeling function* $L$, which assigns a label $L(l, C) \in \{r, b, rb, \bot\}$ to each clause $C$ in a derivation $\Pi$. The leaves are first labeled. Then, the label $L(l, C)$ of a literal $l$ in the conclusion $C$ of an inference with premises $C_0, \ldots, C_{n-1}$ is computed as $L(l, C) = L(l, C_0) \sqcup \cdots \sqcup L(l, C_{n-1})$, where $\sqcup$ is the join operator of the lattice defined by Fig. 5. Labels for the pivots are also computed in this way.

Given an $RB$-refutation $\Pi$, the algorithm of [16] can be summarized as follows:

- If $C$ is a leaf of $\Pi$, then:    $\Phi_1 = \{C|_b\}$, if $R \vdash C$;   $\{\overline{C|_r}\}$, if $B \vdash C$,

where $C|_b$ and $C|_r$ denote the restriction of $C$ to literals with label $b$ and $r$.

- If $C$ is the conclusion of the HR-rule with premises $C_0, \ldots, C_{n-1}$, then, for some literals $p_1, \ldots, p_{n-1}$ and clauses $D_1, \ldots, D_{n-1}, E$, we have $C_0 = \overline{p_1} \vee \cdots \vee \overline{p_{n-1}} \vee E$, $C_1 = D_1 \vee p_1, \ldots,$ $C_{n-1} = D_{n-1} \vee p_{n-1}$, and $C = \bigvee D_i \vee E$. The pivots $p_i$ are assumed to have the same label in [16]. Then:

**Fig. 5.** The Hasse Diagram of $\sqcup$

$$\Phi_2 = \begin{cases} I_{C_0} \vee \bigvee_{i=1}^{n-1} I_{C_i}, & \text{if } L(p_i, D_i \vee p_i) \sqcup L(\overline{p_i}, \bigvee \overline{p_i} \vee E) = r; \\ I_{C_0} \wedge \bigwedge_{i=1}^{n-1} I_{C_i}, & \text{if } L(p_i, D_i \vee p_i) \sqcup L(\overline{p_i}, \bigvee \overline{p_i} \vee E) = b; \\ \begin{cases} (I_{C_0} \vee \bigvee \overline{p_i}) \wedge \bigwedge_{i=1}^{n-1}(p_i \vee I_{C_i}), \\ (I_{C_0} \wedge \bigwedge p_i) \vee \bigvee_{i=1}^{n-1}(\overline{p_i} \wedge I_{C_i}) \end{cases}, & \text{if } L(p_i, D_i \vee p_i) \sqcup L(\overline{p_i}, \bigvee \overline{p_i} \vee E) = rb. \end{cases}$$

*We argue that Alg. 1 in the HR system generalizes the method of [16]; the* behavior of the labeling function on the shared literals can in fact be simulated in our framework, by assigning appropriate sets $\Delta_R^C, \Delta_B^C$ to every clause $C$ in every inference.

*Consider a leaf $C$ of the RB-refutation $\Pi$, such that $C \in \mathcal{L}_R$.* Using [16], the red literals of $C$ are labeled with $r$, and the grey literals with one of the labels $r, b, rb$. The partial interpolant $C|_b$ is thus a sub-clause of $C|_{RB}$. We then fix $\Delta_B^C$ such that $C|_b = C|_{\Delta_B^C}$, and hence our partial interpolant is also a partial interpolant of [16]. A similar argument holds when $C \in \mathcal{L}_B$.

*Consider now an arbitrary HR inference in $\Pi$, with root $C$ and leaves $C_i$.* The relation (d)→(g) can be further exploited to obtain new partial interpolants by removing the colored literals of $D_i$ and $E$ in (d) and $\overline{(g)}$ using the HR rule:

$$\text{(m)} \quad (I_{C_0} \vee E|_{\Delta_R^0} \vee \bigvee \overline{p_i}|_{R\Delta_R^0}) \wedge \bigwedge (I_{C_i} \vee D_i|_{\Delta_R^i} \vee p_i|_{R\Delta_R^i}) \wedge \bigwedge \overline{D_i}|_{\Delta_R^C} \wedge \overline{E}|_{\Delta_R^C};$$

$$\text{(n)} \quad (I_{C_0} \wedge \overline{E}|_{\Delta_B^0} \wedge \bigwedge p_i|_{B\Delta_B^0}) \vee \bigvee (I_{C_i} \wedge \overline{D_i}|_{\Delta_B^i} \wedge \overline{p_i}|_{B\Delta_B^i}) \vee \bigvee D_i|_{\Delta_B^C} \vee E|_{\Delta_B^C},$$

It is always possible to split a HR inference in a sequence of HR inferences so that the labeling of the pivots is achieved as in [16]. In turn, the labeling of [16] allows us to further simplify the formulas (m) and (n) above and deriving the partial interpolants of [16] as special cases of these formulas. For example, if if the label is $r$, then the $\Delta_R, \Delta_B$ sets are chosen so that, if $p_i$ is grey, then $p_i \in \Delta_R^i \setminus \Delta_B^i$ and $\overline{p_i} \in \Delta_R^0 \setminus \Delta_B^0$. In this case, (n) reduces to the formula

$$(I_{C_0} \wedge \overline{E}|_{\Delta_B^0}) \vee \bigvee (I_{C_i} \wedge \overline{D_i}|_{\Delta_B^i}) \vee \bigvee D_i|_{\Delta_B^C} \vee E|_{\Delta_B^C},$$

which generalizes the partial interpolant

$$\bigvee_{i=0}^{n-1} I_{C_i}$$

of [16]. In a similar way, the partial interpolants generalizing the results of [16] are also obtained when considering the label $b$, respectively $rb$, in our framework.

Summarizing, when instantiating Alg. 1 in the HR system, we explore various good interpolants w.r.t. to their logical strength, some of these interpolants generalizing the ones derived in [16].

## 6 Conclusions

In this paper we proposed a new parametric interpolation framework for arbitrary first-order theories and inference systems. The main advantage of our framework is its ability to compute various interpolants of different structure and strength, with or without quantifiers, from the same proof. We described our method in relation with well-known interpolation algorithms, that respectively address local derivations in first-order logic and the propositional hyper-resolution system, and showed that they can be regarded as instantiations of our method.

Our work makes the first step towards a theoretical formalization of a generic interpolation approach, characterizing the notion of a "good" interpolant in terms of structure and logical strength. We believe our parametric interpolation algorithm can be adjusted and instantiated to cover a range of previously proposed systems (some being discussed in the paper) as well as new ones. As future work, we will study the relationships among specific inference systems and theories, and features of the derivations that can be produced; the goal is to obtain efficient interpolation algorithms specialized to various theories. On the practical side, we intend to apply our work on examples coming from bounded model checking and/or invariant discovery, in order to assess the practical impact on concrete verification problems.

**Acknowledgements.** We acknowledge funding from the Austrian FWF grants S11410-N23 and T425-N23, the Austrian WWTF grant ICT C-050, and ICT COST Action IC0901.

# References

1. A Parametric Interpolation Framework for First-Order Theories - Extended Version, http://www.inf.usi.ch/phd/rollini/KRS13ext.pdf
2. Albarghouthi, A., McMillan, K.L.: Beautiful interpolants. In: Sharygina, N., Veith, H. (eds.) CAV 2013. LNCS, vol. 8044, pp. 313–329. Springer, Heidelberg (2013)
3. Craig, W.: Three Uses of the Herbrand-Gentzen Theorem in Relating Model Theory and Proof Theory. Journal of Symbolic Logic 22(3), 269–285 (1957)
4. D'Silva, V., Kroening, D., Purandare, M., Weissenbacher, G.: Interpolant Strength. In: Barthe, G., Hermenegildo, M. (eds.) VMCAI 2010. LNCS, vol. 5944, pp. 129–145. Springer, Heidelberg (2010)
5. Henzinger, T.A., Jhala, R., Majumdar, R., McMillan, K.L.: Abstractions from Proofs. In: POPL, pp. 232–244 (2004)
6. Hoder, K., Kovács, L., Voronkov, A.: Playing in the Grey area of Proofs. In: POPL, pp. 259–272 (2012)
7. Huang, G.: Constructing Craig Interpolation Formulas. In: Li, M., Du, D.-Z. (eds.) COCOON 1995. LNCS, vol. 959, pp. 181–190. Springer, Heidelberg (1995)
8. Jhala, R., McMillan, K.L.: Interpolant-Based Transition Relation Approximation. In: Etessami, K., Rajamani, S.K. (eds.) CAV 2005. LNCS, vol. 3576, pp. 39–51. Springer, Heidelberg (2005)
9. Jhala, R., McMillan, K.L.: A Practical and Complete Approach to Predicate Refinement. In: Hermanns, H., Palsberg, J. (eds.) TACAS 2006. LNCS, vol. 3920, pp. 459–473. Springer, Heidelberg (2006)
10. Kovács, L., Voronkov, A.: Interpolation and Symbol Elimination. In: Schmidt, R.A. (ed.) CADE-22. LNCS, vol. 5663, pp. 199–213. Springer, Heidelberg (2009)
11. Krajícek, J.: Interpolation Theorems, Lower Bounds for Proof Systems, and Independence Results for Bounded Arithmetic. Journal of Symbolic Logic 62(2), 457–486 (1997)
12. McMillan, K.: Interpolation and SAT-Based Model Checking. In: Hunt Jr., W.A., Somenzi, F. (eds.) CAV 2003. LNCS, vol. 2725, pp. 1–13. Springer, Heidelberg (2003)
13. McMillan, K.L.: An Interpolating Theorem Prover. In: Jensen, K., Podelski, A. (eds.) TACAS 2004. LNCS, vol. 2988, pp. 16–30. Springer, Heidelberg (2004)

14. McMillan, K.L.: Quantified Invariant Generation Using an Interpolating Saturation Prover. In: Ramakrishnan, C.R., Rehof, J. (eds.) TACAS 2008. LNCS, vol. 4963, pp. 413–427. Springer, Heidelberg (2008)

15. Pudlák, P.: Lower Bounds for Resolution and Cutting Plane Proofs and Monotone Computations. Journal of Symbolic Logic 62(3), 981–998 (1997)

16. Weissenbacher, G.: Interpolant Strength Revisited. In: Cimatti, A., Sebastiani, R. (eds.) SAT 2012. LNCS, vol. 7317, pp. 312–326. Springer, Heidelberg (2012)

17. Yorsh, G., Musuvathi, M.: A Combination Method for Generating Interpolants. In: Nieuwenhuis, R. (ed.) CADE 2005. LNCS (LNAI), vol. 3632, pp. 353–368. Springer, Heidelberg (2005)

# Dalal's Revision without Hamming Distance

Pilar Pozos-Parra[1], Weiru Liu[2], and Laurent Perrussel[3]

[1] University of Tabasco, Mexico
pilar.pozos@ujat.mx
[2] Queen's University Belfast, UK
w.liu@qub.ac.uk
[3] IRIT - Université de Toulouse, France
laurent.perrussel@univ-tlse1.fr

**Abstract.** A well known strategy for belief revision is the use of an operator which takes as input a belief base and formula and outputs a new consistent revised belief base. Many operators require additional information such as epistemic entrenchment relations, system of spheres, faithful orderings, subformulae relation, etc. However, in many applications this extra information does not exist and all beliefs have to be equally considered. Other operators that can do without background information are dependent on the syntax. Among the few operators that possess both kinds of independence: of extra information and of the syntax, Dalal's operator is the most outstanding. Dalal's revision moves from the models of the base to the models of the input formula which are closest in terms of Hamming distance. A drawback of Dalal's approach is that it fails when faced with inconsistent belief bases. This paper proposes a new method for computing Dalal's revision that avoids the computation of belief bases models. We propose a new distance between formulae based on distances between terms of formulae in DNF and a revision operator based on these distances. The proposed operator produces Dalal's equivalent results when the belief base and new input are both consistent. Moreover, this new operator is able to handle inconsistent belief bases. We also analyze several properties of the new operator. While the input belief base and formula need a compilation to DNF, the operator meets desirable properties making the approach suitable for implementation.

## 1 Introduction

Belief revision is a framework that characterizes the process of belief change in which an agent revises its beliefs when newly received evidence contradicts them. Logic-based belief revision has been studied extensively [1–3]. Usually an agent's beliefs are represented as a theory or base $K$ and a new input is in the form of a propositional formula $\mu$ which must be preserved after the revision. Many belief revision operators $\circ$ have been proposed to tackle the problem, they take the base and the formula as input and reach a new consistent revised belief base $K \circ \mu$ as output. Diverse operators existing in the literature need additional information such as epistemic entrenchment relations [4], system of spheres [5],

F. Castro, A. Gelbukh, and M. González (Eds.): MICAI 2013, Part I, LNAI 8265, pp. 41–53, 2013.
© Springer-Verlag Berlin Heidelberg 2013

faithful orderings [1], subformulae relations[6], etc. However, in most of the cases we do not have this extra information. There exist formula-based belief operators which do not need extra information; however, they are sensitive to the syntax, i.e., two equivalent inputs may produce different outputs. So they lose the desirable property of independence of syntax that is met by most of the operator mentioned previously. Dalal's operator is the most outstanding revision technique that meets both: independence of syntax and independence of extra information. The revision is based on the Hamming distance between interpretations once it is extended to distances between interpretations and bases. Dalal's operator takes the interpretations which are models of the input formula and which are closest to the belief base. In practice this framework entails a costly computation of models. For example, suppose that $K = \{a \to b\}$ and $\mu = a \land \neg c \land d \land e \land f \land g$. The approach needs to consider 96 models for the base and 2 models for the input formula, so the approach calculates 192 distances between interpretations in order to select the models of $\mu$ closest to $K$.

Another drawback of Dalal approach is its inability to revise inconsistent bases. For example suppose an agent who holds the following information: it is raining, if it is raining it is cloudy, it is not cloudy, and the sky is blue, represented by the following base $\{a, a \to b, \neg b, c\}$, now suppose the agent receives the new information: it is cloudy. In this case Dalal revision needs a preprocessing to transform an inconsistent base into a consistent one and then revise by $b$. A possible solution may be to consider each formula as a base and then merge the formulae of the belief base, however, the process became more expensive and the merging phase does not take into account the new information who may be the key to recover consistency.

On the other hand, efforts have been made to reduce the computational costs associated with models by compiling the initial belief base and new input into prime implicant and prime implicate forms [7, 8]. Belief compilation has been proposed recently for dealing with the computational intractability of general propositional reasoning [9]. A propositional theory is compiled off-line into a target language, which is used on-line to answer a large number of queries in polynomial time. The idea behind belief compilation is to push as much of the computational overhead into the off-line phase as possible, as it is then amortized over all on-line queries. Target compilation languages and their associated algorithms allow us to develop on-line reasoning systems requiring fewer resources. Thus, we propose reducing computation by compiling the belief base and formula representing new evidence to their Disjunctive Normal Form (DNF), and then avoiding computation of distances from a interpretation to another by computing a new distance directly between terms of formulae in DNF. The idea behind this new distance is that instead of measuring how different the models of the belief base are from a model of the new evidence, we compute how different the terms of the belief base are from the terms of the formula representing new evidence. This notion of *distance between terms* avoids reaching the level of models and measures distances between sets of models represented by subformulae (terms) instead. In the case of the previous example, the computed distances are only

2 instead of 192, see Section 3 for more details. While the operator based on this new distance meets the desirable properties of independence of syntax and of extra information, a compilation of the belief base and formula to a DNF is required.

Classical belief revision always trust new information and thus revises the current beliefs to accommodate new evidence to reach a consistent belief base. Most studies on belief revision are based on the AGM (Alchourron, Gardenfors & Makinson) postulates [6] which captures this notion of priority and describe minimal properties a revision process should have. The AGM postulates formulated in the propositional setting in [1], denoted as $R_1$-$R_6$, characterize the requirements with which a revision operator should comply. For example, postulate $R_1$, also called the success postulate, captures the priority of new evidence over the belief base, it requires that the revision result of a belief base $K$ by a proposition $\mu$ (new information) should always maintain $\mu$ being believed. $R_3$ is the previously mentioned principle of independence of syntax. In this paper we analyze the satisfaction of $R_1$-$R_6$ by the new operator.

To summarize, the major contribution of this paper is to propose a new method that reproduces Dalal's results and is able to handle two drawbacks of Dalal's revision: the need to compute all the models of formulae and the inability to handle inconsistent belief bases. The new method satisfies postulates $R_1$-$R_6$ when both inputs: the belief base and new evidence are consistent, and it satisfies some of postulates when the inputs are inconsistent. The complexity of the new method, once the formula is in DNF, is polynomial. The rest of the paper is organized as follows. After providing some technical preliminaries and reviewing the characterization of revision process, in Section 3 we introduce the new distance and its respective operator. Then we analyze the satisfaction of the postulates and the complexity issues. Finally, we conclude with some future work.

## 2  Preliminaries

We consider a language $\mathcal{L}$ of propositional logic using a finite ordered set of symbols or atoms $P := \{p_1, p_2, ..., p_n\}$. A belief base/theory $K$ is a finite set of propositional formulae of $\mathcal{L}$ representing the beliefs from a source (we identify $K$ with the conjunction of its elements). A literal $l$ is an atom or the negation of an atom. A term $D$ is a conjunction of literals: $D = l_{r_1} \wedge ... \wedge l_{r_m}$, where, $r_i \in \{1, ..., n\}$ and $l_{r_i}$ concerns atom $p_{r_i}$. A minterm is term in which each atoms of language appears exactly once. A Disjunctive Normal Form of a formula $\phi$ is a disjunction of terms $\text{DNF}_\phi = D_1 \vee ... \vee D_k$ which is equivalent to $\phi$. If a literal $l$ appears in a term $D$, it is denoted by $l \in D$ and if $D$ appears in $\text{DNF}_\phi$, it is denoted by $D \in \text{DNF}_\phi$. If $D$ is a term, $index(D)$ denotes the set of indexes of the literals appearing in $D$. For example, if $D = p_4 \wedge \neg p_2 \wedge p_8$, then $index(D) = \{2, 4, 8\}$.

A set of possible interpretations from $P$ of language $\mathcal{L}$ is denoted as $\mathcal{W}$. $w \in \mathcal{W}$ is denoted as vectors of the form $(w(p_1), ..., w(p_n))$, where $w(p_i) = 1$ or $w(p_i) = 0$

for $i = 1, ..., n$. A interpretation $w$ is a model of $\phi \in \mathcal{L}$ if and only if $\phi$ is true under $w$ in the classical truth-functional manner. The set of models of a formula $\phi$ is denoted by $mod(\phi)$. $K$ is consistent iff there exists model of $K$.

$|X|$ denotes the cardinality of $X$ if $X$ is a set or $|X|$ denotes the number of literals occurring in $X$ if $X$ is a term, finally, it denotes the absolute value of $X$ if $X$ is a number. $|l|_b$ denotes 1 (respectively 0) if $l$ is an atom (respectively the negation of an atom). Let $\leq_\psi$ be a relation over a set of possible interpretations; $x =_\psi y$ is a notation for $x \leq_\psi y$ and $y \leq_\psi x$, and $x <_\psi y$ is a notation for $x \leq_\psi y$ and $y \not\leq_\psi x$.

In [6] eight postulates have been proposed to characterize the process of belief revision, which are known as the AGM Postulates. Assuming a proposition setting, in [10, 1] this characterization is rephrased producing the following R$_1$-R$_6$ postulates, where $K$, $K_1$ and $K_2$ are belief bases to be revised and $\mu$, $\mu_1$ and $\mu_2$ are new evidence:

R$_1$. $K \circ \mu$ implies $\mu$.
R$_2$. If $K \wedge \mu$ is satisfiable, then $K \circ \mu \equiv K \wedge \mu$.
R$_3$. If $\mu$ is satisfiable, then $K \circ \mu$ is also satisfiable.
R$_4$. If $K_1 \equiv K_2$ and $\mu_1 \equiv \mu_2$, then $K_1 \circ \mu_1 \equiv K_2 \circ \mu_2$.
R$_5$. $(K \circ \mu_1) \wedge \mu_2$ implies $K \circ (\mu_1 \wedge \mu_2)$.
R$_6$. If $(K \circ \mu_1) \wedge \mu_2$ is satisfiable, then $K \circ (\mu_1 \wedge \mu_2)$ implies $(K \circ \mu_1) \wedge \mu_2$.

A representational theorem has been provided which shows equivalence between the six postulates and a revision strategy based on total pre-orders. The theorem is based on the notion of *faithful assignment*. The formal definitions are as follows [10]:

**Definition 1.** *Let* $\mathcal{W}$ *be the set of all interpretations of a propositional language* $\mathcal{L}$. *A function that maps each sentence* $\psi$ *in* $\mathcal{L}$ *to a total pre-order* $\leq_\psi$ *on interpretations* $\mathcal{W}$ *is called a faithful assignment if and only if:*

*1. $w_1, w_2 \models \psi$ only if $w_1 =_\psi w_2$;*
*2. $w_1 \models \psi$ and $w_2 \not\models \psi$ only if $w_1 <_\psi w_2$; and*
*3. $\psi \equiv \phi$ only if $\leq_\psi = \leq_\phi$.*

**Theorem 1 (Representation Theorem).** *A revision operator* $\circ$ *satisfies Postulates* R$_1$-R$_6$, *iff there exists a faithful assignment that maps each sentence* $\psi$ *into a total pre-order* $\leq_\psi$ *such that:* $mod(\psi \circ \mu) = min(mod(\mu), \leq_\psi)$.

## 3   Distance between Terms

Without loss of generality we consider only compiled languages so that each belief base is taken as a DNF, and each formula representing new evidence is taken as a DNF too. For example, for the belief base $\{a, a \rightarrow b, \neg b, c\}$, we consider the compiled belief base $(a \wedge \neg a \wedge \neg b \wedge c) \vee (a \wedge b \wedge \neg b \wedge c)$. Moreover, we consider only terms with non repeated literals, then terms such as $a \wedge a \wedge a \wedge b$ will be considered simply as $a \wedge b$.

Classically in Dalal's revision the process uses two type of distances: Hamming distance which is a distance from a interpretation to another one defined as follows: $d(w_1, w_2) = \sum_{p \in P} |w_1(p) - w_2(p)|$ and a distance from a interpretation to a belief base defined as follows: $d(w, K) = min_{w' \in mod(K)} d(w, w')$. The latter distance allows the definition of a pre-order over the models of the input information, $w_1 \leq_K w_2$ _iff_ $d(w_1, K) \leq d(w_2, K)$. The closest interpretations to the belief base are the models of the revision process $mod(K \circ_D \mu) = min(mod(\mu), \leq_K)$. Our proposal of belief revision is quite similar; the process defines a distance between terms as follows:

**Definition 2 (Distance between terms).** _Let_ $D = l_{r_1} \wedge ... \wedge l_{r_m}$ _and_ $D' = l'_{s_1} \wedge ... \wedge l'_{s_k}$ _be two terms, the distance between_ $D$ _and_ $D'$, _denoted_ $d(D, D')$, _is defined as:_ $d(D, D') = \sum_{i \in \{r_1, ..., r_m\}} \left( ||l_i|_b - |l'_i|_b| \quad s.t. \quad i \in \{s_1, ..., s_k\} \right)$.

Or equivalently $d(D, D') = \sum_{i \in index(D)} \left( ||l_i|_b - |l'_i|_b| \quad s.t. \quad i \in index(D') \right)$, when both $D$ and $D'$ are consistent, $d(D, D') = \sum_{i \in index(D) \cap index(D')} ||l_i|_b - |l'_i|_b|$ can be used instead. If both $D$ and $D'$ are minterms, we can consider them as possible interpretations and then recover Hamming distance. Moreover, the following desirable properties are satisfied: $d(D, D') = d(D', D)$ and $d(D, D') = 0$ if $D = D'$.

This term-based distance allows us to define a succinct process to reproduce minimal Hamming distances. Consider the example in the Introduction, where $K = \{\neg a \vee b\}$ and $\mu = a \wedge \neg c \wedge d \wedge e \wedge f \wedge g$. The 96 models of $K$: $\{(0,0,0,0,0,0,0), (0,0,0,0,0,0,1), ..., (0,1,1,1,1,1,1), (1,1,0,0,0,0,0), (1,1,0,0,0,0,1), ..., (1,1,1,1,1,1,1)\}$ can be represented in a succinct form as $(0, x_2, x_3, x_4, x_5, x_6, x_7)$ or $(x'_1, 1, x'_3, x'_4, x'_5, x'_6, x'_7)$ where every $x_i$ and $x'_i$ can take the value 0 or 1. The models of $\mu$ can be represented in a succinct form as $(1, y_2, 0, 1, 1, 1, 1)$ where $y_2$ can take the value 0 or 1. Now, it is easy to verify that a Hamming distance between two interpretations is the number of positions for which the corresponding valuation of symbols is different. In other words, it measures the minimum number of substitutions required to change one interpretation into the other. We want to transform the models of $K$ into models of $\mu$ with minimal change. The notion of minimal change is expressed by substitutions as follows: in order to change a model of $K$ expressed as $(0, x_2, x_3, x_4, x_5, x_6, x_7)$ into a model of $\mu$ expressed as $(1, y_2, 0, 1, 1, 1, 1)$ we need to substitute 0 by 1 in the first position and assign the following values to the variables: $x_2 = y_2$, $x_3 = 0$, $x_4 = 1$, $x_5 = 1$, $x_6 = 1$, and $x_7 = 1$, i.e., the minimal change, the minimal Hamming distance for these two patterns is 1. Considering now the second succinct form of expressing models of $K$: $(x'_1, 1, x'_3, x'_4, x'_5, x'_6, x'_7)$, in order to transform it into the succinct form of models of $\mu$ $(1, y_2, 0, 1, 1, 1, 1)$, no substitution is required, solely an assignment of Boolean variables as follows: $x'_1 = 1$, $x'_3 = 0$, $x'_4 = 1$, $x'_5 = 1$, $x'_6 = 1$, $x'_7 = 1$ and $y_2 = 1$. This means the minimal Hamming distance for these two patterns is 0. Thus, we found the model of $\mu$ $(1,1,0,1,1,1,1)$ that represents the revision of $K$ by $\mu$ in terms of minimal Hamming distance, i.e. the minimal change found is 0: none substitution is required.

The succinct forms of models can be represented by terms of a DNF, hence, $\neg a$ represents $(0, x_2, x_3, x_4, x_5, x_6, x_7)$, $b$ represents $(x'_1, 1, x'_3, x'_4, x'_5, x'_6, x'_7)$ and $a \wedge \neg c \wedge d \wedge e \wedge f \wedge g$ represents $(1, y_2, 0, 1, 1, 1, 1)$. Actually, in this case the models of $\mu$ leave free solely the second position, which means that the models of $K$ can fix a Boolean value only in the second position if it is required to hold a minimal change, in this case the second position is fixed with 1 by the second pattern of $K$. To capture this notion of fixing a model of $\mu$ with the help of literal belonging to the models of $K$, we introduce the notion of extension of terms as follows:

**Definition 3 (Extension of terms).** *The extension of term $D_1$ by a term $D_2$, denoted $ext(D_1, D_2)$, is defined as:* $ext(D_1, D_2) = D_1 \wedge \bigwedge_{l_i \in D_2 | i \notin index(D_1)} l_i$.

I.e. the result of extending a term with a second term is a term that includes all the literals of the former and the literals of the second term that do not consider atoms appearing in the former. Notice that in the running example, $ext(\neg a, a \wedge \neg c \wedge d \wedge e \wedge f \wedge g) = \neg a \wedge \neg c \wedge d \wedge e \wedge f \wedge g$ and $ext(a \wedge \neg c \wedge d \wedge e \wedge f \wedge g, \neg a) = a \wedge \neg c \wedge d \wedge e \wedge f \wedge g$, then the extension of terms is not commutative. This notion of extension can be extended to formulae. Thus, we will be able to extend the terms of $\mu$ by terms of belief base $K$ preserving consistency.

**Definition 4 (Extension of formulae).** *We define the extension of formula $\phi_1$ by a formula $\phi_2$, denoted $ext(\phi_1, \phi_2)$, as the following multiset:*

$$ext(\phi_1, \phi_2) = \{ext(D_1, D_2) | D_1 \in \phi_1 \quad and \quad D_2 \in \phi_2\}.$$

This definition can help us to find the potential extended terms that will form part of the revision result. In the running example considering the term of $\mu$ and the two terms of $K$, we have $ext(\mu, K) = \{a \wedge \neg c \wedge d \wedge e \wedge f \wedge g, a \wedge b \wedge \neg c \wedge d \wedge e \wedge f \wedge g\}$. If we see a term as a subformula, we can find the models of a term. Then $mod(ext(D_1, D_2)) \subseteq mod(D_1)$ and the union of the models of every term appearing in a formula equals the models of the formula: $\cup_{D \in \phi} mod(D) = mod(\phi)$. Thus $\cup_{D \in ext(\mu, K)} mod(D) \subseteq mod(\mu)$, i.e., the models of the extension of $\mu$ by $K$ are a refinement of the models of $\mu$ such that the refinement models are the closest to the models of base $K$, and then the extended terms belonging to such extension are the potential candidates to forming part of the revision result.

Once we compute the potential terms that may be part of the revision result, the question arises of how to select from all the extended terms the ones that will constitute the revision result? A solution is to deploy the notion of minimal change, i.e., minimal substitutions for transforming a model of $K$ into a model of $\mu$. Definition 2 measures the change required for such transformation. Note that the distance between terms is a succinct form of computing Hamming distances where the sum considers solely the atoms appearing in both terms and, as in Hamming distance, the sum increases only when the related literals are opposite. Definition 2 allows us to define a pre-order over the extended terms as follows: $ext(D_1, D_2) \le ext(D_3, D_4)$ *iff* $d(D_1, D_2) \le d(D_3, D_4)$.

Which means that the extension of $D_1$ by $D_2$ is preferred to the extension of $D_3$ by $D_4$. So, finally, the terms forming part of the operator's outcome are the extended terms of $\mu$ by terms of $K$ that required minimal change to transform a model of $K$ into a model of $\mu$, i.e.

**Definition 5 (Dalal's Revision without Hamming distance).** *Let $K$ be a belief base and $\mu$ a formula representing new evidence. The revision of $K$ by $\mu$, $K \circ \mu$, is defined as follows: $K \circ \mu = \bigvee min(ext(\mu, K), \leq)$.*

It should be noted that our process of revision inputs formulae in DNF and outputs formulae in DNF, i.e. we propose a syntactical framework which is desirable for a framework of iterated belief revision: from the second iteration the compilation of formulae to DNF is no longer required. Classical Dalal's revision inputs formulae and outputs models.

*Example 1.* The following example was presented in [8]: $K = (\neg p_2 \wedge \neg p_3) \vee (\neg p_1 \wedge \neg p_3 \wedge p_4) \vee (\neg p_2 \wedge p_4)$ and $\mu = (p_3 \wedge \neg p_4) \vee (p_1 \wedge p_2)$. Dalal's revision must find the models of the result on the models of $\mu$. As we can see in Table 1 the models of $\mu$ that are in the revision result using Dalal $K \circ_D \mu$ are $(0,0,1,0)$, $(1,0,1,0)$, $(1,1,0,0)$, $(1,1,0,1)$ and $(1,1,1,1)$ which minimal Hamming distance is 1. An equivalent result is produced with our operator $K \circ \mu = (\neg p_2 \wedge p_3 \wedge \neg p_4) \vee (\neg p_2 \wedge p_3 \wedge \neg p_4) \vee (p_1 \wedge p_2 \wedge \neg p_3) \vee (p_1 \wedge p_2 \wedge \neg p_3 \wedge p_4) \vee (p_1 \wedge p_2 \wedge p_4)$ by computing solely 6 distances instead of 49 (7 models of $\mu$ by 7 models of $K$), see Table 2.

**Table 1.** Distances between interpretations required for $K \circ_D \mu$

| | $w' \in mod(K)$ | | | | | | |
|---|---|---|---|---|---|---|---|
| | (0,0,0,0) | (0,0,0,1) | (0,0,1,1) | (0,1,0,1) | (1,0,0,0) | (1,0,0,1) | (1,0,1,1) |
| $w \in mod(\mu)$ | $d(w,w')$ | $d(w,w')$ | $d(w,w')$ | $d(w,w')$ | $d(w,w')$ | $d(w,w')$ | $d(w,w')$ |
| (0,0,1,0) | 1 | 2 | 1 | 3 | 2 | 3 | 2 |
| (0,1,1,0) | 2 | 3 | 2 | 2 | 3 | 4 | 3 |
| (1,0,1,0) | 2 | 3 | 2 | 4 | 1 | 2 | 1 |
| (1,1,0,0) | 2 | 3 | 4 | 2 | 1 | 2 | 3 |
| (1,1,0,1) | 3 | 2 | 3 | 1 | 2 | 1 | 2 |
| (1,1,1,0) | 3 | 4 | 3 | 3 | 2 | 3 | 2 |
| (1,1,1,1) | 4 | 3 | 2 | 2 | 3 | 2 | 1 |

**Table 2.** Distances between terms required for $K \circ \mu$

| | $D_1 = p_3 \wedge \neg p_4 \in \mu$ | | $D_1 = p_1 \wedge p_2 \in \mu$ | |
|---|---|---|---|---|
| $D_2 \in K$ | $ext(D_1, D_2)$ | $d(D_1, D_2)$ | $ext(D_1, D_2)$ | $d(D_1, D_2)$ |
| $\neg p_2 \wedge \neg p_3$ | $\neg p_2 \wedge p_3 \wedge \neg p_4$ | 1 | $p_1 \wedge p_2 \wedge \neg p_3$ | 1 |
| $\neg p_1 \wedge \neg p_3 \wedge p_4$ | $\neg p_1 \wedge p_3 \wedge \neg p_4$ | 2 | $p_1 \wedge p_2 \wedge \neg p_3 \wedge p_4$ | 1 |
| $\neg p_2 \wedge p_4$ | $\neg p_2 \wedge p_3 \wedge \neg p_4$ | 1 | $p_1 \wedge p_2 \wedge p_4$ | 1 |

*Example 2.* In [7] the following example is presented: $K = a \vee (a \wedge b) \vee (a \wedge c) \vee (b \wedge c)$ and $\mu = \neg a \wedge \neg b$. From now we suppose that atoms are ordered alphabetically. The models of $\mu$ are $(0, 0, 1)$ and $(0, 0, 0)$. As we can see in Table 3 the models of $K \circ_D \mu$ are $(0, 0, 0)$ and $(0, 0, 1)$ too. Given 5 models of K, the number of Hamming distances computed is 10. An equivalent result is found with our operator $K \circ \mu = (\neg a \wedge \neg b) \vee (\neg a \wedge \neg b \wedge c) \vee (\neg a \wedge \neg b \wedge c)$, which computes only 4 distances between terms.

<table>
<tr><td colspan="2" align="center">**Table 3.** $K \circ_D \mu$</td><td colspan="2" align="center">**Table 4.** $K \circ \mu$</td></tr>
<tr><td>$w \in mod(\mu)$</td><td>$d(w, K)$</td><td>$ext(D_1, D_2) \in ext(\mu, K)$</td><td>$d(D_1, D_2)$</td></tr>
<tr><td>(0,0,0)</td><td>1</td><td>$\neg a \wedge \neg b$</td><td>1</td></tr>
<tr><td>(0,0,1)</td><td>1</td><td>$\neg a \wedge \neg b$</td><td>2</td></tr>
<tr><td></td><td></td><td>$\neg a \wedge \neg b \wedge c$</td><td>1</td></tr>
<tr><td></td><td></td><td>$\neg a \wedge \neg b \wedge c$</td><td>1</td></tr>
</table>

As we can see in Table 4 the extension of terms of $\mu$ by terms of $K$ can hold repeated elements as a result of Definition 4 where a multiset is considered instead of a set. However, the repeated elements do not necessarily hold the same distance; we may compute different distances for repeated elements of the multiset given that the repeated elements come from different extensions to different terms. In this case the extended terms $ext(\neg a \wedge \neg b, a)$ and $ext(\neg a \wedge \neg b, a \wedge b)$ hold the same result $\neg a \wedge \neg b$, even when the second operand is not the same in both cases. Indeed, this difference is the cause of producing a different distance between the corresponding terms: $d(\neg a \wedge \neg b, a) = 1$ and $d(\neg a \wedge \neg b, a \wedge b) = 2$. This means that any model represented[1] by $a$ needs 1 substitution for transforming it to a model represented by $\neg a \wedge \neg b$ while any model represented by $a \wedge b$ needs 2 substitutions for transforming it to a model represented by $\neg a \wedge \neg b$, see 2nd and 3rd rows in Table 4. Actually, it is simpler considering the terms as subformulae, then we can say the models of $a$ need at least 1 substitution for being transformed to models of $\neg a \wedge \neg b$, while the models of $a \wedge b$ need at least 2 substitutions for being transformed to models of $\neg a \wedge \neg b$.

Although the notion of multiset helps to define the process, this notion leads into duplicate terms in the final result. Then, an elimination phase of repeated terms will be desirable. A simple transformation from a multiset to a set will be enough for erasing the repeated elements. However, there are non-desirable elements as $\neg a \wedge \neg b \wedge c$ that is model inclusion subsumed by $\neg a \wedge \neg b$, i.e. $mod(\neg a \wedge \neg b \wedge c) \subseteq mod(\neg a \wedge \neg b)$. Thus, we propose cleaning the result as follows: first create a set with terms that are not model inclusion subsumed by other terms, $\mathsf{NonSubsum}(K \circ \mu) = \{D \in K \circ \mu | \forall_{D' \in K \circ \mu} mod(D') \subseteq mod(D)\}$, then take the disjunction of such set $\mathsf{Clean}(K \circ \mu) = \vee_{D \in \mathsf{NonSubsum}(K \circ \mu)} D$. We can argue about the necessity of computing models but actually this set can be defined through indexes sets as follows: $\mathsf{NonSubsum}(\phi) = \{D \in \phi | \forall_{D' \in \phi | index(D) \subseteq index(D')} |D| \leq$

---

[1] Recall, $a$ representing a model means $a$ represents the model pattern $(1, x_2, x_3)$ where $x_2$ and $x_3$ can take value of 1 or 0.

$|D'|$ and $\forall_{l\in D}l \in D'\}$. I.e., if two or more terms share the same literals the set will keep only the term that has the minimal number of literals. So, $K \circ \mu = (\neg a \wedge \neg b) \vee (\neg a \wedge \neg b \wedge c) \vee (\neg a \wedge \neg b \wedge c)$ can be written in an equivalent form as $\mathsf{Clean}(K \circ \mu) = (\neg a \wedge \neg b)$ which makes more apparent the equivalence with Dalal's result: $mod(K \circ_D \mu) = \{(0,0,0),(0,0,1)\}$.

*Example 3.* Let us now consider the inconsistent base presented at the beginning of this section $K = (a \wedge \neg a \wedge \neg b \wedge c) \vee (a \wedge b \wedge \neg b \wedge c)$ and suppose that the new evidence $b$ is received, then as we can see in Table 5 the models of $\mu$ can be computed, however, there are no models of $K$, which disqualify Dalal's revision: the Hamming distances cannot be computed. The result of our operator is $\mathsf{Clean}(K \circ \mu) = a \wedge b \wedge c$ which means the agent gives up its belief concerning $\neg b$ but keeps the rest. The process transforms the inconsistent base $K$ into a consistent base $K \circ \mu$ with a minimal change. Notice that the extended term $a \wedge \neg a \wedge b \wedge c$ is model inclusion subsumed by $a \wedge b \wedge c$, due to an inconsistent term being subsumed by a consistent one.

<table>
<tr><td colspan="2">**Table 5.** $K \circ_D \mu$</td></tr>
<tr><td>$w \in mod(\mu)$</td><td>$d(w,K)$</td></tr>
<tr><td>(0,1,0)</td><td>?</td></tr>
<tr><td>(0,1,1)</td><td>?</td></tr>
<tr><td>(1,1,0)</td><td>?</td></tr>
<tr><td>(1,1,1)</td><td>?</td></tr>
</table>

<table>
<tr><td colspan="2">**Table 6.** $K \circ \mu$</td></tr>
<tr><td>$ext(D_1,D_2) \in ext(\mu,K)$</td><td>$d(D_1,D_2)$</td></tr>
<tr><td>$a \wedge \neg a \wedge b \wedge c$</td><td>1</td></tr>
<tr><td>$a \wedge b \wedge c$</td><td>1</td></tr>
</table>

Our operator can deal with inconsistent beliefs bases, which do not have any models; in contrast Dalal's operator does not operate without belief base models. Some authors such as [11] consider $K \circ_D \mu = \mu$ when $K$ is inconsistent, however, the revised result loses too much consistent information which can be retained. Let $K = a \wedge \neg a \wedge b \wedge c \wedge \neg c$ and new evidence $\mu = c$, the revised result is $K \circ_D \mu = c$, which is consistent but the revision itself violates the minimal change principle. The agent actually gives up all the previous information keeping on the new information. Iteratively, an agent would forget everything every time it has inconsistent information and retains only the newest information. Notice that between the inconsistencies there is consistent information about $b$ which is lost. The result of our approach conserves as much as possible the information of $K$, i.e. $K \circ \mu = a \wedge \neg a \wedge b \wedge c$, even when the result is inconsistent, the agent keeps the information concerning $b$, gives up the contradiction about $c$ and retains the contradiction about $a$. Actually, the method can be easily extended for recovering consistency when the result is not consistent: merely erasing the contradictory information; then for this example the result would be $b \wedge c$.

## 4   Postulates and Complexity

We show now that the newly proposed operator satisfies postulates $R_1$-$R_6$. In [10] the representation theorem is used for proving Dalal's operator satisfies the postulates, therefore, we show our proposal and Dalal's revision provide equivalent results.

**Proposition 1.** *If both $K$ and $\mu$ are consistent formulae in DNF, then $K \circ_D \mu \equiv K \circ \mu$ where $\circ_D$ denotes Dalal's revision operator and $\circ$ denotes terms distance-based revision operator.*

*Proof.* First, if a interpretation $w$ belongs to the set of models of formula $\phi$: $w \in mod(\phi)$, there exists at least one term $D \in \phi$ such that $w \in mod(D)$.
($\Rightarrow$) Let $w \in mod(K \circ_D \mu)$ iff $w \in mod(\mu)$ and $\forall_{w' \in mod(\mu)} \ w \leq_K w'$, then $\forall_{w' \in mod(\mu)} \ min_{x \in mod(K)} d(w, x) \leq min_{x \in mod(K)} d(w', x)$. Let $x' \in mod(K)$ such that $d(w, x') = min_{x \in mod(K)} d(w, x)$ and call $m$ the Hamming distance between $w$ and $x'$, i.e. $d(w, x') = m$; note that $m$ is the minimal Hamming distance between $w$ and base $K$, in other interpretations the minimal change for transforming a model of $K$ into a model of $\mu$ is $m$. Now, we use the notation introduced above: $p_i = 1$ and $\neg p_i = 0$, where $p_i$ is an atom and $i = 1, ..., n$, then $w$ can be seen as $(l_1, ..., l_n)$ and $x'$ can be seen as $(l'_1, ..., l'_n)$ where $l_i = p_i$ if $w(p_i) = 1$ and $l_i = \neg p_i$ if $w(p_i) = 0$ and similarly for the $l'_i$s. Notice that there are $m$ opposite literals between $w$ and $x'$, i.e. Hamming distance between $w$ and $x'$ can be calculated by $\sum_{i=1}^{n} ||l_i|_b - |l'_i|_b| = m$.

Also, it is worth to note that for every term $D_1 \in \mu$ such that $w \in mod(D_1)$ it must be satisfied that if $l \in D_1$, $l \in \{l_1, ..., l_n\}$, similarly, for every term $D_2 \in K$ such that $x' \in mod(D_2)$ it must be satisfied that if $l \in D_2$, $l \in \{l'_1, ..., l'_n\}$; thus $\sum_{i \in index(D_1) \cap index(D_2)} ||l_i|_b - |l'_i|_b| \leq \sum_{i=1}^{n} ||l_i|_b - |l'_i|_b| = m$, i.e. $d(D_1, D_2) \leq m$. Now, suppose that $d(D_1, D_2) < m$, then there exists a model of $K$ that can be transformed to a model of $\mu$ with strictly less substitutions than $m$, contradicting the fact that $m$ is the minimal Hamming distance. Therefore, $d(D_1, D_2) = m$, which means that all the opposite literals appear in both terms, thus $ext(D_1, D_2)$ extends $D_1$ with literals of $D_2$ that do not oppose the literals of $D_1$, therefore if $l \in D_2$ and $l \in ext(D_1, D_2)$ then $l \in \{l_1, ..., l_n\}$, which means that $w \in ext(D_1, D_2)$. Now, suppose that there is a $ext(D_3, D_4) \in ext(\mu, K)$ such that $ext(D_3, D_4) < ext(D_1, D_2)$, then $d(D_3, D_4) < d(D_1, D_2)$, i.e., we can find a model of $D_4$ (model of $K$) that can be transformed into a model of $D_3$ (model of $\mu$) with strictly less substitutions than $m$, which is not possible. Therefore, $\forall_{ext(D_3, D_4) \in ext(\mu, K)} \ ext(D_1, D_2) \leq ext(D_3, D_4)$ and given that $w \in ext(D_1, D_2)$, we can conclude that $w \in mod(K \circ \mu)$.
($\Leftarrow$) The proof in the other direction is straightforward. Let $w \in mod(K \circ \mu)$, then there exist $k$ terms $D'_1, ..., D'_k$ in $\mu$ such that $w \in mod(D'_i)$, $i = 1, ...k$. Let's take $D_1 \in \{D'_1, ..., D'_k\}$, $D_2 \in K$ such that $w \in ext(D_1, D_2)$ and $\forall_{ext(D_3, D_4) \in ext(\mu, K)} \ ext(D_1, D_2) \leq ext(D_3, D_4)$, notice that we assure the existence of such $D_1$ and $D_2$, given that $w \in mod(K \circ \mu)$. Thus $\forall_{ext(D_3, D_4) \in ext(\mu, K)} \ d(D_1, D_2) \leq d(D_3, D_4)$, which means that the minimal change for transforming a model of $K$ into a model of $\mu$ is the same distance required for transforming a model of $D_2$ into $w$, which in terms of Hamming distance is expressed as $\forall_{w' \in mod(\mu)} \ min_{x \in mod(D_2)} d(w, x) \leq min_{x \in mod(K)} d(w', x)$. Given that $mod(D_2) \subseteq mod(K)$, $\forall_{w' \in mod(\mu)} \ min_{x \in mod(K)} d(w, x) \leq min_{x \in mod(K)} d(w', x)$ holds, which means that

$\forall_{w' \in mod(\mu)}$ $w \leq_K w'$, clearly $w \in mod(\mu)$ and finally, we can conclude that $w \in mod(K \circ_D \mu)$.

□

Thus, we can be sure that the distance-based operator $\circ$ based on terms satisfies postulates $R_1$-$R_6$ when both the belief base and new evidence are consistent. When the belief base or the new evidence are inconsistent, then only some of the properties are satisfied. For instance, it is evident $R_2$ is satisfied, however, $R_1$ and $R_3$ are not satisfied, let's take $K = \neg a \wedge a$ and $\mu = b$ then $K \circ \mu = \neg a \wedge a \wedge b$, which intuitive interpretation is if the agent holds inconsistent beliefs concerning $a$ and he receives information concerning $b$ he keeps holding its inconsistency concerning $a$ because the new information does not help him to give up the inconsistency. $R_4$ is not satisfied, we can find inconsistent belief bases or formulae for which results are not equivalent. Finally, our operator satisfy $R_5$ and $R_6$, for the sake of space we omit the proofs.

*Complexity:* An important issue is the computational complexity of the operators, even when the revision methods are intractable in the general case, it is not clear under which restrictions the methods would became tractable. The most widely investigated computational task in the literature is deciding the following relation: $K \circ \mu \models \phi$ where $K$, $\mu$ and $\phi$ are inputs. I.e., Given a knowledge base $K$, a new formula $\mu$ and a formula query $\phi$, decide whether $\phi$ is a logical consequence of the revised belief base $K \circ \mu$. The complexity of Dalal's revision operator belongs to, in the general case, $P^{NP[O(log\ n)]}$-complete (the class of problems solvable in polynomial time using a logarithmic number of calls to an NP oracle, where an NP oracle is a subroutine solving an NP-complete problem) [11]. Another problem studied is the complexity of model checking for belief revision: given a knowledge base $K$, a new formula $\mu$ and a interpretation $w$, decide if $w \in mod(K \circ \mu)$. The complexity of Dalal's revision in this case is in $P^{NP[O(log\ n)]}$-complete too [12]. The authors in both cases have proved that the complexity remains the same whether inputs are restricted to those in Horn format (conjunctions of Horn clauses) or not. However, as far as we know there is no formal analysis when inputs are restricted to those in the dual format (disjunctions of terms) even when it is evident that the problem of determining the satisfiability of a Boolean formula in DNF is polynomial time.

Once the inputs are in DNF the proposed method can be implemented in polynomial time. The extension of terms can be computed in $n_1 * n_2 * n_3$, where $n_1$ is the number of terms in $K$, $n_2$ is the number of terms in $\mu$ and $n_3$ is the maximum number of literals appearing in a term, if both $K$ and $\mu$ are consistent $n_3$ is the number of atoms of the language. Thus, for realistic implementations we propose maintaining an algorithm in class polynomial using a method that transforms a formula to its DNF, we know that the worst case, when the input is a formula in Conjunctive Normal Form (CNF), has exponential complexity. However, given the quantity of research about SAT problems, we can find many efficient examples in the literature transforming a formula to CNF, which can be adapted distributing conjunction over disjunctions rather than disjunctions over conjunctions in the final step of the conversion and then obtain an algorithm for dealing with realistic scenarios, in particular we are interested in adapting the algorithm used in [13].

# 5   Conclusion

One of the most established methods of revising belief bases without extra information is Dalal's operator, which takes as input a belief base $K$ and a formula $\mu$ and gives as result a revised consistent belief base. Suitable implementations of Dalal's operator must deal with the calculation of belief base models. In this paper, we have proposed a new method for computing Dalal's revision which does not need to compute Hamming distances and calculates distance between terms instead. Given that the classical revision framework gives priority to new evidence, the proposed method uses definitions considering this principle, thus the extension of formulae gives priority to the new formula $\mu$ keeping all the literals of $\mu$ and complementing the term with literals of $K$. However, there are some attempts that consider $\mu$ should not have the priority, and our approach is flexible enough that Definition 3 can be easily adapted in order to take extensions of $K$ by $\mu$ instead of $\mu$ by $K$ or we can consider a weighted formulae to compute the extension. The operator meets the desirable properties of $R_1$-$R_6$ when both inputs are consistent. When the belief base or new information is inconsistent some properties are satisfied such as $R_2$, $R_4$, $R_5$, independence of extra information and the first property of iterated belief revision framework [2]. Properties $R_1$, $R_3$ and $R_4$ cannot be accomplished for inconsistent inputs, however, the results seem intuitive.

Our method has another advantage over Dalal's result: its representational succinctness at once erasing both repeated and subsumed terms. As future work, a deep analysis of the definitions will be carried out in order to combine this approach with an algorithm transforming formulae to its DNF and solve realistic cases. Moreover, an analysis and extension of the proposal will be considered in order to satisfy the four properties of iterated belief revision framework.

# References

1. Katsuno, H., Mendelzon, A.O.: Propositional knowledge base revision and minimal change. Artif. Intell. 52, 263–294 (1992)
2. Darwiche, A., Pearl, J.: On the logic of iterated belief revision. Artif. Intell. 89, 1–29 (1997)
3. Ma, J., Liu, W., Benferhat, S.: A belief revision framework for revising epistemic states with partial epistemic states. In: AAAI (2010)
4. Gardenfors, P.: Knowledge in Flux: Modeling the Dynamics of Epistemic States. MIT Press (1988)
5. Grove, A.: Two modellings for theory change. Journal of Philosophical Logic, 157–170 (1988)
6. Alchourron, C., Gardenfors, P., Makinson, D.: On the logic of theory change: Partial meet contraction and revision functions. Journal of Symbolic Logic, 510–530 (1985)
7. Bienvenu, M., Herzig, A., Qi, G.: Prime implicate-based belief revision operators. In: Proceedings of the 2008 Conference on ECAI 2008: 18th European Conference on Artificial Intelligence, pp. 741–742. IOS Press, Amsterdam (2008)

8. Marchi, J., Bittencourt, G., Perrussel, L.: Prime forms and minimal change in propositional belief bases. Ann. Math. Artif. Intell. 59, 1–45 (2010)
9. Darwiche, A., Marquis, P.: A knowledge compilation map. CoRR abs/1106.1819 (2011)
10. Katsuno, H., Mendelzon, A.O.: A unified view of propositional knowledge base updates. In: Proceedings of IJCAI 1989, pp. 1413–1419. Morgan Kaufmann (1989)
11. Eiter, T., Gottlob, G.: On the complexity of propositional knowledge base revision, updates, and counterfactuals. Artif. Intell. 57, 227–270 (1992)
12. Liberatore, P., Schaerf, M.: The complexity of model checking for belief revision and update. In: AAAI/IAAI, vol. 1, pp. 556–561. AAAI Press / The MIT Press (1996)
13. McAreavey, K., Liu, W., Miller, P., Meenan, C.: Tools for finding inconsistencies in real-world logic-based systems. In: STAIRS, pp. 192–203 (2012)

# Default Assumptions and Selection Functions: A Generic Framework for Non-monotonic Logics*

Frederik Van De Putte

Centre for Logic and Philosophy of Science, Ghent University, Belgium
frvdeput.vandeputte@ugent.be

**Abstract.** We investigate a generalization of so-called *default-assumption consequence relations*, obtained by replacing the consequence relation of classical logic with an arbitrary supraclassical, compact Tarski-logic, and using arbitrary selection functions on sets of sets of defaults. Both generalizations are inspired by various approaches in non-monotonic logic and belief revision. We establish some meta-theoretic properties of the resulting systems. In addition, we compare them with two other frameworks from the literature on non-monotonic logic, viz. adaptive logics and selection semantics.

## 1 Introduction

This paper concerns a line of research proposed in [1, Chapter 2]. In this book, David Makinson introduces the reader to the very broad and diverse field of non-monotonic logics. He does so by means of three prototypical classes of consequence relations, showing how these can be further refined, thus giving rise to the most well-known approaches in this domain. The first of these three prototypes are called *Default Assumption Consequence Relations* (henceforth DACRs).

DACRs are not only interesting didactically, but can also be seen as a bridge between philosophical work on defeasible reasoning and more AI-oriented approaches to human reasoning. That is, DACRs strike a nice middle ground between conceptual elegance, metatheoretic well-behavedness, and ease of implementation. The latter feature is due to the fact that DACRs are defined syntactically, where their non-monotonic behavior depends essentially on the treatment of a specific set of (explicitly represented) assumptions (see Sect. 2).

Our aim is to investigate a generalized version of the DACR-format, which allows for a greater range of applications, yet preserves the core ideas behind DACRs. In this paper, we report some first results, paving the way for more detailed work. In addition, we spell out some questions that are raised by our preliminary insights.

*Outline.* In Sect. 2, we give the exact definition of DACRs and explain how we generalize these. In the remaining sections of this paper, we present a number of results that revolve around three main topics. As far as we were able to check, none of these have been mentioned previously in the literature. In Sect. 3, we investigate the main metatheoretic properties of $\mathrel{|\!\sim}^{\mathsf{DA}}_{\Delta,\varphi}$ and give some basic

---

* I am indebted to David Makinson for comments on a previous version of this paper.

F. Castro, A. Gelbukh, and M. González (Eds.): MICAI 2013, Part I, LNAI 8265, pp. 54–67, 2013.

representation theorems for it. In Sect. 4, we show how it can be characterized in terms of a certain type of constrained derivations. Finally, Sect. 5 compares DACRs to selection semantics in the vein of [2].

To keep the paper reader-friendly, we introduce our notation gradually and sometimes implicitly throughout this introduction. The reader may find an overview of notational conventions in the appendix.

# 2    Generalized DACRs

*The Original Definition.* DACRs are defined on the basis of classical propositional logic (henceforth **CL**). The basic idea behind their construction is that, when reasoning non-monotonically, we rely on a set of assumptions $\Delta$ in the object language of **CL**. These are used to generate conclusions in as far as they are consistent with our premise set $\Gamma$. That is, we reason on the basis of maximal subsets of $\Delta$ consistent with $\Gamma$, and intersect the resulting consequence sets.

This idea is made formally precise in Definition 1, which defines a consequence relation $\vdash_{\Delta}^{\mathsf{DA}}$ for every set of assumptions $\Delta$. Here, $\Phi$ denotes the set of all formulas in **CL**, $\vdash_{\mathbf{CL}}$ denotes the consequence relation of **CL**, and $\perp$ denotes the logical falsum.

**Definition 1 (DACRs, original form).** *Where $\Gamma \cup \Delta \subseteq \Phi$, let $\mathcal{S}_{\Delta}^{\mathbf{CL}}(\Gamma)$ be the set of all $\Delta' \subseteq \Delta$ such that $\Gamma \cup \Delta' \nvdash_{\mathbf{CL}} \perp$. Let $\max_{\subset}(\mathcal{S}_{\Delta}^{\mathbf{CL}}(\Gamma))$ be the set of all $\subset$-maximal members of $\mathcal{S}_{\Delta}^{\mathbf{CL}}(\Gamma)$.*
*Where $\Gamma \cup \Delta \subseteq \Phi$, $\Gamma \vdash_{\Delta}^{\mathsf{DA}} A$ ($A \in C_{\Delta}(\Gamma)$) iff for all $\Delta' \in \max_{\subset}(\mathcal{S}_{\Delta}^{\mathbf{CL}}(\Gamma))$, $\Gamma \cup \Delta' \vdash_{\mathbf{CL}} A$.*

As shown in [1], every consequence relation $\vdash_{\Delta}^{\mathsf{DA}}$ satisfies a large number of well-known metatheoretic properties such as left and right absorption, reflexivity, and cumulativity – all of these are defined in Sect. 3 below.

*Generalized DACRs.* The class of logics which we will study in this paper is given by Definition 3. This is obtained from Definition 1 by (i) replacing $\vdash_{\mathbf{CL}}$ with an arbitrary consequence relation $\vdash$ satisfying certain basic properties; and (ii) replacing the function $\max_{\subset}$ with an arbitrary selection function $\varphi$, where

**Definition 2.** *$f : X \to Y$ is a selection function iff for all $x \in X$, $f(x) \subseteq x$.*

**Definition 3 (DACRs, generalized).** *Let $\mathbf{L}$ be an arbitrary compact, supraclassical Tarski-logic with consequence relation $\vdash \subseteq \wp(\Phi) \times \Phi$. Where $\Gamma \cup \Delta \subseteq \Phi$, let $\mathcal{S}_{\Delta}(\Gamma) = \{\Delta' \subseteq \Delta \mid \Gamma \cup \Delta' \nvdash \perp\}$. Let $\mathbb{S}_{\Delta} = \{\mathcal{S}_{\Delta}(\Gamma) \mid \Gamma \subseteq \Phi\}$.*
*Where $\varphi : \mathbb{S}_{\Delta} \to \wp(\wp(\Delta))$ is a selection function, let $\Gamma \vdash_{\Delta,\varphi}^{\mathsf{DA}} A$ ($A \in C_{\Delta,\varphi}(\Gamma)$) iff for all $\Delta' \in \varphi(\mathcal{S}_{\Delta}(\Gamma))$, $\Gamma \cup \Delta' \vdash A$.*

In the remainder of this introduction, we briefly motivate the generalizations mentioned under (i) and (ii) above.

The motivation for (i) is rather straightforward. This generalization is very common in non-monotonic logic and belief revision (see [3] and [4] respectively).

Moreover, the same move is made in [5], where also a generalized version of DACRs is studied (we return to this paper below).

From the viewpoint of applications, there are also obvious reasons why we would use richer systems than **CL** as the monotonic core of our non-monotonic logic. To give but one example, one may find it useful to distinguish beliefs from (contextual) certainties, and apply a defeasible mechanism to the former of the type: "where $A$ is a belief, infer $A$ unless this leads to triviality". One may even want to distinguish between different degrees or types of belief. Similarly, moving to the predicative level seems to be indispensable if one wants to model default information about certain classes of objects in a natural way.

So let us focus instead on point (ii). As will become clear in Sect. 3, moving from $\mathsf{max}_\subset$ to arbitrary selection functions results in the loss of some quite important properties. Consequently, metatheoretic investigations of the more general format focus on conditions on $\varphi$ which allow us to preserve some of the meta-properties.

The main idea behind using selection functions is that not all $\Delta' \in \mathcal{S}_\Delta(\Gamma)$ have the same status, and hence we have reasons for using only some of them to generate consequences. Makinson explains this in [1], and refers to [5], where a selection function is used to select a subset of $\mathsf{max}_\subset(\mathcal{S}_\Delta(\Gamma))$.

In the current paper, we take a yet more general perspective, also allowing for sets to be selected that are not $\subset$-maximal. This move can be motivated in various, more or less independent ways. In the remainder of this introduction, we give three examples.

First, suppose that we use a partial order $\prec$ on $\wp(\Delta)$ which expresses informational content – such an approach would be similar to Levi's recent approach to belief contraction [6].[1] This partial order may be based on various criteria, such as simplicity, explanatory power, likelihood, etc. Logical strength may be just one of those criteria, and even if it would receive the highest priority, this would still not imply that only $\subset$-maximal sets are selected. One may well prefer smaller sets $\Delta'$ if these carry the same logical content, over the $\subset$-maximal ones.[2]

Second, one may combine a preference relation $\prec$ on $\wp(\Delta)$ with an indifference relation $\sim$ on $\wp(\Delta)$. Here $\Delta' \sim \Delta''$ expresses that both sets are equally important, and hence that if one is selected, so should the other. This again echoes an idea from the logic of belief revision – see [7]. The combination of $\prec$ and $\sim$ into a single selection function $\varphi$ may take several forms. Examples are:

(a)  $\varphi(X) = \{x \in X \mid x \sim y \text{ for some } y \in \mathsf{min}_\prec(X)\}$.
(b)  $\varphi(X) = \mathsf{min}_{\prec'}(X)$, where $\prec' = \prec \setminus \sim$.

It can be easily checked that under both approaches, we may end up selecting $\Delta'$ which are not $\subset$-maximal.

---

[1] Makinson points out that one may apply Levi's idea to obtain a generalization of DACRs as well. See [1, Chapter 2, pp. 47-49].

[2] This remark holds in particular for cases where $\Delta$ is closed under $\vdash$. In this case, the $\subset$-maximal members of $\mathcal{S}_\Delta(\Gamma)$ will contain many redundant formulas.

A third motivation is the following: suppose that we use a preference relation $\prec$, and that for some $\Delta' \in \max_\prec(\mathcal{S}_\Delta(\Gamma))$, $A \in \Delta - \Delta'$. Then one may reason as follows: given that $A$ is not included in *every* $\prec$-maximal subset of $\Delta$ consistent with $\Gamma$, there is at least some reason to be suspicious about this assumption. Hence, we should not rely on it when inferring anything from $\Gamma$. This idea is akin to Horty's *direct skeptical approach* to default logic, where only those default rules are applied which are a member of *every* maximal extension – see e.g. [8].

The selection function which implements this idea would look as follows:

$$\varphi(X) = \bigcap \max_\prec(X) \cap X$$

Whenever $X = \mathcal{S}_\Delta(\Gamma)$ and $\max_\prec(X) \neq \emptyset$, it can easily be shown that $\varphi(X) \neq \emptyset$.[3]

By now, the reader should be convinced that there are at least some interesting constructions which fall under the generic format given by Definition 3. However, it remains an open question how such logics behave in general, which properties they satisfy, and how they compare to other formalisms in the field of non-monotonic logic. Rather than studying each of the above constructions separately, we shall start from their common structure and try to see how much can be obtained at this abstract level.

# 3   Some Conditions on DACRs

In this section, we investigate the metatheoretic behavior of DACRs. We focus on six key properties which are familiar from the literature. This results in a number of representation theorems, linking those properties to conditions on the selection function $\varphi$. The conditions are exactly the same as those used in [2], where so-called selection semantics are studied – see also Section 5.

In the remainder, let $Cn(\Gamma) = \{A \mid \Gamma \vdash A\}$. Where $\mathrel{\vert\!\sim} \subseteq \wp(\Phi) \times \Phi$ is arbitrary, let $C(\Gamma) = \{A \mid \Gamma \mathrel{\vert\!\sim} A\}$.

*DACRs versus Inference Relations.* The first thing to observe about DACRs is that they are *inference relations* in the sense of [2]. That is, when $\mathrel{\vert\!\sim} = \mathrel{\vert\!\sim}^{DA}_{\Delta,\varphi}$ for a $\Delta \subseteq \Phi$ and a selection function $\varphi : \mathbb{S}_\Delta \to \wp(\wp(\Delta))$, each of the following holds:

*Reflexivity*         $\Gamma \subseteq C(\Gamma)$.
*Left Absorption*    $C(Cn(\Gamma)) = C(\Gamma)$.
*Right Absorption*  $C(\Gamma) = Cn(C(\Gamma))$.

Reflexivity is immediate in view of the reflexivity of **L** and Definition 3. For *Left Absorption*, we rely on the Tarski-properties of $\vdash$ and the fact that $\mathcal{S}_\Delta(\Gamma) = \mathcal{S}_\Delta(Cn(\Gamma))$. *Right Absorption* is immediate in view of the fact that the intersection of a set of sets $Cn(\Theta)$ is itself closed under $Cn$.

Perhaps more surprisingly, the class of all DACRs is fully characterized by these three properties:

---

[3] This holds since $\mathcal{S}_\Delta(\Gamma)$ is closed under intersection.

**Theorem 1.** $\succ$ *satisfies reflexivity, left and right absorption iff there is a* $\Delta \subseteq \Phi$ *and a* $\varphi : \mathbb{S}_\Delta \to \wp(\wp(\Delta))$ *such that* $\succ \ = \ \succ^{DA}_{\Delta,\varphi}$.

*Proof.* It suffices to check the left-right direction. So suppose the antecedent holds. Let $\Delta = \Phi$. Note that, for all $\Gamma \subseteq \Phi$, $\max_\subset(\mathcal{S}_\Delta(\Gamma))$ is the set of all $\subset$-maximal $\Gamma' \supseteq \Gamma$ such that $\Gamma' \not\vdash \bot$. Hence, for all $\Gamma$ such that $\Gamma \not\vdash \bot$, (a) $\bigcap \max_\subset(\mathcal{S}_\Delta(\Gamma)) = Cn(\Gamma)$. Note also that (b) $\mathcal{S}_\Delta(\Gamma) = \emptyset$ iff $Cn(\Gamma) = C(\Gamma) = \Phi$.

Where $X \in \mathbb{S}_\Delta$, let $\Theta_X = \bigcap \max_\subset(X)$ if $X \neq \emptyset$, and $\Theta_X = \Phi$ otherwise. By (a), (b) and left absorption,

$$C(\Theta_X) = C(Cn(\Gamma)) = C(\Gamma) \tag{1}$$

Where $X \in \mathbb{S}_\Delta$, let $\varphi(X) = \{\Theta \mid C(\Theta_X) \subseteq \Theta \subseteq \Phi\} \cap X$. By (1),

$$\varphi(\mathcal{S}_\Delta(\Gamma)) = \{\Theta \mid C(\Gamma) \subseteq \Theta \subseteq \Phi\} \cap \mathcal{S}_\Delta(\Gamma) \tag{2}$$

In the remainder we show that, for all $\Gamma \subseteq \Phi$, $C(\Gamma) = C_{\Delta,\varphi}(\Gamma)$.

Case 1: $Cn(\Gamma) = \Phi$. By left absorption and reflexivity, $C(\Gamma) = \Phi$. Also, $\mathcal{S}_\Delta(\Gamma) = \emptyset$, and hence $\varphi(\mathcal{S}_\Delta(\Gamma)) = \emptyset$. Consequently, $C_{\Delta,\varphi}(\Gamma) = \Phi$.

Case 2: $Cn(\Gamma) \neq \Phi$. Case 2.1: $C(\Gamma) = \Phi$. By (2), by the construction and since each $\Delta' \in \mathcal{S}_\Delta(\Gamma)$ is consistent, $\varphi(\mathcal{S}_\Delta(\Gamma)) = \emptyset$. It follows that $C_{\Delta,\varphi}(\Gamma) = \Phi$.

Case 2.2: $C(\Gamma) \neq \Phi$. By right absorption, $C(\Gamma) \not\vdash \bot$. By reflexivity, $\Gamma \cup C(\Gamma) \not\vdash \bot$. Hence, $C(\Gamma) \in \mathcal{S}_\Delta(\Gamma)$. By (2), $\varphi(\mathcal{S}_\Delta(\Gamma)) \neq \emptyset$. Hence, $C_{\Delta,\varphi}(\Gamma) = \bigcap_{C(\Gamma) \subseteq \Delta'} Cn(\Gamma \cup \Delta') = Cn(\Gamma \cup C(\Gamma)) = C(\Gamma)$. □

*Consistency Preserving DACRs.* One natural property of non-monotonic consequence relations is the following:

*Consistency Preservation*    If $\Gamma \succ \bot$ then $\Gamma \vdash \bot$.

It can be easily observed that this property does not hold for all relations $\succ^{DA}_{\Delta,\varphi}$. It may well be that, although $\mathcal{S}_\Delta(\Gamma) \neq \emptyset$ (and hence $\Gamma \not\vdash \bot$), the selection function is defined in such a way that $\varphi(\mathcal{S}_\Delta(\Gamma)) = \emptyset$, and hence, $\Gamma \succ^{DA}_{\Delta,\varphi} \bot$. In particular, where $\varphi = \min_\prec$, this is the case whenever there are infinite descending chains of ever better members of $\mathcal{S}_\Delta(\Gamma)$, or when $\prec$ is cyclic over $\mathcal{S}_\Delta(\Gamma)$.

So the relations $\succ^{DA}_{\Delta,\varphi}$ which preserve consistency constitute a proper subclass of inference relations. This class is characterized by the following condition:

(CP)  If $X \neq \emptyset$, then $\varphi(X) \neq \emptyset$.

**Theorem 2.** $\succ$ *satisfies reflexivity, left and right absorption and consistency preservation iff there is a* $\Delta \subseteq \Phi$ *and a* $\varphi : \mathbb{S}_\Delta \to \wp(\wp(\Delta))$ *which satisfies (CP), such that* $\succ \ = \ \succ^{DA}_{\Delta,\varphi}$.

*Proof.* As before, we leave the right-left direction to the reader. The proof of left to right is already implicit in the proof of the left-right direction for Theorem 1. That is, let $\Delta$ and $\varphi$ be constructed as in that proof. We know that $C(\Gamma) = C_{\Delta,\varphi}(\Gamma)$ for all $\Gamma \subseteq \Phi$. Suppose now that $\mathcal{S}_\Delta(\Gamma) \neq \emptyset$. It follows that $\bot \notin Cn(\Gamma)$. By consistency preservation, $\bot \notin C(\Gamma)$. Hence, $C(\Gamma) \neq \Phi$. So we are in case 2.2 of that proof, and hence $\varphi(\mathcal{S}_\Delta(\Gamma)) \neq \emptyset$. □

*Cumulativity.* The property *Cumulativity* was introduced by Gabbay in his [9], where it is assumed to be a fundamental property of any sensible non-monotonic inference relation. Intuitively, it says that whenever we add a consequence to our premise set, this should not make a difference with regards to the overall conclusions we may draw. From the point of view of applications, this property is important, since it allows us to rely on previously established consequences, when trying to find out whether a different formula also follows from the premises.

Cumulativity is usually divided into two components, which may be formulated as follows:

*Cautious Monotonicity.*   If $\Gamma \subseteq \Gamma' \subseteq C(\Gamma)$, then $C(\Gamma) \subseteq C(\Gamma')$.
*Cumulative Transitivity.*   If $\Gamma \subseteq \Gamma' \subseteq C(\Gamma)$, then $C(\Gamma') \subseteq C(\Gamma)$.

The sets of all relations $\vDash_{\Delta,\varphi}^{DA}$ which satisfy cautious monotonicity, resp. cumulative transitivity, are characterized by the following conditions on $\varphi$: where $X, Y \in \mathbb{S}_\Delta$,

(CM)   If $\varphi(X) \subseteq Y \subseteq X$, then $\varphi(Y) \subseteq \varphi(X)$
(CT)   If $\varphi(X) \subseteq Y \subseteq X$, then $\varphi(X) \subseteq \varphi(Y)$

**Fact 1.** $\mathcal{S}_\Phi(\Gamma) \subseteq \mathcal{S}_\Phi(\Gamma')$ iff $Cn(\Gamma') \subseteq Cn(\Gamma)$.

**Theorem 3.** $\vDash$ *satisfies reflexivity, left and right absorption and cautious monotonicity iff there is a $\Delta \subseteq \Phi$ and a $\varphi : \mathbb{S}_\Delta \to \wp(\wp(\Delta))$ which satisfies (CM), such that* $\vDash = \vDash_{\Delta,\varphi}^{DA}$.

*Proof.* ($\Rightarrow$) It suffices to check that the $\varphi$ from the proof of Theorem 1 satisfies (CM) whenever $\vDash$ is cautiously monotonic. To see why this is so, suppose $\varphi(X) \subseteq Y \subseteq X$, where $X, Y \in \mathbb{S}_\Delta$. Let $\Gamma$ and $\Gamma'$ be such that $X = \mathcal{S}_\Delta(\Gamma)$ and $Y = \mathcal{S}_\Delta(\Gamma')$. By Fact 1, $Cn(\Gamma) \subseteq Cn(\Gamma')$.

Suppose now that $A \notin C(Cn(\Gamma))$. By left and right absorption, $A \notin Cn(C(\Gamma))$. Let $\Theta = C(\Gamma) \cup \{\neg A\}$. Note that $\Theta \nvdash \bot$, and by the reflexivity of $C$, $\Gamma \subseteq \Theta$. It follows that $\Theta \in \mathcal{S}_\Delta(\Gamma)$. By the construction, $\Theta \in \varphi(\mathcal{S}_\Delta(\Gamma))$. Hence $\Theta \in \varphi(X)$, and hence $\Theta \in Y$. So $\Gamma' \cup \Theta \nvdash \bot$. By monotonicity of $\vdash$, $\Gamma' \nvdash A$, or equivalently, $A \notin Cn(\Gamma')$.

So we have shown that

$$Cn(\Gamma) \subseteq Cn(\Gamma') \subseteq C(Cn(\Gamma)) \tag{3}$$

By (3) and cautious monotonicity, $C(Cn(\Gamma)) \subseteq C(Cn(\Gamma'))$, whence by left absorption, $C(\Gamma) \subseteq C(\Gamma')$. Relying on (2), we have: $\varphi(\mathcal{S}_\Delta(\Gamma')) = \{\Theta \mid C(\Gamma') \subseteq \Theta \subseteq \Phi\} \cap \mathcal{S}_\Delta(\Gamma') \subseteq \{\Theta \mid C(\Gamma) \subseteq \Theta \subseteq \Phi\} \cap \mathcal{S}_\Delta(\Gamma') \subseteq \{\Theta \mid C(\Gamma') \subseteq \Theta \subseteq \Phi\} \cap \mathcal{S}_\Delta(\Gamma) = \varphi(\mathcal{S}_\Delta(\Gamma))$.

($\Leftarrow$) Suppose that $\Gamma \subseteq \Gamma' \subseteq C(\Gamma)$. It follows that $\mathcal{S}_\Delta(\Gamma') \subseteq \mathcal{S}_\Delta(\Gamma)$. Let $\Delta' \in \varphi(\mathcal{S}_\Delta(\Gamma))$. It follows that $\Delta'$ is consistent with $C(\Gamma)$. Hence $\Delta'$ is also consistent with $\Gamma'$, whence $\Delta' \in \mathcal{S}_\Delta(\Gamma')$. So we have:

$$\varphi(\mathcal{S}_\Delta(\Gamma)) \subseteq \mathcal{S}_\Delta(\Gamma') \subseteq \mathcal{S}_\Delta(\Gamma)$$

By (CM), $\varphi(\mathcal{S}_\Delta(\Gamma')) \subseteq \varphi(\mathcal{S}_\Delta(\Gamma))$. Since also $\Gamma \subseteq \Gamma'$, it follows at once that $C_{\Delta,\varphi}(\Gamma) \subseteq C_{\Delta,\varphi}(\Gamma')$.   $\square$

**Theorem 4.** $\hspace{-0.3em}\mathrel{|\!\sim}$ *satisfies reflexivity, left and right absorption and cumulative transitivity iff there is a* $\Delta \subseteq \Phi$ *and a* $\varphi : \mathbb{S}_\Delta \to \wp(\wp(\Delta))$ *which satisfies (CT), such that* $\mathrel{|\!\sim} = \mathrel{|\!\sim}^{DA}_{\Delta,\varphi}$.

*Proof.* ($\Rightarrow$) The proof is identical to the one for Theorem 3 above, except for the last paragraph. By the cumulative transitivity of $\mathrel{|\!\sim}$, we can derive that $C(Cn(\Gamma')) \subseteq C(Cn(\Gamma))$. By left absorption, $C(\Gamma') \subseteq C(\Gamma)$. It follows that every consistent extension of $C(\Gamma)$ is also a consistent extension of $\Gamma'$. Hence,

$$\mathcal{S}_\Delta(\Gamma) \cap \{\Theta \mid C(\Gamma) \subseteq \Theta \subseteq \Phi\} \subseteq \mathcal{S}_\Delta(\Gamma') \tag{4}$$

By (4) and (2), $\varphi(\mathcal{S}_\Delta(\Gamma)) = \{\Theta \mid C(\Gamma) \subseteq \Theta \subseteq \Phi\} \cap \mathcal{S}_\Delta(\Gamma) \subseteq \{\Theta \mid C(\Gamma) \subseteq \Theta \subseteq \Phi\} \cap \mathcal{S}_\Delta(\Gamma') \subseteq \{\Theta \mid C(\Gamma') \subseteq \Theta \subseteq \Phi\} \cap \mathcal{S}_\Delta(\Gamma') = \varphi(\mathcal{S}_\Delta(\Gamma'))$.

($\Leftarrow$) By the same reasoning as for the right-left direction of Theorem 3, we can derive that $\varphi(\mathcal{S}_\Delta(\Gamma)) \subseteq \mathcal{S}_\Delta(\Gamma') \subseteq \mathcal{S}_\Delta(\Gamma)$. By (CT),

$$\varphi(\mathcal{S}_\Delta(\Gamma)) \subseteq \varphi(\mathcal{S}_\Delta(\Gamma')) \tag{5}$$

Suppose now that $A \in C_{\Delta,\varphi}(\Gamma')$. Hence $A \in \bigcap_{\Delta' \in \varphi(\mathcal{S}_\Delta(\Gamma'))} Cn(\Gamma' \cup \Delta')$. Since $\Gamma' \subseteq C(\Gamma)$, also $A \in \bigcap_{\Delta' \in \varphi(\mathcal{S}_\Delta(\Gamma'))} Cn(C(\Gamma) \cup \Delta')$. By (5),

$$A \in \bigcap_{\Delta' \in \varphi(\mathcal{S}_\Delta(\Gamma))} Cn(C(\Gamma) \cup \Delta') \tag{6}$$

Note that for all $\Delta' \in \varphi(\mathcal{S}_\Delta(\Gamma))$, $C(\Gamma) \subseteq Cn(\Gamma \cup \Delta')$. Hence

$$A \in \bigcap_{\Delta' \in \varphi(\mathcal{S}_\Delta(\Gamma))} Cn(\Gamma \cup \Delta') = C_{\Delta,\varphi}(\Gamma) \tag{7}$$

$\square$

*Open Problems.* As indicated before, we inspected only a limited number of meta-theoretic properties. One important property which was left outside the scope of this paper is the so-called *Disjunction Property* – see [3] for its definition –, and related properties that concern the behavior of $\mathrel{|\!\sim}$ with respect to (classical) disjunction and implication. In this context, it seems less straightforward to apply the same conditions as studied in [2], let alone to obtain representation theorems of the type given above. Similarly, other conditions from [3] such as *Loop* and *Rational Monotony* need further study in the context of (generalized) DACRs.

In view of the construction used in the proof of Theorem 1 (which is called upon in all subsequent proofs of this section), the framework of DACRs is very liberal. In particular, letting $\Phi$ play the role of the set of assumptions can be viewed as way of turning upside down the whole idea behind DACRs, in order to obtain the above representation theorem. This in turn explains how it is possible to obtain at least some results that run parallel to those from [2], where the selection functions operate on models instead (see also Sect. 5).

Still, one may ask whether stronger results can be obtained, by restricting the sets of assumptions $\Delta$ under consideration. For instance, one may require $\Delta$ to be consistent and perhaps even closed under $Cn$. In a more restricted setting, such conditions are studied in [5]. However, in the general case we have not come accross any syntactic properties of $\sim$ which would single out the class of all DACRs based on such consistent $\Delta$.

## 4   DACRs and Adaptive Logics

In [10] and earlier work, Batens developed a so-called *standard format of adaptive logics* (henceforth ALs). ALs have been developed for various purposes: to model reasoning with inconsistent information, to capture the dynamics inherent to belief revision, to obtain conflict-tolerant deontic logics, as an alternative foundation of mathematics, etc.[4] The standard format unifies these different systems in terms of one basic underlying structure, thereby allowing us to study their generic properties. In addition, it provides us with a simple recipe to develop new such logics, and immediately equips them with a rich metatheory.

Adaptive logics in standard format are similar to DACRs in their original form, in the sense that they are also defined on the basis of a supra-classical compact Tarski-logic and a specific set of assumptions. However, there is also an important difference, in that in ALs the assumptions have a negative character – in this context, one often speaks of abnormal formulas, or simply abnormalities.

In this paper, we will focus on the characterization of a specific type of ALs, viz. those that use the so-called minimal abnormality strategy. As we will show, this characterization can be generalized in the same way as was done with DACRs in Sect. 1. More importantly, the resulting logics display a simple, one-to-one correspondence with DACRs.[5]

*Generalized ALs.* Let $\Omega \subseteq \Phi$ denote a set of *abnormalities*, i.e. formulas which are assumed to be false unless the premises tell us otherwise. We use $\neg$ and $\vee$ to denote classical negation, resp. disjunction. Where $\Lambda \subseteq_f \Phi$, let $\bigvee \Lambda$ denote the disjunction of the members of $\Lambda$.[6]

The basic idea behind ALs is the following. Suppose that $\Gamma \vdash A \vee \bigvee \Upsilon$ for some $\Upsilon \subseteq_f \Omega$. Then, assuming that the abnormalities in $\Upsilon$ are false, we can apply disjunctive syllogism, and hence derive $A$ in a proof from $\Gamma$.

In the AL proof theory, this idea is made explicit by adding to each step in a proof a so-called condition $\Upsilon \subseteq_f \Omega$. Using a specific rule, the reasoner may "push" abnormalities to the condition whenever they are derivable in disjunction with other formulas. This mimics the fact that when reasoning defeasibly, we "jump" to a certain conclusion which does not follow by **L** alone.

Obviously, such an inferential system would make little sense, unless it is accompanied by some way of constraining derivations, in view of conflicts between

---

[4] This list is by far not exhaustive. See [11] For a longer list and numerous references.

[5] Batens himself notes the correspondence between the original DACRs and ALs that use the *minimal abnormality strategy* in the forthcoming book [12]. We return to this point at the end of this section.

[6] Here and below, $X \subseteq_f Y$ denotes that $X$ is a finite subset of $Y$.

our (negative) assumptions and the premise set. In the AL terminology, this mechanism is called *marking*: lines are marked at a certain point in the proof, when it turns out that their conditions are problematic in view of the premises. Marks may come and come as a proof proceeds, whence the AL proof theory is called *dynamic*.

To avoid going into the details of this marking mechanism and the corresponding adaptive consequence relation, we shall characterize this relation in a more static fashion here. The interested reader is referred to [10] for the official definition, and the proof that our definition is equivalent to it.[7]

Let $\mathcal{T}_\Omega(\Gamma)$ denote the set of all $\Delta \subseteq \Omega$ such that $\Gamma \vdash \bigvee \Delta$. So $\Gamma$ informs us that at least one of the members of each $\Delta \in \mathcal{T}_\Omega(\Gamma)$ is true. This information is taken into account by quantifying over so-called *choice sets* of $\mathcal{T}_\Omega(\Gamma)$. These are sets $\Theta \subseteq \Omega$ such that $\Theta \cap \Delta = \emptyset$ for all $\Delta \in \mathcal{T}_\Omega(\Gamma)$. Let henceforth $\mathcal{R}_\Omega(\Gamma)$ denote the set of all choice sets of $\mathcal{T}_\Omega(\Gamma)$.

It is the set $\mathcal{R}_\Omega(\Gamma)$ which provides us with the constraint on the derivations that are allowed for in an adaptive logic based on $\Omega$. That is, a derivation of $A$ from $\Gamma$ is only warranted if, for each $\Theta \in \min_\subset(\mathcal{R}_\Gamma(\Omega))$, one may derive $A$ on a condition $\Upsilon$ that has an empty intersection with $\Theta$. Formally:

**Definition 4.** $\Gamma \mathrel{\vertbar\!\sim}^{AL}_\Omega A$ *iff for every* $\Theta \in \min_\subset(\mathcal{R}_\Gamma(\Omega))$, *there is a* $\Upsilon \subseteq \Omega - \Theta$ *such that* $\Gamma \Vdash A \vee \bigvee \Upsilon$.

The generalization we mentioned above is obtained by replacing the function $\min_\subset$ in Definition 4 with an arbitrary selection function with an appropriate domain. So we obtain the following definition:

**Definition 5.** *Where* $\Omega \subseteq \Phi$, *let* $\mathbb{U}_\Omega = \{\mathcal{R}_\Omega(\Gamma) \mid \Gamma \subseteq \Phi\}$. *Let* $\chi : \mathbb{U}_\Omega \to \wp(\wp(\Omega))$ *be a selection function.*
$\Gamma \mathrel{\vertbar\!\sim}^{AL}_{\Omega,\chi} A$ *iff for every* $\Theta \in \chi(\mathcal{R}_\Omega(\Gamma))$, *there is a* $\Upsilon \subseteq \Omega - \Theta$ *such that* $\Gamma \vdash A \vee \bigvee \Upsilon$.

*Representation Theorem.* The correspondence between DACRs and ALs follows from a deeper connection between the sets $\mathcal{S}_\Delta(\Gamma)$ and $\mathcal{R}_\Omega(\Gamma)$, which we spell out first. Where $\Delta \subseteq \Phi$, let $\Delta^\neg = \{\neg A \mid A \in \Delta\}$. We have:

**Theorem 5.** *If* $\Gamma \nvdash \bot$, *then*

1. $\mathcal{S}_\Delta(\Gamma) = \{\Delta - \Theta \mid \Theta^\neg \in \mathcal{R}_{\Delta^\neg}(\Gamma)\}$ *and*
2. $\mathcal{R}_\Delta(\Gamma) = \{\Delta - \Theta \mid \Theta^\neg \in \mathcal{S}_{\Delta^\neg}(\Gamma)\}$.

*Proof. Ad 1.* ($\subseteq$) Let $\Delta' \in \mathcal{S}_\Delta(\Gamma)$. Let $\Theta = \Delta - \Delta'$, whence $\Delta' = \Delta - \Theta$. Assume that $\Theta^\neg \notin \mathcal{R}_{\Delta^\neg}(\Gamma)$. It follows that, for some $\Psi^\neg \in \mathcal{T}_{\Delta^\neg}(\Gamma)$, $\Theta^\neg \cap \Psi^\neg = \emptyset$. Hence $\Theta \cap \Psi = \emptyset$, and hence $\Psi \subseteq \Delta'$. Note that, since $\Gamma \vdash \bigvee \Psi^\neg$, $\Gamma \cup \Psi \vdash \bot$. Hence also $\Gamma \cup \Delta' \vdash \bot$, which contradicts the fact that $\Delta' \in \mathcal{S}_\Delta(\Gamma)$.

($\supseteq$) Let $\Theta^\neg \in \mathcal{R}_{\Delta^\neg}(\Gamma)$. Let $\Delta' = \Delta - \Theta$. Suppose that $\Delta' \notin \mathcal{S}_\Delta(\Gamma)$. It follows that $\Gamma \cup \Delta' \vdash \bot$. Hence, $\Gamma \vdash \bigvee \Psi^\neg$ for a $\Psi \subseteq \Delta'$. But then $\Psi^\neg \in \mathcal{T}_{\Delta^\neg}(\Gamma)$. Since $\Psi \subseteq \Delta'$, $\Psi^\neg \cap \Theta^\neg = \emptyset$. Hence $\Theta^\neg$ is not a choice set of $\mathcal{T}_{\Delta^\neg}(\Gamma)$ — a contradiction.
*Ad 2.* Similar to the first item and therefore safely left to the reader. □

---

[7] See [10, Sect. 3] and [10, Theorem 8] respectively.

To obtain the correspondence between DACRs and the AL-proof theory, we need some more notational conventions. Where $\varphi : \mathbb{S}_\Delta \to \wp(\wp(\Delta))$ is a selection function, define the selection function $\varphi^\neg : \mathbb{U}_{\Delta^\neg} \to \wp(\wp(\Delta^\neg))$ as follows:

$$\varphi^\neg(X) =_{df} \{\Theta^\neg \in X \mid \Delta - \Theta \in \varphi(\{\Delta - \Theta' \mid (\Theta')^\neg \in X\})\}$$

Using the same equation, we can define a selection function $\chi^\neg : \mathbb{S}_{\Delta^\neg} \to \wp(\wp(\Delta^\neg))$ for every selection function $\chi : \mathbb{U}_\Delta \to \wp(\wp(\Delta))$; it suffices to replace $\varphi$ with $\chi$.

**Theorem 6.** *Each of the following hold:*

1. $\vdash^{DA}_{\Delta,\varphi} = \vdash^{AL}_{\Delta^\neg,\varphi^\neg}$.
2. $\vdash^{AL}_{\Omega,\chi} = \vdash^{DA}_{\Omega^\neg,\chi^\neg}$.

*Proof. Ad 1.* We prove that, for all $\Gamma \cup \{A\} \subseteq \Phi$, $\Gamma \vdash^{DA}_{\Delta,\varphi} A$ iff $\Gamma \vdash^{AL}_{\Delta^\neg,\varphi^\neg} A$. The case where $\Gamma \vdash \bot$ is trivial in view of Definitions 3 and 5 respectively. So suppose that $\Gamma \nvdash \bot$. We have: $\Gamma \vdash^{DA}_{\Delta,\varphi} A$ iff for all $\Delta' \in \varphi(\mathcal{S}_\Delta(\Gamma))$, $\Gamma \cup \Delta' \vdash A$ iff [by compactness and the deduction theorem] for all $\Delta' \in \varphi(\mathcal{S}_\Delta(\Gamma))$, $\Gamma \vdash A \vee \bigvee(\Delta'')^\neg$ for some finite $\Delta'' \subseteq \Delta'$ iff [by Theorem 5 and the definition of $\varphi^\neg$], for all $\Theta^\neg \in \varphi^\neg(\mathcal{R}_{\Delta^\neg}(\Gamma))$, there is a $(\Delta'')^\neg \subseteq \Delta^\neg - \Theta^\neg$ such that $\Gamma \vdash A \vee \bigvee(\Delta'')^\neg$ iff [by Definition 5] $\Gamma \vdash^{AL}_{\Delta^\neg,\varphi^\neg} A$.

*Ad 2.* Similar and hence left to the reader.     □

In other words, abnormalities, as conceived in the generalized AL framework, behave exactly as negative assumptions, as conceived in the generalized DACR-framework (and vice versa). It should however be noted that this property relies essentially on the presence of a classical negation and disjunction in the object language of **L**.

Where $\sigma \in \{\varphi, \chi\}$, it can be easily verified that $\sigma = \mathsf{max}_C$ iff $\sigma^\neg = \mathsf{min}_C$. Hence, relying on Theorem 6, we obtain a one-to-one correspondence between the original DACR-framework and ALs that use the minimal abnormality strategy:

**Corollary 1.** *Each of the following holds:*

1. $\vdash^{DA}_{\Delta,\mathsf{max}_C} = \vdash^{AL}_{\Delta^\neg,\mathsf{min}_C}$.
2. $\vdash^{AL}_{\Omega,\mathsf{min}_C} = \vdash^{DA}_{\Omega^\neg,\mathsf{max}_C}$.

*Open Problem: Complexity of DACRs.* Various complexity results have been obtained for ALs that use the minimal abnormality strategy – see [13–15] in particular. Complexity reductions in this area are usually conditional on certain restrictions on the sets $\mathcal{R}_\Omega(\Gamma)$ and $\mathsf{min}_C(\mathcal{R}_\Omega(\Gamma))$. For instance, when $\mathcal{R}_\Omega(\Gamma)$ is finite, then the adaptive consequence set (given the minimal abnormality strategy) is decidable. Or, when $\mathsf{min}_C(\mathcal{R}_\Omega(\Gamma))$ consists of finite sets only, then the adaptive consequence set is in $\Sigma^0_2$.

Hence, one interesting line of research consists in generalizing these results to the case where we use arbitrary selection functions. In view of Theorem 6, this would at once give us complexity results on generalized DACRs as well.

# 5   DACRs versus Selection Semantics

In his [2], Lindström studies non-monotonic reasoning from a semantic viewpoint. The idea is that from the set of all models of our premise set, we select a subset using a selection function. A formula is a consequence of $\Gamma$, given this selection function, iff it holds in all the selected models of $\Gamma$. In this section, we investigate the relation between this construction and our generalized form of DACRs.

*Selection Semantics.* Consider a set $\mathcal{M}$ of models (states, points), and a validity relation $\models \ \subseteq \mathcal{M} \times \Phi$. $\mathcal{M}(\Gamma)$ denotes the set of all models of $\Gamma$, i.e. the set of all $M \in \mathcal{M}$ such that $M \models A$ for all $A \in \Gamma$. Semantic consequence is defined as follows: $\Gamma \Vdash A$ iff $M \models A$ for all $M \in \mathcal{M}(\Gamma)$. In the remainder, we assume that $\mathcal{M}$ and $\models$ are such that $\Vdash \ = \ \vdash$.

A *semantic selection function* $f$ is one that selects an $\mathcal{M}' \subseteq \mathcal{M}(\Gamma)$ for each $\Gamma \subseteq \Phi$. Given such an $f$, we define the consequence relation $\vdash^s_f$ as follows:

**Definition 6.** $\Gamma \vdash^s_f A$ *iff* $M \models A$ *for all* $M \in f(\mathcal{M}(\Gamma))$

As shown in [2], the class of all relations $\vdash^s_f$ coincides with the class of all inference relations (see Sect. 3 where this class was defined). By Theorem 1, every relation $\vdash^s_f$ is equivalent to a relation $\vdash^{DA}_{\Delta,\varphi}$ and vice versa.

There is however a deeper connection between selection semantics and (generalized) DACRs. To explain this, we first define a more specific class of selection semantics.

*Assumption-based Selection Functions.* Where $\Delta \subseteq \Phi$, let $\Delta(M) = \{A \in \Delta \mid M \models A\}$. Let $\mathbb{V}_\Delta(\Gamma) = \{\Delta(M) \mid M \in \mathcal{M}(\Gamma)\}$ and $\mathbb{V}_\Delta = \{\mathbb{V}_\Delta(\Gamma) \mid \Gamma \subseteq \Phi\}$. Note that $\mathbb{V}_\Delta \subseteq \wp(\wp(\Delta))$.

Consider a selection function $\psi : \mathbb{V}_\Delta \to \wp(\wp(\Delta))$. From it, we can define a semantic selection function $f_\psi$ as follows:

$$f_\psi(\mathcal{M}(\Gamma)) = \{M \in \mathcal{M}(\Gamma) \mid \Delta(M) \in \psi(\mathbb{V}_\Delta(\Gamma))\}$$

As a result, $\psi$ immediately gives us an inference relation $\vdash^s_{\Delta,\psi} \ =_{df} \ \vdash^s_{f_\psi}$, which is characterized by a selection semantics. In the remainder, we will focus on the relation between the class of consequence relations $\vdash^s_{\Delta,\psi}$ and $\vdash^{DA}_{\Delta,\varphi}$. In particular, we will check whether, given a fixed $\Delta$, the former can be translated into the latter and vice versa.

*From DACRs to Assumption-based Selection Semantics.* A first question is whether in general, the domain $\mathbb{S}_\Delta$ of the selection function $\varphi$ used in the definition of a DACR coincides with the domain $\mathbb{V}_\Delta$ of the selection function $\psi$. In general, this is not the case, as the following example shows:

*Example 1.* Let **L** = **CL**. Let $\Delta = \{p, q\}$. Let $\Gamma_a = \{\neg p \vee \neg q\}$ and $\Gamma_b = \{\neg p \vee \neg q, p \vee q\}$. We have:

$$\mathcal{S}_\Delta(\Gamma_a) = \mathcal{S}_\Delta(\Gamma_b) = \{\{p\}, \{q\}, \emptyset\}$$
$$\mathcal{V}_\Delta(\Gamma_a) = \{\{p\}, \{q\}, \emptyset\}$$
$$\mathcal{V}_\Delta(\Gamma_b) = \{\{p\}, \{q\}\}$$

As a consequence, one cannot simply use the same selection function $\varphi$ to define an assumption-based selection semantics. Nevertheless, there is a very simple connection between both. Where $X$ is a set of sets $x$, let $I_\subseteq(X) = \{y \subseteq x \mid x \in X\}$. We have:

**Lemma 1.** $\mathcal{S}_\Delta(\Gamma) = I_\subseteq(\mathcal{V}_\Delta(\Gamma))$.

*Proof.* ($\subseteq$) Let $\Delta' \in \mathcal{S}_\Delta(\Gamma)$. Hence $\Gamma \cup \Delta' \nvdash \bot$. Let $M$ be a model of $\Gamma \cup \Delta'$. It follows that $\Delta' \subseteq \Delta(M)$. Hence, $\Delta' \in I_\subseteq(\mathcal{V}_\Delta(\Gamma))$.
($\supseteq$) Let $\Delta' \in I_\subseteq(\mathcal{V}_\Delta(\Gamma))$. Hence for an $M \in \mathcal{M}(\Gamma)$, $\Delta(M) \supseteq \Delta'$. It follows that $\Gamma \cup \Delta \nvdash \bot$. Hence also $\Gamma \cup \Delta' \nvdash \bot$, and hence $\Delta' \in \mathcal{S}_\Delta(\Gamma)$.  $\square$

As a result, one may easily obtain $\mathcal{S}_\Delta(\Gamma)$ from $\mathcal{V}_\Delta(\Gamma)$. This is, essentially, the motor behind the proof of the following theorem:

**Theorem 7.** *For every $\Delta \subseteq \Phi$ and selection function $\varphi : \mathbb{S}_\Delta \to \wp(\wp(\Delta))$, there is a selection function $\psi : \mathbb{V}_\Delta \to \wp(\wp(\Delta))$ such that $\vdash^{DA}_{\Delta,\varphi} = \vdash^s_{\Delta,\psi}$.*

*Proof.* Where $\Gamma \cup \Delta \subseteq \Phi$, let

$$\psi(\mathcal{V}_\Delta(\Gamma)) =_{df} \{\Theta \subseteq \Delta \mid \Theta \supseteq \Pi \text{ for a } \Pi \in \varphi(I_\subseteq(\mathcal{V}_\Delta(\Gamma)))\} \cap \mathcal{V}_\Delta(\Gamma) \quad (8)$$

We have: $\Gamma \vdash^s_{\Delta,\psi} A$ iff for every $M \in \mathcal{M}(\Gamma)$ with $\Delta(M) \in \psi(\mathcal{V}_\Delta(\Gamma))$, $M \models A$ iff [by the definition of $\psi$] for every $M \in \mathcal{M}(\Gamma)$ with $\Delta(M) \supseteq \Pi$ for a $\Pi \in \varphi(I_\subseteq(\mathcal{V}_\Delta(\Gamma)))$, $M \models A$ iff [by Lemma 1] for every $M \in \mathcal{M}(\Gamma)$ with $\Delta(M) \supseteq \Pi$ for a $\Pi \in \varphi(\mathcal{S}_\Delta(\Gamma))$, $M \models A$ iff [by soundness and completeness] for all $\Pi \in \varphi(\mathcal{S}_\Delta(\Gamma))$, $\Gamma \cup \Pi \vdash A$ iff [by Definition 3] $\Gamma \vdash^{DA}_{\Delta,\varphi} A$.  $\square$

*From Assumption-based Selections to DACRs.* Characterizing assumption-based selection semantics by means of DACRs turns out to be less straightforward. The main problem is that $\mathcal{V}_\Delta(\Gamma)$ is not a function of $\mathcal{S}_\Delta(\Gamma)$. This follows immediately from Example 1 above. In fact, using this example we can show a stronger fact:

**Theorem 8.** *There are $\Delta \subseteq \Phi$ and selection functions $\psi : \mathbb{V}_\Delta \to \wp(\wp(\Delta))$ such that, for no $\varphi : \mathbb{S}_\Delta \to \wp(\wp(\Delta))$, $\vdash^s_{\Delta,\psi} = \vdash^{DA}_{\varphi,\psi}$.*

*Proof.* Let $\Delta$, $\Gamma_a$ and $\Gamma_b$ be as in Example 1. Let $\psi$ be defined as follows. If $\emptyset \in \mathcal{V}_\Delta(\Gamma_a)$, let $\psi(\mathcal{V}_\Delta(\Gamma_a)) = \{\emptyset\}$. If $\emptyset \notin \mathcal{V}_\Delta(\Gamma_a)$, let $\psi(\mathcal{V}_\Delta(\Gamma_a)) = \{\{p\}\}$ if $\{p\} \in \mathcal{V}_\Delta(\Gamma_a)$ and let $\psi(\mathcal{V}_\Delta(\Gamma_a)) = \mathcal{V}_\Delta(\Gamma_a)$ otherwise. It follows that $C^s_{\Delta,\psi}(\Gamma_a) = Cn(\Gamma_a)$ and $C^s_{\Delta,\psi}(\Gamma_b) = Cn(\{p, \neg q\})$.
Assume now that $\varphi : \mathbb{S}_\Delta \to \wp(\wp(\Delta))$ is a selection function such that $\sim^{DA}_{\varphi,\Delta} = \vdash^s_{\Delta,\psi}$. It follows that $C_{\Delta,\varphi}(\Gamma_a) = Cn(\Gamma_a)$ and $C_{\Delta,\varphi}(\Gamma_b) = Cn(\{p, \neg q\})$. Hence, for all $\Delta' \in \varphi(\mathcal{S}_\Delta(\Gamma_b))$, $p \in \Delta'$. But then, since $\mathcal{S}_\Delta(\Gamma_b) = \mathcal{S}_\Delta(\Gamma_a)$, also $p \in C_{\Delta,\varphi}(\Gamma_a)$ — a contradiction.  $\square$

*Open Problem: Conditions for Adequacy.* This negative result motivates further research on conditions on $\psi$ or $\Delta$ which ensure that $\mathrel{|\!\!\!\sim}^{\mathsf{DA}}_{\Delta,\psi} = \mathrel{|\!\!\!\sim}^{\mathsf{s}}_{\Delta,\psi}$. For instance, one may easily prove that where $\psi = \sigma(\mathsf{max}_{\mathsf{C}})$ for an arbitrary selection function $\sigma$, $\mathrel{|\!\!\!\sim}^{\mathsf{DA}}_{\Delta,\psi} = \mathrel{|\!\!\!\sim}^{\mathsf{s}}_{\Delta,\psi}$. More general conditions, including cases for which $\varphi(X) \not\subseteq \mathsf{max}_{\mathsf{C}}(X)$, are yet to be established.

The advantage of this work is twofold. First, it allows us to characterize assumption-based selection semantics in terms of DACRs, and hence to reduce reasoning in terms of (possibly complex, infinite) models to reasoning in terms of (simple, finite) sets of formulas. Second, it allows us to carry over all the metatheoretic results on selection semantics from [2] immediately to DACRs, whenever the aforementioned conditions hold.

# 6    Conclusion

We have argued that DACRs provide an elegant framework for modeling reasoning on the basis of defeasible assumptions. In particular, given the generalization in terms of selection functions we proposed, one can let various parameters determine which assumptions are used in cases of conflict. We established general conditions on the selection functions which warrant well-behavior of DACRs, and compared them to adaptive logics and selection semantics.

As mentioned at the start of this paper, this is but a first step in the investigation of the generalized form of DACRs. In addition to the open question mentioned in previous sections, one may investigate more specific constructions of selections functions, such as those mentioned in Section 2. How exactly should one make the notion of "informational content" formally precise in this context? And what behavior of $\varphi$, and hence the resulting DACR, does this result in?

# References

1. Makinson, D.: Bridges from Classical to Nonmonotonic Logic. Texts in Computing, vol. 5. King's College Publications, London (2005)
2. Lindström, S.: A semantic approach to nonmonotonic reasoning: inference operations and choice. Uppsala Prints and Reprints in Philosophy 10 (1994)
3. Makinson, D.: General patterns in nonmonotonic reasoning. In: Handbook of Logic in Artificial Intelligence and Logic Programming, vol. III. Clarendon Press (1994)
4. Alchourrón, C., Gärdenfors, P., Makinson, D.: On the logic of theory change: Partial meet contraction and revision functions. Journal of Symbolic Logic 50, 510–530 (1985)
5. Gärdenfors, P., Makinson, D.: Nonmonotonic inference based on expectations. Artificial Intelligence 65, 197–245 (1994)
6. Levi, I.: Mild Contraction. Evaluating Loss of Information due to Loss of Belief. Clarendon Press (2004)
7. Rott, H., Pagnucco, M.: Severe withdrawal (and recovery). Journal of Philosophical Logic 29, 501–547 (2000)
8. Horty, J.F.: Reasons as Defaults. Oxford University Press (2012)

9. Gabbay, D.M.: Theoretical foundations for nonmonotonic reasoning inexpert systems. In: Apt, K. (ed.) Logics and Models of Concurrent Systems. Springer (1985)
10. Batens, D.: A universal logic approach to adaptive logics. Logica Universalis 1, 221–242 (2007)
11. Straßer, C.: Adaptive Logic and Defeasible Reasoning. Applications in Argumentation, Normative Reasoning and Default Reasoning. Springer (201x)
12. Batens, D.: Adaptive Logics and Dynamic Proofs. Mastering the Dynamics of Reasoning, with Special Attention to Handling Inconsistency (in Progress)
13. Horsten, L., Welch, P.: The undecidability of propositional adaptive logic. Synthese 158, 41–60 (2007)
14. Verdée, P.: Adaptive logics using the minimal abnormality strategy are $\Pi_1^1$-complex. Synthese 167, 93–104 (2009)
15. Odintsov, S., Speranski, S.: Computability issues for adaptive logics in expanded standard format. Studia Logica (in print, 2013)

# Appendix: Notational Conventions

We use $X, Y, \ldots$ for arbitrary sets and $f$ to for arbitrary functions. Where $\prec$ is a partial order on $X$, let $\mathsf{max}_{\prec}(X) = \{x \in X \mid$ for no $y \in X, x \prec y\}$. Similarly, $\mathsf{min}_{\prec}(X) = \{x \in X \mid$ for no $y \in X, y \prec x\}$. Where $X$ is a set, $\wp(X)$ denotes the power set of $X$. $X \subseteq_f Y$ means that $X$ is a finite subset of $Y$.

We use $\mathbf{L}$ to refer to a fixed (arbitrary) supraclassical, compact Tarski-logic. $\vdash$ denotes the consequence relation of $\mathbf{L}$ and $\Phi$ its set of well-formed formulas. We use upper case letters $A, B, \ldots$ for formulas and upper case Greek letters $\Gamma, \Delta, \ldots$ for sets of formulas.

Let $Cn(\Gamma) = \{A \mid \Gamma \vdash A\}$ and let $C_{X,f} = \{A \mid \Gamma \hspace{0.2em}\vdash\hspace{-0.8em}\sim_{X,f} A\}$. Where $\hspace{0.2em}\vdash\hspace{-0.8em}\sim$ is an unspecified non-monotonic consequence relation, $C(\Gamma) = \{A \mid \Gamma \hspace{0.2em}\vdash\hspace{-0.8em}\sim A\}$.

Caligraphic letters $\mathcal{S}, \mathcal{T}, \ldots$ are used for sets of sets of formulas, and $\mathbb{S}, \mathbb{T}, \ldots$ for sets of sets of sets of formulas. Functions of the the type $\mathbb{S} \to \mathbb{S}'$ are denoted by small Greek letters $\varphi, \chi, \ldots$.

# Soft Constraints for Lexicographic Orders*

Fabio Gadducci[1], Mattias Hölzl[2], Giacoma V. Monreale[1], and Martin Wirsing[2]

[1] Dipartimento di Informatica, Università di Pisa, Pisa
[2] Institut für Informatik, LMU, München

**Abstract.** While classical Constraint Satisfaction Problems (CSPs) concern the search for the boolean assignment of a set of variables that has to satisfy some given requirements, their soft variant considers ordered domains for assignments, thus modeling preferences: the aim is to provide an environment where suitable algorithms (e.g. on constraint propagation) can be stated and proved, and inherited by its instances.

Besides their flexibility, these formalisms have been advocated for their modularity: suitable operators can be defined, in order to manipulate such structures and build new ones. However, some intuitive constructions were given less attention, such as lexicographic orders.

Our works explores such orders in three instances of the soft CSP framework. Our results allow for a wider application of the formalism, and it is going to be pivotal for the use of constraints in modeling scenarios where the features to be satisfied are equipped with a fixed order of importance.

**Keywords:** Soft constraints, lexicographic orders.

## 1  Introduction

Classical Constraint Satisfaction Problems (CSPs) concern the search for those assignments to a set of variables that may satisfy a family of requirements [17]. In order to decrease the complexity of such a search, various heuristics have been proposed. One of such families is labelled as "constraint propagation": it refers to any reasoning that consists of explicitly forbidding some values or their combinations for the variables of a problem because a subset of its constraints would not be satisfied otherwise. A standard technique for implementing constraint propagation is represented by local consistency algorithms [17, § 3].

The soft framework extends the classical constraint notion in order to model preferences: the aim is to provide a single environment where suitable properties (best known so far are those concerning local consistency [9], and recently also on bucket partitioning [16]) can be proven and inherited by all the instances. Technically, this is done by adding to the classical CSP notion a representation of the levels of satisfiability of each constraint. Albeit appearing with alternative presentations in the literature, the additional component consists of a poset

---

* Partly supported by the EU FP7-ICT IP ASCEns and by the MIUR PRIN CINA.

F. Castro, A. Gelbukh, and M. González (Eds.): MICAI 2013, Part I, LNAI 8265, pp. 68–79, 2013.

(stating the desirability among levels) equipped with a binary operation (defining how two levels can be combined): see e.g [5,19] for two seminal accounts.

The use of these soft formalisms has been advocated for two main reasons. First of all, for their flexibility: their abstract presentation allows for recasting many concrete cases previously investigated in the literature. A bird-view of the expressiveness of the approach can be probably glimpsed at [1]. As important as flexibility is modularity: suitable operators can be defined, in order to manipulate such structures and build new ones that verify the same properties, hence, which are still amenable to the same tools and techniques.

Two classical proposals are based on valuation structures, where the values associated to each constraint are taken respectively from a totally ordered monoid [19] and a c-semiring [5]. Also, a novel and more general formalism based on families of partially ordered monoids was introduced in [13], specifically targeted to tackle operators representing lexicographic orders. The correspondence between the former two proposals was identified early on [2]. The aim of the paper is to recast the latter approach in the standard mold of soft constraints technology. To this end, it provides a novel classification of those three formalisms in terms of ordered monoids, which allows to relate them uniformly. The wealth of techniques introduced in each single approach can then be easily transferred among them. As a main testbed, the paper explores the ability of the three approaches in modeling lexicographic orders.

Our proposal pushes partially ordered valuation structures as a more general proposal for soft constraints, which precisely corresponds to what are called ic-monoids in [13] (§ 2). We first consider a few instances, and a case study illustrating the various constructions (§ 3). We then investigate the definition of operators representing lexicographic orders (§ 4 and § 5), proving some properties for them (§ 6) and applying the formalism to the case study (§ 7). A concluding section recalls the rationale of our work and wraps up the paper (§ 8).

## 2   Three Domains for Assignments

This section considers three different proposals for the domain of values in the soft constraint framework, and establishes some connections among them. First, however, it recalls some basic mathematical notions.

**Definition 1.** *A partial order (PO) is a pair $\langle A, \leq \rangle$ such that $A$ is a set of values and $\leq \, \subseteq A \times A$ is a reflexive, transitive, and anti-symmetric relation. A partial order with top (POT) is a triple $\langle A, \leq, \top \rangle$ such that $\langle A, \leq \rangle$ is a PO, $\top \in A$ and $\forall a \in A. a \leq \top$. A join semi-lattice (JSL) is a POT such that for each finite, not-empty set $X \subseteq A$ there exists a least upper bound (LUB) $\bigvee X$.*

Should we also include the LUB for the empty set, $\bigvee \emptyset$ would coincide with the bottom element $\bot$ of the PO, i.e., $\forall a \in A. \bot \leq a$.

A PO is a total order (TO) if either $a \leq b$ or $b \leq a$ holds for all $a, b \in A$.

**Definition 2.** *A commutative monoid with identity (CMI) is a triple $\langle A, \otimes, 1 \rangle$ such that $A$ is a set of values and $\otimes : A \times A \to A$ is an associative and commutative function with $1$ as identity, i.e., $\forall a \in A. a \otimes 1 = a$.*

An example of CMI is represented by natural numbers with addition $\langle \mathbb{N}, +, 0 \rangle$.

## 2.1   The Domains . . .

We open with a novel structure that adapts to the standard soft constraints technology the proposal concerning what are called ic-monoids in [13].

**Definition 3.** *A* partially-ordered valuation structure *(PVS) is a 4-tuple* $G = \langle A, \leq, \otimes, \top \rangle$ *such that* $G^{\leq} = \langle A, \leq, \top \rangle$ *is a POT,* $G^{\otimes} = \langle A, \otimes, \top \rangle$ *is a CMI, and* monotonicity *holds.*
*A PVS G is* bounded *if* $G^{\leq}$ *has bottom element* $\perp$.

Stating that the monoidal operator is monotone means that $a \leq b \Rightarrow a \otimes c \leq b \otimes c$ holds for all $a, b, c \in A$. Also note that if $G$ is bounded then the bottom is the (necessarily unique) absorbing element for $\otimes$, i.e., $a \otimes \perp = \perp$ for all $a \in A$.
We now recall the formalism advanced by [19][1].

**Definition 4.** *A* valuation structure *(VS) is a PVS G such that* $G^{\leq}$ *is a TO.*

Finally, we recall the definition of absorptive semirings (also c-semirings [5]), recasting it in terms of suitable POs (see also [3]).

**Definition 5.** *A* semiring valuation structure *(SVS) is a 4-tuple* $G = \langle A, \leq, \otimes, \top \rangle$ *such that* $G^{\leq} = \langle A, \leq, \top \rangle$ *is a JSL,* $G^{\otimes} = \langle A, \otimes, \top \rangle$ *is a CMI, and* distributivity *holds.*

The monoidal operator $\otimes$ is distributive if $a \otimes \bigvee X = \bigvee \{ a \otimes x \mid x \in X \}$ holds for any finite, non-empty subset $X$ of $A$. Also, recall that if $G$ is bounded, then the LUB exists also for the empty set, and the law trivially holds for that case.

## 2.2   . . . and Their Connections

We now turn our attention to the relationship between the three proposals.

**Lemma 1.** *Let G be a SVS. Then, it is also a PVS.*

Indeed, from distributivity it easily follows that the tensor operator is monotone, thus implying the lemma above.

In turn, both PVSs and SVSs generalise VSs, replacing their TO with a PO and a JSL, respectively. Moreover, SVSs are well-known as an alternative presentation for c-semirings, as shown e.g. in [3] (where they are referred to with their classical name of absorptive semirings). Indeed, the relationship between VSs and SVSs is even tighter, as stated by the lemma below (see [2, Section 4]).

**Lemma 2.** *Let G be a VS. Then, it is also a SVS.*

Indeed, in a TO each finite set $X$ admits a maximum, i.e., $\bigvee X \in X$. It is easy to check that this fact and monotonicity imply distributivity.
The relationship among the three domains is summed up in Fig. 1.

---

[1] The reader should be advised that the chosen order for VSs is the dual of the one adopted in the valuation structure literature. It is clearly an equivalent formalism: our choice allows for a simpler comparison with PVSs and SVSs (see below).

---

VS (TOT, monotone) [19] $\subseteq$ SVS (JSL, distributive) [5] $\subseteq$ PVS (POT, monotone) [13]

---

**Fig. 1.** Relationships among the three domains (for TOT a TO with top)

## 3    Instances and Examples

This section shows some domains for preferences adopted in the soft constraint literature, as well as some examples of the operators on VSs and SVSs defined there. It is further shown that these domains and operators can be instantiated also for the PVSs formalisms, and later on they are applied in a quite simple case study, which has been adapted from [13].

### 3.1    Some Instances ...

The starting point is represented by the results in Section 2, relating VSs and SVSs as instances of the more general notion of PVSs.

*A few VSs.* We thus first recall some instances of VSs.

The simplest example is the boolean algebra $B = \langle \{\bot, \top\}, \Rightarrow, \vee, \top \rangle$.

Possibly, the most prominent example of a VS is the so-called tropical semiring $T = \langle \mathbb{N}, \geq, +, 0 \rangle$, with $\geq$ the inverse of the usual order notion on naturals, thus such that 0 is the top element [15]. It is used for modelling problems where a cost has to be minimised, as in shortest path scenarios under the name of weighted constraint satisfaction [14].

Another variant considers a truncated segment of the natural numbers: $T_n = \langle [0, n], \geq, +_t, 0 \rangle$, such that $m +_t o$ is either $m + o$ or, should it be that $m + o \geq n$, just $n$. Both variants have been extensively studied, since most VSs can be reconnected to these case studies (see e.g. [8]).

Otherwise, the monoidal operator can be replaced by the standard natural multiplication, for $M = \langle \mathbb{N}^+, \geq, \cdot, 1 \rangle$, with $\mathbb{N}^+$ the positive natural numbers. The complementary segment $[0, 1]$ over the rational numbers (possibly extending to the real ones) defines the probabilistic VS $F = \langle [0, 1], \leq, \cdot, 1 \rangle$ [7].

*A few operators for PVSs.* The most standard operator for SVSs is the cartesian product: applied to SVSs $G_0$ and $G_1$, it returns a SVS whose set of elements is the cartesian product $A_0 \times A_1$, while the other components are obviously defined. As for most operators (a notable exception being the lexicographic order in Section 5), the class of VSs is not closed under it.

As a side remark, it is often the case that it is not possible to decompose an SVS as the product of two or more VSs: as a counterexample, it suffices to consider two VSs $G_0$ and $G_1$ and the lifting $(G_0 \times G_1)_\bot$, adding a new bottom element (see also the final remark on Section 6).

Most important is the case of multi-criteria SVSs, as considered in e.g. [4]. Let us start by considering an SVS $G = \langle A, \leq, \otimes, \top \rangle$: let $H(A)$ be the Hoare power-domain, i.e., the set of down-closed (with respect to $\leq$) subsets of $A$, and $\leq_H$ the order $S_1 \leq_H S_2$ if $S_1 \subseteq S_2$. In other terms, the usual powerset construction for $A$, up-to removing some of its subsets. Now, for an SVS $G = \langle A, \leq, \otimes, \top \rangle$, its power-domain $H(G)$ is defined as $\langle H(A), \leq_H, \otimes_H, \{\top\} \rangle$, for $\otimes_H$ the obvious extension to sets. The LUB is just set union, and furthermore it is easy to show that distributivity holds, so that $H(G)$ is also an SVS.

In the case study we will consider precisely those two operators we just described. It is relatively simple to show that the class of PVSs is closed under them. Additionally, it behaves better with yet another operator, the lexicographic one, which is also going to be needed for the case study. The main properties for the latter operator will be described in the following sections.

## 3.2    . . . and a Simple Example

The running example in [13] models a scenario concerning the scheduling of meetings. Among other requirements, each person has to express a possible degree of preference for a given date, and s/he must moreover explicitly state how much her/his presence is actually crucial for that meeting.

We can revise and enrich the original example, using some of the instances and operators just defined. We may assume to have three meetings to organise, each one of them among five possible dates. Some dates might not be compatible, since they overlap (at least, each date overlaps with itself) or because some people are not willing to have too close meetings. For the three meetings, each date (in fact, also each pair and each triple of dates) has associated a set of possible values, representing e.g. the interest and willingness of the persons to be in. The problem is to find the set of three dates maximising such features.

Summing up, each value states how much a person is crucial for a meeting, and her/his willingness to appear in a given date. Also, we may record the status of a person among the group of the possible attendees of the meetings (e.g., the position in a firm or the level of expertise in a technical team).

The last feature can be modelled by $T$, with 0 the top, and it is an important condition to guarantee. Instead, the statement of the relevance of a person for a meeting can be expressed as $B$, and its willingness by $F$.

In order to model the preference domain for this scenario we have to take into account the three features, by attaching more importance to the last two, i.e., the relevance of a person for a meeting and her/his willingness to participate. Indeed, a meeting should be scheduled in the date for which the willingness of relevant people is maximal, while the status of any person should just influence the quality of the best solutions with respect to the other two parameters.

As we will show later on in Section 7, the situation could be modelled by using a lexicographic operator between the two PVSs $B \times F$ and $T$.

# 4  Deriving Lexicographic Orders

Building on some classical results for partial orders (see e.g. [11]), we are now going to introduce the key operator for the lexicographic operator of PVSs: it is used in later sections to take two PVSs and to build a new one whose order corresponds to the lexicographic ordering of the two underlying structures.

## 4.1  Some Facts on Lexicographic Orders for Cartesian Products

This section states some (mostly well-known) properties of lexicographic orders: the characterization of such orders for PVSs is built upon these results.

**Definition 6.** *Let $\langle A_0, \leq_0 \rangle$ and $\langle A_1, \leq_1 \rangle$ be POs. Then, the associated lexicographic order $\leq_l$ on $A_0 \times A_1$ is given by*

$$\langle a_0, a_1 \rangle \leq_l \langle b_0, b_1 \rangle \ if \ \begin{cases} a_0 <_0 b_0 & or \\ a_0 =_0 b_0 \ \& \ a_1 \leq_1 b_1 \end{cases}$$

*with $a < b$ meaning that $a \leq b$ and $a \neq b$.*

It is easy to see that the order $\leq_l$ is a partial one, and that the occurrence of either top or bottom elements is preserved.

**Lemma 3.** *Let $P_0 = \langle A_0, \leq_0 \rangle$ and $P_1 = \langle A_1, \leq_1 \rangle$ be POs. Then, also $P_0 \times_l P_1 = \langle A_0 \times A_1, \leq_l \rangle$ is so. Moreover, if both $P_0$ and $P_1$ are either POTs or bounded, then also $P_0 \times_l P_1$ is so.*

A tighter property holds if the underlying orders are total.

**Lemma 4.** *Let $\langle A_0, \leq_0 \rangle$ and $\langle A_1, \leq_1 \rangle$ be TOs. Then, also $\langle A_0 \times A_1, \leq_l \rangle$ is so.*

With some calculations, it can be shown that the lexicographic order forms a JSL if both underlying orders are so, and the latter is bounded.

**Proposition 1.** *Let $\langle A_0, \leq_0 \rangle$ and $\langle A_1, \leq_1 \rangle$ be JSLs such that $\langle A_1, \leq_1 \rangle$ is bounded. Then, also $\langle A_0 \times A_1, \leq_l \rangle$ is a JSL.*

*Proof.* The first step is to provide an explicit candidate for the LUB operator. So, let $X \subseteq A_0 \times A_1$ be a finite set, $X_i = \{a_i \mid \langle a_0, a_1 \rangle \in X\}$ the projection of $X$ on the $i$-th component, and $m(X) = \{a_1 \in X_1 \mid \langle \bigvee X_0, a_1 \rangle \in X\}$. Then

$$\bigvee X = \langle \bigvee X_0, \bigvee m(X) \rangle$$

Note that $m(X)$ might be empty, should $\bigvee X_0 \notin X_0$, thus the LUB would be $\langle \bigvee X_0, \perp_1 \rangle$, hence the requirement that $\langle A_1, \leq_1 \rangle$ must be bounded.

Now, let us consider an element $\langle c_0, c_1 \rangle$ that is an upper bound of $X$, i.e., such that $\forall \langle a_0, a_1 \rangle \in X.\langle a_0, a_1 \rangle \leq_l \langle c_0, c_1 \rangle$: this means that $\bigvee X_0 \leq_0 c_0$. The proof then proceeds by case analysis. If $\bigvee X_0 <_0 c_0$, it is straightforward. If instead $\bigvee X_0 = c_0$, then it holds $\bigvee m(X) \leq_1 c_1$: by definition of $\leq_l$, should $\bigvee X_0 \in X_0$, and by the presence of $\perp_1$ in the second component of $\bigvee X$, otherwise.

## 4.2   Choosing the Right Carrier

Building on this, we can finally consider the structure that we are going to adopt for lexicographic PVSs. We further need an additional definition, in order to manipulate (and restrict) the cartesian product of the carriers of two POs.

**Definition 7.** *Let* $G = \langle A, \leq, \otimes, \top \rangle$ *be a PVS. The set* $C(A)$ *of its collapsing elements is defined as* $\{c \in A \mid \exists a, b \in A. a < b \wedge a \otimes c = b \otimes c\}$.

Note that if $G$ is bounded, then clearly $\bot \in C(A)$. In the following, we define $A^C$ as the set of those elements of $A$ that are not collapsing, i.e., $A^C = A \setminus C(A)$.

We can now define the construction we intend to exploit for obtaining PVSs representing lexicographic orders.

**Definition 8.** *Let* $G_0 = \langle A_0, \leq_0, \otimes_0, \top_0 \rangle$ *and* $G_1 = \langle A_1, \leq_1, \otimes_1, \top_1 \rangle$ *be PVSs such that* $G_1$ *is bounded. Then, the associated lexicographic carrier is defined as*

$$A_0 \times_l A_1 = (A_0^C \times A_1) \cup (C(A_0) \times \{\bot_1\})$$

In other terms, we restrict our attention to those pairs whose first components is not collapsing, with the exception of those whose second component is the bottom (thus including the bottom element $\langle \bot_0, \bot_1 \rangle$, should $G_0$ be bounded).

Given the results in the previous section for lexicographic orders over cartesian products, equivalent properties can be stated also for the smaller carrier.

**Proposition 2.** *Let* $G_0 = \langle A_0, \leq_0, \otimes_0, \top_0 \rangle$ *and* $G_1 = \langle A_1, \leq_1, \otimes_1, \top_1 \rangle$ *be PVSs such that* $G_1$ *is bounded and both* $\langle A_0, \leq_0 \rangle$ *and* $\langle A_1, \leq_1 \rangle$ *are POs (bounded POs, POTs, TOs, JSLs). Then, also* $\langle A_0 \times_l A_1, \times_l \rangle$ *is so.*

*Proof.* All proofs are straightforward, except the one for JSLs. The candidate LUB for a finite set $X \subseteq A_0 \times_l A_1$ is still the same as in the proof of Proposition 1. Should $\bigvee X_0$ be not collapsing, or $m(X)$ empty, obviously $\langle \bigvee X_0, \bigvee m(X) \rangle \in A_0 \times_l A_1$. Otherwise, let $\bigvee X_0 \in X_0$ be collapsing. In this case, though, it must be that $m(X) = \{\bot_1\}$, thus the result holds.

We close this section by establishing some closure properties for the set $A^C$ that are going to be needed later on.

**Lemma 5.** *Let* $\langle A, \leq, \otimes, \top \rangle$ *be a PVS. Then,* $a \otimes b \in C(A)$ *iff* $\{a, b\} \cap C(A) \neq \emptyset$.

In other terms, for any PVS both sets $C(A)$ and $A^C$ are closed under the monoidal operator. Moreover, if $a \otimes b \in A^C$, then $\{a, b\} \subseteq A^C$.

## 5   Deriving Valuation Structures

Building on the characterization results stated in the previous section, we are now ready to move to define the lexicographic operators for PVSs.

First of all, we recall that given two monoids $\langle A_0, \otimes_0, \top_0 \rangle$ and $\langle A_1, \otimes_1, \top_1 \rangle$, the cartesian product of their carriers $A_0 \times A_1$ can obviously be equipped with a monoidal tensor $\otimes_p$ that is defined point-wise, with $\langle \top_0, \top_1 \rangle$ as the identity.

**Definition 9.** $G_0 = \langle A_0, \leq_0, \otimes_0, \top_0 \rangle$ and $G_1 = \langle A_1, \leq_1, \otimes_1, \top_1 \rangle$ be PVSs such that $G_1$ is bounded. Then, the lexicographic structure is defined as

$$Lex(G_0, G_1) = \langle A_0 \times_l A_1, \leq_l, \otimes_p, \langle \top_0, \top_1 \rangle \rangle$$

Recall that $A_0 \times_l A_1$ discards all the elements $\langle a_0, a_1 \rangle$ of the cartesian product $A_0 \times A_1$ such that $a_0$ is collapsing and $a_1 \neq \perp_1$. The intuition for it is rather straightforward. Should any collapsing element appear in the first component, there would no chance for $\otimes_p$ to be monotone, unless, of course, the second is the absorbing element $\perp_1$.

**Proposition 3.** Let $G_0$ and $G_1$ be PVSs such that $G_1$ is bounded. Then, also $Lex(G_0, G_1)$ is a PVS.

*Proof.* The crucial observation is that the triple $\langle A_0 \times_l A_1, \otimes_p, \langle \top_0, \top_1 \rangle \rangle$ is a monoid, i.e., that it is closed under the monoidal operator $\otimes_p$. Indeed, the only problem may occur for those pairs $\langle a_0, a_1 \rangle$ and $\langle b_0, b_1 \rangle$ such that either $a_0$ or $b_0$ belongs to $C(A_0)$. Suppose that $a_0 \in C(A_0)$ and $b_0 \in A_0^C$. By Lemma 5, also $a_0 \otimes_0 b_0 \in C(A_0)$, so $a_1 \otimes_1 b_1$ must be equal to $\perp_1$. It is indeed so: since $a_0 \in C(A_0)$, then $a_1 = \perp_1$ and so is $\perp_1 \otimes b_1$, hence no problem arises. $\square$

As noted in the previous section, the lexicographic order associated to two total orders is also total. This property also holds for VSs.

**Proposition 4.** Let $G_0$ and $G_1$ be VSs such that $G_1$ is bounded. Then, also $Lex(G_0, G_1)$ is a VS.

The theorem does not hold for SVSs since in general distributivity fails. We are however able to state a weaker result, which we consider an interesting contribution to the literature on semiring-based formalisms.

**Theorem 1.** Let $G_0$ be a VS and $G_1$ a bounded SVS. Then, also $Lex(G_0, G_1)$ is an SVS.

*Proof.* As it often occurs in these situations, the only property that is difficult to check is distributivity: explicitly, taking into account the definition of the monoidal operator $\otimes_p$, it must be shown that for any finite, non-empty subset $X \subseteq A_0 \times_l A_1$ the equality below holds

$$\langle a_0, a_1 \rangle \otimes_p \bigvee_l X = \bigvee_l \{\langle a_0 \otimes_0 b_0, a_1 \otimes_1 b_1 \rangle \mid \langle b_0, b_1 \rangle \in X\}$$

Now, since $G_0$ is a VS, for any finite, non-empty set $X_0$ we have $\bigvee X_0 \in X_0$ and moreover, since $\otimes_0$ is also monotone, $a_0 \otimes_0 \bigvee X_0 = \bigvee\{a_0 \otimes_0 b_0 \mid b_0 \in X_0\}$.

Thus, should $\bigvee X_0$ be collapsing, also $a_0 \otimes_0 \bigvee X_0$ is so, thus $\bigvee m(X) = \perp_1$ and the equality immediately holds.

If instead $\bigvee X_0$ is not collapsing, recall that either $a_0$ is collapsing and $a_1 = \perp_1$ or $a_0$ is not collapsing. In the first case, also $a_0 \otimes_0 \bigvee X_0$ is collapsing, and the equality holds, since the second component is always $\perp_1$. In the second case, $a_0 \otimes_0 \bigvee X_0$ is not collapsing and the equality holds by distributivity of $\otimes_1$.

# 6  Some Alternative Properties

In this section we are going to investigate some properties of the structure of the set of collapsing elements of a PVS.

*On (weakly) strict PVSs.* We start considering a counterpart property with respect to the set of collapsing elements.

**Definition 10.** *Let* $G = \langle A, \leq, \otimes, \top \rangle$ *be a PVS. We say that it is* strict *if* $C(A) = \emptyset$; *it is* weakly strict *if it is bounded and* $C(A) = \{\bot\}$.

Thus, if a PVS $G_0$ is strict, then $A_0 \times_l A_1$ turns out to coincide with $A_0 \times A_1$, and no pair has to be discarded. Should instead $G_0$ be weakly strict, we have that $A_0 \times_l A_1$ is $((A_0 \setminus \{\bot_0\}) \times A_1) \cup \{\langle \bot_0, \bot_1 \rangle\}$. Indeed, many PVS instances are going to fall into this situation.

Note how strictness can be rephrased in terms of a standard notion concerning the monoidal operator. We say that a monoidal operator $\otimes$ is strictly monotone if $a < b$ implies $a \otimes c < b \otimes c$ for all elements $a, b, c \in A$; it is weakly so if the property holds whenever $c \neq \bot$.

**Lemma 6.** *Let* $G = \langle A, \leq, \otimes, \top \rangle$ *be a PVS. It is* strict *if the monoidal operator* $\otimes$ *is strictly monotone. It is* weakly strict *if it is bounded and the monoidal operator* $\otimes$ *is weakly strict monotone.*

*On cancellative PVSs.* In the soft constraint literature, weakly strict VSs are called strictly monotonic VSs [7]. An alternative characterisation for such structures that is simpler to verify can be found below. As before, we say that a monoidal operator $\otimes$ is cancellative if $a \otimes c = b \otimes c$ implies $a = b$ for all elements $a, b, c \in A$; it is weakly so if the property holds whenever $c \neq \bot$.

**Definition 11.** *Let* $G = \langle A, \leq, \otimes, \top \rangle$ *be a PVS. We say that it is* cancellative *if the monoidal operator* $\otimes$ *is so. It is* weakly cancellative *if it is bounded and the monoidal operator* $\otimes$ *is weakly so.*

Note that any (weakly) cancellative PVS is (weakly) strict. The vice versa does not hold in general, except for VSs (see [3]).

**Lemma 7.** *Let* $G$ *be a VS. If it is (weakly) strict, then it is also (weakly) cancellative.*

It follows by the fact that in a VS we have $a \vee b \in \{a, b\}$ for any element $a, b \in A$: thus, if $a \otimes c = b \otimes c$ it must be that $a = b$, since the alternative $a < b$ (or its symmetric choice) would imply that also $a \otimes c \neq b \otimes c$.

*On idempotent monoids.* The situation is quite less convenient for those PVSs such that the monoidal operator $\otimes$ is idempotent, i.e., such that $a \otimes a = a$ for all $a \in A$. In this case $C(A) = A$, since $a \otimes b$ is the greatest lower bound of $a$ and $b$ (see [5]). Thus, if $G_0$ is idempotent we have that $A_0 \times_l A_1$ coincides with $A_0 \times \{\bot_1\}$, hence with $A_0$.

*On adding bounds to monoids.* Finally, let us consider structures possibly lacking the bottom element. Such a requirement has to be enforced in some situations, e.g. when requiring a PVS to be strict. However, removing and later adding a bottom element is never a problem. Indeed, it is easy to show that for any PVS $G$ a new one $G_\perp$ can be obtained, such that $A_\perp = A \uplus \{\perp\}$ and furthermore $\perp \leq_\perp a$ and $a \otimes_\perp \perp = \perp$ for all $a \in A$.

There are two relevant properties of the lifting. First of all, it adds no identification among the elements of the original PVS: $a \leq b$ iff $a \leq_\perp b$ for all $a, b \in A$. Hence, any PVS can become bounded without any loss in the precision of the order on the preferences. Related to this fact, the lifting also inherits the relevant properties we discussed in this section so that if $G$ is either strict or cancellative, then it is also weakly so.

# 7  Applying the Lexicographic Operator

The scheduling example introduced in Section 3.2 shows the usefulness of the lexicographic operator. We can indeed use this operator to model the preference domain for the scenario we described.

As said previously, we have to take into account three features: for each person the relevance for a meeting and the willingness, which can be modelled by $B \times F$, ans well as the status, which can be modelled by $T$.

As observed in Section 3.1, $T$ is a VS. Differently from $T_n$, it is cancellative, so the good properties discussed in the previous section hold. In particular, it can be always used as the first component of any lexicographic construction. However, in order to use it as the second component, as it is necessary in the scheduling example, its bounded version $T_\infty$ has to be considered, obtained by adding the infinite $\infty$ as the bottom element.

We also know that the cartesian product applied to SVSs $B$ and $F$ returns a new SVS $B \times F$, therefore we can model the preference domain for the scheduling scenario as $Lex(B \times F, T_\infty)$. Clearly, the unique collapsing element of SVS $B \times F$ is the bottom $\langle \perp, 0 \rangle$, hence, since $T_\infty$ is a bounded VS, then $Lex(B \times F, T_\infty)$ is a PVS, with carrier $((\{\perp, \top\} \times [0,1]) \setminus \{\langle \perp, 0 \rangle\}) \times T_\infty$ plus the bottom $\langle \perp, 0, \infty \rangle$.

In this case, note that preference values $\langle \langle \top, 0 \rangle, 0 \rangle$ and $\langle \langle \perp, 1 \rangle, 0 \rangle$ are not comparable, since the first component is so: $\top$ dominates $\perp$ but 0 does not dominate 1. As it can occur with POs, no value is better than the other: the LUB of these two elements is indeed different from both of them. However, usually one would like to retain the information on all these alternative solutions, and not the LUB of these which could correspond to no real solution. This is the classical situation of multi-criteria constraint satisfaction: we can then exploit the Hoare power-domain (see section 3.1), thus modeling the preference domain of our example as $H(Lex(B \times F, T_\infty))$.

# 8  Conclusions and Future Works

In this paper we presented three possible preference domains to be adopted in the soft constraint techniques. Two of them (VSs and SVSs) were well-known, while the other one (PVSs) has been adapted to the standard soft constraint mold from the ordered monoids proposal in [13]. We studied their connections, and we investigated which of them is best suited for capturing the lexicographic operator. Finally, we discussed some instances of VSs, and a few operators for SVSs, relating them to PVSs, and rounding up the section with a simple example to illustrate the use of the lexicographic order.

Each one of those approaches has its own strength. The complexity of local consistency is actually one of the key issues in the work of VSs, as an intuitive generalization of weighted CSPs [6]. What this paper has shown is that PVSs are the most flexible proposal, as far as modularity is concerned. SVSs instead represent an intermediate stage, as far as expressiveness and (possibly) efficiency is concerned, yet they still allows for suitable constraint propagation techniques whose feasibility has still to be checked for PVSs.

Indeed, the introduction of PVSs might be the starting point on a reflection about the overall properties that are required for the domain of preferences in a soft constraint satisfaction problem. We recall that the soft framework has been introduced in order to provide a single environment where suitable properties (e.g. on constraint propagation or on branch&bound resolution techniques) of constraint satisfaction problems can be proved once and for all the instances. In [13], it has been shown that standard branch&bound techniques can be applied to constraint satisfaction problems whose preference domain is a PVS. When originally introduced, both VSs and SVSs were defined for idempotent monoidal operators, and this allows for the application of a simple constraint propagation algorithm based on arc consistency [12,18]. Later, both structures were extended with a notion of *residuation*, assuming the existence of a partial inverse operator (whenever $a \leq b$, then an element $a \ominus b$ is defined, satisfying $(a \ominus b) \otimes b = a$), such that a more complex variant of the same propagation algorithm can be applied [10,3,9]. It has to be proved that the same algorithm can be used for idempotent or (suitable variants of) residuated PVSs, even if these structures lack the distributivity law.

# References

1. Bistarelli, S.: Semirings for Soft Constraint Solving and Programming. LNCS, vol. 2962. Springer, Heidelberg (2004)
2. Bistarelli, S., Fargier, H., Montanari, U., Rossi, F., Schiex, T., Verfaillie, G.: Semiring-based CSPs and Valued CSPs: Frameworks, properties, and comparison. Constraints 4(3), 199–240 (1999)
3. Bistarelli, S., Gadducci, F.: Enhancing constraints manipulation in semiring-based formalisms. In: Brewka, G., Coradeschi, S., Perini, A., Traverso, P. (eds.) ECAI 2006. FAIA, vol. 141, pp. 63–67. IOS Press, Amsterdam (2006)
4. Bistarelli, S., Gadducci, F., Larrosa, J., Rollon, E., Santini, F.: Local arc consistency for non-invertible semirings, with an application to multi-objective optimization. Expert Systems with Applications 39(2), 1708–1717 (2012)
5. Bistarelli, S., Montanari, U., Rossi, F.: Semiring-based constraint solving and optimization. Journal of ACM 44(2), 201–236 (1997)

6. Cohen, D.A., Cooper, M.C., Jeavons, P., Krokhin, A.A.: The complexity of soft constraint satisfaction. Artificial Intelligence 170(11), 983–1016 (2006)
7. Cooper, M.C.: Reduction operations in fuzzy or valued constraint satisfaction. Fuzzy Sets and Systems 134(3), 311–342 (2003)
8. Cooper, M.C.: High-order consistency in valued constraint satisfaction. Constraints 10(3), 283–305 (2005)
9. Cooper, M.C., de Givry, S., Sanchez, M., Schiex, T., Zytnicki, M., Werner, T.: Soft arc consistency revisited. Artificial Intelligence 174(7-8), 449–478 (2010)
10. Cooper, M.C., Schiex, T.: Arc consistency for soft constraints. Artificial Intelligence 154(1-2), 199–227 (2004)
11. Geil, O., Pellikaan, R.: On the structure of order domains. Finite Fields and Their Applications 8(3), 369–396 (2002)
12. Van Hentenryck, P., Deville, Y., Teng, C.-M.: A generic arc-consistency algorithm and its specializations. Artificial Intelligence 57(2-3), 291–321 (1992)
13. Hölzl, M.M., Meier, M., Wirsing, M.: Which soft constraints do you prefer? In: Rosu, G. (ed.) WRLA 2008. ENTCS, vol. 283(2), pp. 189–205. Elsevier, Amsterdam (2009)
14. Larrosa, J., Schiex, T.: In the quest of the best form of local consistency for Weighted CSP. In: Gottlob, G., Walsh, T. (eds.) IJCAI 2003, pp. 239–244. Morgan Kaufmann, San Francisco (2003)
15. Pin, J.-E.: Tropical semirings. In: Gunawardena, J. (ed.) Idempotency, pp. 50–69. Cambridge University Press, Cambridge (1998)
16. Rollon, E., Larrosa, J., Dechter, R.: Semiring-based mini-bucket partitioning schemes. In: IJCAI 2013. Morgan Kaufmann, San Francisc (2013)
17. Rossi, F., van Beek, P., Walsh, T.: Handbook of Constraint Programming. Foundations of Artificial Intelligence. Elsevier, Amsterdam (2006)
18. Schiex, T.: Arc consistency for soft constraints. In: Dechter, R. (ed.) CP 2000. LNCS, vol. 1894, pp. 411–424. Springer, Heidelberg (2000)
19. Schiex, T., Fargier, H., Verfaillie, G.: Valued constraint satisfaction problems: Hard and easy problems. In: IJCAI 1995, pp. 631–637. Morgan Kaufmann, San Francisco (1995)

# Expressive Reasoning on Tree Structures: Recursion, Inverse Programs, Presburger Constraints and Nominals

Everardo Bárcenas[1] and Jesús Lavalle[2]

[1] Universidad Politécnica de Puebla
`ismael.barcenas@uppuebla.edu.mx`
[2] Universidad Autónoma de Puebla
`jlavalle@cs.buap.mx`

**Abstract.** The Semantic Web lays its foundations on the study of graph and tree logics. One of the most expressive graph logics is the fully enriched $\mu$-calculus, which is a modal logic equipped with least and greatest fixed-points, nominals, inverse programs and graded modalities. Although it is well-known that the fully enriched $\mu$-calculus is undecidable, it was recently shown that this logic is decidable when its models are finite trees. In the present work, we study the fully-enriched $\mu$-calculus for trees extended with Presburger constraints. These constraints generalize graded modalities by restricting the number of children nodes with respect to Presburger arithmetic expressions. We show that the logic is decidable in EXPTIME. This is achieved by the introduction of a satisfiability algorithm based on a Fischer-Ladner model construction that is able to handle binary encodings of Presburger constraints.

## 1 Introduction

The $\mu$-calculus is an expressive propositional modal logic with least and greatest fixed-points, which subsumes many temporal, modal and description logics (DLs), such as the Propositional Dynamic Logic (PDL) and the Computation Tree Logic (CTL) [2]. Due to its expressive power and nice computational properties, the $\mu$-calculus has been extensively used in many areas of computer science, such as program verification, concurrent systems and knowledge representation. In this last domain, the $\mu$-calculus has been particularly useful in the identification of expressive and computationally well-behaved DLs [2], which are now known the standard ontology language OWL for the W3C. Another standard for the W3C is the XPath query language for XML. XPath also takes an important role in many XML technologies, such as XProc, XSLT and XQuery. Due to its capability to express recursive and multi-directional navigation, the $\mu$-calculus has also been successfully used as a framework for the evaluation and reasoning of XPath queries [1,4]. Since the $\mu$-calculus is as expressive as the monadic second order logic (MSOL), it has been also successfully used in the XML setting in the description of schema languages [1], which can be seen as the tree version of regular expressions. Analogously as regular expressions are interpreted as sets

F. Castro, A. Gelbukh, and M. González (Eds.): MICAI 2013, Part I, LNAI 8265, pp. 80–91, 2013.

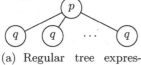
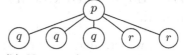

(a) Regular tree expression: $p(q^\star)$

(b) Non-regular tree expression for a balanced tree: $p(q > r)$

**Fig. 1.** Tree expressions

of strings, XML schemas (regular tree expressions) are interpreted as sets of unranked trees (XML documents). For example, the expression $p(q^\star)$ represents the sets of trees rooted at $p$ with either none, one or more children subtrees matching $q$. See figure 1(a) for an interpretation of $p(q^\star)$. However, it is well-known that expressing arithmetical constraints goes beyond regularity [1]. For instance, $p(q > r)$ denotes the trees rooted at $p$ with more $q$ children than $r$ children. In figure 1(b) is depicted an interpretation of $p(q > r)$. In the present work, we study an extension of the $\mu$-calculus for trees with Presburger constraints that can be used to express arithmetical restrictions on regular (tree) languages.

**Related Work.** The extension of the $\mu$-calculus with nominals, inverse programs and graded modalities is known as the fully enriched $\mu$-calculus [2]. Nominals are intuitively interpreted as singleton sets, inverse programs are used to express past properties (backward navigation along accesability relations), and graded modalities express numerical constraints on the number immediate successors nodes [2]. All of them, nominals, inverse programs and graded modalities are present in OWL. However, the fully enriched $\mu$-calculus was proven by Bonatti and Peron to be undecidable [3]. Nevertheless, Bárcenas et al. [1] recently showed that the fully enriched $\mu$-calculus is decidable in single exponential time when its models are finite trees. Graded modalities in the context of trees are used to constrain the number of children nodes with respect to constants. In this work, we introduce a generalization of graded modalities. This generalization considers numerical bounds on children with respect to Presburger arithmetical expressions, as for instance $\phi > \psi$, which restricts the number of children where $\phi$ holds to be strictly greater than the number of children where $\psi$ is true. Other works have previously considered Presburger constraints on tree logics. MSOL with Presburger constraints was shown to be undecidable by Seidl et al. [9]. Demri and Lugiez proved a PSPACE bound on the propositional modal logic with Presburger constraints [5]. A tree logic with a fixed-point and Presburger constraints was shown to be decidable in EXPTIME by Seidl et al. [10]. In the current work, we push further decidability by allowing nominals and inverse programs in addition than Presburger constraints.

**Outline.** We introduce a modal logic for trees with fixed-points, inverse programs, nominals and Presburger constraints in Section 2. Preliminaries of the satisfiability algorithm for the logic are described in Section 3. In Section 4, an EXPTIME satisfiability algorithm is described and proven correct. A summary together with a discussion of further research is reported in Section 5.

## 2   A Tree Logic with Recursion, Inverse, Counting and Nominals

In this section, we introduce an expressive modal logic for finite unranked tree models. The tree logic (TL) is equipped with operators for recursion ($\mu$), inverse programs (I), Presburger constraints (C), and nominals (O).

**Definition 1 ($\mu$TLICO syntax).** *The set of $\mu TLICO$ formulas is defined by the following grammar:*

$$\phi := p \mid x \mid \neg\phi \mid \phi \vee \phi \mid \langle m \rangle \phi \mid \mu x.\phi \mid \phi - \phi > k$$

Variables are assumed to be bounded and under the scope of a modal ($\langle m \rangle \phi$) or a counting formula ($\phi - \psi > k$).

Formulas are interpreted as subset tree nodes: propositions $p$ are used to label nodes; negation and disjunction are interpreted as complement and union of sets, respectively; modal formulas $\langle m \rangle \phi$ are true in nodes, such that $\phi$ holds in at least one accessible node through adjacency $m$, which may be either $\downarrow$, $\rightarrow$, $\uparrow$ or $\leftarrow$, which in turn are interpreted as the children, right siblings, parent and left siblings relations, respectively; $\mu x.\phi$ is interpreted as a least fixed-point; and counting formulas $\phi - \psi > k$ holds in nodes, such that the number of its children where $\phi$ holds minus the number of its children where $\psi$ holds is greater than the non-negative integer $k$. Consider for instance the following formula $\psi$:

$$p \wedge (q - r > 0)$$

This formula is true in nodes labeled by $p$, such that the number of its $q$ children is greater than the number of its $r$ children. $\psi$ actually corresponds to the example of Section 1 about a balanced tree: $p(q > r)$. In Figure 2 there is a graphical representation of a model for $\psi$. Due to the fixed-points in the logic, it is also possible to perform recursive navigation. For example, consider the following formula $\phi$:

$$\mu x.\psi \vee \langle \downarrow \rangle x$$

$\phi$ is true in nodes with at least one descendant where $\psi$ is true, that is, $\phi$ recursively navigates along children until it finds a $\psi$ node. A model for $\phi$ is depicted in Figure 2. Backward navigation may also be possible to express with the help of inverse programs (converse modalities). For instance, consider the following formula $\varphi$:

$$\mu x.t \vee \langle \uparrow \rangle x$$

$\varphi$ holds in nodes with an ancestor named $t$, that is, $\varphi$ recursively navigates along parents until it finds a $t$ node. A model for $\varphi$ is depicted in Figure 2.

In order to provide a formal semantics, we need some preliminaries. A tree structure $\mathcal{T}$ is a tuple $(P, \mathcal{N}, \mathcal{R}, L)$, where: $P$ is a set of propositions; $\mathcal{N}$ is a finite set of nodes; $\mathcal{R} : \mathcal{N} \times M \times \mathcal{N}$ is relation between nodes and modalities $M$ forming a tree, written $n \in \mathcal{R}(n, m)$; and $L : \mathcal{N} \times P$ is a labeling relation, written $p \in L(n)$.

Given a tree structure, a valuation $V$ of variables is defined as a mapping from the set variables $X$ to the nodes $V : X \mapsto \mathcal{N}$.

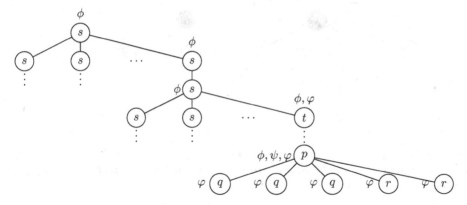

**Fig. 2.** A model for $\psi \equiv (p \wedge [q - r > 0])$, $\phi \equiv \mu x.\psi \vee \langle\downarrow\rangle x$ and $\varphi \equiv \mu x.t \vee \langle\uparrow\rangle x$

**Definition 2 ($\mu$TLICO semantics).** *Given a tree structure $\mathcal{T}$ and a valuation $V$, $\mu$TLICO formulas are interpreted as follows:*

$$[\![p]\!]_V^{\mathcal{T}} = \{n \mid p \in L(n)\} \qquad\qquad [\![x]\!]_V^{\mathcal{T}} = V(x)$$

$$[\![\neg\phi]\!]_V^{\mathcal{T}} = \mathcal{N} \setminus [\![\phi]\!]_V^{\mathcal{T}} \qquad\qquad [\![\phi \vee \psi]\!]_V^{\mathcal{T}} = [\![\phi]\!]_V^{\mathcal{T}} \cup [\![\psi]\!]_V^{\mathcal{T}}$$

$$[\![\langle m\rangle\phi]\!]_V^{\mathcal{T}} = \{n \mid \mathcal{R}(n, m) \cap [\![\phi]\!]_V^{\mathcal{T}} \neq \emptyset\} \quad [\![\mu x.\phi]\!]_V^{\mathcal{T}} = \bigcap \{\mathcal{N}' \subseteq \mathcal{N} \mid [\![\phi]\!]_{V[\mathcal{N}'/x]}^{\mathcal{T}} \subseteq \mathcal{N}'\}$$

$$[\![\phi - \psi > k]\!]_V^{\mathcal{T}} = \{n \mid |\mathcal{R}(n, \downarrow) \cap [\![\phi]\!]_V^{\mathcal{T}}| - |\mathcal{R}(n, \downarrow) \cap [\![\psi]\!]_V^{\mathcal{T}}| > k\}$$

We also use the following notation: $\top = p \vee \neg p$, $\phi \wedge \psi = \neg(\neg\phi \vee \neg\psi)$, $[m]\phi = \neg\langle m\rangle\neg\phi$, $\nu x.\phi = \neg\mu x.\neg\phi\,[^x/_{\neg x}]$, $(\phi-\psi \leq k) = \neg(\phi-\psi > k)$, $\phi-\psi \,\#k$ for $\# \in \{\leq, >\}$ and $(\phi_1 + \phi_2 + \ldots + \phi_n - \psi_1 - \psi_2 - \ldots - \psi_m \,\#k) = (\bigcup_i^n \phi_i - \bigcup_j^m \psi_j \,\#k)$. Note that $\top$ is true in every node, conjunction $\phi \wedge \psi$ holds whenever both $\phi$ and $\psi$ are true, $[m]\phi$ holds in nodes where $\phi$ is true in each accessible node through $m$, $\nu x.\phi$ is a greatest fixed-point, $\phi - \psi \leq k$ holds in nodes where the number of its $\phi$ children nodes minus the number of its $\psi$ children is less than the constant $k$, and $\phi_1 + \phi_2 + \ldots + \phi_n - \psi_1 - \psi_2 - \ldots - \psi_m \,\#k$ is true in nodes where the sum of its $\phi_i$ $(i = 1, \ldots, n)$ children minus the sum of its $\psi_j$ $(j = 1, \ldots, m)$ children satisfies $\#k$.

The interpretation of nominals is a singleton, that is, nominals are formulas which are true in exactly one node in the entire model [2]. Now, is easy to see that $\mu$TLICO can navigate recursively thanks to the fixed-points, and in all directions thanks to inverse programs. Hence, $\mu$TLICO can then express for a formula to be true in one node while being false in all other nodes of the model.

**Definition 3 (Nominals).** *Nominals are defined as follows:*

$$nom(\phi) = \phi \wedge siblings(\neg\phi) \wedge ancestors(\neg\phi) \wedge descendants(\neg\phi)$$

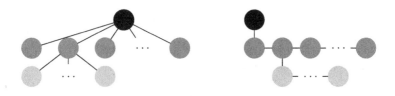

**Fig. 3.** Bijection of $n$-ary and binary trees

*where siblings($\neg\phi$), ancestors($\neg\phi$), and descendants($\neg\phi$) are true, if and only if, $\phi$ is not true in all siblings, ancestors and descendants, respectively, and they are defined as follows:*

$$siblings(\phi) = [\rightarrow]\phi \wedge [\leftarrow]\phi$$
$$ancestors(\phi) = [\uparrow](\mu x.\phi \wedge siblings(\phi) \wedge [\uparrow]x)$$
$$descendants(\phi) = [\downarrow](\mu x.\phi \wedge [\downarrow]x)$$

## 3  Syntactic Trees

In this Section, we give a detailed description of the syntactic version of tree models used by the satisfiability algorithm.

We first introduce some preliminaries. There is well-known bijection between binary and $n$-ary unranked trees [7]. One adjacency is interpreted as the first child relation and the other adjacency is for the right sibling relation. In Figure 3 is depicted an example of the bijection. Hence, without loss of generality, from now on, we consider binary unranked trees only. At the logic level, formulas are reinterpreted as expected: $\langle\downarrow\rangle\phi$ holds in nodes such that $\phi$ is true in its first child; $\langle\rightarrow\rangle\phi$ holds in nodes where $\phi$ is satisfied by its right (following) sibling; $\langle\uparrow\rangle\phi$ is true in nodes whose parent satisfies $\phi$; and $\langle\leftarrow\rangle\phi$ satisfies nodes where $\phi$ holds in its left (previous) sibling.

For the satisfiability algorithm we consider formulas in negation normal form only. The negation normal form (NNF) of $\mu$TLIC formulas is defined by the usual De Morgan rules and the following ones: nnf($\langle m\rangle\phi$) = $\langle m\rangle\neg\phi \vee \neg\langle m\rangle\top$, nnf($\mu x.\phi$) = $\mu x.\neg\phi\,[^x/_{\neg x}]$, nnf($\phi - \psi > k$) = $\phi - \psi \leq k$, and nnf($\phi - \psi \leq k$) = $\phi - \psi > k$. Hence, negation in formulas in NNF occurs only in front of propositions and formulas of the form $\langle m\rangle\top$. Also notice that we consider an extension of $\mu$TLIC formulas consisting of conjunctions, $\phi - \psi \leq k$ and $\top$ formulas, with the expected semantics.

We now consider a binary encoding of natural numbers. Given a finite set of propositions, the binary encoding of a natural number is the boolean combination of propositions satisfying the binary representation of the given number. For example, number 0 is written $\bigwedge_{i\geq 0}\neg p_i$, and number 7 is $p_2 \wedge p_1 \wedge p_0 \wedge \bigwedge_{i>2}\neg p_i$ (111 in binary). The binary encoding of constants is required in the definition of counters, which are used in the satisfiability algorithm to verify counting subformulas. Given a counting formula $\phi - \psi \#k$, counters $C(\phi) = k_1$ and $C(\psi) =$

$k_2$ are the sequence of propositions occurring positively in the binary encoding of a constants $k_1$ and $k_2$, respectively. We write $C_i(\phi) = k$ to refer to an individual of the sequence. A formula $\phi$ induces a set of counters corresponding to its counting subformulas. The bound in the amount of counter propositions is given by the constant $K(\phi)$, which is defined as the sum of the constants of the counting subformulas, more precisely: $K(p) = K(x) = K(\top) = 0$, $K(\langle m \rangle \phi) = K(\neg \phi) = K(\mu x.\phi) = K(\phi)$, $K(\phi \vee \psi) = K(\phi \wedge \psi) = K(\phi) + K(\psi)$, and $K(\phi - \psi \# k) = K(\phi) + K(\psi) + k + 1$.

Nodes in syntactic trees are defined as sets of subformulas. These subformulas are extracted with the help of the Fischer-Ladner Closure. Before defining the Fischer-Ladner Closure, consider the Fischer-Ladner relation $R^{\text{FL}}$ for $i = 1, 2$, $\circ = \vee, \wedge$ and $j = 1, \ldots, \log(K(\phi))$:

$$R^{\text{FL}}\left(\psi, \text{nnf}(\psi)\right), \qquad\qquad R^{\text{FL}}\left(\psi_1 \circ \psi_2, \psi_i\right),$$
$$R^{\text{FL}}\left(\langle m \rangle \psi, \psi\right), \qquad\qquad R^{\text{FL}}\left(\mu x.\psi, \psi\left[{}^{\mu x.\psi}/{}_x\right]\right),$$
$$R^{\text{FL}}\left(\psi_1 - \psi_2 \# k, \psi_i\right), \qquad R^{\text{FL}}\left(\psi_1 - \psi_2 \# k, \langle \downarrow \rangle \mu x.\psi_i \vee \langle \rightarrow \rangle x\right),$$
$$R^{\text{FL}}\left(\psi_1 - \psi_2 \# k, C_j(\psi_i) = K(\phi)\right), \quad R^{\text{FL}}\left(\neg \psi, \psi\right).$$

**Definition 4 (Fischer-Ladner Closure).** *Given a formula $\phi$, the Fischer-Ladner Closure of $\phi$ is defined as $CL^{FL}(\phi) = CL_k^{FL}(\phi)$, such that $k$ is the smallest positive integer satisfying $CL_k^{FL}(\phi) = CL_{k+1}^{FL}(\phi)$, where for $i \geq 0$:*

$$CL_0^{FL}(\phi) = \{\phi\}; \quad CL_{i+1}^{FL}(\phi) = CL_i^{FL}(\phi) \cup \{\psi \mid R^{FL}(\psi', \psi), \psi' \in CL_i^{FL}(\phi)\}.$$

*Example 1.* Consider the formula $\phi = p \wedge [(q - r) > 1] \wedge r > 0$, then for $j = 1, 2$, we have that

$$\text{CL}^{\text{FL}}(\phi) = \{p \wedge [(q - r) > 1] \wedge (r > 0)), p \wedge [(q - r) > 1], (r > 0), p, [(q - r > 1)],$$
$$q, r, C_j(q) = 3, C_j(r) = 3, \langle \downarrow \rangle \mu x.q \vee \langle \rightarrow \rangle x, \langle \downarrow \rangle \mu x.r \vee \langle \rightarrow \rangle x\} \cup \text{CL}^{\text{FL}}(\text{nnf}(\phi))$$

We are now ready to define the lean set for nodes in syntactic trees. The lean set contains the propositions, modal subformulas, counters and counting subformulas of the formula in question (for the satisfiability algorithm). Intuitively, propositions will serve to label nodes, modal subformulas contain the topological information of the trees, and counters are used to verify the satisfaction of counting subformulas.

**Definition 5 (Lean).** *Given a formula $\phi$, its lean set is defined as follow*

$$lean(\phi) = \left\{p, \langle m \rangle \phi, \psi_1 - \psi_2 \# k \in CL^{FL}(\phi)\right\} \cup \left\{\langle m \rangle \top, p'\right\},$$

*provided that $p'$ does not occur in $\phi$ and $m = \downarrow, \rightarrow, \uparrow, \leftarrow$.*

*Example 2.* Consider again the formula $\phi = p \wedge [(q-r) > 1] \wedge r > 0$ of Example 1, then for $j = 1, 2$, we have that:

$$lean(\phi) = \{p, q, r, C_j(q) = 3, C_j(r) = 3, \langle \downarrow \rangle \psi_j, \langle \rightarrow \rangle \psi_j, \langle \downarrow \rangle \text{nnf}(\psi_j), \langle \rightarrow \rangle \text{nnf}(\psi_j)$$
$$(q - r) \# 1, r \# 0, \langle m \rangle \top, p'\},$$

where $\psi_1 = \mu x.q \vee \langle \rightarrow \rangle x$ and $\psi_2 = \mu x.r \vee \langle \rightarrow \rangle x$. Recall that $C_j(\psi) = k$ are the corresponding propositions, required to define the binary encoding of $k$.

A $\phi$-node $n^\phi$ is defined as a subset of the lean, such that: at least one proposition (different from the counter propositions) occurs in $n^\phi$; if a modal subformula $\langle m \rangle \psi$ occurs in $n^\phi$, then $\langle m \rangle \top$ also does; and $n^\phi$ can be either the root, a children or a sibling. More precisely, the set of $\phi$-nodes is defined as follows:

$$\mathcal{N}^\phi = \{n^\phi \in \text{lean}(\phi) \mid p \in n^\phi, \langle m \rangle \psi \in n^\phi \Rightarrow \langle m \rangle \top \in n^\phi, \langle \uparrow \rangle \top \in n^\phi \Leftrightarrow \langle \leftarrow \rangle \top \notin n^\phi\}$$

When it is clear from the context, $\phi$-nodes are called simply nodes.

We are finally ready to define $\phi$-trees. A $\phi$-tree is defined either as empty $\emptyset$, or as a triple $(n^\phi, T_1^\phi, T_2^\phi)$, provided that $n^\phi$ is a $\phi$-node and $T_i^\phi$ ($i = 1, 2$) are $\phi$-trees. The root of $(n^\phi, T_1^\phi, T_2^\phi)$ is $n^\phi$. We often call $\phi$-trees simply trees.

*Example 3.* Consider the formula $\phi = p \wedge [(q - r) > 1] \wedge r > 0$. Then $T = (n_0, (n_1, \emptyset, (n_2, \emptyset, (n_3, \emptyset, (n_4, \emptyset, \emptyset)))), \emptyset)$ is a $\phi$-tree, where

$$n_0 = \{p, C(q) = 0, C(r) = 0, (q - r) > 1, r > 0, \langle \downarrow \rangle \psi_1, \langle \downarrow \rangle \psi_2, \langle \downarrow \rangle \top\},$$
$$n_1 = \{q, C(q) = 3, C(r) = 1, (q - r) \leq 1, r \leq 0, \langle \rightarrow \rangle \psi_1, \langle \rightarrow \rangle \psi_2, \langle \uparrow \rangle \top, \langle \rightarrow \rangle \top\}$$
$$n_2 = \{q, C(q) = 2, C(r) = 1, (q - r) \leq 1, r \leq 0, \langle \rightarrow \rangle \psi_1, \langle \rightarrow \rangle \psi_2, \langle \leftarrow \rangle \top, \langle \rightarrow \rangle \top\}$$
$$n_3 = \{q, C(q) = 1, C(r) = 1, (q - r) \leq 1, r \leq 0, \langle \rightarrow \rangle \psi_2, \langle \leftarrow \rangle \top, \langle \rightarrow \rangle \top\}$$
$$n_4 = \{r, C(q) = 0, C(r) = 1, (q - r) \leq 1, r \leq 0, \langle \leftarrow \rangle \top\}.$$

$\phi$-nodes $n_i$ ($i = 0, \ldots, 4$) are defined from the lean of $\phi$ (Example 2). In Figure 4 is depicted a graphical representation of $T$. Notice that counters in the root $n_0$ are set to zero $0$. This is because counters are intended to count on the siblings only. For instance, counters in $n_1$ are set to 3 and 1 for $q$ and $r$, respectively, because there are three $q$'s and one $r$ in $n_1$ and its siblings. Counting formulas occur positively only at the root $n_0$, because they are intended to be true when the counters in the children of $n_0$ satisfy the Presburger constraints. Since $n_i$ ($i > 0$) does not have children, then counting formulas occur negatively in these nodes. Finally, notice that modal subformulas define the topology of the tree.

## 4   Satisfiability

In this section we define a satisfiability algorithm for the logic $\mu$TLIC following the Fischer-Ladner method [1,5]. Given an input formula, the algorithm decides whether or not the formula is satisfiable. The algorithm builds $\phi$-trees in a bottom-up manner. Starting from the leaves, parents are iteratively added until a satisfying tree with respect to $\phi$ is found.

Algorithm 1 describes the bottom-up construction of $\phi$-trees. The set $Init(\phi)$ gathers the leaves. The satisfiability of formulas with respect to $\phi$-trees is tested with the entailment relation $\vdash$. Inside the loop, the $Update$ function consistently adds parents to previously build trees until either a satisfying tree is found or

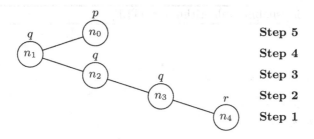

Step 5

Step 4

Step 3

Step 2

Step 1

**Fig. 4.** $\phi$-tree model for $\phi = p \wedge [(q - r) > 1] \wedge (r > 0)$ built by the satisfiability algorithm in 5 steps

no more trees can be built. If a satisfying tree is found, the algorithm returns that the input formula is satisfiable, otherwise, the algorithm returns that the input formula is not satisfiable.

*Example 4.* Consider the formula $\phi = p \wedge [(q - r) > 1] \wedge (r > 0)$. The $\phi$-tree $T$, described in Example 3, is built by the satisfiability algorithm in 5 steps. All leaves are first defined by $Init(\phi)$: notice that $n_4$ is a leaf because it does not contain downward modal formulas. Once in the cycle, parents and previous siblings are iteratively added to previously built trees, which by the second step consists of leaves only: it is easy to see that $n_3$ can be a previous sibling of $n_4$, and the same for $n_2$ and $n_3$, and $n_1$ and $n_2$, respectively; also it is clear that $n_0$ can be a parent of $n_1$. Notice that $n_0$ is the root due to the absence of upward modal formulas. The construction of $T$ is graphically represented in Figure 4.

We now give a detailed description of the algorithm components.

**Definition 6 (Entailment).** *The entailment relation is defined as follows:*

$$\frac{}{n \vdash \top} \qquad \frac{\phi \in n}{n \vdash \phi} \qquad \frac{\phi \notin n}{n \vdash \neg\phi} \qquad \frac{n \vdash \phi \quad n \vdash \psi}{n \vdash \phi \wedge \psi}$$

$$\frac{n \vdash \phi}{n \vdash \phi \vee \psi} \qquad \frac{n \vdash \psi}{n \vdash \phi \vee \psi} \qquad \frac{n \vdash \phi[^{\mu x.\phi}/_x]}{n \vdash \mu x.\phi}$$

*If there is node $n$ in a tree $T$, such that $n$ entails $\phi$ ($n \vdash \phi$) and formulas $\langle\uparrow\rangle\top$ and $\langle\leftarrow\rangle\top$ does not occur in the root of $T$, we then say that the tree $T$ entails $\phi$, $T \vdash \phi$. Given a set of trees $X$, if there is a tree $T$ in $X$ entailing $\phi$ ($T \vdash \phi$), then $X$ entails $\phi$, $X \vdash \phi$. Relation $\nvdash$ is defined in the obvious manner.*

Leaves are $\phi$-nodes without downward adjacencies, that is, formulas with the form $\langle\downarrow\rangle\psi$ or $\langle\rightarrow\rangle\psi$ do not occur in leaves. Also, counters are properly initialized, that is, for each counting subformula $\psi_1 - \psi_2 \#k$ of the input formula, if a leaf satisfies $\psi_i$ ($i = 1, 2$), then $C(\psi_i) = 1$ is contained in the leaf, otherwise $C(\psi_i) = 0$, that is, no counting proposition corresponding to $\psi_i$ occurs in the leaf. The set of leaves is defined by the $Init$ function.

---

**Algorithm 1.** Satisfiability algorithm for $\mu$TLIC

---

$Y \leftarrow \mathcal{N}^\phi$
$X \leftarrow Init(\phi)$
$X' \leftarrow \emptyset$
**while** $X \nvdash \phi$ and $X \neq X'$ **do**
$\quad X' \leftarrow X$
$\quad X \leftarrow Update(X', Y)$
$\quad Y \leftarrow Y \setminus root(X)$
**end while**
**if** $X \vdash \phi$ **then**
$\quad$ **return** $\phi$ is satisfiable
**end if**
**return** $\phi$ is not satisfiable

---

**Definition 7 (Init).** *Given a formula $\phi$, its initial set is defined as follows:*

$$
\begin{aligned}
Init(\phi) =\{n^\phi \in \mathcal{N}^\phi \mid &\langle\downarrow\rangle\top, \langle\rightarrow\rangle\top \notin n^\phi, \\
&[\psi_1 - \psi_2 \,\#k] \in lean(\phi), \psi_i \in n^\phi \Rightarrow [C(\psi_i) = 1] \in n^\phi, \\
&[\psi_1 - \psi_2 \,\#k] \in lean(\phi), \psi_i \notin n^\phi \Rightarrow [C(\psi_i) = 0] \in n^\phi\}
\end{aligned}
$$

Notice that, from definition of $\phi$-nodes, if formulas of the forms $\langle\downarrow\rangle\top$ and $\langle\rightarrow\rangle\top$ does not occur in leaves, then neither formulas of the forms $\langle\downarrow\rangle\psi$ and $\langle\rightarrow\rangle\psi$.

*Example 5.* Consider again the formula $\phi$ of Example 3. It is then easy to see that $n_4$ is a leaf. $n_4$ does not contain downward modal formulas $\langle\downarrow\rangle\psi$ and $\langle\rightarrow\rangle\psi$. Also, counters are properly initialized in $n_4$, i.e., $C(r) = 1$ occurs in $n_4$.

Recall that the *Update* function consistently adds parents to previously built trees. Consistency is defined with respect to two different notions. One notion is with respect to modal formulas. For example, a modal formula $\langle\downarrow\rangle\phi$ is contained in the root of a tree, if and only if, its first children satisfies $\phi$.

**Definition 8 (Modal Consistency).** *Given a $\phi$-node $n^\phi$ and a $\phi$-tree $T$ with root $r$, $n^\phi$ and $T$ are $m$ modally consistent $\Delta_m(n^\phi, T)$, if and only if, for all $\langle m\rangle\psi, \langle\overline{m}\rangle\phi$ in $lean(\phi)$, we have that*

$$
\langle m\rangle\psi \in n^\phi \Leftrightarrow r \vdash \psi,
$$

$$
\langle\overline{m}\rangle\psi \in r \Leftrightarrow n^\phi \vdash \psi.
$$

*Example 6.* Consider $\phi$ of Figure 4. In step 2, it is easy to see that $n_3$ is modally consistent with $n_4$: formula $\langle\rightarrow\rangle\mu x.r \vee \langle\rightarrow\rangle x$ is clearly true in $n_3$, because $r$ occurs in $n_4$. In the following steps, $n_i$ is clearly modally consistent with $n_{i+1}$.

The other consistency notion is defined in terms of counters. Since the first child is the upper one in a tree, it must contain all the information regarding counters, i.e., each time a previous sibling is added by the algorithm, counters must be updated. Counter consistency must also consider that counting formulas occurs in the parents, if and only if, the counters of its first child are consistent with the constraints in counting subformulas.

**Definition 9 (Counter Consistency).** *Given a $\phi$-node $n^\phi$ and trees $T_1$ and $T_2$, we say that $n^\phi$ and $T_i$ are counter consistent $\Theta(n^\phi, T_1, T_2)$, if and only if, for the root $r_i$ of $T_i$ and $\forall [\psi_1 - \psi_2 \,\#k] \in lean(\phi)$ ($i = 1, 2$):*

$$[C(\psi_i) = k'] \in n^\phi, n^\phi \vdash \psi_i \Leftrightarrow [C(\psi_i) = k' - 1] \in r_2$$
$$[C(\psi_i) = k'] \in n^\phi, n^\phi \nvdash \psi_i \Leftrightarrow [C(\psi_i) = k'] \in r_2$$
$$[\psi_1 - \psi_2 \,\#k] \in n^\phi \Leftrightarrow [C(\psi_i) = k_i] \in r_1, k_1 - k_2 \,\#k$$

*Example 7.* Consider the formula $\phi$ of Example 3 and Figure 4. In steps 2, 3 and 4, since previous siblings are added, counters for $q$ are incremented in $n_3$, $n_2$ and $n_1$, respectively. In step 5, the counting formulas $q - r > 1$ and $r > 0$ are present in the root $n_0$, due to the fact that counters, in the first child, satisfy the Presburger constraints.

*Update* function gathers the notions of counter and modal consistency.

**Definition 10 (Update).** *Given a set of $\phi$-trees $X$, the update function is defined as follow for $i = 1, 2$:*

$$Update(X, Y) = \{(n^\phi, T_1, T_2) \mid T_i \in X, n^\phi \in Y, \Delta_i(n^\phi, T_i), \Theta(n^\phi, T_1, T_2)\}$$

We finally define the function $root(X)$, which takes as input a set of $\phi$-trees and returns a set with the roots of the $\phi$-trees.

We now show that the algorithm is correct and terminates. It is clear that the algorithm terminates due to the facts that set of $\phi$-nodes is finite and that the *Update* function is monotone. Algorithm correctness is shown by proving that the algorithm is sound and complete.

**Theorem 1 (Soundness).** *If the satisfiability algorithm returns that $\phi$ is satisfiable, then there is tree model satisfying $\phi$.*

*Proof.* Assume $T$ is the $\phi$-tree that entails $\phi$. Then we construct a tree model $\mathcal{T}$ isomorphic to $T$ as follows: the nodes of $\mathcal{T}$ are the $\phi$-nodes; for each triple $(n, T_1, T_2)$ in $T$, $n_1 \in \mathcal{R}(n, \downarrow)$ and $n_2 \in \mathcal{R}(n, \rightarrow)$, provided that $n_i$ are the roots of $T_i$ ($i = 1, 2$); and if $p \in n$, then $p \in L(n)$. We now show by induction on the structure of the input formula $\phi$ that $\mathcal{T}$ satisfies $\phi$. All cases are immediate. In the case of fixed-points, we use the fact that there is an equivalent finite unfolding $\mu x.\psi \equiv \psi \left[ ^{\mu x.\psi} / _x \right]$.

**Theorem 2 (Completeness).** *If there is a model satisfying a formula $\phi$, then the satisfiability algorithm returns that $\phi$ is satisfiable.*

*Proof.* The proof is divided in two main steps: first we show that there is a lean labeled version of the satisfying model; and then we show that the algorithm actually builds the lean labeled version.

Assume $\mathcal{T}$ satisfies the formula $\phi$. We construct a lean labeled version $T$ of $\mathcal{T}$ as follows: the nodes and shape of $T$ are the same than $\mathcal{T}$; for each $\psi \in \text{lean}(\phi)$, if $n$ in $\mathcal{T}$ satisfies $\psi$, then $\psi$ is in $n$ of $T$; and the counters are set in the nodes in $T$ as the algorithm does in a bottom-up manner.

It is now shown by induction on the derivation of $T \vdash \phi$ that $T$ entails $\phi$. By the construction of $T$ and by induction most cases are straightforward. For the fixed-point case $\mu x.\psi$, we proceed by induction on the structure of the unfolding $\psi\left[\mu x.\psi / x\right]$. This is immediate since variables and hence unfolded fixed-points occur in the scope of modal or counting formulas only.

Before proving that the algorithm builds $T$, we need to show that there are enough $\phi$-nodes to construct $T$. That is, counter formulas may enforce the duplication of nodes in order to be satisfied. Counters are used to distinguish potentially identical nodes. We then show that counters are consistent. More precisely, we will show that provided that $\phi$ is satisfied, then there is a $\phi$-tree entailing $\phi$, such that each $\phi$-node has no identical children. This is shown by contradiction. We assume that there is no tree with non-identical children entailing $\phi$. Assume that $T$ entails $\phi$, such that $T$ has identical children. We now prune $T$ to produce a tree $T'$ by removing the duplicated children. It is now shown that $T'$ also entails $\phi$ by induction on the derivation $T' \vdash \phi$. Most cases are trivial. Consider now the case of counting subformulas $\psi_1 - \psi_2 \# k$. We need to ensure that counted nodes (the ones that satisfy $\psi_i$ for $i = 1, 2$) were not removed in the pruning process. This is not possible since only identical nodes were removed, and hence removed nodes share the same counters.

We are now ready to show that the algorithm builds the lean labeled version $T$ of the satisfying model $\mathcal{T}$. It is proceed by induction on the height of $\mathcal{T}$. The base case is trivial. Consider now the induction step. By induction, we know that the left and right subtrees of $T$ were built by the algorithm, we now show that the root $n$ of $T$ can be joined to the previously built left and right subtrees. This is true due to the following: $\Delta(n, n_i)$ is consistent with $\mathcal{R}$, where $i = 1, 2$ and $n_i$ are the roots of the left and right subtrees, respectively; and $K(\phi)$ is consistent with the satisfaction of the counting subformulas.

**Theorem 3 (Complexity).** *The satisfiability algorithm takes at most single exponential time with respect to the size of the input formula.*

*Proof.* We first show that the lean set of the input formula $\phi$ has linear size with respect to the size of $\phi$. This is easily proven by induction on the structure $\phi$. We then proceed to show that the algorithm is exponential with respect to the size of the lean. Since the number of $\phi$-nodes is single exponential with respect to lean size, then there are at most an exponential number of steps in the loop of the algorithm. It remains to prove that each step, including the ones inside the loop, takes at most exponential time: computing $Init(\phi)$ implies the traversal of $\mathcal{N}^\phi$ and hences takes exponential time; testing $\vdash$ takes linear time with respect to the node size, and hence its cost is exponential with respect to the set of trees; and since the cost of relations of modal and counter consistency $\Delta_m$ and $\Theta$ is linear, then the $Update$ functions takes exponential time.

## 5    Discussion

We introduced a modal logic for trees with least and greatest fixed-points, inverse programs, nominals and Presburger constraints ($\mu$TLICO). We showed that the logic is decidable in single exponential time, even if the Presbuger constraints are in binary. Decidability was shown by a Fischer-Ladner satisfiability algorithm. We are currently exploring symbolic techniques, such as Binary Decision Diagrams, to achieve an efficient implementation of the satisfiability algorithm.

The fully enriched $\mu$-calculus for trees has been previously used as a reasoning framework for the XPath query language enhanced with a limited form of counting (numerical constraints) [1]. Bárcenas et al. [1] also showed that XML schemas (regular tree languages) with numerical constraints can be succinctly expressed by the fully enriched $\mu$-calculus. An immediate application of $\mu$TLICO is its use as a reasoning framework for XPath and XML schemas with a more general form of counting (arithmetical constraints). In another setting, arithmetical constraints on trees have been also successfully used in the verification of balanced tree structures such as AVL or red-black trees [8,6]. We believe that another field of application for the logic presented in the current work is in the verification of balanced tree structures.

## References

1. Bárcenas, E., Genevès, P., Layaïda, N., Schmitt, A.: Query reasoning on trees with types, interleaving, and counting. In: Walsh, T. (ed.) IJCAI, pp. 718–723. IJCAI/AAAI (2011)
2. Bonatti, P.A., Lutz, C., Murano, A., Vardi, M.Y.: The complexity of enriched $\mu$-calculi. In: Bugliesi, M., Preneel, B., Sassone, V., Wegener, I. (eds.) ICALP 2006. LNCS, vol. 4052, pp. 540–551. Springer, Heidelberg (2006)
3. Bonatti, P.A., Peron, A.: On the undecidability of logics with converse, nominals, recursion and counting. Artif. Intell. 158(1), 75–96 (2004)
4. Calvanese, D., Giacomo, G.D., Lenzerini, M., Vardi, M.Y.: Node selection query languages for trees. In: Fox, M., Poole, D. (eds.) AAAI. AAAI Press (2010)
5. Demri, S., Lugiez, D.: Complexity of modal logics with Presburger constraints. J. Applied Logic 8(3), 233–252 (2010)
6. Habermehl, P., Iosif, R., Vojnar, T.: Automata-based verification of programs with tree updates. Acta Inf. 47(1), 1–31 (2010)
7. Hosoya, H., Vouillon, J., Pierce, B.C.: Regular expression types for XML. ACM Trans. Program. Lang. Syst. 27(1), 46–90 (2005)
8. Manna, Z., Sipma, H.B., Zhang, T.: Verifying balanced trees. In: Artemov, S., Nerode, A. (eds.) LFCS 2007. LNCS, vol. 4514, pp. 363–378. Springer, Heidelberg (2007)
9. Seidl, H., Schwentick, T., Muscholl, A.: Numerical document queries. In: Neven, F., Beeri, C., Milo, T. (eds.) PODS, pp. 155–166. ACM (2003)
10. Seidl, H., Schwentick, T., Muscholl, A., Habermehl, P.: Counting in trees for free. In: Díaz, J., Karhumäki, J., Lepistö, A., Sannella, D. (eds.) ICALP 2004. LNCS, vol. 3142, pp. 1136–1149. Springer, Heidelberg (2004)

# Completion-Based Automated Theory Exploration

Omar Montano-Rivas*

Universidad Politécnica de San Luis Potosí,
Academia de Tecnologías de Información y Telemática,
Urbano Villalón 500, 78362 San Luis Potosí, S.L.P., México
omar.montano@upslp.edu.mx
http://atit.upslp.edu.mx/index.php/planta-docente/ptc/omar-montano

**Abstract.** Completion-based automated theory exploration is a method to explore inductive theories with the aid of a convergent rewrite system. It combines a method to synthesise conjectures/definitions in a theory with a completion algorithm. Completion constructs a convergent rewrite system which is then used to reduce redundancies and improve prove automation during the exploration of the theory. However, completion does not always succeed on a set of identities and a reduction ordering. A common failure occurs when an initial identity or a normal form of a critical pair cannot be oriented by the given ordering. A popular solution to this problem consists in using the instances of those rules which can be oriented for rewriting, namely ordered rewriting. Extending completion to ordered rewriting leads to 'unfailing completion'. In this paper, we extend the class of theories on which the completion-based automated theory exploration method can be applied by using unfailing completion. This produce stronger normalization methods compared to those in [20,21]. The techniques described are implemented in the theory exploration system *IsaScheme*.

**Keywords:** theory exploration, completion, ordered rewriting.

## 1 Introduction

Automated theory exploration includes the invention of definitions, conjectures, theorems, examples, counter-examples, problems, and algorithms for solving those problems. Automating these discovery processes is an exciting area for research with applications to automated theorem proving [10,25], formal methods [8,16,15,14], algorithm synthesis [5,6], and others [13,9,19].

A central problem of automated theory exploration is how to exploit discovered theorems to reduce redundant ones and improve prove automation. Collecting specialised versions of theorems can be unwieldy and does not add anything

---

* This work has been supported by Universidad Politécnica de San Luis Potosí and SEP-PROMEP. Thanks to Moa Johansson and Lucas Dixon for feedback on an earlier draft.

F. Castro, A. Gelbukh, and M. González (Eds.): MICAI 2013, Part I, LNAI 8265, pp. 92–109, 2013.

new to the discovery process. The theory formation system HR uses its *surprisingness* heuristic to avoid making tautologies of a particular type. For example, for any $A$ and $p$, the conjecture

$$\neg(\neg(p\ A)) \leftrightarrow p\ A$$

is always going to be true. HR rejects this tautology by using an ad-hoc technique called *forbidden paths* (see [9] pg. 111). Forbidden paths are construction path segments (supplied to HR prior to theory-formation) HR is not allowed to take. For example, it is not allowed to follow a negation step with another negation step, hence avoiding the above tautology.

A more powerful and general technique to avoid redundancies is using rewrite systems to generate only *irreducible* theorems (w.r.t. previously discovered ones). This technique was described in [11] and implemented in the IsaCoSy system. In IsaCoSy, the above tautology is stored as a rewrite rule:

$$\neg(\neg(P)) \rightarrow P$$

which is used to *normalise* new conjectures. Moreover, the lemmata discovered during the exploration of the theory are used to avoid further redundancies such as the one originated with the above tautology. This technique however, still generates many different versions of the same theorem. The culprit is that the rewrite system IsaCoSy generates is not confluent and thus, a theorem could have different normal forms. For example, IsaCoSy was used to synthesise properties about tail recursive reverse in a theory of lists with append (@), reverse (*rev*) and tail recursive reverse (*qrev*). For this theory, IsaCoSy built a rewrite system with 24 rewrite rules (plus 6 rules from definitions) and synthesised 45 conjectures it could not prove[1]. This could have been improved with the convergent rewrite system from table 1 which consists of 5 rewrite rules (plus 4 rules from definitions as tail recursive reverse is redefined in terms of reverse). This shorter complete rewrite system proves all 24 theorems IsaCoSy synthesises including the 45 unfalsified and unproved conjectures (it rewrites the theorems and conjectures to a term of the form $t = t$, which is trivially proved using reflexivity of equality).

The technique described in [11] was refined in the IsaScheme system (see [20,21]) to produce convergent systems of equations (when possible) using completion of rewrite systems, thus producing the rules of table 1 with the above theory of lists. However, completion does not always succeed on a set of identities and a reduction ordering. A common failure occurs when an initial identity or a normal form of a critical pair cannot be oriented by the given ordering. For example, an attempt to run the completion algorithm with a set of equations containing a permutative rule such as commutativity $f\ X\ Y = f\ Y\ X$ is bound to fail as there is no rewrite ordering $\succ$ such that $f\ X\ Y \succ f\ Y\ X$. A popular solution to this problem consists in using the instances of those rules which can

---

[1] See http://dream.inf.ed.ac.uk/projects/lemmadiscovery/
results/List_rev_qrev.txt for details.

**Table 1.** Convergent rewrite system about append (@), reverse (*rev*) and tail recursive reverse (*qrev*) in the theory of lists

| No. | Theorem |
|-----|---------|
| Def | $[\,] @ l = l$ |
| Def | $(h \mathbin{\#} t) @ l = h \mathbin{\#} (t @ l)$ |
| Def | $rev\ [\,] = [\,]$ |
| Def | $rev\ (h \mathbin{\#} t) = (rev\ t) @ (h \mathbin{\#} [\,])$ |
| 1 | $rev\ (rev\ z) = z$ |
| 2 | $rev\ (z @ x) = rev\ x @ rev\ z$ |
| 3 | $x @ [\,] = x$ |
| 4 | $(z @ y) @ x = z @ (y @ x)$ |
| 5 | $qrev\ z\ x = rev\ z @ x$ |

be oriented for rewriting, namely *ordered rewriting*. The rewrite relation under ordered rewriting needs a reduction order $\succ$ as in termination. Termination is enforced by admitting a rewrite step only if it decreases the term w.r.t. $\succ$. Identities can be used in both directions because termination is enforced in each rewrite step (provided the order decreases). The requirement for $\succ$ is that it needs to be total on ground terms. This does not pose any problem rewriting terms with variables because we can always replace all variables by new free constants [2]. Thus for example,

$$x * y = y * x$$

cannot be oriented, but if $a$, $b$ are constants with $b * a \succ a * b$ we may rewrite

$$b * a \to a * b.$$

Extending completion to ordered rewriting leads to 'unfailing completion'. This extended completion algorithm does not fail because it can handle non-orientable identities (although it could generate non-terminating executions). In this paper we propose a theory exploration algorithm based on unfailing completion with the aim to get a rewrite system that is terminating and confluent on ground terms, and thus, improving on previous attempts to exploit non-orientable equations.

The organisation of the paper is as follows. We present some background material relevant to this paper in Section 2. Section 3 describes our theory-formation algorithm with two case studies showing its applicability and higher-order capabilities. Section 5 presents details regarding the design and implementation of our approach. The limitations and future work is discussed in Section 6 and the conclusions in Section 7.

## 2    Preliminaries

### 2.1    Notations

We mainly follow the notation in [18]. In this paper, we also assume the use of a linear well-founded AC-compatible ordering for higher-order terms [24,26,2].

A *signature* is a set of typed *function symbols* denoted by $\mathcal{F}$. Terms are generated from a set of typed *variables* $\mathcal{V}$ and a signature $\mathcal{F}$ by $\lambda$-abstraction and application and are denoted by $\mathcal{T}(\mathcal{F}, \mathcal{V})$.

When ambiguities arise, variables inside terms begin with capital letters and lower case letters stand for function symbols. We differentiate *free variables* from *bound variables* in that the latter are bound by $\lambda$-abstraction. The sets of function symbols, free variables and bound variables in a term $t$ are denoted by $\mathcal{F}(t)$, $\mathcal{V}(t)$ and $\mathcal{B}(t)$, respectively. We denote the set of pure lambda terms as $\Lambda = \mathcal{T}(\emptyset, \mathcal{V})$. If $\mathcal{V}(M) = \emptyset$, then we say that $M$ is *closed*. We denote $\Lambda^{\emptyset} := \{M \in \Lambda \,|\, M \text{ is closed}\}$ as the set of pure closed lambda terms. If $M \in \Lambda^{\emptyset}(A)$, then we say that $M$ *has type* $A$ or $A$ *is inhabited* by $M$. The inhabitants of $A$ whose size is smaller than or equal to $i$ is denoted by $\Lambda_i^{\emptyset}(A) := \{M \in \Lambda_i^{\emptyset}(A) \,|\, size(M) \leq i\}$ where the size is defined inductively as:

$$size(M) := \begin{cases} 1 & \text{if } M \text{ is variable,} \\ 1 + size(N) + size(P) & \text{if } M \equiv (N\,P), \\ 1 + size(N) & \text{if } M \equiv (\lambda x.N) \end{cases}$$

Positions are strings of positive integers. $\varepsilon$ and $\cdot$ denote the empty string (root position) and string concatenation. $\mathcal{P}os(t)$ is the set of positions in term $t$. The *subterm* of $t$ at position $p$ is denoted $t|_p$. The result of replacing $t|_p$ at position $p$ in $t$ by u is written $t[u]_p$.

A *substitution* $\sigma : \mathcal{V} \to \mathcal{T}(\mathcal{F}, \mathcal{V})$ is a finite mapping from variables into terms of the same type. For $\sigma = \{x_1 \mapsto t_1, \ldots, x_n \mapsto t_n\}$ we define $Dom(\sigma) = \{x_1, \ldots, x_n\}$ and $Cod(\sigma) = \{t_1, \ldots, t_n\}$. The application of a substitution to a term is defined by

$$\sigma(t) := (\lambda \overline{x_k}.\, t)(\overline{t_n}) {\Uparrow}_{\beta}^{\eta}$$

If there is a substitution $\sigma$ such that $\sigma(s) = \sigma(t)$ we say $s$ and $t$ are *unifiable*. If there is a substitution $\sigma$ such that $\sigma(s) = t$ we say that s *matches* the term $t$. The list of bound variables in a term $t$ at position $p \in \mathcal{P}os(t)$ is denoted as

$$\begin{aligned} \mathcal{B}(t, \varepsilon) &= [\,] \\ \mathcal{B}((t_1\ t_2),\ i \cdot p) &= \mathcal{B}(t_i, p) \\ \mathcal{B}(\lambda x.\, t,\ 1 \cdot p) &= x \cdot \mathcal{B}(t, p) \end{aligned}$$

A *renaming* $\rho$ is an injective substitution with $Cod(\rho) \in \mathcal{V}$ and $Dom(\rho) \cap Cod(\rho) = \{\}$. An $\overline{x_k}-lifter$ of a term $t$ away from $W$ is a substitution $\sigma = \{F \to (\rho F)(\overline{x_k}) | F \in \mathcal{V}(t)\}$ where $\rho$ is a renaming with $Dom(\rho) = \mathcal{V}(t), Cod(\rho) \cap W = \{\}$ and $\rho F : \tau_1 \to \ldots \tau_k \to \tau$ if $x_1 : \tau_1, \ldots, x_k : \tau_k$ and $F : \tau$. An example is $\sigma = \{F \mapsto G\ x, S \mapsto T\ x\}$ which is an $x - lifter$ of $f\ (\lambda y.\ g\ (F\ y))\ S$ away from any $W$ not containing $G$ or $T$ (the corresponding renaming is $\rho = \{F \mapsto G, S \mapsto T\}$).

*Patterns* are $\lambda$-terms in which the arguments of a free variable are ($\eta$-equivalent to) pairwise distinct bound variables. For instance, $(\lambda x\, y\, z.\ f\ (H\ x\ y)\ (H\ x\ z))$, $(\lambda x.\ c\ x)$ and $(\lambda x.\ F\ (\lambda z.\ x\ z))$ are patterns, while $(\lambda x\, y.\ G\ x\ x\ y)$, $(\lambda x\, y.\ F\ y\ c)$ and $(\lambda x\, y.\ H\ (F\ x)\ y)$ are not patterns.

A pair $(l, r)$ of terms such that $l \notin \mathcal{V}$, $l$ and $r$ are of the same type and $\mathcal{V}(r) \subseteq \mathcal{V}(l)$ is called a *rewrite rule*. We write $l \to r$ for $(l, r)$. A *higher-order rewrite system* (HRS for short) $\mathcal{R}$ is a set of rewrite rules. A set of rewrite rules whose left-hand sides are patterns is called a *pattern rewrite system* (PRS). The rewrite rules of a HRS $\mathcal{R}$ define a reduction relation $\to_{\mathcal{R}}$ on $\mathcal{T}(\mathcal{F}, \mathcal{V})$ in the usual way.

$$s \to_{\mathcal{R}} t \Leftrightarrow \exists (l \to r) \in \mathcal{R},\ p \in \mathcal{P}os(s),\ \sigma.\ s|_p = \sigma(l) \wedge t = s[\sigma(r)]_p$$

An *ordered rewrite system* is a pair $(E, \succ)$ where $E$ is a set of equations and $\succ$ is a reduction ordering. The ordered rewrite system relation is defined by

$$s \to_{(E)\succ} t \Leftrightarrow \exists (l = r) \in E,\ p \in \mathcal{P}os(s),\ \sigma.\ s|_p = \sigma(l), \sigma(l) \succ \sigma(r) \wedge t = s[\sigma(r)]_p$$

The notation $s \doteq t \in E$ is short for $s = t \in E \vee t = s \in E$. If for some $l \doteq r \in E$ we have $\sigma(l) \succ \sigma(r)$ for all substitutions $\sigma$ we write $l \to r$ and call it a *rule*. Given the relation $\to$, $\overset{*}{\to}$ denotes the transitive and reflexive closure of $\to$. Two terms are called *joinable*, written $s \downarrow t$, if there is a term $u$ such that $s \overset{*}{\to} u$ and $t \overset{*}{\to} u$. They are called *ground joinable*, written $s \Downarrow t$, if for all ground substitution $\sigma$, $\sigma(s)$ and $\sigma(t)$ are joinable. An ordered rewriting system is called *ground terminating* if there is no sequence of ground terms $\{a_i | i \in \mathbb{N}\}$ such that $a_i \to a_{i+1}$ for all $i$. An ordered rewriting system is called *ground confluent* if whenever $r$, $s$, $t$ are ground terms with $r \overset{*}{\to} s$ and $r \overset{*}{\to} t$ then $s \downarrow t$. An ordered rewriting system which is ground terminating and ground confluent is called *ground convergent* or *ground complete*. It follows from Newman's lemma that if $(E, \succ)$ is ground complete then each ground term $s$ has a unique normal form.

In general, the problem of deciding whether an ordered rewriting system is ground confluent is undecidable. However, ground confluence is decidable for ground terminating finite ordered rewriting systems by checking whether all so called *critical pairs* are ground joinable.

**Definition 1.** *Let $l_1 \to r_1$ and $l_2 \to r_2$ be two rewrite rules and $p \in \mathcal{P}os(l_1)$ such that:*

- $\mathcal{V}(l_1) \cap \mathcal{B}(l_1) = \{\ \}$,
- *the head of $l_1|_p$ is not a free variable in $l_1$, and*
- *the two patterns $\lambda\overline{x_k}.\,(l_1|_p)$ and $\lambda\overline{x_k}.\,(\sigma(l_2))$ where $\{\overline{x_k}\} = \mathcal{B}(l_1, p)$ and $\sigma$ is an $\overline{x_k} - lifter$ of $l_2$ away from $\mathcal{V}(l_1)$, have a most general unifier $\theta$.*

*Then the pattern $l_1$ overlaps the pattern $l_2$ at position $p$. The rewrite rules yield the **critical pair** $< \theta(r_1), \theta(l_1[\sigma(r_2)]_p) >$.*

## 2.2 Proving Ground Joinability

We can distinguish between two approaches to prove ground joinability: semantic and syntactic. The semantic approach guarantees ground joinability of an equation at hand by a semantic-based test for the given theory. This is possible, for example, for AC-theories where the semantics of the theory tells us that ground joinability test reduces to sorting and testing for identity [1]. To go beyond fixed theories, Martin and Nipkow developed a syntactic criterion [17]. Informally, let $\mathcal{F}$ be a finite signature and $>$ be a strict order on $\mathcal{F}$. Let $s, t \in \mathcal{T}(\mathcal{F}, \mathcal{V})$ and suppose $s = t$ is the equation to be tested for ground joinability and $\mathcal{V}(s) \cup \mathcal{V}(t) = \{x_1, \ldots, x_n\}$. Now consider any ordering relation $>'$, namely all linear orderings $\sigma(x_{i1}) \sim_1 \cdots \sim_{n-1} \sigma(x_{in}), \sim_i \in \{>, \equiv\}$, between ground instances $\sigma(x_{i1}), \ldots, \sigma(x_{in})$ and try to prove $s \downarrow t$ under $\succ$ where $\succ$ is the induced ordering on ground terms by $> \cup >'$ using an AC-compatible version of the *lexicographic path ordering* or the *Knuth-Bendix ordering*.

*Example 1.* Let $\mathcal{R}$ be the following rewrite system:

$$R = \left\{ \begin{array}{l} 0 + y = y, \\ x + y = y + x \end{array} \right\}$$

Also let $\succ$ be a rewrite order (for example the lexicographic path order) such that $0 + y \succ y$. Lexicographic orders have the subterm property and thus $0 + y \succ y$ it is always the case (let assume we choose $0 < +$). Note that neither $x + y \succ y + x$ nor $y + x \succ x + y$, otherwise we could erroneously prove termination of commutativity. Now assume we want to prove that $y + 0$ and $y$ are ground joinables given $\mathcal{R}$. To prove this, we could try to use the order $\succ$ (in fact, we could try any rewrite order).

Martin and Nipkow suggested to extend the order $\succ$ to include variable $y$ as constant (as $y$ is the only variable in terms $y + 0$ and $y$). This yields the following orders:

- The lexicographic order induced by $y < 0 < +$.
- The lexicographic order induced by $y = 0 < +$.
- The lexicographic order induced by $0 < y < +$.
- The lexicographic order induced by $0 < y = +$.
- The lexicographic order induced by $0 < + < y$.

Now we check joinability of $y + 0$ and $y$ with all extended orders. If $y + 0$ and $y$ are joinables with every extended order then that implies ground joinability. Otherwise we just can't tell whether $y + 0$ and $y$ are ground joinables and probably we should try another order or even other class of orders (polynomial orders, knuth-bendix orders, lexicographic orders with status, etc)[2]. For the example above, the joinability test fails with the lexicographic order induced by $y = 0 < +$ as we can not rewrite $y + 0$ into $0 + y$ using commutativity because $y + 0 \not\succ 0 + y$.

---

[2] This constitutes the undecidability of ground joinability which is inherited from the termination problem.

## 3  Theory Exploration

Automated theory-exploration consists not only of inventing mathematical theorems from a set of axioms. Among other activities, it also includes the discovery of new concrete notions or definitions. This activity helps with the development of the theory in a coherent and natural way in which exploration proceeds in layers. For example, starting from the concepts of zero and succesor we can define addition. Once this new concept of interest is added to the theory, we can start guessing its (equational) properties by conjecturing statements about it. Proved conjectures or theorems are then used to construct a ground convergent system which can be used to find new irreducible conjectures or for theorem proving. Afterwards, we begin a new layer in which multiplication is defined in terms of addition, followed by another layer with exponentiation using the definition of multiplication and so on. This process is similar to the well-known programming paradigm in computer science that programs should be developed incrementally. In this paradigm, a programmer defines a collection of data structures and basic functions and then proceeds by defining new functions in terms of the given ones. Eventually, the extended system acts itself as a base system which is further extended by new functions and so on.

Formally this can be expressed as a set of inference rules as follows:

**Definition 2.** *Given an initial theory $\Gamma$, a total ordering on ground terms $\succ$ and a set of equations $E$ (possibly empty),* **theory exploration** *can be described with the inference rules of table 2:*

**Table 2.** The inference rules for theory exploration

| | | |
|---|---|---|
| Invention: | $\dfrac{\Gamma \vdash E}{\Gamma, Def \vdash E}$ | if $Def$ is normal form of $\rightarrow_{(E)\succ}$ |
| Discover: | $\dfrac{\Gamma \vdash E}{\Gamma \vdash E \cup \{s \doteq t\}}$ | if $s$ and $t$ are normal forms of $\rightarrow_{(E)\succ}$ and $\Gamma \vdash s = t$ |
| Deduction: | $\dfrac{\Gamma \vdash E}{\Gamma \vdash E \cup \{s \doteq t\}}$ | if $s = t$ is a critical pair of $E$ and not $s \Downarrow_E t$ |
| Simplification: | $\dfrac{\Gamma \vdash E \cup \{s \doteq t\}}{\Gamma \vdash E \cup \{u \doteq t\}}$ | if $s \rightarrow_{(E)\succ} u$ and $s \doteq t \notin E$ |
| Deletion: | $\dfrac{\Gamma \vdash E \cup \{s = t\}}{\Gamma \vdash E}$ | if $s \Downarrow_E t$ |

There is room for flexibility in how the inference rules are applied. One simple version of theory exploration mixes the above inference rules according to the following strategy:

$$((((Simplification + Deletion)^*; Deduction)^*; Discover)^*; Invention)^*$$

The *Invention* rule can be seen as adding an axiom/definition to the theory. For example, let $\Gamma_N$ be the theory of natural numbers in which we already have the constant function zero $(0)$, the unary function successor $(suc)$ and the induction rule on the naturals. An application of *Invention* is needed to invent the definition for addition:

$$\frac{\Gamma_N \vdash \{\}}{\Gamma_N,\ 0 + y = y \ \wedge\ suc\ x + y = suc\ (x + y) \vdash \{\}}.$$

Notice that the signature of the theory is potentially updated with every application of the *Invention* rule as there is an implicit creation of new function symbols. Therefore, there is also an implicit update to the ordering relation $\succ$ which is not reflected in the rules shown in table 2. Also note that we must guarantee that the axioms or new definitions are shown to be consistent w.r.t. the current theory. For example, in the Isabelle prover the function package (see [12]) can be used to make sure consistency is not broken[3].

Now that we have invented the definition for addition we use the *Discover* rule to create new theorems. For example, let $\Gamma_+$ be the theory $\Gamma_N$ augmented with the definition for addition. Two applications of *Discover* yields

$$\Gamma_+ \vdash \left\{ \begin{array}{c} 0 + y = y, \\ suc\ x + y = suc\ (x + y) \end{array} \right\}.$$

The defining equations for addition constitute a ground convergent system and thus, irreducible terms are unique. Note that commutativity and associativity properties of addition are not (rewriting) consequences of the defining equations, as there are models of the equations which do not satisfy the aforementioned properties. For instance, consider the interpretation $I$ whose domain is the two elements set $\{0, a\}$ and such that $suc_I$, the interpretation of $suc$ in $I$, is the identity $suc_I\ 0 = 0$, $suc_I\ a = a$ and $+_I$, the interpretation of $+$ in $I$, is the second projection: $u +_I v = v$. Then the defining equations are satisfied in $I$. However, $x + y = y + x$ is not valid in $I$, since $x + y = y$ in $I$ and $y + x = x$ in $I$. This suggests we should device some mechanism to *synthesise* non-rewriting consequences in the theory and then prove them. There are several techniques to perform this task and any of them are compatible with the rest of the paper (see [20,21,11] for further details). In inductive theories, we can use induction[4] to prove new theorems such as commutativity of addition. The synthesis of conjectures and the discharge of proof obligations by induction can be seen as an application of *Discover*:

$$\Gamma_+ \vdash \left\{ \begin{array}{c} 0 + y = y, \\ suc\ x + y = suc\ (x + y), \\ x + y = y + x \end{array} \right\}.$$

---

[3] By using existing definitional tools we ensured that IsaScheme is conservative by construction, and thus offered a maximum of safety from unsoundness [12].

[4] There is also available the proof method *inductionless induction* or *proof by consistency* (Hubert comon, D. Kapur and D. Musser).

The produced rewrite system is no longer ground convergent as there are non-ground joinable critical pairs, e.g. $y + 0 = y$. To prove $y + 0 \Downarrow y$ we must show $\sigma(y + 0) \downarrow \sigma(y)$ for each ground substitution $\sigma$. For the case in which $\sigma(y + 0) \succ \sigma(0 + y)$ this is easily proved with the following reduction steps: $\sigma(y + 0) \rightarrow_{(E)\succ} \sigma(0 + y) \rightarrow_{(E)\succ} \sigma(y)$. However, for the case in which $\sigma(y + 0) \not\succ \sigma(0 + y)$ we can not prove the equation to be joinable. Here we can apply the rules *Deduction*, *Simplification* and *Deletion* to generate again a ground convergent system. Note that these three rules constitute a ground completion algorithm as described in [17]. An application of *Deduction* generates the non-ground joinable critical pair $y + 0 = y$.

$$\Gamma_+ \vdash \left\{ \begin{array}{c} 0 + y = y, \\ suc\ x + y = suc\ (x + y), \\ x + y = y + x, \\ y + 0 = y \end{array} \right\}.$$

Another critical pair is produced with $suc\ x + y = suc\ (x + y)$ and $x + y = y + x$, and yields

$$\Gamma_+ \vdash \left\{ \begin{array}{c} 0 + y = y, \\ suc\ x + y = suc\ (x + y), \\ x + y = y + x, \\ y + 0 = y, \\ y + suc\ x = suc\ (x + y) \end{array} \right\}.$$

If we assume that the implicit ordering $\succ$ satisfy $0 + y \succ y$, $suc\ x + y \succ suc\ (x + y)$ and $y + 0 \succ y$ but $y + suc\ x \not\succ suc\ (x + y)$ then we can use the later equation to generate a new critical pair $y + suc\ x = suc\ (y + x)$ which can be oriented by a recursive path ordering as $y + suc\ x \succ suc\ (x + y)$ producing.

$$\Gamma_+ \vdash \left\{ \begin{array}{c} 0 + y = y, \\ suc\ x + y = suc\ (x + y), \\ x + y = y + x, \\ y + 0 = y, \\ y + suc\ x = suc\ (x + y), \\ y + suc\ x = suc\ (y + x) \end{array} \right\}.$$

Finally, an application of *Deletion* yields

$$\Gamma_+ \vdash \left\{ \begin{array}{c} 0 + y = y, \\ suc\ x + y = suc\ (x + y), \\ x + y = y + x, \\ y + 0 = y, \\ y + suc\ x = suc\ (y + x) \end{array} \right\}.$$

This rewrite system is ground convergent again, however it does not include the associativity property of addition. Again, note that associativity of addition is not a rewriting consequence of the previous equations. Here a discovery process is needed once more to uncover the associativity property of addition and induction is needed again to prove it. An application of *Discover* yields

$$\Gamma_+ \vdash \left\{ \begin{array}{c} 0 + y = y, \\ suc\ x + y = suc\ (x + y), \\ x + y = y + x, \\ y + 0 = y, \\ y + suc\ x = suc\ (y + x), \\ (x + y) + z = x + (y + z) \end{array} \right\},$$

This again produces a rewrite system which is no longer ground convergent. However, an application of *Deduction*, *Simplification* and *Deletion* produces the ground convergent system:

$$\Gamma_+ \vdash \left\{ \begin{array}{c} 0 + y = y, \\ suc\ x + y = suc\ (x + y), \\ x + y = y + x, \\ y + 0 = y, \\ y + suc\ x = suc\ (y + x), \\ (x + y) + z = x + (y + z), \\ x + (y + z) = y + (x + z) \end{array} \right\}.$$

## 4 Higher Order Example

Let $\Gamma_G$ be the theory $\Gamma_N$ (see section 3) augmented with Gödel's recursor for natural numbers:

$$rec\ 0\ y\ F = y$$
$$rec\ (suc\ x)\ y\ F = F\ x\ (rec\ x\ y\ F)$$

Two application of *Discover* yields:

$$\Gamma_G \vdash \left\{ \begin{array}{c} rec\ 0\ y\ F = y \\ rec\ (suc\ x)\ y\ F = F\ x\ (rec\ x\ y\ F) \end{array} \right\}.$$

An application of *Invention* is needed to invent the definition for addition.

$$\frac{\Gamma_G \vdash \left\{ \begin{array}{c} rec\ 0\ y\ F = y \\ rec\ (suc\ x)\ y\ F = F\ x\ (rec\ x\ y\ F) \end{array} \right\}}{\Gamma_G,\ \oplus = \lambda x\, y.\ rec\ x\ y\ (\lambda u\, v.\ suc\ v) \vdash \left\{ \begin{array}{c} rec\ 0\ y\ F = y \\ rec\ (suc\ x)\ y\ F = F\ x\ (rec\ x\ y\ F) \end{array} \right\}}$$

Now assume $\Gamma_\oplus$ is the theory $\Gamma_G$ with the definition of $\oplus$. We create a new theorem with the application of *Discover*.

$$\Gamma_\oplus \vdash \left\{ \begin{array}{c} rec\ 0\ y\ F = y \\ rec\ (suc\ x)\ y\ F = F\ x\ (rec\ x\ y\ F) \\ \oplus = \lambda x\, y.\ rec\ x\ y\ (\lambda u\, v.\ suc\ v) \end{array} \right\}.$$

One application of discover yields the theorem $rec\ x\ 0\ (\lambda u.\ suc) = x$.

$$\Gamma_\oplus \vdash \left\{ \begin{array}{l} rec\ 0\ y\ F = y \\ rec\ (suc\ x)\ y\ F = F\ x\ (rec\ x\ y\ F) \\ \qquad\qquad \oplus = \lambda x\,y.\ rec\ x\ y\ (\lambda u\,v.\ suc\ v) \\ rec\ x\ 0\ (\lambda u.\ suc) = x \end{array} \right\}.$$

The rewrite system has the critical pair $suc\ (rec\ x\ 0\ (\lambda u.\ suc)) = suc\ x$ which can be easily proved to be ground joinable. An application of *Discover* synthesises the theorem $rec\ y\ x\ (\lambda u.\ suc) = rec\ x\ y\ (\lambda u.\ suc)$ (the normal form of the commutativity property of $\oplus$).

$$\Gamma_\oplus \vdash \left\{ \begin{array}{l} rec\ 0\ y\ F = y \\ rec\ (suc\ x)\ y\ F = F\ x\ (rec\ x\ y\ F) \\ \qquad\qquad \oplus = \lambda x\,y.\ rec\ x\ y\ (\lambda u\,v.\ suc\ v) \\ rec\ x\ 0\ (\lambda u.\ suc) = x \\ rec\ y\ x\ (\lambda u.\ suc) = rec\ x\ y\ (\lambda u.\ suc) \end{array} \right\}.$$

The produced rewrite system is no longer ground convergent as there are non-ground joinable critical pairs, e.g. $rec\ y\ (suc\ x)\ (\lambda u.\ suc) = suc\ (rec\ y\ x\ (\lambda u.\ suc))$. Therefore, an application of *Deduction* produces the ground convergent rewrite system:

$$\Gamma_\oplus \vdash \left\{ \begin{array}{l} rec\ 0\ y\ F = y \\ rec\ (suc\ x)\ y\ F = F\ x\ (rec\ x\ y\ F) \\ \qquad\qquad \oplus = \lambda x\,y.\ rec\ x\ y\ (\lambda u\,v.\ suc\ v) \\ rec\ x\ 0\ (\lambda u.\ suc) = x \\ rec\ y\ x\ (\lambda u.\ suc) = rec\ x\ y\ (\lambda u.\ suc) \\ rec\ y\ (suc\ x)\ (\lambda u.\ suc) = suc\ (rec\ y\ x\ (\lambda u.\ suc)) \end{array} \right\}.$$

An application of *Discover* synthesises the (normal form of the) associativity property of $\oplus$.

$$rec\ x\ (rec\ y\ z\ (\lambda u.\ suc))\ (\lambda u.\ suc) = rec\ y\ (rec\ x\ z\ (\lambda u.\ suc))\ (\lambda u.\ suc)$$

This yields:

$$\Gamma_\oplus \vdash \left\{ \begin{array}{l} rec\ 0\ y\ F = y \\ rec\ (suc\ x)\ y\ F = F\ x\ (rec\ x\ y\ F) \\ \qquad\qquad \oplus = \lambda x\,y.\ rec\ x\ y\ (\lambda u\,v.\ suc\ v) \\ rec\ x\ 0\ (\lambda u.\ suc) = x \\ rec\ y\ x\ (\lambda u.\ suc) = rec\ x\ y\ (\lambda u.\ suc) \\ rec\ y\ (suc\ x)\ (\lambda u.\ suc) = suc\ (rec\ y\ x\ (\lambda u.\ suc)) \\ rec\ x\ (rec\ y\ z\ (\lambda u.\ suc))\ (\lambda u.\ suc) = rec\ y\ (rec\ x\ z\ (\lambda u.\ suc))\ (\lambda u.\ suc) \end{array} \right\}.$$

This again produces a rewrite system which is already ground convergent.

# 5   Automating Theory Exploration

IsaScheme is an automated theory exploration system for the interactive theorem prover Isabelle. IsaScheme is implemented in Standard ML (SML) where most of the functions used are supplied by Isabelle's ML function library. These functions are broadly composed by unification and matching for terms and types, type inference, parsing facilities for terms, types and tactics, parsing facilities for new user defined Isar commands, access to definitional packages such as the function package [12] and access to counter-example checkers such as Quickcheck [7], Nitpick [4] and Refute.

The architecture and design of IsaScheme closely follows the presentation of the theory detailed in section 3 and is ilustrated in figure 1. Control flows between three core modules that implement the synthesis of conjectures and definitions (Synthesis module), normalisation of terms and the associated ground completion algorithm (Normalisation module), and the filtering of conjectures and definitions using subsumption and counter-example checking (Identification module).

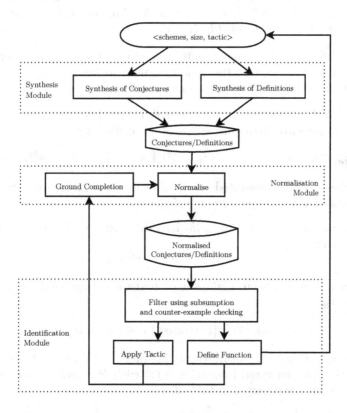

**Fig. 1.** The flow control between modularised components in IsaScheme

## 5.1   Synthesis of Conjectures and Definitions

Our implementation of the synthesis of conjectures and definitions is based on *schemes*. A scheme is a higher-order formula intended to generate, via substitution, new definitions of the underlying theory and conjectures about them. However, not every higher-order formula is a scheme. Here, we formally define schemes.

**Definition 3.** *A* **scheme** *$s$ is a (non-recursive) constant definition of a proposition in HOL, $s_n \equiv \lambda \overline{x}. t$, which we write in the form $s_n \ \overline{x} \equiv t$.*

For the scheme $s_n \ \overline{x} \equiv t$, $\overline{x}$ are free variables and $t : bool$ does not contain $s_n$, does not refer to undefined symbols and does not introduce extra free variables. The scheme (where $dvd$ means "divides") $prime \ P \equiv 1 < P \wedge ((dvd \ M \ P) \rightarrow M = 1 \vee M = P)$ is flawed because it introduces the extra free variable $M$ on the right hand side. The correct version is $prime \ P \equiv 1 < P \wedge (\forall m. (dvd \ m \ P) \rightarrow m = 1 \vee m = P)$ assuming that all symbols are properly defined.

**Definition 4.** *We say that a scheme $s := s_n \ \overline{x} \equiv t$ is a* **definitional scheme** *if $t$ has the form $\exists \overline{f} \ \forall \overline{y} \ \wedge_{i=1}^{m} l_i = r_i$ and the head of each $l_i \in \overline{f}$. The* **defining equations** *of $s$ are then denoted by $l_1 = r_1, \ldots, l_m = r_m$.*

See [20,21] for examples (and counter-examples) of schemes and definitional schemes. In order to describe the technique used to instantiate schemes automatically, here we define some preliminary concepts.

**Definition 5.** *For a scheme $s := u \equiv v$ with $\mathcal{V}(s) = \{x_1 : A_1, \ldots, x_n : A_n\}$, the set of* **schematic substitutions** *with size $i$ is defined by:*

$$Sub(s, i) := \{\sigma \mid \sigma = \{x_1 \mapsto t_1 \in \Lambda_i^{\emptyset}(A_1), \ldots, x_n \mapsto t_n \in \Lambda_i^{\emptyset}(A_n)\}\}.$$

For a scheme $s$, the generated schematic substitutions are used to produce instantiations of $s$; i.e. conjectures or definitions.

**Definition 6.** *Given $\sigma \in Sub(s, i)$, the* **instantiation of the scheme** *$s := u \equiv v$ with $\sigma$ is defined by*

$$inst(u \equiv v, \sigma) := \sigma(v).$$

**Definition 7.** *For a scheme $s$, the* **set of instantiations** *$Insts(s, i)$ with size $i$ is denoted by*

$$Insts(s, i) := \{inst(s, \sigma) \mid \sigma \in Sub(s, i)\}.$$

*Example 2.* Let $\mathcal{F}$ be a signature consisting of $\mathcal{F} = \{+ : nat \rightarrow nat \rightarrow nat\}$. The instantiations generated from scheme (1) with $P : ((nat \rightarrow nat \rightarrow nat) \rightarrow nat \rightarrow nat \rightarrow nat$ are depicted in table 3.

$$\begin{pmatrix} scheme \ P \ \equiv \\ \forall x \, y. \ x + y = P \ x \ y \ + \end{pmatrix} \tag{1}$$

**Table 3.** The instantiations induced by scheme (1) with size 8

| $Sub(s, X)$ | $Insts(s, X)$ |
|---|---|
| $\sigma_1 = \{P \mapsto (\lambda x\, y\, z.\, x)\}$ | $\forall x\, y.\ x + y = x$ |
| $\sigma_2 = \{P \mapsto (\lambda x\, y\, z.\, y)\}$ | $\forall x\, y.\ x + y = y$ |
| $\sigma_3 = \{P \mapsto (\lambda x\, y\, z.\, z\, x\, x)\}$ | $\forall x\, y.\ x + y = x + x$ |
| $\sigma_4 = \{P \mapsto (\lambda x\, y\, z.\, z\, y\, y)\}$ | $\forall x\, y.\ x + y = y + y$ |
| $\sigma_5 = \{P \mapsto (\lambda x\, y\, z.\, z\, x\, y)\}$ | $\forall x\, y.\ x + y = x + y$ |
| $\sigma_6 = \{P \mapsto (\lambda x\, y\, z.\, z\, y\, x)\}$ | $\forall x\, y.\ x + y = y + x$ |

**Table 4.** The instantiations induced by definitional scheme (2) with size 8

| $Sub(s, X)$ | $Insts(s, X)$ |
|---|---|
| $\sigma_1 = \{P \mapsto (\lambda x\, y\, z.\, x)\}$ | $\exists f.\ \forall x\, y.\ \bigwedge \begin{cases} f\ 0\ y\ = y \\ f\ (s\ x)\ y = s\ x \end{cases}$ |
| $\sigma_2 = \{P \mapsto (\lambda x\, y\, z.\, y)\}$ | $\exists f.\ \forall x\, y.\ \bigwedge \begin{cases} f\ 0\ y\ = y \\ f\ (s\ x)\ y = s\ y \end{cases}$ |
| $\sigma_3 = \{P \mapsto (\lambda x\, y\, z.\, z\, x\, x)\}$ | $\exists f.\ \forall x\, y.\ \bigwedge \begin{cases} f\ 0\ y\ = y \\ f\ (s\ x)\ y = s\ (f\ x\ x) \end{cases}$ |
| $\sigma_4 = \{P \mapsto (\lambda x\, y\, z.\, z\, y\, y)\}$ | $\exists f.\ \forall x\, y.\ \bigwedge \begin{cases} f\ 0\ y\ = y \\ f\ (s\ x)\ y = s\ (f\ y\ y) \end{cases}$ |
| $\sigma_5 = \{P \mapsto (\lambda x\, y\, z.\, z\, x\, y)\}$ | $\exists f.\ \forall x\, y.\ \bigwedge \begin{cases} f\ 0\ y\ = y \\ f\ (s\ x)\ y = s\ (f\ x\ y) \end{cases}$ |
| $\sigma_6 = \{P \mapsto (\lambda x\, y\, z.\, z\, y\, x)\}$ | $\exists f.\ \forall x\, y.\ \bigwedge \begin{cases} f\ 0\ y\ = y \\ f\ (s\ x)\ y = s\ (f\ y\ x) \end{cases}$ |

*Example 3.* Let $\mathcal{F}$ be a signature consisting of $\mathcal{F} = \{0 : nat, s : nat \to nat\}$. The instantiations generated from definitional scheme (2) with $P : (nat \to nat \to (nat \to nat \to nat) \to nat$ are depicted in table 4.

$$\left( \begin{array}{l} def\text{-}scheme\ P \equiv \\[4pt] \quad \exists f.\ \forall x\, y.\ \bigwedge \begin{cases} f\ 0\ y\ = y \\ f\ (s\ x)\ y = s\ (P\ x\ y\ f) \end{cases} \end{array} \right) \tag{2}$$

## 5.2   Normalization Module

The normalisation module consists of two main components. A component responsible for the normalisation of instantiations and a component that performs the ground completion of a rewrite system.

The normalisation of instantiations component takes as input an instantiation generated by the technique described in Section 5.1. This instantiation is then normalised w.r.t. a rewrite system generated by the component that performs completion. The normalisation process consists on exhaustive rewriting using Isabelle's Simplifier [23]. Ordered rewriting is performed by simplification procedures. Simplification procedures, also called simprocs, implement custom simplification procedures that are triggered by the Simplifier on a specific term-pattern and rewrite a term according to a theorem. IsaScheme uses simprocs to handle permutative rules as they potentially loops.

The component performing the ground completion algorithm of a rewrite system takes as input a set of equations (possibly empty) and a new theorem/equation to be added to the rewrite system. All function symbols $c_1, c_2, \ldots, c_n$ are then extracted from the equations and a precedence on the set of equations (discarding permutative rules) $c_1' \sim_1 c_2' \ldots \sim_{n-1} c_n', \sim_i \in \{>, \equiv\}$ is found such that the induced recursive path ordering is compatible with the equations.

Instead of enumerating all possible precedences of $n$ function symbols, namely all linear orderings, we encode the problem into a set of linear inequalities in HOL and then we call the counter-example checker Refute to determine the satisfiability of the formula. Refute then translates the formula into propositional logic and calls different SAT Solvers which usually solve the satisfiability problem in under a second. Empirical results show the efficiency of the approach as opposed to enumerating the possible precedences.

The inference rules *Deduction*, *Simplification* and *Deletion* for ground completion from Section 3 are then applied to the set of equations using the recursive path ordering found by the SAT Solvers. IsaScheme mixes the inference rules according to the strategy $((Simplification + Deletion)^*; Deduction)^*$. If the exhaustive application of the inference rules succeeds then a ground convergent rewrite system $R$ is produced. The rewrite system $R$ is then stored globally so that other modules and components of the system can access the ground convergent rewrite system.

The ground completion algorithm, described in Section 3, is potentially non-terminating as is shown in Section 6. IsaScheme uses timeouts in this critical execution part to avoid non-termination. If a timeout in completion is reached, IsaScheme runs completion without the *Deduction* rule, thus producing a potentially non-ground convergent rewrite system.

### 5.3   Identification Module

Our implementation of the Identification Module is mainly composed by three components: filtering of conjectures and definitions, the application of tactics, and the definition of new recursive functions.

Two different schematic substitutions $\sigma_1$ and $\sigma_2$ can produce equivalent instantiations. For this reason IsaScheme stores the normal forms of the instantiations produced by the synthesis Module. Whenever a new normalised instantiation is produced, IsaScheme checks if the instantiation was not previously generated and filters it accordingly. IsaScheme uses existing Isabelle tools such as discrimination nets and matching to provide a fast and economic subsumption of instantiations. All instances of already proved theorems are discarded by IsaScheme.

Counter-example checking is then applied at non-filtered conjectures. For this we use Quickcheck and Nitpick as they usually provide a good range of applicability for conjectures involving recursive functions and datatypes. In case a conjecture is not rejected by counter-example checking a proof attempt is performed with a tactic supplied by the user. IsaScheme uses existing Isabelle parsers to parse proof methods and they are then used to discharge proof obligations. These proof obligations include the conjectures not filtered by subsumption and counter-example checking, the detection of *argument neglecting functions* and the detection of *equivalent definitions* (see [20,21]) during the exploration of the theory. Unfalsified and unproven conjectures are kept in cache and they are revisited every time a new proof is found.

As described in Section 5.1, definitional schemes are used to generate new recursive definitions. However, definitional schemes could generate non-terminating functions. For this reason, IsaScheme uses Isabelle's function package to safely define general recursive function definitions.

Definitional instantiations not filtered by subsumption are sent to the function package to test for well-definedness. Since the exploration process could generate a substantial number of definitions and each of them could potentially produce a multitude of conjectures, IsaScheme filters out recursive functions that ignore one or more of their arguments, so call *argument neglecting functions*. IsaScheme also checks whether the new definition is equivalent to a previously defined function and discards it accordingly. The defining equations of not filtered well-defined functions are then added to the global rewrite system to exploit them during normalisation.

# 6    Limitations and Further Work

The completion algorithm described in section 3 attempts to construct a ground convergent rewrite system from a given set of equations. However, completion can fail in an infinite execution of rules *Deduction, Simplification* and *Deletion*. An example of non-termination of completion is described with the theory $\{f\ (g\ (f\ x)) = f\ (g\ x)\}$ and the recursive path ordering $\succ$ induced by the precedence $g > f$. Here, rules *Deduction, Simplification* and *Deletion* are non-terminating and yield an incremental rewrite system of the form

$$\left\{ \begin{array}{c} f\ (g\ (f\ x)) = f\ (g\ x) \\ \vdots \\ f\ (g^n\ (f\ x)) = f\ (g^n\ x) \end{array} \right\}.$$

Another example of non-termination of completion is described with the theory $\{(x * y) * z = x * (y * z),\ x * y = y * x,\ i\ (x * x) = 1\}$ as there is no equivalent ground complete ordered rewriting system as any such system would have to contain infinitely many equations to deal with $i\ (a * a)$, $i\ (a * (a * (b * b)))$, $i\ (a * (a * (a * (a * (b * b)))))$ and so on.

In fact, IsaScheme uses timeouts in critical executions parts such as completion to avoid non-termination. If a timeout in completion is reached, IsaScheme runs completion without the *Deduction* rule, thus producing a potentially non-ground convergent rewrite system. Better strategies to deal with non-termination of completion such as infinitary rewriting [3] are, however, interesting further work.

# 7  Conclusion

We have outlined a theory exploration algorithm based on ground completion [17] capable of dealing with higher-order rewrite systems. It uses Martin's syntactic criterion to prove ground joinability [17] and Mayr's notion of higher-order critical pair [18]. This improves previous attempts to exploit non-orientable equations which results in the production of stronger normalization methods compared to those in [20,21]. We have implemented the aforementioned techniques in a tool called IsaScheme developed on top of Isabelle/HOL [22].

# References

1. Avenhaus, J., Hillenbrand, T., Löchner, B.: On using ground joinable equations in equational theorem proving. Journal of Symbolic Computation 36(1-2), 217–233 (2003); First Order Theorem Proving.
2. Baader, F., Nipkow, T.: Term Rewriting and All That. Cambridge University Press (1998)
3. Bahr, P.: Partial order infinitary term rewriting and böhm trees. In: Lynch, C. (ed.) Proceedings of the 21st International Conference on Rewriting Techniques and Applications, Dagstuhl, Germany. Leibniz International Proceedings in Informatics (LIPIcs), vol. 6, pp. 67–84. Schloss Dagstuhl–Leibniz-Zentrum fuer Informatik (2010)
4. Blanchette, J.C., Nipkow, T.: Nitpick: A counterexample generator for higher-order logic based on a relational model finder. In: Kaufmann, M., Paulson, L.C. (eds.) ITP 2010. LNCS, vol. 6172, pp. 131–146. Springer, Heidelberg (2010)
5. Buchberger, B.: Algorithm Invention and Verification by Lazy Thinking. In: Petcu, D., Negru, V., Zaharie, D., Jebelean, T. (eds.) Proceedings of SYNASC 2003, 5th International Workshop on Symbolic and Numeric Algorithms for Scientific Computing Timisoara, Timisoara, Romania, October 1-4, pp. 2–26. Mirton Publisher (2003)
6. Buchberger, B., Craciun, A.: Algorithm synthesis by lazy thinking: Using problem schemes. In: Petcu, D., Negru, V., Zaharie, D., Jebelean, T. (eds.) Proceedings of SYNASC 2004, 6th International Symposium on Symbolic and Numeric Algorithms for Scientific Computing, Timisoara, Romania, pp. 90–106. Mirton Publisher (2004)
7. Claessen, K., Hughes, J.: Quickcheck: a lightweight tool for random testing of Haskell programs. In: ICFP 2000: Proceedings of the Fifth ACM SIGPLAN International Conference on Functional Programming, pp. 268–279. ACM, New York (2000)
8. Claessen, K., Johansson, M., Rosén, D., Smallbone, N.: Automating inductive proofs using theory exploration. In: Bonacina, M.P. (ed.) CADE 2013. LNCS, vol. 7898, pp. 392–406. Springer, Heidelberg (2013)

9. Colton, S.: Automated Theory Formation in Pure Mathematics. PhD thesis, Division of Informatics, University of Edinburgh (2001)
10. Johansson, M.: Automated Discovery of Inductive Lemmas. PhD thesis, School of Informatics, University of Edinburgh (2009)
11. Johansson, M., Dixon, L., Bundy, A.: Conjecture synthesis for inductive theories. Journal of Automated Reasoning (2010) (accepted for publication, to appear)
12. Krauss, A.: Automating Recursive Definitions and Termination Proofs in Higher-Order Logic. PhD thesis, Dept. of Informatics, T. U. München (2009)
13. Lenat, D.B.: AM: An artificial intelligence approach to discovery in mathematics as heuristic search. In: Knowledge-Based Systems in Artificial Intelligence. McGraw Hill, New York (1982); Stanford as TechReport AIM 286
14. Lin, Y., Bundy, A., Grov, G.: The use of rippling to automate event-b invariant preservation proofs. In: Goodloe, A.E., Person, S. (eds.) NFM 2012. LNCS, vol. 7226, pp. 231–236. Springer, Heidelberg (2012)
15. Llano, M.T., Ireland, A., Pease, A.: Discovery of invariants through automated theory formation. In: Refine, pp. 1–19 (2011)
16. Maclean, E., Ireland, A., Grov, G.: The core system: Animation and functional correctness of pointer programs. In: International Conference on Automated Software Engineering, pp. 588–591 (2011)
17. Martin, U., Nipkow, T.: Ordered rewriting and confluence. In: Stickel, M.E. (ed.) CADE 1990. LNCS, vol. 449, pp. 366–380. Springer, Heidelberg (1990)
18. Mayr, R., Nipkow, T.: Higher-order rewrite systems and their confluence. Theoretical Computer Science 192, 3–29 (1998)
19. McCasland, R., Bundy, A., Smith, P.: Ascertaining mathematical theorems. In: Carette, J., William, W., Farmer, M. (eds.) Proceedings of Calculemus 2005, Newcastle, UK (2005)
20. Montano-Rivas, O., McCasland, R., Dixon, L., Bundy, A.: Scheme-based synthesis of inductive theories. In: Sidorov, G., Hernández Aguirre, A., Reyes García, C.A. (eds.) MICAI 2010, Part I. LNCS, vol. 6437, pp. 348–361. Springer, Heidelberg (2010)
21. Montano-Rivas, O., McCasland, R., Dixon, L., Bundy, A.: Scheme-based theorem discovery and concept invention. Expert Systems with Applications 39(2), 1637–1646 (2012)
22. Nipkow, T., Paulson, L.C., Wenzel, M.T.: Isabelle/HOL. LNCS, vol. 2283. Springer, Heidelberg (2002)
23. Paulson, L.C.: A higher-order implementation of rewriting. Science of Computer Programming 3, 119–149 (1983)
24. Rubio, A., Nieuwenhuis, R.: A total ac-compatible ordering based on rpo. Theoretical Computer Science 142, 209–227 (1995)
25. Sutcliffe, G., Gao, Y., Colton, S.: A Grand Challenge of Theorem Discovery (June 2003)
26. Walukiewicz, D.: A total AC-compatible reduction ordering on higher-order terms. In: Larsen, K.G., Skyum, S., Winskel, G. (eds.) ICALP 1998. LNCS, vol. 1443, pp. 530–542. Springer, Heidelberg (1998)

# Possibilistic Minimal Models for Possibilistic Normal Programs

Rubén Octavio Vélez Salazar, José Arrazola Ramírez,
and Iván Martínez Ruiz

Benémerita Universidad Autónoma de Puebla

**Abstract.** In this paper we present possibilistic minimal models for possibilistic normal programs, we relate them to the possibilistic $C_\omega$ logic, $PC_\omega L$, and to minimal models of normal logic programs. Possibilistic stable models for possibilistic normal programs have been presented previously, but we present a more general type. We also characterize the provability of possibilistic atoms from possibilistic normal programs in terms of $PC_\omega L$.

## 1 Introduction

Minimal models have been thoroughly studied. In fact, there are subclasses of these models: the subclass of Answer Set Programming [6,4] and the subclass of Pstable models [9], which have been widely accepted by researchers who develop Logic Programming. Their success lies in the fact that they have constituted a suitable formalism in representing a wide variety of problems in Artificial Intelligence which include incomplete information, non-monotonic reasoning, etc. They have also turned out to be an excellent paradigm in solving combinatoric problems [1]. The main idea in using minimal models is to obtain the essential information modeled by a logic program. In this paper, we generalize the concept of minimal models to the field of possibilistic logic by defining possibilistic minimal models for possibilistic normal logic programs, adding the ability to handle uncertainty in the information modeled by the logic programs.

Uncertainty is an attribute of information. The pioneering work of Claude Shannon [17] on Information Theory led to the universal acceptance that information is statistical in nature. As a consequence, dealing with uncertainty was confined to the Theory of Probability.

Tversky and Kahneman observed in [18], that many decisions we make in our common life are based on beliefs concerning the likelihood of uncertain events. In fact, we commonly use statements such as "I think that...", "chances are...", "it is probable that...", "it is plausible that...", etc., for supporting our decisions. In these kinds of statements we usually appeal to our experience or our commonsense. It is not surprising to think that a reasoning based on these kinds of statements could reach biased conclusions. However, these conclusions could also reflect the experience or commonsense of an expert.

F. Castro, A. Gelbukh, and M. González (Eds.): MICAI 2013, Part I, LNAI 8265, pp. 110–119, 2013.

Pelletier and Elio [15] pointed out that people simply have tendencies to ignore certain information because of the (evolutionary) necessity to make decisions quickly. This gives rise to biases in judgments concerning what they really want to do. In view of the fact that we know that a reasoning based on statements which are quantified by relative likelihoods could capture our experience or our commonsense, the question is: how could these statements be captured by real application systems, like Multi Agent Systems? For those steeped in probability, Halpern [7] has remarked that probability has its problems.

Didier Dubois et. al. [3] presented *Possibilistic Logic*, which enables handling information with uncertainty. Their logic is based on the Theory of Possibility of Zadeh [19]. The paper by Dubois et. al. [3], included an axiomatization for Possibilistic Logic and an extended resolution-based method which is viable for computer implementation.

According to Nicolas et. al. [11], Possibilistic Logic provides a sound and complete machinery for handling qualitative uncertainty with respect to a semantics expressed by means of possibility distributions which rank order the possible interpretations. Nicolas mentions that in possibilistic logic one deals with uncertainty by means of classical two-valued (true or false) interpretations that can be more or less certain, more or less possible. Possibilistic Logic is not concerned to deal with vague representations in a multi-valued framework but instead, it stays in the framework of classical logic to which it adds a way to graduate the confidence it has in each proposed information[11].

Also in [11], a combination between Answer Set Programming (ASP) [1] and Possibilistic Logic [3] was proposed. This framework is able to deal with reasoning that is non-monotonic as well as uncertain. Nicolas' approach is based on the concept of a possibilistic stable model which defines a semantics for possibilistic normal logic programs. One weak point of this approach is that it relies on the expressiveness of normal logic programs.

Paraconsistent Logic has become important to the area of computer science since the publication of a paper by David Pearce [14], in which a link between the class of intermediate logics and Answer Set Programming (ASP) is established[10], [12].

Considering the importance of the minimal models in combination with its usefulness within the context of paraconsistent logic $C_\omega$, and the need for a better way of handling uncertain information we present the *Possibilistic $C_\omega$ Logic.*

First in Section 2, we present some background on both $C_\omega$ Logic and Possibilistic $C_\omega$ Logic. Then, in Section 3, we present some known results on normal logic programs and the deduction of atoms. On Section 4 we discuss briefly some consequences and applications of previous results to possibilistic normal programs. Finally, in Section 5 we give the conclusions and present some ideas for future work.

# 2    Background

In this section we first introduce the syntax of logic formulas considered in this paper. Then we present a few basic definitions of how logics can be built to interpret the meaning of such formulas in order to, finally, give a brief introduction to several of the logics that are relevant for the results of our later sections.

## 2.1    Syntax of Formulas

We consider a formal (propositional) language built from: an enumerable set $L$ of elements called *atoms* (denoted $a$, $b$, $c$, ...); the binary connectives $\land$ (*conjunction*), $\lor$ (*disjunction*) and $\rightarrow$ (*implication*); and the unary connective $\neg$ (*negation*). Formulas (denoted $A$, $B$, $C$, ...) are constructed as usual by combining these basic connectives together.

A *theory* is just a set of formulas and, in this paper, we only consider finite theories. Moreover, if $T$ is a theory, we use the notation $\mathscr{L}_T$ to stand for the set of atoms that occur in the theory $T$.

Note, however, that the logic connectives that we have just introduced have no meaning by themselves. The names of the connectives (e.g. "disjunction" or "negation") do state some intuition of what the symbol is *intended* to mean, but their *formal meaning* can only be given through a formally defined semantics. Even more confusingly, different semantics might assign different meanings to the same symbol. To avoid possible ambiguities, we sometimes use subscripts to distinguish such connectives, e.g. the symbols $\land_X$ and $\land_Y$ are two different conjunction connectives as defined by the logics $X$ and $Y$ respectively. The subscript might be dropped if the relevant logic is clear by context, or if the formula is actually parametrized by an unspecified logic and is intended to be evaluated under several different semantics.

## 2.2    Logic Systems

We consider a *logic* simply as a set of formulas that, moreover, satisfies the following two properties: (i) is closed under *modus ponens* (i.e. if $A$ and $A \rightarrow B$ are in the logic, then also $B$ is) and (ii) is closed under substitution (i.e. if a formula $A$ is in the logic, then any other formula obtained by replacing all occurrences of an atom $b$ in $A$ with another formula $B$ is still in the logic). The elements of a logic are called *theorems* and the notation $\vdash_X A$ is used to state that the formula $A$ is a theorem of $X$ (i.e. $A \in X$). We say that a logic $X$ is *weaker than or equal to* a logic $Y$ if $X \subseteq Y$, similarly we say that $X$ is *stronger than or equal to* $Y$ if $Y \subseteq X$.

*Hilbert Style Proof Systems.* There are many different approaches that have been used to specify the meaning of logic formulas or, in other words, to define *logics*. In Hilbert style proof systems, also known as axiomatic systems, a logic is specified by giving a set of axioms (which is usually assumed to be closed by substitution). This set of axioms specifies, so to speak, the "kernel" of the logic. The actual logic is obtained when this "kernel" is closed with respect to the inference rule of modus ponens.

The notation $\vdash_X F$ for provability of a logic formula $F$ in the logic $X$ is usually extended within Hilbert style systems, given a theory $T$, using $T \vdash_X F$ to denote the fact that the formula $F$ can be derived from the axioms of the logic and the formulas contained in $T$ by a sequence of applications of modus ponens.

### 2.3 Brief Survey of Logics

In this subsection we present a Hilbert style definition of the paraconsistent logic $C_\omega$, with a few notes.

**Definition 1.** $C_\omega$ *is defined by the following set of axioms and modus ponens as the only rule of inference:*

*Pos 1:* $A \rightarrow (B \rightarrow A)$
*Pos 2:* $(A \rightarrow (B \rightarrow C)) \rightarrow ((A \rightarrow B) \rightarrow (A \rightarrow C))$
*Pos 3:* $A \wedge B \rightarrow A$
*Pos 4:* $A \wedge B \rightarrow B$
*Pos 5:* $A \rightarrow (B \rightarrow (A \wedge B))$
*Pos 6:* $A \rightarrow (A \vee B)$
*Pos 7:* $B \rightarrow (A \vee B)$
*Pos 8:* $(A \rightarrow C) \rightarrow ((B \rightarrow C) \rightarrow (A \vee B \rightarrow C))$ $C_\omega 1$: $A \vee \neg A$
$C_\omega 2$: $\neg\neg A \rightarrow A$

The $C_\omega$ logic is considered the weakest paraconsistent logic, see [2]. Let us note that $A \vee \neg A$ is a theorem of $C_\omega$ (it is even an axiom of the logic), while the formula $(\neg A \wedge A) \rightarrow b$ is not. This non-theorem shows one of the motivations of paraconsistent logics: they allow some degree of inconsistency.

### 2.4 Possibilistic $C_\omega$ Logic ($PC_\omega L$)

The following definitions can be found in [3], to which the reader is referred for further details.

A *necessity-valued* formula is a pair $(A\ \alpha)$, where $A$ is a classical propositional formula and $\alpha \in (0, 1]$. $(A\ \alpha)$ expresses that $A$ is certain to the extent $\alpha$, that is, $N(A) \geq \alpha$, where $N$ is a necessity measure which models our state of knowledge. The constant $\alpha$ is known as the *valuation* of the formula and is represented as $val(A)$.

A necessity valued knowledge base (or simply, a possibilistic knowledge base) $\mathcal{F}$ is defined as a finite set (that is, a conjunction) of necessity valued formulas. We denote by $\mathcal{F}^*$ the set of classical formulas obtained from $\mathcal{F}$ by ignoring the weights of the formulas, that is, if $\mathcal{F} = \{(A_i\ \alpha_i) : i = 1, \ldots, n\}$ then, $\mathcal{F}^* = \{A_i : i = 1, \ldots, n\}$. We call $\mathcal{F}^*$ the *classical projection* of $\mathcal{F}$.

In [3], an axiomatic system for Possibilistic Logic ($PL$) is proposed. We now present the axioms for Possibilistic Paraconsistent $C_\omega$-Logic ($PC_\omega L$).

**Definition 2.** *We define Possibilistic Paraconsistent $C_\omega$-Logic ($PC_\omega L$) by means of the set of axioms $\{(A\ 1) \mid A$ is an axiom of $C_\omega\}$, together with the following rules of inference:*

$$(GMP)\ (A\ \alpha), (A \to B\ \beta) \vdash_{PC_\omega L} (B\ \min\{\alpha, \beta\})$$
$$(S)\ \ \ \ (A\ \alpha) \vdash_{PC_\omega L} (A\ \beta)\ \text{if } \alpha \geq \beta.$$

It is not difficult to verify that $(A \wedge B \to C\ \alpha) \equiv (B \to (A \to C)\ \alpha)$ in $PC_\omega L$ and that the transitivity of implication is also valid in $PC_\omega L$, i.e.

$$(A \to B\ \ \alpha), (B \to C\ \ \beta) \vdash_{PC_\omega L} (A \to C\ \ \min\{\alpha, \beta\}).$$

## 3 Normal Programs

A Normal Logic Program or Normal Program is a finite set of normal clauses, which are formulas that have the form:

$$\bigwedge_{j=1}^{m} b_j \wedge \bigwedge_{k=1}^{l} \neg c_k \to a,$$

where $a$, $b_j$ and $c_k$ are atoms.

A Possibilistic Normal Program is a finite set of possibilistic normal clauses, which are possibilistic formulas that have the form: $(A\ \alpha)$, where $A$ is a normal clause and $\alpha \in (0, 1]$.

### 3.1 Resolution

*Resolution* is an inference rule that generalizes *modus ponens*. For propositional formulas in conjunctive normal form, it is based on just one inference rule namely:

$$\frac{A \vee c \quad B \vee \neg c}{A \vee B}\ Res$$

The following inference rules appear when we study resolution techniques applied to normal programs.

**Definition 3.** *[8] The following are rules of inference for Normal Programs known as Rule G, Rule Ca and Rule R, respectively.*

$$\frac{A \wedge d \to x \quad B \to d}{A \wedge B \to x}\ G \qquad \frac{A \wedge c \to x \quad B \wedge \neg c \to x}{A \wedge B \to x}\ Ca$$

$$\frac{A \wedge c \to x \quad B \wedge \neg c \to y}{\neg y \wedge A \wedge B \to x}\ R$$

*where $x$, $y$, $c$ and $d$ are atoms, and the formulas $A, B$ represent arbitrary conjunctions of literals.*

In the following theorems [8], let $C$ denote classical logic and let $\vdash_{GCaR}$ denote deduction using the rules written in the subscript.

**Theorem 1.** *[8] Let $P$ be a Normal Program and let $A$ be a normal formula. Then $P \vdash_C A$ if and only if $P \vdash_{GCaR} A$.*

**Theorem 2.** *[8] Let $P$ be a Normal Program and let $a$ be an atom. If $P \vdash_{GCaR} a$ then $P \vdash_{GCa} a$.*

Therefore, if $a$ is an atom then $P \vdash_C a$ if and only if $P \vdash_{GCaR} a$. So, combining these two theorems we have $P \vdash_C a$ if and only if $P \vdash_{GCa} a$.

In [16], the authors relate Rule G and Rule Ca to the paraconsistent logic $C_\omega$.

**Theorem 3.** *[16] Let $x$, $y$, $c$ and $d$ be atoms, and let the formulas $A, B$ represent an arbitrary conjunction of literals. Then*

$$A \wedge d \rightarrow x, B \rightarrow d \vdash_{C_\omega} A \wedge B \rightarrow x \text{ and}$$

$$A \wedge c \rightarrow x, B \wedge \neg c \rightarrow x \vdash_{C_\omega} A \wedge B \rightarrow x$$

**Corollary 1.** *If $P$ is a Normal Program and $a$ is an atom then $P \vdash_C a$ if and only if $P \vdash_{C_\omega} a$.*

*Proof.* The proof follows from Theorem 3 and the previous comments.

Our goal is to extend this result to the possibilistic case, which we do in Section 4.

### 3.2 Minimal Models for Normal Programs

Given the class of Normal Programs, a *semantic operator* is a function that assigns to each Normal Program $P$, some subset of $2^{\mathscr{L}_P}$, the power set of $\mathscr{L}_P$. These sets of atoms, which are called the *semantic models* of the program $P$, are usually some "preferred" subset of the classical (two-valued) models of $P$.

The simplest example of a semantic operator is the one of *classical models*, which merely maps each program to its standard two-valued models. Another more interesting example is the semantics of minimal models, see [?].

**Definition 4.** *Let $P$ be a Normal Program. A set of atoms $M$ is a minimal model of $P$ if $M$ is a classical model of $P$ and is minimal (with respect to set inclusion) among the other classical models of $P$. We use Min to denote the semantic operator of minimal models, i.e. $\text{Min}(P)$ is the set of minimal models of $P$.*

Minimal models for Normal Programs are characterized by the following result [13]], in which we write $\widetilde{M}$ to denote the complement of $M$, and define $\neg\widetilde{M} = \{\neg a \mid a \in \widetilde{M}\}$.

**Theorem 4.** *Let $P$ be a Normal Program and $M$ a set of atoms in $\mathscr{L}_P$. Then $M$ is a minimal model of $P$ if and only if $P \cup \neg\widetilde{M} \vdash_C M$.*

## 4    Contribution

We will extend results in the previous sections to possibilistic logics.

### 4.1    Normal Programs and the Provability of Possibilistic Atoms

We can extend the inference rules $G$ and $Ca$ in the following way, towards $PC_\omega L$ and normal logic programs:

**Theorem 5**

$$\frac{(A \wedge d \to x \ \alpha) \quad (B \to d \ \beta)}{(A \wedge B \to x \ min\{\alpha, \beta\})} \ G$$

$$\frac{(A \wedge c \to x \ \alpha) \quad (B \wedge \neg c \to x \ \beta)}{(A \wedge B \to x \ min\{\alpha, \beta\})} \ Ca$$

*where $x$, $y$, $c$ and $d$ are atoms, the formulas $A, B$ represent arbitrary conjunctions of literals and $\alpha, \beta$ in $(0, 1]$.*

*Proof.* The proof of the rule $G$ is as follows:

1. $(A \wedge d \to x \ \ \alpha)$                     Hypothesis
2. $(B \to d \ \ \beta)$                              Hypothesis
3. $(d \to (A \to x) \ \ \alpha)$                    Equivalence(1)
4. $(B \to (A \to x) \ \ min\{\alpha, \beta\})$      Transitivity(2,3)
5. $(A \wedge B \to x \ \ min\{\alpha, \beta\})$     Equivalence(4)

Now, we verify that the rule $Ca$ is also valid in $PC_\omega L$:

1. $(A \wedge c \to x \ \ \alpha)$                                                            Hypothesis
2. $(B \wedge A \wedge c \to A \wedge c \ \ 1)$                                               (Pos 4 1)
3. $(A \wedge B \wedge c \to x \ \ \alpha)$                                                   Transitivity(2,1)
4. $(B \wedge \neg c \to x \ \ \beta)$                                                        Hypothesis
5. $(A \wedge B \wedge \neg c \to B \wedge \neg c \ \ 1)$                                     (Pos 4 1)
6. $(A \wedge B \wedge \neg c \to x \ \ \beta)$                                               Transitivity(5,4)
7. $((A \wedge B \wedge c \to x) \to$
    $((A \wedge B \wedge \neg c \to x) \to ((A \wedge B \wedge c) \vee (A \wedge B \wedge \neg c) \to x)) \ \ 1)$ (Pos8 1)
8. $((A \wedge B \wedge \neg c \to x) \to ((A \wedge B \wedge c) \vee (A \wedge B \wedge \neg c) \to x) \ \ \alpha)$ GMP(3,7)
9. $((A \wedge B \wedge c) \vee (A \wedge B \wedge \neg c) \to x \ \ min\{\alpha, \beta\})$   GMP(6,8)
10. $((A \wedge B) \wedge (c \vee \neg c) \to x \ \ min\{\alpha, \beta\})$                    Distributive Property
11. $((c \vee \neg c) \to ((A \wedge B) \to x) \ \ min\{\alpha, \beta\})$                     Equivalence
12. $(c \vee \neg c \ 1)$                                                                     $(C_\omega 1 \ 1)$
13. $(A \wedge B \to x \ \ min\{\alpha, \beta\})$                                             GMP(11,12)

By Theorem 5 and Corollary 1 we have the following result, in which $PL$ denotes the standard Possibilistic Logic:

**Corollary 2.** *Let $P$ be a Possibilistic Normal Program and let $a$ be an atom. Then $P \vdash_{PL} (a \ \alpha)$ if and only if $P \vdash_{PC_\omega L} (a \ \alpha)$.*

## 4.2  Possibilistic Minimal Models for Possibilistic Normal Programs

We use the following concepts, which were presented in [5].

**Definition 5.** *Given a Possibilistic Normal Program $P$ and two subsets $M_1$ and $M_2$ of $\mathscr{L}_P$ (possibilistidc atoms), we say that $M_1 \preceq M_2$ if the following two conditions hold:*

1. *$M_1^* \subseteq M_2^*$,*
2. *For every $(a\ \alpha) \in M_2$, if $(a\ \beta) \in M_1$ then $\alpha < \beta$.*

One can verify that $\preceq$ is a partial order in $2^{\mathscr{L}_P}$.

**Definition 6.** *Given a Possibilistic Normal Program $P$ we define the inconsistency degree of $P$ by $Incon(P) = max\ \{\alpha : P \vdash_{PC_\omega L} (\perp \alpha)\}$, where $\perp$ is the logical constant bottom. When $Incon(P) = 0$ we say that $P$ is consistent (or $PC_\omega L$ consistent).*

**Definition 7.** *Given a Possibilistic Normal Program $P$ and a subset $M$ of $\mathscr{L}_P$, we say that $M$ is a Possibilistic Minimal Model of $P$,*

1. *For any $(a\ \alpha), (a\ \beta) \in M$, we have $\alpha = \beta$.*
2. *$Incons(P \cup (\neg\widetilde{M^*}\ 1)) = 0$, and $P \cup (\neg\widetilde{M^*}\ 1) \vdash_{PC_\omega L} M$.*
3. *If $M$ is minimal with respect to the relation $\preceq$ among all the sets of atoms that satisfy the previous two conditions.*

We use $PMin$ to denote the semantic operator of possibilistic minimal models, i.e. $PMin(P)$ is the set of minimal models of possibilistic normal program $P$.

**Theorem 6.** *If $P$ is a Possibilistic Normal Program and $M \subseteq \mathscr{L}_P$, then $M \in PMin(P)$ implies that $M^* \in Min(P^*)$.*

*Proof.* Let $M \in PMin(P)$. By Definition 7, we have $P \cup (\neg\widetilde{M^*}\ 1) \vdash_{PC_\omega L} M$, which implies that $P^* \cup \neg\widetilde{M^*} \vdash_{C_\omega} M^*$. Now, by Theorem 4 we have that $M^*$ is a minimal model of $P^*$, so $M^* \in Min(P^*)$.

The reciprocal of the previous theorem is not true. If

$$P = \{(\neg a \to b\ 0.6), (\neg b \to a\ 0.3)\}$$

and $M = \{(a\ 0.7)\}$, then $M^*$ is a minimal model of $P^*$, but $P \cup (\neg\widetilde{M^*}\ 1) \nvdash_{PC_\omega L} (a\ 0.7)$. Nevertheless, we may construct a possibilisitic model of $P$ the following way.

**Theorem 7.** *Let $P$ be a Possibilistic Normal Program and $M \subseteq \mathscr{L}_P$ such that $M^* \in Min(P^*)$. If*

$$N = \{(a\ \alpha) \mid a \in M \text{ and } \alpha = max\{\beta \mid P \cup (\neg\widetilde{M^*}\ 1) \vdash_{PC_\omega L} (a\ \beta)\}\}$$

*then $N \in PMin(P)$.*

*Proof.* Let $N$ be defined as above.

1. By the definition of $N$ we have that for any $(a\ \alpha), (a\ \beta) \in N$, we have $\alpha = \beta$.
2. By the hypothesis and Theorem 4 we have that $P^* \cup \neg \widetilde{M}^*$ is consistent. Therefore, $\mathrm{Incons}\left(P \cup (\neg \widetilde{N^*}\ 1)\right) = 0$, since $N^* = M^*$. Also, by the definition of $N$, we have that $P \cup (\neg \widetilde{N^*}\ 1) \vdash_{PC_\omega L} N$.
3. By the definition of $N$, there is no $N_1 \in \mathscr{L}_P$ such that for any $(a\ \alpha) \in M$ we have $P \cup (\neg \widetilde{N_1^*}\ 1) \vdash_{PC_\omega L} (a\ \alpha)$ and $N_1 \preceq N$. Therefore, $N$ is $\preceq$ – minimal.

## 5   Conclusion

We have defined the concept of possibilistic minimal models for possibilistic normal programs, establishing a methodology to find them, by generalizing the rules $Ca$ and $G$. Also, we have proved the non-existence of a bijective correspondence between the possibilistic minimal models for possibilistic normal programs and the minimal models for normal programs. Our next step is to extend our results to stable and Pstable semantics for possibilistic logic programs.

**Acknowledgements.** The authors wish to acknowledge support from Vicerrectoría de Investigación y Posgrado de la Benemérita Universidad Autónoma de Puebla, under the project named "Aplicaciones de Teoría de Modelos en Lógica y Topología."

## References

1. Baral, C.: Knowledge representation, reasoning and declarative problem solving. Cambridge University Press (2003)
2. da Costa, N.C.A.: On the theory of inconsistent formal systems. Notre Dame Journal of Formal Logic 15(4), 497–510 (1974)
3. Dubois, D., Lang, J., Prade, H.: Possibilistic logic. In: Handbook of Logic in Artificial Intelligence and Logic Programming, vol. 3, pp. 439–513. Oxford University Press, Inc., New York (1994)
4. Erdogan, S.T., Lifschitz, V.: Definitions in answer set programming. In: Lifschitz, V., Niemelä, I. (eds.) Proceedings of International Conference on Logic Programming and Nonmonotonic Reasoning (LPNMR), pp. 114–126 (2004)
5. Estrada-Estrada, O.H., Arrazola-Ramírez, J.R.E., Osorio-Galindo, M.J.: Possibilistic intermediate logic. Int. J. Adv. Intell. Paradigms 4(2), 149–167 (2012)
6. Gelfond, M., Lifschitz, V.: The stable model semantics for logic programming, pp. 1070–1080. MIT Press (1988)
7. Halpern, J.: Reasoning about uncertainty. Massachusetts Institue of Technology (2003)
8. Arrazola, J., Borja, V., Osorio, M., Navarro, J.: Ground non-monotonic modal logic s5: new results. Journal of Logic and Computation 15, 787–813 (2005)
9. Arrazola, J., Borja, V., Osorio, M., Navarro, J.: Logics with common weak completions. Journal of Logic and Computation 16, 867–890 (2006)

10. Marek, V.W.: Stable models and an alternative logic programming paradigm. In: In The Logic Programming Paradigm: a 25-Year Perspective, pp. 375–398. Springer (1999)
11. Nicolas, P., Garcia, L., Stéphan, I., Lefèvre, C.: Possibilistic uncertainty handling for answer set programming. Annals of Mathematics and Artificial Intelligence 47(1-2), 139–181 (2006)
12. Niemela, I.: Logic programs with stable model semantics as a constraint programming paradigm (1998)
13. Osorio, M., Pérez, J.A.N., Arrazola, J.: Applications of intuitionistic logic in answer set programming. CoRR, cs.LO/0305046 (2003)
14. Pearce, D.: Stable inference as intuitionistic validity. The Journal of Logic Programming 38, 79–91 (1999)
15. Pelletier, F., Elio, R.: Scope of Logic, Methodology and Philosophy of Science. Kluwer Academic Press (2002)
16. Zepeda, C., Dávila, R., Osorio, M. (eds.): Programas Logicos Disyuntivos y la demostrabilidad en $C_\omega$. Workshop in Logic, Language and Computation 2006. CEUR Workshop Proceedings (November 2006)
17. Shannon, C.: A mathematical theory of communication. The Bell System Technical Journal 27, 379–423 (1948)
18. Tversky, A., Kahneman, D.: Judgment under uncertainty: Heuristics and biases. Science 185(4157), 1124–1131 (1974)
19. Zadeh, L.A.: Fuzzy sets as a basis for a theory of possibility. Fuzzy Sets Syst. 100, 9–34 (1999)

# Estimating the Number of Test Cases for Active Rule Validation

Lorena Chavarría-Báez[1], Xiaoou Li[2], and Rosaura Palma-Orozco[1]

[1] Instituto Politécnico Nacional - Escuela Superior de Cómputo
[2] Centro de Investigación y de Estudios Avanzados del IPN
{lchavarria,rpalma}@ipn.mx, lixo@cs.cinvestav.mx

**Abstract.** One of the most important steps in the validation of active rules is the generation of test cases. In this paper we introduce a way to estimate the total number of test cases needed to validate the rule base completely. Using this value it is possible to get an objective validation level of the rule base.

## 1 Introduction

*Active rules* are a powerful mechanism to create reactive (active) systems. Before an active system starts working, its rule base must be *validated* in order to ensure that the system does what it should do according to user's expectation and knowledge [1]. Steps of the validation are: 1) *test case generation*, identifies test data that simulate system's inputs, 2) *test case experimentation*, exercises the set of test data by both the system and the set of experts, 3) *evaluation*, interprets the result of the previous step and reports system's errors, 4) *validity assessment*, provides a conclusion about the validity of the system, and 5) *system refinement*, provides a guidance on how to correct the errors [1], [2]. Test case generation (TCG) is one of the most important steps in this process since the lack of errors in a system not always means that it is right, but it could reflect the inability to create enough and/or proper test cases that demonstrate the system's failures. TCG involves two principal elements: *how many* and *which* test cases have to be executed in the system. This paper is centered on the first aspect.

So far, most of the research work on rule validation has been focused on validating production rule-based systems by using measures to determine the accuracy of the system's responses to given inputs [1], [2], [3]. In order to do so, authors of those proposals describe a strategy that has two parts: first, they create a minimal set of test inputs, and second, they apply a Turing Test-like evaluation methodology. One of the principal problems of those works lays on the first point: in order to create test cases, authors generate a "quasi exhaustive" set of test cases, and then they reduce it to a "reasonable" set of test cases by using both user-defined and domain-specific validation criteria. Since validation criteria are subjective, they may vary from an expert to another, this way to determine the number of test cases required for rule validation is not completely suitable.

F. Castro, A. Gelbukh, and M. González (Eds.): MICAI 2013, Part I, LNAI 8265, pp. 120–131, 2013.
© Springer-Verlag Berlin Heidelberg 2013

In this paper, we propose a novel manner, inspired by the cyclomatic complexity metric and using the Conditional Colored Petri Net (CCPN), to estimate the total number of test cases for active rule-based systems validation based on the counting of the linearly independent paths through the CCPN. Since cyclomatic complexity requires both a unique entry/exit node, we introduce them in the CCPN using virtual places. Then, we compute a modified version of the cyclomatic complexity formula to give an evaluation. Our work has the following advantages: 1) as far as we know, it is the first one addressing validation of active rules (a more comprehensive kind of rules than production rules due to the event part), 2) it gets the total number of test cases to validate the complete active rule base, and 3) unlike existing proposals for validating production rules, our measure can be used as a quantitative indicator of the active rule base' validation level since it can be expressed as a ratio between the number of test cases performed and the total number of test cases.

The rest of the paper is organized as follows: Section 2 describes the fundamentals of active rules, and their modeling using the CCPN. Section 3 shows our motivation, the representation of the elements of our cyclomatic complexity version on the CCPN and the estimation of the number of test cases. Section 4 gives details of the computation using an example. Finally, conclusion and future work are delineated in Section 5.

## 2  Active Rules

An active rule has the following general syntax [4]: **ON** *event* **IF** *condition* **THEN** *action* which is interpreted as *when an event happens if the condition is true then the action is performed automatically*. An event is something that occurs at a point in time. It can be of two types: primitive (atomic), or composite (a combination of primitive or composite events using operators of a given event algebra) [4]. The condition examines the context in which the event has taken place. The action describes the task to be carried out by the rule.

In the following there is a set of active rules, taken from [5], defined on the relations `account`(*num, name, balance, rate*) and `low-acc`(*num, start, end*), which contain information about bank's accounts, and a history of all time periods in which an account had a low balance, respectively.

**Example 1.** Bank's policies and active rules for managing customers' accounts.
1) When an account's interest rate is modified, if that account has a balance less than 500 and an interest rate greater than 0%, then that account's interest is lowered to 0%.
2) When a new account is registered, if the account has an interest rate greater than 1% but less than 20%, then that account's interest rate is raised to 2%.
$r_1$
ON update `account.`*rate*
IF *balance* < 500 and *rate* > 0
THEN update `account` set *rate* = 0 where *balance* < 500 and *rate* > 0

$r_2$
ON insert `account`
IF $rate > 1$ and $rate < 2$
THEN update `account` set $rate = 2$ where $rate > 1$ and $rate < 2$

## 2.1    Execution Model

The steps of this model specify how active rules are treated at runtime [4]. *Signaling*, refers to the appearance of an event occurrence caused by an event source. *Triggering*, takes the events produced thus far, and triggers the corresponding rules. *Evaluation*, evaluates the condition of the triggered rules. The rule conflict set is formed from all the rules whose condition is satisfied. *Scheduling*, indicates how the rule conflict set is processed. *Execution*, carries out the actions of the chosen rules. During the action execution other events can, in turn, be signaled which may produce a cascade rule firing.

From above process, we distinguish two types of rules: 1) those triggered *if and only if* the user explicitly executes the task described in their events (*anchor rules*), and 2) those whose event is also raised as consequence of rule interaction.

**Example 2.** Execution of the rule base of Example 1.

Let's suppose that user inserts a new account with the values (1, 'x', 400, 1.3) (*signaling*). Then, $r_2$, an anchor rule, is *triggered*. Since its condition is true (*evaluation*), its action is carried out (*execution*), which, in turn, causes that $r_1$ triggers. Due to $r_1$'condition is true the event update `account`.*rate* is raised again, so $r_1$ triggers one more time, but, in this occasion the condition is false. Then, rule execution finishes.

In order to an active rule base starts working, it is imperative user participation through generating different event combinations. We call such combinations *entry* or *starting points*. For each entry point, there is a final state (or *exit point*) in which no more rules are triggered (that is true whenever there are no loops). Therefore, an active rule base can have more than one entry point and zero or more exit points.

## 2.2    Rule Modeling

The Conditional Colored Petri Net (CCPN) is a PN extension to symbolize and analyze active rules. We don't elaborate on its formalism but for a complete description of it, see reference [6]. Fig. 1 shows the graphical items of CCPN. Events and places are related in the following way: a *primitive place*, represents a primitive event. A composite event, such as *conjunction*, is depicted by a *composite place*. A *copy place*, which contains the same information as its original one, is used when one event triggers two or more rules. A *virtual place*, acts as an event warehouse.

Rules and transitions have the following relationship: *Rule transitions*, represent rules and stores their conditions. *Composite transitions*, are useful to define composite events. For example, to construct the conjunction of events $e_1$ and $e_2$,

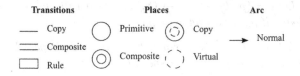

**Fig. 1.** Basic CCPN elements

a composite transition would hold $AND(e_1, e_2)$. *Copy transitions*, duplicate one event for each triggered rule. Its condition is always true.

As in PN, places and transitions, and vice versa, are connected by a *directed arc*.

Sets of primitive, composite, copy, and virtual places are denoted by $P_{prim}$, $P_{comp}$, $P_{copy}$, and $P_{virtual}$, respectively. $T_{rule}$, $T_{comp}$, and $T_{copy}$ indicate the collections of rule, composite and copy transitions, respectively. Finally, $A$, is the set of arcs.

In CCPN, an active rule is mapped to a rule transition, event and action parts are mapped to input and output places of the transition, respectively (see Fig. 2(a)). Whenever an event triggers two or more rules it has to be duplicated by means the copy structure depicted in Fig. 2(b). Composite events formation is considered in CCPN using the composite structure drawn in Fig. 2(c). Composite transition's input places represent all the events needed to form a composite event while its output place corresponds to the whole composite event. Virtual place of Fig. 2(d) represents an event repository. The CCPN model of a set of active rules is formed by connecting those places that represent both the action of one rule and the event of another one.

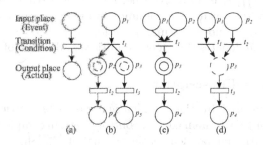

**Fig. 2.** CCPN structures: (a) Basic (b) Copy (c) Composite (d) Virtual

As in traditional PN notation, $\cdot t$ denotes the input places of transition $t$. We use $^*t$ to refer to the set of primitive input places of a composite transition $t$. We introduce the following definitions to describe some special elements of the CCPN.

**Definition 1.** *Let $p \in P_{prim}$ be an initial (final) place if $\cdot p = \emptyset$ ($p\cdot = \emptyset$).*

**Definition 2.** *Let $c = (p_i, t_j) \rightarrow \ldots \rightarrow (t_m, p_n)$ be a path, $p_i, p_n \in P_{prim}$. $c$ is a circular path (loop) if $p_n^{\cdot} = t_n$ and $t_n^{\cdot} = p_i$.*

**Definition 3.** *Let $p \in P_{prim}$ be a reachable place if it is possible to get to it, through the links in the graph, from a specific place.*

**Definition 4.** *Let $c$ be a circular path, and $P_c$ be the set of primitive places of $c$. $c$ is reachable if $\exists p_j \mid p_j \in P_c, \mid {\cdot}p_j \mid > 1$, and $p_j$ is reachable. In other case, $c$ is non-reachable.*

**Example 3.** CCPN of the rule base of Example 1.

In Fig. 3, transitions $t_1$, and $t_2$ depict rules $r_1$, and $r_2$, respectively. $p_1$ represents rule 1's event and $p_2$ stands for its action. Similar reasoning applies for $t_2$.

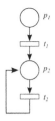

**Fig. 3.** CCPN of Example 1

## 3     Estimation of the Number of Test Cases

The following notation will be used through the rest of the paper:

- $R = \{r_1, r_2, \ldots, r_j\}$, $r_i$ is an active rule. Each $r_i$ is a triplet $(e, c, a)$ where: $e$ is either a primitive event or a conjunction of them, $c$ is a single condition or a composite one, and $a$ is a unique action.
- $r_i.e$, $r_i.c$, and $r_i.a$ denotes the event, condition, and action of $r_i$, respectively.

### 3.1     Motivation and Description

Our proposal is inspired by the *cyclomatic complexity* metric, developed by Thomas McCabe in 1976 to manage and control program complexity by counting the number of linearly independent paths through it [7], [8].

Given a program, a directed graph, G, called the *program control graph*, in which each node represents a block of code and each edge stands for the sequential flow between blocks of code, is associated with it. All the nodes are attainable from a single one (*entry*) and all of them reach a unique node (*exit*). Cyclomatic complexity, $v$, of G is computed using the formula:

$$v = e - n + 2 \tag{1}$$

where $e$ is the number of edges, $n$ is the number of nodes and 2 is a constant value.

Since CCPN describes both the structure and relationships among active rules, we propose to use it to estimate the number of test cases needed to perform a complete rule validation based on the concept of the cyclomatic complexity. However, it is necessary to find those rules which can be connected to a unique entry/exit node so that, from the entry one, all the rules can be triggered, and the exit node can be reached. Below we introduce the basis to do this work.

**Entry Node.** Taking into account that all entry points of active rules happens by user participation, it is possible to consider that all of them have a common source (entry node). The question is: *What are the rules that must be connected to an entry node so that the complete rule base can be fired, at least, once?* It is clear that one option is to admit all of them; however, this is not suitable since some rules can also be triggered as consequence of rule interaction. So, we focus on the following types of rules: 1) anchor rules, and 2) those with composite events. Rules in the former case are important since there is no other way in which they can perform their action. In the latter case, such rules must be analyzed in order to ensure that their primitive events are reached and, in consequence, they will be triggered.

**Exit Node.** After a rule performs its action, it meets its goal. Since all the rules are supposed to be triggered at least once, then all of them converge to a common state (although not at the same time) when their execution finishes. So, it is possible to consider that active rules have an exit point. To identify the rules linked up to the exit node, we examine if the execution of the rule base finishes using the following definitions.

**Definition 5.** *Let $r_i$ be a final rule if $r_i.a \notin \bigcup_{i=0}^{i=|R|} r_i.e$.*

**Definition 6.** *Let $r_i \to r_j \ldots \to r_n$ be a circular sequence of rules if $r_n.a = r_i.e$.*

If there aren't circular sequences of rules in the rule base, rule execution ends. Therefore, all the actions of final rules are eligible to be connected with the exit node. If it is not the case, for any circular sequence, we randomly select a rule to be connected with the exit node as if it were a final rule. This process does not affect rule behavior since it is done for validation purposes which is performed off-line.

## 3.2   Formalization on CCPN

Sections before we conclude that active rules have a single entry/exit point. Fig. 4 shows our proposal to delineate this conclusion in the CCPN.

**Entry Node.** Rules described in Section 3.1 correspond with transitions in CCPN with the following characteristics: 1) rule transitions with initial places ($t_1$ in Fig. 5), and rule transitions which are part of a non-reachable circular path ($t_3$ and $t_5$ in Fig. 5), and 2) composite transitions. To answer the question raised in Section 3.1 we need to analyze the afore mentioned rule transitions and to select those whose primitive input places must be linked up to transition $t_{entry}$.

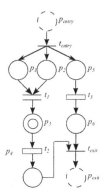

**Fig. 4.** Our proposal

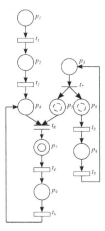

**Fig. 5.** An example of CCPN

For example, in Fig. 5 we can see that the ocurrence of the events described in places $(p_1, p_3)$ or $(p_1, p_8)$ is enough to guarantee that all rule transitions will be triggered. The demanding task is to compute the set of *linked input places, LIP*. We propose the Algorithm 1 in order to compute such places. Our algorithm receives a CCPN model and reckons the set of: 1) initial places (line 2), 2) non-reachable circular paths (line 3), 3) primitive input places of composite transitions (line 4), and 4) reachable places from initial nodes (line 5). Then it checks if all the primitive places are attainable from the set of initial places (line 7). If it is true, all the initial places are considered as linked ones (line 8). In other case, it analyzes, by means of Function *SimplifiedPaths*, only the primitive input places of composite transitions which have not been examined (line 11) and verifies if there exists any relationship between them and the primitive places of non-reachable circular paths (line 12) so that only the essential places are considered. Finally, in this case, the set of linked places is formed by the set of

---

**Algorithm 1.** LinkedInputPlaces($CCPN$)

---

**Input**: A CCPN model.
**Output**: The set of CCPN linked input places.

(1) **begin**
(2)      $IP \longleftarrow \bigcup p_i \mid p_i$ is an initial place;
(3)      $NP \longleftarrow \bigcup c_i \mid c_i$ is a non-reachable path;
(4)      $CTIP \longleftarrow \bigcup {}^*t_i \mid t_i \in T_{comp}$;
(5)      $RP \longleftarrow \bigcup p_i \mid p_i \in P_{prim}$ and $p_i$ is reachable from $IP$;
(6)      $LP \leftarrow SP \leftarrow \emptyset$;
(7)      **if** $(IP \cup RP = P_{prim})$ **then**
(8)      $\quad \mid\ LP \longleftarrow IP$;
(9)      **end**
(10)     **else**
(11)     $\quad \mid\ CTIP \leftarrow CTIP - (IP \cup RP)$;
(12)     $\quad \mid\ SP \leftarrow \texttt{SimplifiedPaths}(CTIP, NP)$;
(13)     $\quad \mid\ LP \leftarrow IP \cup SP$;
(14)     **end**
(15) **end**
(16) **return** $LP$;

---

initial ones and the places representing the tasks that the user must perform to ensure that all the transitions will be triggered.

Once the set of linked places is complete, it is possible to create a CCPN with a unique entry node. We developed the Algorithm 2 to perform this task. Lines 2 to 4 create the entry node, $p_{entry}$, the transition $t_{entry}$, and the arc from $p_{entry}$ to $t_{entry}$. The set of linked places is computed in line 6, and lines 7 and 8 creates the arcs from $t_{entry}$ to each linked place.

**Exit Node.** To create the exit node it is necessary to inspect: 1) the final rules, and 2) the circular sequences of rules. In CCPN, a final rule is characterized by a rule transition with a final place, and a circular sequence of rules is described by a circular path. Examination of such elements produces the set of *linked output places, LOP*.

To construct a CCPN with a unique exit node, all final places must be input places of $t_{exit}$. When there are not such places, in order to simulate rule termination, for any circular path, $c$, we choose a place $p \in P_c$ and we create an arc from it and $t_{exit}$. Algorithm 3 performs this task.

Lines (2) - (4) creates the elements $p_{exit}$, $t_{exit}$ and the arc $(t_{exit}, p_{exit})$. Line (5) computes the set of final places. If it is empty, then lines (7) and (8) analyze any circular path and extract a primitive place which is added to the set of linked output places. Finally, lines (10) and (11) generate the arc between each linked output place and $t_{exit}$.

**Path.** We use the notion of *simple path* as measurement unit for computing the number of test cases on CCPN.

---

**Function** SimplifiedPaths($CTIP$, $NP$)

---

**Input**: $CTIP$, and $NP$, the set of primitive input places of composite transitions, and the set of non-reachable paths, respectively.

**Output**: $F$, a subset of linked places.

(1) **begin**
(2) $\quad$ $N \leftarrow CP \leftarrow I \leftarrow P_I \leftarrow F \leftarrow c \leftarrow \emptyset$;
(3) $\quad$ **for** $i \leftarrow 1$ **to** $\mid NP \mid$ **do**
(4) $\quad\quad$ $c \leftarrow NP[i]$;
(5) $\quad\quad$ **if** $(P_c \notin N)$ **then**
(6) $\quad\quad\quad$ $N[i] \leftarrow P_c$;
(7) $\quad\quad$ **end**
(8) $\quad$ **end**
(9) $\quad$ $CP \leftarrow N$;
(10) $\quad$ **for** $i \leftarrow 1$ **to** $\mid N \mid$ **do**
(11) $\quad\quad$ **for** $j \leftarrow i + 1$ **to** $\mid N \mid$ **do**
(12) $\quad\quad\quad$ **if** $(N[i] \cap N[j] \neq \emptyset)$ **then**
(13) $\quad\quad\quad\quad$ $I \leftarrow N[i] \cap N[j]$;
(14) $\quad\quad\quad\quad$ $CP \leftarrow CP - N[i]$;
(15) $\quad\quad\quad\quad$ $CP \leftarrow CP - N[j]$;
(16) $\quad\quad\quad\quad$ $CTIP \leftarrow CTIP - \{N[i] \cup N[j]\}$;
(17) $\quad\quad\quad\quad$ $P_I \leftarrow P_I \cup p \mid p \in I$;
(18) $\quad\quad\quad$ **end**
(19) $\quad\quad$ **end**
(20) $\quad$ **end**
(21) $\quad$ **for** $i \leftarrow 1$ **to** $\mid CP \mid$ **do**
(22) $\quad\quad$ $F \leftarrow F \cup p \mid p \in CP[i]$;
(23) $\quad$ **end**
(24) $\quad$ $F \leftarrow F \cup P_I \cup CTIP$
(25) **end**
(26) **return** $F$;

---

---

**Algorithm 2.** CCPN with a single entry place

---

**Input**: $CCPN$, a CCPN model.

**Output**: A CCPN with a single entry place.

(1) **begin**
(2) $\quad$ $p_{entry} \leftarrow p \mid p \in P_{virtual}$;
(3) $\quad$ $t_{entry} \leftarrow t \mid t \in T_{copy}$;
(4) $\quad$ $A \leftarrow A \cup (p_{entry}, t_{entry})$;
(5) $\quad$ $LIP \leftarrow \emptyset$;
(6) $\quad$ $LIP \leftarrow \texttt{LinkedInputPlaces}(CCPN)$;
(7) $\quad$ **for** $i \leftarrow 1$ **to** $\mid LIP \mid$ **do**
(8) $\quad\quad$ $A \leftarrow A \cup (t_{entry}, LIP[i])$
(9) $\quad$ **end**
(10) **end**
(11) **return**;

---

---

**Algorithm 3.** CCPN with a single exit place

---

**Input:** $CCPN$, a CCPN model.
**Output:** A CCPN with a single exit place.

(1) **begin**
(2)     $p_{exit} \leftarrow p \mid p \in P_{virtual}$;
(3)     $t_{exit} \leftarrow t \mid t \in T_{copy}$;
(4)     $A \leftarrow A \cup (t_{exit}, p_{exit})$;
(5)     $LOP \leftarrow \bigcup p_i \mid p_i{}^\cdot = \emptyset$;
(6)     **if** $(LOP = \emptyset)$ **then**
(7)        $CP \leftarrow c \mid c$ is a circular path;
(8)        $LOP \leftarrow p \mid p \in P_{CP}$;
(9)     **end**
(10)    **for** $i \leftarrow 1$ **to** $\mid LOP \mid$ **do**
(11)       $A \leftarrow A \cup (LOP[i], t_{exit})$;
(12)    **end**
(13) **end**

---

**Definition 7.** *Let* $s = (p_i, t_j) \to (t_j, p_m)$ *be a simple path,* $p_i, p_m \in P_{prim}$, *and* $t_j \in T_{rule}$.

**Definition 8.** *Let* $s_1 = (p_i, t_j) \to (t_j, p_m)$, $s_2 = (p_j, t_q) \to (t_q, p_n)$ *be simple paths.* $s_1$, $s_2$ *are different if* $t_j \neq t_q$.

In Fig. 5 there are six simple paths since, according to Definition 8, $(p_4, t_4) \to (t_4, p_9)$, and $(p_3, t_4) \to (t_4, p_9)$, are not different.

For the computation of the number of test cases, we need to know all the simple paths of a CCPN.

**Definition 9.** *Given a CCPN model, then* $SP$ *represents the set of all different simple paths computed from* $p_{entry}$ *to* $p_{exit}$.

## 3.3   Computing the Number of Test Cases

In order to compute the number of test cases for active rules validation on CCPN we need to find the sets LIP, LOP, and SP. We distinguish two cases of application on the CCPN.

- Case 1: There is, at least, one final place.
  In this case it is not necessary to simulate an exit point, then our CCPN is similar to a program control graph and the number of test cases, $v$, is obtained as in (1), where $e = \mid SP \mid + \mid LIP \mid + \mid LOP \mid$, and $n = \mid P_{prim} \mid +2$. The number 2 is added to consider the places $p_{entry}$ and $p_{exit}$.
- Case 2: There is not any final place.
  In this case we simulate an exit point and it does not have to be considered as part of the test cases, then $v$ is calculated as:

$$v = e - n + 1 \tag{2}$$

where $e$ and $n$ are obtained as in Case 1.

## 4   Example

Let's consider the CCPN of Fig. 6, which was created with a special software system [9]. Using Algorithm 3 and after creating the structure of the *entry node*, we have to find the LIP set. We compute: $IP \leftarrow \{p_{14}, p_4\}$; $NP \leftarrow \{(p_{18}, t_{11}) \rightarrow (t_{11}, p_{19}) \rightarrow (p_{19}, t_{12}) \rightarrow (t_{12}, p_{18}); (p_1, t_{13}) \rightarrow (t_{13}, p_3) \rightarrow (p_3, t_1) \rightarrow (t_1, p_5) \rightarrow (p_5, t_{14}) \rightarrow (t_{14}, p_7) \rightarrow (p_7, t_3) \rightarrow (t_3, p_8) \rightarrow (p_8, t_{15}) \rightarrow (t_{15}, p_9) \rightarrow (p_9, t_4) \rightarrow (t_4, p_1); (p_2, t_{13}) \rightarrow (t_{13}, p_3) \rightarrow (p_3, t_1) \rightarrow (t_1, p_5) \rightarrow (p_5, t_{14}) \rightarrow (t_{14}, p_7) \rightarrow (p_7, t_3) \rightarrow (t_3, p_8) \rightarrow (p_8, t_{15}) \rightarrow (t_{15}, p_{10}) \rightarrow (p_{10}, t_5) \rightarrow (t_5, p_{11}) \rightarrow (p_{11}, t_{16}) \rightarrow (t_{16}, p_{12}) \rightarrow (p_{12}, t_6) \rightarrow (t_6, p_2)\}$; $CTIP = \{p_1, p_2, p_5, p_6\}$; $RP = \{p_6, p_{15}, p_{16}, p_{17}\}$. Since $IP \cup RP \neq P_{prim}$ we have: $CTIP \leftarrow \{p_1, p_2, p_5\}$, $LIP \leftarrow \{p_{14}, p_4, p_{18}, p_5\}$. When Function *SimplifiedPaths* is executed, the following tasks are performed: $CP \leftarrow N \leftarrow \{\{p_{18}, p_{19}\}, \{p_1, p_5, p_8\}, \{p_2, p_5, p_8, p_{11}\}\}$. When $i = 2$, and $j = 3$, $N[i] \cap N[j] \neq \emptyset$ and $I \leftarrow \{p_5, p_8\}$, $CP \leftarrow \{\{p_{18}, p_{19}\}\}$, $CTIP \leftarrow \emptyset$, $P_I \leftarrow \{p_5\}$, and $F \leftarrow \{p_{18}\}$. $F \leftarrow \{p_{18}, p_5\}$. Finally, $LIP \leftarrow \{p_4, p_{14}\} \cup \{p_{18}, p_5\}$, and an arc from $t_{entry}$ to each place in $LIP$ can be drawn.

Using Algorithm 3 we generate the structure of the exit node in CCPN. Then, since $LOP \leftarrow p_{17}$, an arc from $p_{17}$ to $t_{exit}$ is drawn.

It is clear that if we follow the links in the resulting CCPN from $p_{entry}$ to $p_{exit}$, all the rule transitions are reachable and we have 14 different simple paths. Finally, we have $LIP = 4$, $LOP = 1$, $SP = 14$, $e = 14 + 4 + 1 = 19$, and $n = 13 + 2 = 15$ which produces:

$$v(CCPN) = 19 - 15 + 2 = 6 \tag{3}$$

In order to examine the rule base *completely* it is necessary to design 6 test cases. Each one of them involves the following rule transitions: $tc_1 = \{t_{11}, t_{12}\}$, $tc_2 = \{t_8, t_9, t_{10}\}$, $tc_3 = \{t_2\}$, $tc_4 = \{t_{14}, t_3, t_5, t_7\}$, $tc_5 = \{t_{14}, t_3, t_5, t_6\}$, $tc_6 = \{t_{14}, t_3, t_4, t_{13}, t_1\}$.

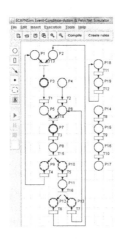

**Fig. 6.** CCPN for Case 1

If rule designer decides, using some reduction technique, to perform only 4 test cases, then the validation level of the rule base can be expressed as 4:6 which is a more objective indicator than those reported thus far.

## 5    Conclusion and Future Work

Validation is a mandatory process for any system, including those based on active rules. In this paper, we present a CCPN-based way to find the total number of test cases needed to inspect all the active rules in a rule base. Unlike existing proposals, our work can give a more objective criterion to indicate the validation level of the rule base since we always find the exact number of test cases. In the future we are going to detail the following steps involved in rule validation.

**Acknowledgments.** Authors recognize the support provided by CONACYT and IPN for the development of this work.

## References

1. Knauf, R., Gonzalez, A.J., Abel, T.: A framework for validation of rule-based systems. IEEE Transactions on Systems, Man and Cybernetics - Part B: Cybernetics 32, 281–295 (2002)
2. Knauf, R., Tsuruta, S., Gonzalez, A.J.: Toward reducing human involvement in validation of knowledge-based systems. IEEE Transactions on Systems, Man and Cybernetics - Part A: Systems and Humans 37, 120–131 (2007)
3. González, A.J., Dankel, D.D.: Prentice-Hall (1993)
4. Paton, N., Díaz, O.: Active database systems. ACM Computing Surveys 31, 62–103 (1999)
5. Baralis, E., Widom, J.: An algebraic approach to static analysis of active database rules. ACM Trans. on Database Systems 25, 269–332 (2000)
6. Li, X., Medina-Marín, J., Chapa, S.: Applying petri nets on active database systems. IEEE Trans. on System, Man, and Cybernetics, Part C: Applications and Reviews 37, 482–493 (2007)
7. MacCabe, T.J.: A complexity measure. IEEE Transactions on Software Engineering SE-2, 308–320 (1976)
8. MacCabe, T.J.: Cyclomatic complexity and the year 2000. IEEE Software 13, 115–117 (1996)
9. Chavarría-Báez, L., Li., X.: Ecapnver: A software tool to verify active rule bases. In: Proc. of the 22nd Intl. Conf. on Tools with Artificial Intelligence, Arras, France, pp. 138–141 (2010)

# A Dynamic Multi-Expert Multi-Criteria Decision Making Model for Risk Analysis

Yeleny Zulueta[1], Vladimir Martell[1], Juan Martínez[2], and Luis Martínez[2]

[1] University of Informatics Science, Cuba
[2] University of Jaen, Spain

**Abstract.** Risks behavior may vary over time. New risks may appear, secondary risks may arises from the treatment of initial risks and the project managers may decide to ignore some insignificant risks. These facts demand to perform Risk Analysis in a dynamic way to support decisions by an effective and continuous process instead of single one. Risk Analysis is usually solved using Multi-Criteria Decision Making methods that are not efficient in handling the changes of risks exposure values during different periods. Therefore, our aim in this contribution is to propose a Dynamic Multi-Expert Multi-Criteria Decision Making Model for Risk Analysis, which allows not only to integrate the traditional dimensions of risks (probability and impact), but also to consider the current and past performances of risks exposure values in the project life cycle.

**Keywords:** risk analysis, dynamic multi-criteria decision making, aggregation operators.

## 1 Introduction

Project Risk Management (PRM) is a critical issue in success of projects and businesses due to they are exposed to risks which are the combination of the probability of an event and its consequences [1]. That is why PRM has become a rapidly developing discipline, receiving more and more attention in modern society. Stakeholders demand more effective methods to cover themselves against negative risk consequences as well as to provide a forwardlooking radar, identifying threats to be avoided and providing early indicators of potential problems.

In the literature can be found different approaches for PRM [2–4]. Traditional PRM process is comprised of four major phases: risk identification, risk analysis, risk response planning, and risk monitoring and control [4], all of them related with the communication.

In this contribution we are focus on the Risk Analysis (RA) phase due to it allows evaluating and prioritizing risks and providing the information for managing the right risks.

RA is usually modeled as a Multi-Criteria Decision Making (MCDM) problem in which experts express their preferences for each risk, over two traditional criteria: probability and impact. Traditional RA approaches, obtain an overall rating by calculating the risk exposure, which is the product of the likelihood

F. Castro, A. Gelbukh, and M. González (Eds.): MICAI 2013, Part I, LNAI 8265, pp. 132–143, 2013.
© Springer-Verlag Berlin Heidelberg 2013

of an unsatisfactory outcome (probability) and the loss to the parties affected when the outcome is unsatisfactory (impact). Then risks are ranked considering the rating values, the most serious risk item will be addressed first. Such a prioritization is required in order to provide focus for real important risks.

During the project life cycle, some risks are treated but not eliminated and new risks may appear in different moments; while secondary risks may arise from the management of initial risks; simultaneously, the project managers may ignore or accept some of the trivial risks. As a result, RA must be an iterative process requiring commitment and continuous responses from the project team because overall risks behavior may vary over time.

Previous elements arise the necessity of improve MCDM methods for RA in a dynamic way, in order to support decisions by an effective and continuous process instead of single one.

However, classical MCDM [5] models focus towards the selection of the best alternative from a finite number of feasible solutions, according to a set of criteria, but without considering the temporal performance of such alternatives during different time periods. That means that they are not effective in handling the challenge of dynamic RA during the project life cycle.

We believe that currently there are dynamic techniques allowing us to handle decisions in dynamic contexts and their promising results, is a real reason to continue working in this direction. For instance, Dynamic Multi-Criteria Decision Making (DMCDM) is able to support interdependent decisions in an evolving environment, in which both criteria and alternatives may change, and later decisions need to take into account feedback from previous ones [6].

On account of this, the application of DMCDM to traditional RA allows to consider the current and past performances of risks in the project.

To achieve this aim, in this contribution a new DMCDM approach for RA is introduced. It supports prioritization of risks in RA decision situations requiring either ordered risk rankings at different moments of the project life cycle, or just one at the end of a decision process but always considering the current and past performances of risks exposure.

The remaining of this paper is organized as follows. Section 2 briefly reviews the DMCDM issue. Section 3 introduces the new DMCDM model for RA. Section 4 presents an illustrative example and Section 5 concludes the paper.

## 2   Background on DMCDM

Main features of a DMCDM problem include, on the one hand, the dynamic nature of the set of alternatives and the set of criteria assessed in each considered decision moment, and on the other hand, the temporal profile of an alternative matters for comparison with other alternatives [6]. In dynamic decision making environments, alternatives may evolve during different periods along with decision makers preferences for them, therefore different and continuous responses are needed across the time [7].

The surveyed literature indicates that most research in dynamic decision making, model the problem as a three-dimensional decision matrix which is first transformed into conventional two-dimensional decision matrix by aggregating the time dimension, and secondly solved through classical MCDM methods. Some approaches [8–12] follow the scheme of the Technique for Order Preference by Similarity to Ideal Solution (TOPSIS) [13] while in others [14, 15], alternatives are ranked using mathematical programming models considering the priorities of criteria calculated in the multiple periods using the Analytic Hierarchy Process (AHP) [16]. In general, preferences are gathered at different periods and the final decision is accomplished at the end of the process.

However, none of these approaches is general enough to model other MCDM problems in which both criteria and alternatives change and separated but interlinked decisions are taken either frequently, or just at the end of the decision process, considering feedback from previous ones [6].

In that respect, Campanella and Ribeiro [17] properly formalized the DMCDM in a general framework that extends the classic MCDM model. The resolution process in the framework can be summarized in three phases at each period [17]:

1. Computing non-dynamic ratings.
2. Computing dynamic ratings.
3. Ranking alternatives according to their historical information, which is updated for new iterations.

The selection of an appropriate associative aggregation operator for accomplishing the second step is critical due to its properties can highly modify the computing cost as well as the results. The associativity property avoids dealing with all past alternatives rating values (dynamic and non-dynamic) while the type of reinforcement [18] reflected by the aggregation operator allows to manipulate the tendency of low or high non-dynamic ratings. However, using any associative aggregation operator, there are situations where equal dynamic ratings values are generated regardless of temporal performance of alternatives.

To remedy this drawback, in [19] the resolution procedure for DMCDM was improved by performing a new aggregation step for computing a *discriminative dynamic index* that allows to handle ties in the dynamic ratings of the alternatives, on the basis of differences in their temporal trends and consequently obtain rankings for supporting dynamic decisions. Due to our proposal take it as base, this approach is revised in the next section.

## 2.1 Improved DMCDM Approach

To support consistent decisions in cases in which the DMCDM framework in [17] is not effective, a discriminative dynamic index was introduced obtaining the general resolution procedure for DMCDM [19] depicted in Figure 1.

The first step is essentially developed following MCDM traditional models. Let $T = \{1, 2, \ldots\}$ be the (possibly infinite) set of discrete decision moments,

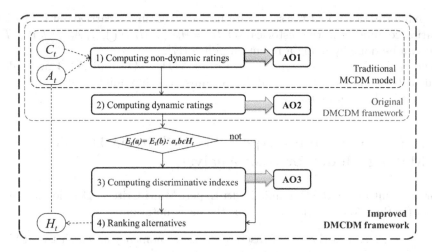

**Fig. 1.** Improved DMCDM resolution procedure

and $A_t$ the set of available alternatives at each decision moment $t \in T$. At each time period $t \in T$, for each available alternative $a \in A_t$, a *non-dynamic rating* $R_t(a) \in [0,1]$ is computed by usually using an aggregation operator **AO1** : $[0,1]^n \to [0,1]$, that combines the assessments of all criteria, $C_t = \{c_1, ..., c_n\}$ $\forall t \in T$.

The second step lies on the DMCDM framework presented in [17]. The dynamic nature of the decision process is supported by an evaluation function $E_t : A_t \cup H_{t-1} \to [0,1]$ which is defined for each $t \in T$ as:

$$
E_t(a) = \begin{cases} R_t(a), & a \in A_t \setminus H_{t-1} \\ \mathbf{AO2}(E_{t-1}(a), R_t(a)), & a \in A_t \cap H_{t-1} \\ E_{t-1}(a), & a \in H_{t-1} \setminus A_t \end{cases} \quad (1)
$$

The third step consists of computing a discriminative dynamic index which is performed just if equal dynamic ratings values are generated in the second step. The discriminative dynamic index $I_t : A_t \cup H_{t-1} \to [-1,1]$, which represents the rating behavior of the alternative until $t$, is defined as:

$$
I_t(a) = \begin{cases} D_t(a), & a \in A_t \setminus H_{t-1} \\ \mathbf{AO3}(I_{t-1}(a), D_t(a)), & a \in A_t \cap H_{t-1} \\ I_{t-1}(a), & a \in H_{t-1} \setminus A_t, \end{cases} \quad (2)
$$

where the rating change, $D_t(a)$, is the difference between the ratings at the current and previous period such that $D_t(a) = R_t(a) - R_{t-1}(a), t > 1$ and $D_1 = 0$.

These tree steps will eventually enable to obtain a final ranking of alternatives. If different alternatives obtain equal dynamic rating, $E_t(\cdot)$ at a period $t$, the final ranking will be generated considering the discriminative dynamic index values $I_t(\cdot)$ that will reflect a *dynamic perspective*.

The information about the set of alternatives over time is carried out from one iteration to another in the historical set $H_0 = \emptyset$, $\qquad H_t = \bigcup_{t' \leq t} A_{t'}$, $\quad t, t' \in T$. That can be done by fixing a retention policy [17].

The choices of the aggregation operators **AO1**, **AO2** and **AO3** are independent since they are used for different aims and they might reflect different attitudes in decision making.

## 3    A Dynamic Multi-Expert Multi-Criteria Decision Making Model for Risk Analysis

In order to introduce the Dynamic Multi-Expert Multi-Criteria Decision Making Model for Risk Analysis, let us present the basic notation:

- $T = \{1, 2, \ldots\}$ is the set of discrete decision moments in which the RA is performed in the project.
- $\mathfrak{R}_t = \{r_i | i \in (1, ..., m)\}$ is the set of available risks to be analyzed at each decision moment $t \in T$.
- Each risk is assessed according to the set of criteria $C_t = \{c_j | j \in (1, ..., n)\}$ which weights are given by the vector $W_t = \{w_j | j \in (1, ..., n)\}$ with $w_j \in [0, 1]$, $\sum_{j=1}^{n} w_j = 1, \forall t \in T$.
- The set of experts evaluating risks is $E_t = \{e_k | k \in (1, ..., p)\}$.
- The preference provided by expert $e_k \in E$ over criterion $c_j \in C$ for risk $r_i \in \mathfrak{R}_t$ is represented by $x_i^{jk}$.

Additionally, the proposed model has the following features:

- Its goal is to support prioritization of risks in decision situations requiring either ordered ranking lists at different moments of the project life cycle, or just one at the end of a decision process but always considering the current and past performances of risks.
- It is based on the original DMCDM framework in [17] as well as in its improvement introduced in [19].
- It extends the previous approaches to deal with the preferences provided by multiple experts.
- It flexibly allows to incorporate not only probability and impact as criteria but also other criteria according to the necessities of the project as well as to set the importance of these criteria in the overall result.
- It consists of six steps:
  **1** Gathering experts preferences.
  **2** Computing risk exposure.
  **3** Computing dynamic risk exposure.
  **4** Computing dynamic discriminative index.
  **5** Ranking risks.

In the following, an explanation of each step is given.

### 3.1  Gathering Experts Preferences

Each expert provides $e_k$ her/his preferences over criteria for each risk, by means of assessment vectors $X_i^k = \{x_i^{1k}, ..., x_i^{nk}\}$.

### 3.2  Computing Risk Exposure

At each time period, $t \in T$, the risk exposure value of each risk, $RE_i^t$, is computed by a two-step aggregation process instead of a single operator **AO1**:

1. Computing collective criteria values:
   The assessment of all experts about each criterion is denoted as $x_i^j$ and it is computed using the mean aggregation operator $\Omega$ such that:

$$x_i^j = \Omega(x_i^{j1}, ..., x_i^{jp}) = \frac{1}{p}\sum_{k=1}^{p} x_i^{jk}. \tag{3}$$

2. Computing risk exposure:
   The overall risk exposure of a risk $r_i$ is denoted as $RE_i^t$ and it is computed using the weighted sum aggregation operator $\Theta$ such that:

$$RE_i^t = \Theta(x_i^1, ..., x_i^n) = \sum_{j=1}^{n} w_j \cdot x_i^j. \tag{4}$$

### 3.3  Computing Dynamic Risk Exposure

At each time period, $t \in T$, the dynamic risk exposure value of each risk, denoted by $RE_i^t$, is computed using Equation (1) as:

$$DRE_i^t = \begin{cases} RE_i^t & \text{if } r_i \in \mathfrak{R}_t \setminus \mathfrak{H}_{t-1} \\ \dfrac{0.5 \cdot DRE_i^{t-1} \cdot RE_i^t}{DRE_i^{t-1} \cdot RE_i^t + 0.5 \cdot (1 - DRE_i^{t-1} - RE_i^t)} & \text{if } r_i \in \mathfrak{R}_t \cap \mathfrak{H}_{t-1} \\ DRE_i^{t-1} & \text{if } r_i \in \mathfrak{H}_{t-1} \setminus \mathfrak{R}_t \end{cases} \tag{5}$$

The performance of the dynamic risk exposure computation depends on the risk, $r_i$ as:

- for $r_i$ belonging only to the current set of risks, its dynamic risk exposure corresponds to its non-dynamic rating,
- for $r_i$ belonging only to the historical set of risks, its dynamic risk exposure is equal to the dynamic risk exposure in the previous period and
- for $r_i$ belonging to both (current and historical sets of risks), its dynamic risk exposure is obtained by aggregating its non-dynamic risk exposure with its dynamic risk exposure in the previous decision period. Due to we are interested in reinforcing the tendency of low and high risk exposure values, we have set **AO2** as the uninorm operator $\Phi_{SP}$.

Uninorms were introduced by Yager and Rybalov [20] as a generalization of t-norms and t-conorms. They are commutative, associative and increasing binary operators with a neutral element $e \in [0,1]$. In this case we have selected $e = 0.5$ with the purpose of modeling the reinforcement in such way that:

- An upward reinforcement when $RE_i^t > 0.5$ and $DRE_i^{t-1} > 0.5$.
- A downward reinforcement when contrarily $RE_i^t < 0.5$ and $DRE_i^{t-1} < 0.5$.
- A full reinforcement when one value is higher and the other is lower than 0.5.

### 3.4  Computing Dynamic Discriminative Index

At each time period, $t \in T$, if there exist equal dynamic risk exposure values for risks, their dynamic discriminative indexes are computed using Equation (2) as:

$$I_i^t = \begin{cases} D_i^t & \text{if } r_i \in \mathfrak{R}_t \setminus \mathfrak{H}_{t-1} \\ I_i^{t-1} & \text{if } r_i \in \mathfrak{H}_{t-1} \setminus \mathfrak{R}_t \\ \Psi(D_i^t, I^{t-1}) & \text{if } r_i \in \mathfrak{R}_t \cap \mathfrak{H}_{t-1} \end{cases} \tag{6}$$

where the risk exposure change, $D_i^t$, is the difference between the ratings at the current and previous period such that $D_i^t = RE_i^t - RE_i^{t-1}, t > 1$ and $D_i^1 = 0$. The index $I_i^t$ performance depends on the risk, $r_i$ as:

- for $r_i \in \mathfrak{R}_t \setminus \mathfrak{H}^{t-1}$, its discriminative dynamic index $I_i^t$, is the rating change $D_i^t$,
- for $r_i \in \mathfrak{H}_{t-1} \setminus \mathfrak{R}^t$, its discriminative dynamic index is obtained from previous iteration, $I_i^t = I_i^{t-1}$.
- for $r_i \in \mathfrak{R}_t \cap \mathfrak{H}^{t-1}$, its discriminative dynamic index is computed by aggregating the discriminative dynamic index in the previous iteration with the current risk exposure change. For computing the dynamic discriminative index, $I_i^t$, we set **AO3** as the Van Melle's combining function modified in [21], such that:

$$\Psi(D_i^t, I^{t-1}) = \begin{cases} D_i^t + I_i^{t-1} - D_i^t \cdot I_i^{t-1} & \text{if} \quad \min\{D_i^t, I_i^{t-1}\} \geq 0 \\ D_i^t + I_i^{t-1} + D_i^t \cdot I_i^{t-1} & \text{if} \quad \max\{D_i^t, I_i^{t-1}\} \leq 0 \\ \frac{D_i^t + I_i^{t-1}}{1 - \min\{|D_i^t|, |I_i^{t-1}|\}} & \text{otherwise} \end{cases} \tag{7}$$

Such an aggregation operator allows to model the index performance according to the desired *attitudes to deal with the risk exposure changes* [19]:

- Optimistic: when both values are positive the aggregation acts as an upward reinforcement.
- Pessimistic: when both values are negative, it acts as a downward reinforcement.
- Averaging: when one value is negative and the another positive, it acts as an averaging operator.

Table 1. Key features of the aggregation operators

| Operator | Definition | Properties |
|---|---|---|
| $\Omega, \Theta$ | $[0,1]^n \to [0,1]$ | |
| $\Phi_{SP}$ | $[0,1]^2 \to [0,1]$ | Associativity, Full Reinforcement |
| $\Psi$ | $[-1,1]^2 \to [-1,1]$ | Associativity, Bipolarity, Full Reinforcement |

Table 1 summarizes the key features of aggregation operators used in the aggregation steps of the proposed model. Note that although the associativity and reinforcement properties characterized $\Phi_{SP}$ and $\Psi$ operators, the former is defined on $[0,1]$ while the second is defined on $[-1,1]$ since we need to manage decrements and increments in risk exposure.

### 3.5   Ranking Risks

In this phase, a list of ordered risks is obtained according to the decreasing order of all values $DRE_i^t$. For coincidences in $DRE_i^t$ values, the order is determined by the dynamic discriminative index, that is, the larger $DRE_i^t$ the most critical is the risk.

## 4   An Illustrative Example

To better explain our proposed contributions to deal with RA in dynamic multi-experts environments, we introduce an example in which a list of risks is required at three different moments, $T = \{1, 2, 3\}$, in the project life cycle, regarding the behavior of the risk exposure values:

- $\Re_1 = \{r_1, r_2, r_3, r_4, r_5\}$ is the initial set of risks to be analyzed.
- $E = \{e_1, e_2\}, \forall t \in T$ is the set of two experts providing their opinions at the three decision moments.
- $C = \{c_1, c_2\}, \forall t \in T$ is the set of criteria being $c_1$ the probability and $c_2$ the impact of risks.
- All the risks are carried in the historical set from one period to the next due to the small number of risks and periods and managers are interested in to consider much information as possible.

### 4.1   Computations of Risk Exposure, Dynamic Risk Exposure and Dynamic Discriminative Index

Below we present the resolution procedure and results obtained in the Steps 1 to 4 the model. Also we provide computation examples in order to illustrate the performance of the different aggregation operators and their influence in results.

Tables 2 to 4 show the gathered opinions as well as the generated values for risk exposure, dynamic risk exposure and dynamic discriminative index.

1. In Period $t = 1$, just the risk exposure is computed. It is not necessary to compute the dynamic risk exposure since there is no historical information of risks.
2. In Period $t = 2$, a new risk $r_6$ was identified and analyzed. Once obtained risk exposure values, dynamic risk exposure values are also computed for each risk as in the following examples:
   - For risk $r_1$, since the previous and current values of risk exposure are respectively lower and higher than the neutral element 0.5, the corresponding dynamic risk exposure value is between these values. These average behavior is also reflected for $r_3$ and $r_4$.

$$RE_1^2 = \Phi_S P(RE_1^1, RE_1^2)$$
$$= \frac{0.5 \cdot RE_1^1 \cdot RE_1^2}{RE_1^1 \cdot RE_1^2 + 0.5 \cdot (1 - RE_1^1 - RE_1^2)}$$
$$= \frac{0.5 \cdot 0.3000 \cdot 0.7000}{0.3000 \cdot 0.7000 + 0.5 \cdot (1 - 0.3000 - 0.7000)}$$
$$= 0.5000$$

   - For risk $r_2$, since the previous and current values of risk exposure are lower than the neutral element 0.5, the resulting dynamic risk exposure value is pushed down.
   - Conversely for risk $r_5$, since the previous and current values of risk exposure are higher than the neutral element 0.5, the computed dynamic risk exposure value is pushed up.

   After computing dynamic risk exposure values, note that $DRE_1^2 = DRE_3^2 = DRE_4^2$, in consequence the computation of dynamic discriminative index is required to discriminate the order of risks $r_1, r_3$ and $r_4$. In second period, dynamic discriminative index values of risks are equal to their change in risk exposure values.
3. In Period t=3, the risk analyst decided not to evaluate risk $r_2$ due to its low previous values of dynamic risk exposure. After computing risk exposure and dynamic risk exposure, equal values ($DRE_1^3 = DRE_6^3$ and $DRE_3^3 = DRE_4^3$) are obtained, hence the index is computed as in the following examples:

- For risk $r_1$, with an increment of risk exposure from the previous period to current period and a positive value of dynamic discriminative index in the previous period, the index performance is an upward reinforcement:

$$DRE_1^3 = \Psi(D_1^3, I_1^2)$$
$$= D_1^3 + I_1^2 - D_1^3 \cdot I_1^2$$
$$= 0.2000 + 0.4000 - 0.2000 \cdot 0.4000$$
$$= 0.5200 > 0.4000$$

**Table 2.** Results at period t=1

|  | $r_1$ | | $r_2$ | | $r_3$ | | $r_4$ | | $r_5$ | |
|---|---|---|---|---|---|---|---|---|---|---|
|  | $c_1$ | $c_2$ | $c_1$ | $c_2$ | $c_1$ | $c_2$ | $c_1$ | $c_2$ | $c_1$ | $c_2$ |
| $e_1$ | 0.1 | 0.6 | 0.3 | 0.1 | 0.8 | 1.0 | 0.1 | 0.3 | 0.9 | 0.5 |
| $e_2$ | 0.1 | 0.4 | 0.1 | 0.1 | 0.2 | 0.6 | 0.1 | 0.3 | 0.5 | 0.3 |
| $x_i^j$ | 0.1 | 0.5 | 0.2 | 0.1 | 0.5 | 0.8 | 0.1 | 0.3 | 0.7 | 0.4 |
| $RE_i^t$ | 0.3000 | | 0.1500 | | 0.6500 | | 0.2000 | | 0.5500 | |

**Table 3.** Results at period t=2

|  | $r_1$ | | $r_2$ | | $r_3$ | | $r_4$ | | $r_5$ | | $r_6$ | |
|---|---|---|---|---|---|---|---|---|---|---|---|---|
|  | $c_1$ | $c_2$ | $c_1$ | $c_2$ | $c_1$ | $c_2$ | $c_1$ | $c_2$ | $c_1$ | $c_2$ | $c_1$ | $c_2$ |
| $e_1$ | 0.9 | 0.6 | 0.1 | 0.1 | 0.6 | 0.1 | 0.8 | 1.0 | 0.8 | 0.7 | 0.5 | 0.6 |
| $e_2$ | 0.5 | 0.8 | 0.1 | 0.1 | 0.6 | 0.1 | 0.6 | 0.8 | 0.8 | 0.7 | 0.9 | 1.0 |
| $x_i^j$ | 0.7 | 0.7 | 0.1 | 0.1 | 0.6 | 0.1 | 0.7 | 0.9 | 0.8 | 0.7 | 0.7 | 0.8 |
| $RE_i^t$ | 0.7000 | | 0.1000 | | 0.3500 | | 0.8000 | | 0.7500 | | 0.7500 | |
| $DRE_i^t$ | 0.5000 | | 0.0192 | | 0.5000 | | 0.5000 | | 0.7857 | | 0.7500 | |
| $I_i^t$ | 0.4000 | | -0.0500 | | -0.3000 | | 0.6000 | | 0.2000 | | | |

**Table 4.** Results at period t=3

|  | $r_1$ | | $r_3$ | | $r_4$ | | $r_5$ | | $r_6$ | |
|---|---|---|---|---|---|---|---|---|---|---|
|  | $c_1$ | $c_2$ | $c_1$ | $c_2$ | $c_1$ | $c_2$ | $c_1$ | $c_2$ | $c_1$ | $c_2$ |
| $e_1$ | 0.9 | 1.0 | 0.1 | 1.0 | 0.7 | 0.6 | 0.1 | 0.7 | 0.7 | 0.9 |
| $e_2$ | 0.9 | 0.8 | 0.9 | 0.1 | 0.6 | 0.6 | 0.5 | 0.1 | 0.8 | 0.9 |
| $x_i^j$ | 0.9 | 0.9 | 0.5 | 0.6 | 0.5 | 0.6 | 0.3 | 0.4 | 0.6 | 0.9 |
| $RE_i^t$ | 0.9000 | | 0.5500 | | 0.5500 | | 0.3500 | | 0.7500 | |
| $DRE_i^t$ | 0.9000 | | 0.5500 | | 0.5500 | | 0.6638 | | 0.9000 | |
| $I_i^t$ | 0.5200 | | -0.1250 | | 0.4667 | | -0.2500 | | 0.0000 | |

- In contrast, for risk $r_3$, with an increment of risk exposure from the previous period to current period too, but with a negative value of dynamic discriminative index in the previous period. Then the index performance is average:

$$DRE_3^3 = \Psi(D_3^3, I_3^2)$$
$$= \frac{D_3^3 + I_3^2}{1 - \min\{|D_3^3|, |I_3^2|\}}$$
$$= \frac{0.2000 - 0.3000}{1 - 0.2000}$$
$$= -0.1250, 0.2000 > -0.1250 > -0.3000$$

### 4.2   Comparative Analysis of Risk Rankings

Table 5 summarizes the results generated using different approaches:

**A**  The ranking obtained with the traditional RA method (product of impact and probability) which is not suitable for our dynamic problem due to we are interested in the evolution of risks during the project life cycle and in this method the temporal profile of a risk does not matters for comparison with other risks.

**B**  The ranking obtained applying the original DMCDM framework in [17] which obtains in some situations equal dynamic risk exposure for different risks without a solution for discrimination.

**C**  The ranking obtained with the proposed Dynamic Multi-Expert Multi-Criteria Decision Making Model for RA. It enables orders reflecting the risk exposure value behavior, which is the major aim of this contribution.

**Table 5.** Results at period t=3

| | t=1 | t=2 | t=3 |
|---|---|---|---|
| **A** | $r_3 \succ r_5 \succ r_1 \succ r_4 \succ r_2$ | $r_4 \succ r_5 = r_6 \succ r_1 \succ r_3 \succ r_2$ | $r_1 \succ r_6 \succ r_3 = r_4 \succ r_5$ |
| **B** | | $r_5 = r_6 \succ r_3 = r_4 = r_1 \succ r_2$ | $r_1 = r_6 \succ r_5 \succ r_3 = r_4$ |
| **C** | | $r_5 \succ r_6 \succ r_4 \succ r_1 \succ r_3 \succ r_2$ | $r_1 \succ r_6 \succ r_5 \succ r_4 \succ r_3$ |

## 5   Concluding Remarks

In real risk management situations we face the problem of dealing with the dynamic nature of risks due to their performances are not fixed throughout the project life cycle. Risks may remain active even after being treated, other risks may appear in different moments and overall risk exposure behavior may vary over time. To solve above changeable problem, this paper presented a new dynamic multi-expert multi-criteria decision making model for RA. The major value of this work is to formally model the dynamic dimension in the traditional RA process. A very important feature of the model is the use of a bipolar associative aggregation operator to reflect and discriminate the risk exposure performance over time. Furthermore, its functioning has been showed by solving an example and comparing the obtained results.

## References

1. BSI. ISO/IEC Guide 73:2002 Risk Management–Vocabulary–Guidelines for Use in Standards. British Standard Institute, London (2002)
2. IEEE. Standard 1540–2001: Standard for Software Life Cycle Processes–Risk Management. Institute of Electrical and Electronics Engineers, New York (2001)
3. ISO. ISO 10006–Quality Management Systems–Guidelines for Quality Management in Projects, 2nd edn. International Organization for Standardization, Switzerland (2003)

4. PMI. A Guide to the Project Management Body of Knowledge (PMBOK). Project Management Institute, Newton Square, PA, USA (2003)
5. Pedrycz, W., Ekel, P., Parreiras, R.: Models and algorithms of fuzzy multicriteria decision-making and their applications. Wiley, Chichester (2011)
6. Campanella, G., Pereira, A., Ribeiro, R., Varela, M.: Collaborative dynamic decision making: A case study from b2b supplier selection. In: Decision Support Systems–Collaborative Models and Approaches in Real Environments. LNBIP, vol. 121, pp. 88–102. Springer, Heidelberg (2012)
7. Saaty, T.: Time dependent decision-making; dynamic priorities in the ahp/anp: Generalizing from points to functions and from real to complex variables. Mathematical and Computer Modelling 46(7-8), 860–891 (2007)
8. Lin, Y., Lee, P., Ting, H.: Dynamic multi-attribute decision making model with grey number evaluations. Expert Systems with Applications 35, 1638–1644 (2008)
9. Xu, Z.: On multi-period multi-attribute decision making. Knowledge-Based Systems 21(2), 164–171 (2008)
10. Yao, S.: A distance method for multi-period fuzzy multi-attribute decision making (2010)
11. Teng, D.: Topsis method for dynamic evaluation of hi-tech enterprise's strategic performance with intuitionistic fuzzy information. Advances in Information Sciences and Service Sciences (AISS) 3(11), 443–449 (2011)
12. Zhang, L., Zou, H., Yang, F.: A dynamic web service composition algorithm based on topsis. Journal of Networks 6(9), 1296–1304 (2011)
13. Hwang, C., Yoon, K.: Multiple Attribute Decision Making: Methods and Applications. Springer, Berlin (1981)
14. Ustun, O., Demirtas, E.: Multi-period lot-sizing with supplier selection using achievement scalarizing functions. Computers & Industrial Engineering 54(4), 918–931 (2008)
15. Sucky, E.: A model for dynamic strategic vendor selection. Computers and Operations Research 34(12), 3638–3651 (2007)
16. Saaty, T.: The Analytic Hierarchy Process. McGraw-Hill, New York (1980)
17. Campanella, G., Ribeiro, R.: A framework for dynamic multiple-criteria decision making. Decision Support Systems 52(1), 52–60 (2011)
18. Yager, R., Rybalov, A.: Full reinforcement operators in aggregation techniques. IEEE Transactions on Systems, Man, and Cybernetics, Part B: Cybernetics 28(6), 757–769 (1998)
19. Zulueta, Y., Martínez, J., Martínez, L., Espinilla, M.: A discriminative dynamic index based on bipolar aggregation operators for supporting dynamic multi-criteria decision making. In: Aggregation Functions in Theory and in Practise. AISC, vol. 228, pp. 237–248. Springer, Heidelberg (2013)
20. Yager, R., Rybalov, A.: Uninorm aggregation operators. Fuzzy Sets and Systems 80(1), 111–120 (1996)
21. Tsadiras, A., Margaritis, K.: The mycin certainty factor handling function as uninorm operator and its use as a threshold function in artificial neurons. Fuzzy Sets and Systems 93, 263–274 (1998)

# An Architecture for Cognitive Modeling to Support Real-Time Adaptation and Motivational Responses in Video Games

Juan Carlos Conde Ramírez, Abraham Sánchez López,
and Abraham Sánchez Flores

Benemérita Universidad Autónoma de Puebla
Computer Science Department - MOVIS Laboratory
Puebla, Pue., 72000
{juanc.conde,asanchez}@cs.buap.mx, axy72@hotmail.com

**Abstract.** Currently, there are tremendous advances in gaming technologies to improve physical realism of environments and characters. However, game characters are still lacking in the cognitive realism, thus video games and game development tools need to provide functionality to support real-time adaptation and appropriate response to internal motivations. In this paper we propose an architecture for cognitive modeling based on well-known cognitive architectures like ACT-R and Soar. It describes a methodology for developing a behavioral system and it emphasizes an ethological sensing modeling to simulate more realistic behaviors. This methodology serves to develop a component-based system that could improve the ability to create intelligent virtual agents. In this phase of implementation, we present preliminary results of modeling behavior of a fish character in an undersea world using a game engine.

## 1 Introduction

To support functionalities related with generation of complex behaviors on characters, video games will need to implement effective cognitive models that reflect faithfully a particular behavior from a set of requirements obtained in real-time. This paper presents an approach for programming game characters, which demonstrate greater intelligence and realism through their behaviors. Data gathering (physiological, anatomical, ethological, etc.) in experiments with "rational" beings provides the necessary data for generating simulations that can be validated by theoretical models. As mentioned in [1], cognitive modeling may provide not just tools, data generators, instantiations, or integrations, but also theories in full sense of the term. Hence, the proper implementation of the proposed architecture will enable to take one more step towards the creation of behavioral theories, testing and even exploring other cognitive phenomena.

The paper is organized as follows. The Section 2 presents the biological principles considered by an effective behavioral system to generate autonomous cognitive characters. An overview of research in cognitive modeling and a justification of this in video games are presented in Section 3. The Section 4 describes the

F. Castro, A. Gelbukh, and M. González (Eds.): MICAI 2013, Part I, LNAI 8265, pp. 144–156, 2013.

proposal and how it is theoretically supported. The features and results of developing an application which attempts to reproduce the behavior of fish in an undersea world using the methodology proposed are presented in Section 5. Finally, the conclusions and the future work are discussed in Section 6.

## 2   Background

The study of biological systems has inspired the development of a large number of cognitive architectures. According to literature, the most important objectives in living beings, like survive or reproduce, are goals that can be decomposed into other more immediate. To increase the probability of survival, most animals have developed acute perception modalities to detect opportunities and threats in their habitat. The focus of attention is important to behavioral modeling as to gain computational efficiency in sensory processing. Based on the real world, is known that cognitive beings focus their attention in two ways: (1) *using their specialized sense organs*, it is the most common in lower animals and (2) through *cognitive attention* to pay attention only to what is immediately important in your particular situation.

Considering that an animal is a cognitive entity that has the ability of perceiving movement in its environment, some factors must be considered by a system that attempts to simulate such characteristics [2]. **Environment, external stimuli and internal state** let to reflect the physical and mental state (hunger, fatigue, etc.) regarded as the inducer of " motivation" to evoke a particular behavior. The **action selection** occurs after the cognitive entity obtains sensory information about its external world and its internal state, it has to process this information to decide what to do next. And the **behavioral animation** is that in which autonomous models are built by introducing perception and certain behavioral components into the motion control algorithms.

By defining an action as a motor skill, it is necessary to differentiate the *motor control* from the *action selection mechanisms* (see Fig. 1). Motor control mechanisms are responsible for coordinating the actuators (equivalent to muscles) in an agent, this in order to build useful motor skills, i.e. actions. Whilst the action selection mechanisms are only responsible to choose an action without knowing how it is implemented. The action selection mechanism is the key of adaptation and autonomy, as it is a superior control process where the brain can carry out the action selection process on a cognitive or sub-cognitive level.

A. Manning mentions in [3] that *it is often possible to break down complex behavior patterns into smaller units, some of which are immediately equitable with reflexes. Behavior is frequently organized in a hierarchical way... Thus the higher control systems must compete for control for reflexes rather in the manner that reflexes compete for control of muscles.* In practice, there are exclusive actions which use the same actuators and therefore they can not be selected at the same time (walking and sitting). In contrast, the non-exclusive actions can be selected simultaneously (walking and speak).

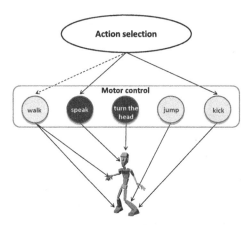

**Fig. 1.** Difference between motor control and action selection mechanisms. This diagram highlights the existence of exclusive and non-exclusive actions.

Thus, the problem of action selection mechanism leads to a design problem and it can be solved by identifying the principles for which living beings select their actions, that is, the priorities for the different behaviors. Therefore, it is clear that the actions selection based on reasoning involves the use of Artificial Intelligence techniques and it is called *task-level motion planning*. Meanwhile the behavior that enables artificial beings become autonomous and "survive" in dynamic environments is a primitive behavior supported in a more primitive and fundamental ability; the reactive or adaptive behavior [3–5].

## 3   Related Work

As mentioned in [6], the study of biological systems has inspired the development of a large number of cognitive architectures in areas such as behavioral animation, artificial life and robotics implementations. Through both experimentation and simulation, biological systems provides means to understand the underlying mechanisms in living organisms while inspiring the development of applications. The work of Ron Sun in [1] explores the view that computational models of cognition may constitute valid theories of cognition. All the discussions point to the position that computational cognitive models can be true theories of cognition.

Moreover, the issues of creating virtual characters with better skeleton and realistic deformable bodies are illustrated in many articles about computer graphics. However, to give a level of believable behavior the challenges are laid on generating on the fly flexible motion and complex behaviors inside of environments using realistic perception capabilities. In this regard, N. Magnenat-Thalmann and D. Thalmann present in [7] research results and future challenges in create realistic and believable virtual humans, where interactivity and group behaviors are also important parameters. The principal conclusion is that the realistic perception of the environment and the internal estate of the "actor" must be reflected affecting its behavior.

The above is important for video games because the study of artificial emotion, from the cognitive psychological perspective, demonstrates that cognitive models in game contents have the most noticeable interaction with users. For example, in [8] it designs an artificial emotion model of the game character. A representative emotion model in the cognitive psychology (OCC) is applied to situations in the game in order to design the CROSS (Character Reaction On Specific Situation) artificial emotion system and to make it as a pre-visualization tool that can be utilized for the stage of planning game. In the same sense, in [9] authors describe their user model for behavioral animation. The model simulates the goals, social traits, perception, and physical behaviors of users in built environments. By inserting virtual users into the environment model and letting them "explore" it on their own volition, their system reveals the interrelationship between the environment and its users.

Nevertheless, there are few works in cognitive architectures for video games specifically, one of them is the RASCALS cognitive architecture presented in [10] which has an high expressive power to building advanced synthetic characters, within the paradigm of logic-based AI. But this is focused in human cognition and the use of an approach to Natural Language Generation (NLG) for the communication *user-character*. In contrast, our work considers the generation of autonomous behaviors endowing characters (no human only) with a certain amount of "common sense" and letting them to generate the boring details from the directives given. The implementation demonstrates the importance of modeling primitive actions properly and shows how to integrate them into motivated complex actions. And it considers the use of simple Fuzzy Cognitive Maps for modeling motivations in a character. It should be emphasized that this model operates within a 3D environment.

## 4  Proposed Architecture for Cognitive Modeling

With the aim of creating an object architecture that could serve as test-bed available and ready to use for testing theories in artificial intelligence, artificial life, but principally cognitive modeling in video games, we propose an hybrid architecture (Fig.2) based on the well-known cognitive architectures ACT-R (Atomic Components of Thought - Rational) and Soar (Historically, State, Operator, And Result, though it is no longer regarded as an acronym). These are the most common in computer science currently. Both provide a conceptual framework for creating models of how performing tasks, they are based on theoretical assumptions sets and have two types of memory; declarative and procedural. However, in ACT-R objectives must be satisfied sequentially while Soar is able to remove (or resolve) intermediate sub-objectives [11].

Both ACT-R and Soar architectures are supported by computer programs that realize these theories of cognition. They both maintain a goal hierarchy where each subsequent sub-goal becomes the focus of the system. Soar was developed by combining three main elements: (a) the heuristic search approach of knowledge-lean and difficult tasks; (b) the procedural view of routine problem solving; and (c) a symbolic theory of bottom-up learning designed to produce the power law of learning. In contrast, ACT-R grew out of detailed phenomena from memory, learning, and problem solving [11, 12].

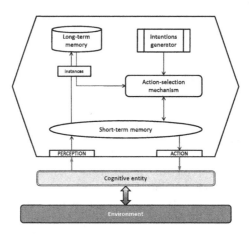

**Fig. 2.** Proposed hybrid architecture for cognitive modeling of game characters

The proposed architecture has two types of memory, declarative (data) and procedural (rules). As Soar and ACT-R, the declarative memory is associated with goals and is removable, therefore this is regarded as a *short-term memory*. Meanwhile, in the procedural memory the rules can be added but not removed in runtime as in a *long-term memory*. Most hybrid architectures are realized in these two ways, but there are also examples where one of the levels is a genetic algorithm, fuzzy logic, or other representation. Reviews of hybrid architectures in [13]. The *Intentions Generator* module is a key component to obtain more complex behaviors, this is the behavior arbitrator whose activation depends on the internal and external state of the cognitive entity. Thus, an effective *Action-selection Mechanism* combines primitive behaviors into motivated behaviors. Finally the situation (internal and external state) and an appropriate response (action) is stored as an *instance* in the long-term memory in similar way as the IBLTool of V. Dutt and C. González performs it in [14]. The correct description of this kind of instances will allow to the action-selection mechanism to obtain better performance and more weighted responses.

### 4.1  Methodology for Developing a Component-Based Behavioral System

The methodology is useful to simulate behavioral systems for testing the different architectures in cognitive modeling (Fig. 3). This is based on the hierarchy of behavioral animation modeling since it has made impressive strides toward autonomy resulting in virtual characters auto-animated endowed of more realistic behaviors [15–18]. It considers three levels of modeling: (1) realistic appearance modeling, (2) realistic smooth and flexible motion modeling and (3) realistic high-level behaviors modeling.

The motor system comprises a dynamic body, actuators and a set of motor controllers. As locomotion is modeled around a mass point that describes the orientation, position, speed and acceleration, thus respective boundaries must be defined.

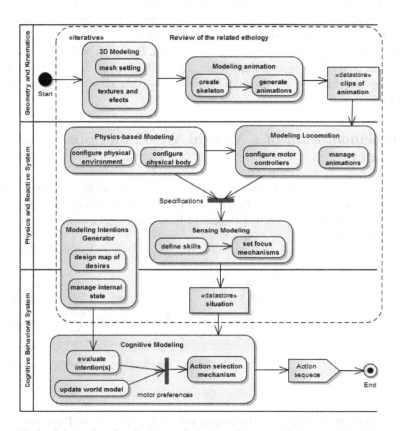

**Fig. 3.** Methodology for developing a behavioral system based on the hierarchy of behavioral animation modeling

Internally, a desire is a potential influence of intention. An agent may have multiple desires, but only those which are the strongest desires will be considered collectively as a specific intention. Finally, additional information should be represented as qualitative recommendations of actions and they are referred as motor preferences. If a sensory stimulus is relevant to an intention occurs, a value will be assigned to the most appropriate motor preference. In this case, the

*short-term memory* represents data obtained in real-time like sensory information and internal states. The *long-term memory* represents *if-then* rules which
determine what can be done and what not, this can not be removed in runtime
(maps of desires, controllers, etc.).

Virtual worlds are fuzzy causal worlds since events cause one another to some
degree, but math models are hard to find, hard to solve and hard to run in
real-time. Therefore, it uses Fuzzy Cognitive Maps (FCMs) for the Intentions
Generator because these can model the desires of a virtual character in its virtual
world in large fuzzy chunks. The causal web is a fuzzy directed graph where the
concept nodes can stand for actions or desires and the causal edges state fuzzy
rules or causal flows between concepts. The justification for using FCMs is that
situated agents with goals can also help choose actions in diverse situations. Each
of these systems keeps the feedforward tree search. But each serial inference uses
only a small part of the stored knowledge. Each FCM input fires all the rules to
some degree. In this way, FCMs model the "circular causality" of real and virtual
worlds [19].

## 5     Implementation of a Virtual World and Simulation Results

Undersea world was selected with the aim of analyzing complex behavior related
to the paradigm of *artificial life*. This consist of fish, plants and different obstacles
to test the inherent cognitive capacities of fish. This world was designed with
the ShiVa3D game engine as seen below.

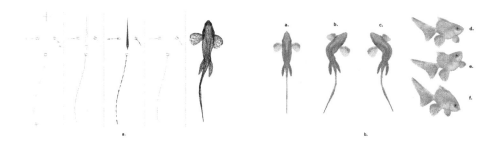

**Fig. 4.** a. Parameter settings for the generation of wave motion. b. Basic movements
idle (a and d), right (b), left (c), up (e), down (f).

The artificial being selected is the goldfish that is a relatively small member
of the carp but it can vary in size and color scheme, and it can be found in most
aquariums. According to the ethology [20], the *carangiform* swimming is the
most appropriate form for this kind of fish. It was modeled as shown in Fig. 4.a.
Combination of atomic actions to generate movement sequences is emphasized by
our implementation. Based on the idea in [21], that behaviors can be either low-
level (common behaviors in most living beings) or high-level (specific behaviors

of a particular creature), we stored 5 atomic actions (Fig. 4.b) into a database of movements where more than one can be executed simultaneously, as long as these are non-exclusive movements.

Fish locomotion is modeled around of a point of mass or center of gravity. Consequently the motor controllers can be classified in displacements and rotations. Displacements are given by the force vector $F$.

$$F = z \cdot \alpha + y \cdot tan(\theta_x) \cdot ||z \cdot \alpha|| \tag{1}$$

where $y, z \in \Re^3$ and they represent the Y and Z axis (in global space) of the body respectively, $\alpha \in \Re$ defines the magnitude of the vector and $\theta \in \Re$ is the angle on the X axis. In turn, rotations on Y axis are given by the 3D matrix rotation. Finally the motor system, which is the core of reactive system, is composed of the following controllers: $M(idle)$, $M(forward)$, $M(backward)$, $M(right)$, $M(left)$, $M(up)$, $M(down)$, $M(brake)$. Needless to explain what each of them performs because its function is trivial.

Furthermore, the hierarchy of intentions considered in the literature [2] provides the theoretical basis for considering the following scheme in this implementation.

Intention to *avoid collision*

⇓

Intention to *run away* from predator

⇓

Intention to *eat* / Intention to *rest*

⇓

Intention to *school*

⇓

Intention to *wander* / Intention to *leave*

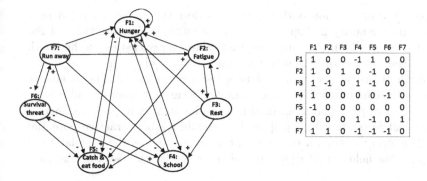

**Fig. 5.** Trivalent fuzzy cognitive map for modeling the intentions generator of a fish. The rules or edges connect causal concepts in a signed connection matrix.

However, due to there are other variables related to these intentions considered as desires (hunger, fatigue or survival threat) which change in an unpredictable manner over time, the implementation of intentions generator requires non-classical techniques of fuzzy logic such as Fuzzy Cognitive Maps. The FCM for a fish is taken up of the work of Julie A. Dickerson and Bart Kosko in [19] and this is shown in Fig.5. But it is clear that the intention to avoid collision is directly related with the data obtained from the sensing system, that is to say, this is part of the reactive system. Finally, intentions to wander and leave are the result of the absence of other desires.

Intentions generator controls, in a high level, perceptual attention focus to filter unnecessary sensory information. Therefore, the sensing system proposed considers four models:

1. Avoidance of collision with terrain.
2. Avoidance of collision with fixed obstacles.
3. Avoidance of collision with dynamic obstacles.
4. Physical touch.

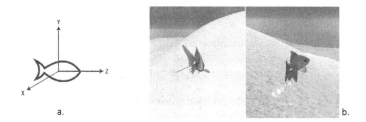

a.                                                                          b.

**Fig. 6.** a. Reference system of the cognitive entity. b. Sensing that defines the reactive behavior with respect to the terrain.

The avoidance of collision with terrain was designed to be activated only when the cognitive entity is displacing. Because intrinsic characteristics of the underwater terrain (Fig. 6), the implementation uses a ray casting method with reference to the lower coordinates of the bounding box of the fish's 3D model and it draws a distinction between go forward and go backward. The avoidance of collision with fixed obstacles is more complex because it must consider some approaches used in path planning. Real fish use landmarks to generate mental maps of geometric relationships [22], so the calculation of attractive potential field (eq. 2) allows to define a target in the space as well as the calculation of repulsive potential field (eq. 3) allows to avoid known obstacles (see Fig. 7.a, 7.b).

$$U_+(q) = \xi \rho_g(q) \tag{2}$$

$$U_-(q) = \begin{cases} \frac{1}{2}\eta(\frac{1}{\rho(q)} - \frac{1}{\rho_0}) & \text{if } \rho(q) \le \rho_0 \\ 0 & \text{otherwise} \end{cases} \tag{3}$$

This is calculated for each point $q \in \Re^3$ where the gradient of $U$ at $q$ is in general $U = U_-(q) + U_+(q)$. $\rho(q)$ is the minimum distance from the point $q$ to the obstacle. The threshold is defined by $\rho_0$, such that beyond this distance the obstacle has no influence. The above for some attractive constant $\xi$ and an repulsive constant $\eta$.

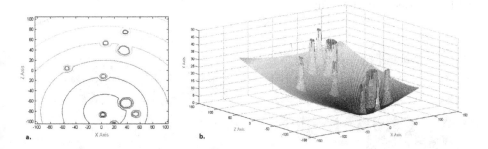

**Fig. 7.** a. Orthogonal view of potential fields calculated for the scene and a temporary target. b. Perspective view of potential fields where the towers represent the repulsive potential field.

Fuzzy Logic is a common resource for solving control problems. In this case, the fuzzy logic facilitates control over the orientation of the artificial fish in Y axis towards a target. The related procedure using the slope between the fish and the target as indicator to determinate if the relative height of the entity is *high*, *medium* or *low* and so make a decision. It uses the membership functions *gama* ($\Gamma$), *lambda* ($\Lambda$) and *function L* as shown in Fig.8.a.

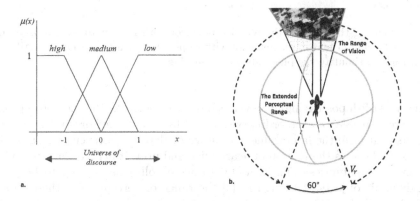

**Fig. 8.** a. Fuzzy logic sets defined by the linguistic variable "relative height". b. Sensing models which attempt to simulate perceptual abilities of real fish. $V_r$ determines the length of the ray and it is limited by an angle of $60°$ (visual range).

However, in the real world exist unknown obstacles which must be considered by the cognitive entity, even it should be able to go over an obstacle relatively large with a small height. Hence, the recalculation of repulsive potential field for an unknown obstacle at runtime is not viable. We implement the ray casting with two rays (right and left) in order to identify the borders of an obstacle and to decide which way to turn; based on the smallest angle determined by the last ray traced (Fig. 9.a). One third ray can be activated to be traced upward to determine whether it is feasible to move up additively or even only move up, and this works in similar way.

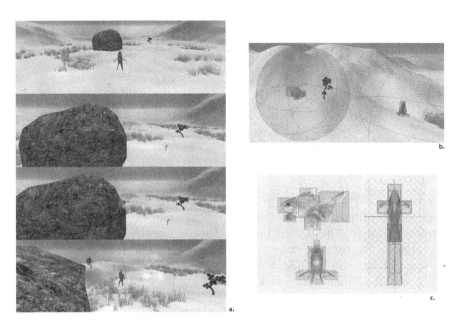

**Fig. 9.** a. Sensing that defines the reactive behavior with respect to fixed objects. b. Sensing that defines the reactive behavior with respect to dynamic objects. c. Artificial fish's ragdoll to simulate the physical contact sensing.

Since most fish possess highly developed sense organs, like the chemoreceptors that are responsible for extraordinary senses of taste and smell or other sensitive receptors that form the lateral line system which detects gentle currents and vibrations, and senses the motion of nearby fish and prey, it is necessary to model this sensory capabilities. This is useful to avoid collisions or even to keeping track dynamic objects. Although in [2] the range of perception of these capabilities, named *the extended perceptual range*, is larger than *the range of vision*, we believe the opposite because the implementation must keep balance between cognitive abilities and unpredictable factors. In Fig. 8.b is shown our proposal wherein the extended perceptual range is a spherical sensor that detects other similar sensors. The visual perception model and the extended perception model together can detecting dynamic objects, and even other cognitive entities (Fig. 9.b). Subsequently, is necessary to simulate physical contact, this in order to define more complex behaviors. For example, assigning the predator-prey roles, or assigning male-female roles in a mating situation. So an "ragdoll" is used to cover the most important parts of the fish (Fig. 9.c).

The updating process of cognitive entity's world model is also a primitive action. In turn, this primitive action requires sensing actions where the reasoning system selects which to execute; this through the behavior arbitrator referred earlier as intentions generator. The reactive system is responsible for executing motor controls efficiently, but this works with the intentions generator and action selection mechanisms to manage the suitable perception model and the activated motor controls to satisfy current intention(s) and thus generate more complex behaviors.

## 6   Conclusions and Future Work

This paper concentrates the most important researches in cognitive modeling for intelligent virtual agents. It also provides an overview of the cognitive architectures ACT-R and Soar, which are the most important currently for computer sciences. In addition, this paper justifies the usefulness of the architecture proposed for cognitive modeling, in a theoretical and technical way. With this progress of the implementation, it has been proved the usability of the methodology. This is used for developing virtual worlds and characters with cognitive behavior, where modeling motor skills and realistic capabilities of sensing are the basis for the reasoning component makes motivated decisions in real-time.

According to literature, the possible applications of our proposal can include test of cognitive models in robotics, experiments to compare similar goal-oriented tasks, design of context-driven controllers, development of procedures for characterization of behavior, test of new sensing mechanisms, on-line path planning and definition of non-deterministic behaviors at runtime.

Future work is to test the cognitive capabilities of agents or characters in complex situations and establish metrics for statistics, and then compare the results of the architecture proposed with any other. This with the aim of improving response time associating "familiar" situations, this approach is based on the Instance-Based Learning (IBL) theory.

## References

1. Sun, R.: Theoretical status of computational cognitive modeling. Cogn. Syst. Res. 10, 124–140 (2009)
2. Tu, X.: Artificial animals for computer animation: biomechanics, locomotion, perception, and behavior. Springer, Heidelberg (1999)
3. Manning, A., Dawkins, M.: An Introduction to Animal Behaviour. Cambridge University Press (1998)
4. Tinbergen, N.: The study of instinct. Clarendon Press (1951)
5. McFarland, D.: Animal behaviour: psychobiology, ethology, and evolution. Longman Scientific and Technical (1993)

6. Weitzenfeld, A.: From brain theory to autonomous robotic agents. In: Mizoguchi, R., Slaney, J.K. (eds.) PRICAI 2000. LNCS, vol. 1886, pp. 351–361. Springer, Heidelberg (2000)
7. Magnenat-Thalmann, N., Thalmann, D.: Virtual humans: thirty years of research, what next? The Visual Computer 21, 997–1015 (2005)
8. Kim, M.: The artificial emotion model of game character through analysis of cognitive situation. In: Proceedings of the 2009 Fourth International Conference on Computer Sciences and Convergence Information Technology, ICCIT 2009, pp. 489–493. IEEE Computer Society, Washington, DC (2009)
9. Yan, W., Kalay, Y.: Geometric, cognitive and behavioral modeling of environmental users. In: Gero, J. (eds.) Design Computing and Cognition 2006, pp. 61–79. Springer (2006)
10. Bringsjord, S., Khemlani, S., Arkoudas, K., Mcevoy, C., Destefano, M., Daigle, M.: Advanced synthetic characters, evil. In: Game-On 2005, 6th International Conference on Intelligent Games and Simulation (M. Al-Akaidi and, European Simulation Society), pp. 31–39 (2005)
11. Ritter, F.E.: Two cognitive modeling frontiers: Emotions and usability. Transactions of the Japanese Society for Artificial Intelligence 24, 241–249 (2009)
12. Anderson, J.: The Architecture of Cognition. Cognitive science series. Lawrence Erlbaum Associates (1996)
13. Kandel, A., Langholz, G.: Hybrid Architectures for Intelligent Systems. CRC Press, Incorporated (1992)
14. Dutt, V., Gonzalez, C.: Making Instance-based Learning Theory usable and understandable: The Instance-based Learning Tool. Comput. Hum. Behavior 28, 1227–1240 (2012)
15. Funge, J.D.: Making them behave: cognitive models for computer animation. PhD thesis, University of Toronto, Toronto, Ont., Canada (1998)
16. Funge, J., Tu, X., Terzopoulos, D.: Cognitive modeling: knowledge, reasoning and planning for intelligent characters. In: Proceedings of the 26th Annual Conference on Computer Graphics and Interactive Techniques, SIGGRAPH 1999, pp. 29–38. ACM Press/Addison-Wesley Publishing Co., New York (1999)
17. Funge, J.: Cognitive modeling for games and animation. Commun. ACM 43, 40–48 (2000)
18. Dannenmann, P., Barthel, H., Hagen, H.: Multi level Control of Cognitive Characters in Virtual Environments. In: Proceedings of the 14th IEEE Visualization 2003 (VIS 2003), p. 92. IEEE Computer Society, Washington, DC (2003)
19. Dickerson, J.A., Kosko, B.: Virtual Worlds as Fuzzy Cognitive Maps. Presence 3, 173–189 (1994)
20. Stephens, K., Pham, B., Wardhani, A.: Modelling fish behaviour. In: Proceedings of the 1st International Conference on Computer Graphics and Interactive Techniques, GRAPHITE 2003, pp. 71–78. ACM, New York (2003)
21. Barthel, H., Dannenmann, P., Hagen, H.: Towards a General Framework for Animating Cognitive Characters. In: Proceedings of the 3rd IASTED International Conference on Visualization, Imaging, and Image Processing, VIIP 2003, Benalmádena, Spain (2003)
22. Chung, S.: Appropriate maze methodology to study learning in fish. University of Toronto Journal of Undergraduate Life Sciences 2 (2009)

# Semantic Representation of CAD Models
# Based on the IGES Standard

Nestor Velasco Bermeo[1], Miguel González Mendoza[1], and Alexander García Castro[2]

[1] ITESM Campus Estado de México, Computer Science Department
[2] Florida State University
{nestorvb,alexgarciac}@gmail.com, mgonza@itesm.mx

**Abstract.** The design process of a product is iterative due to a series of changes that range from client specifications to quality defects. From each of such changes, designers end up with a considerable amount of design files, additionally, if files have to be exchanged with other partners they have to be translated based on the available neutral file formats. In order to identify specific elements stored on the resulting translated files, the designer needs to make use of a CAD system. If the amount of files to consult is significant, the task becomes excessively time consuming. The approach presented here, focuses on the creation of semantic models providing the user; query capabilities over a collection of CAD models in order to identify a specific design based on particular conditions along with exploration capabilities to detect key elements from any IGES CAD file. Both capabilities possible without the need of using a CAD system.

**Keywords:** RDF, CAD, IGES, semantic representation, Ontology.

## 1 Introduction

Product development focuses on tools such as Computer Aided Design (CAD), Computer Aided Engineering (CAE) as well as Computer Aided Manufacturing (CAM). They all systematically contribute to the innovation capabilities of a business [1] and its integration into a global market. Product design follows a process as shown in Figure 1. All products start from a need that derives from either a client specification or market research that denotes such need. During the design process there are two main sub processes; Synthesis and Analysis. The former aims determining its functionality by means of drafts and drawings that denote the relations between the different parts of the product, the latter aims at provide context to the design within the pertinent engineering sciences (mechanical, electrical, etc.) in order to formerly evaluate the product performance (by means of simulation and modeling). The resulting outcomes of the Analysis process are the product's engineering drawings.

F. Castro, A. Gelbukh, and M. González (Eds.): MICAI 2013, Part I, LNAI 8265, pp. 157–168, 2013.
© Springer-Verlag Berlin Heidelberg 2013

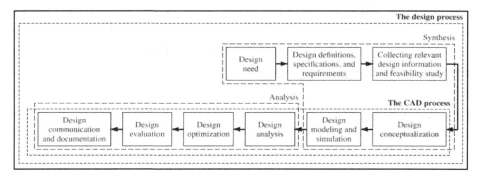

**Fig. 1.** Product Design process. [2][3]

The Design process invariably iterates [4][5] from steps 4 to 9 (as depicted on Figure 1) due to the fact that the deriving drawings don't fulfill the original requirements and specifications. Some of the changes that occur during such iterations are a result of client changes of the product specifications [6] or for quality defects on the resulting product [7]. From the Product's Life Cycle perspective the amount of changes a design undergoes occur mainly on its first Phase as show on Figure 2.

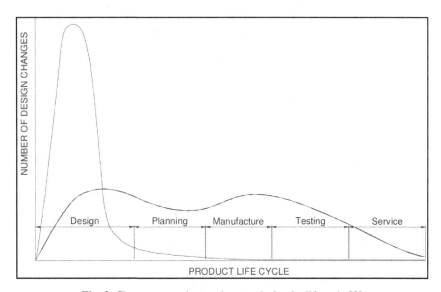

**Fig. 2.** Changes a product undergoes during its lifecycle [8]

From the above described design process it is important to consider that Organizations don't have all the knowledge and expertise to completely produce a product. Specifically whether the design process occurs completely within the company or in conjunction with a series of partners, such partners can be scattered across the globe and that condition itself generates complications in the data exchange process along with the use of different CAD systems.

Data Interoperability problems derive from the high heterogeneity in CAD file formats since each partner might use a different CAD system to create their corresponding designs of the product. Currently the widespread technique of CAD Software integration relies on exporting the original CAD file onto one of the two main neutral formats; the **Standard for the Exchange of Product Data Model** (STEP) [9] and the **Initial Graphics Exchange Specification** (IGES) [10]. Each neutral file format has the capacity of translating geometric model information along with additional product information.

With the use of neutral file formats for CAD system integration the file exchange problem is solved but designers face another complication. That is due to the amount of design files they have to manage and deal for each product which are around an average of 50 to 100 designs (including intermediate drafts and work-in-progress versions). To administrate such files sometimes a firm relies on Document Management System [11] or dedicated systems like Engineering Document Management System [12] which aim at handling data and information related to a design or product from diverse sources and types such as quality requirements or reports, simulation results, geometry data and models, etc. Other management systems commonly used are the Product Data Management (PDM) [13][14].

Those data and file management systems aim at indexing and querying all the files stored within but fail at dealing with neutral CAD files. Commercial solutions focus on their proprietary file formats and provide search and index services but can't provide the same support and capabilities for STEP and IGES files. According to Sheth [15] Heterogeneous sources cause most of the interoperability conflicts whereas such heterogeneity can occur at different levels. For instance in a scenario as described above a company faces a Syntactic heterogeneity which refers to the difference in data formats (for instance if a company has STEP, IGES, NX, PRT files) along with the structural heterogeneity which refers to the differences in representation schema. Finally Semantic heterogeneity is present too when facing differences in the meaning of entities used among the different CAD solutions.

The approach described in this paper focuses on the IGES neutral CAD file format for two main reasons:

1. It can store and represent not only 3D model data but also information from different types of applications such as: Finite Element, Plant Design, Mechanical and Electrical data, etc.
2. Contrary to STEP, IGES has its full specification documentation available and free of charge, whereas STEP is divided upon Application Protocols (AP) and the documentation for each AP has variable costs.

The goal is to create a semantically rich model that represents all the elements and describes the relationships of an IGES CAD file so that designers (or any other involved participant in the product design process) will be able to identify particular information or details of a specific IGES file from a collection of files based on specific criteria.

The rest of the paper is organized as follows; in Section 2 similar approaches focusing on neutral CAD formats are addressed, Section 3 presents the highlights of the IGES standard whereas in Section 4 the main elements and considerations of the semantic models are described. Finally in Section 5 concluding remarks about the semantic representation are presented along with the discourse of future work.

# 2     Related Work

The presented works are centered on the STEP specification, since there is no current efforts that center on IGES the works are relevant because they focus on three main aspect that are as well the driving intentions of the present paper. Those aspects focus on: semantic representation of CAD neutral file exchange format, product description enhancement and a formal ontology for STEP. All works aim at extending the interoperability capabilities of the original neutral file format they worked on.

In terms of semantically modeling the work presented by [16] is an effort to enable the STEP AP 203 (EXPRESS schema) and Part 21 (Geometry data Detailed information) files into OWL models, the work centers on improving STEP's product data interoperability by defining in a formal logic way the semantics of STEP models. The approach centers on the EXPRESS language, by shaping and formulating its structure and semantics according to OWL-DL specifications to achieve consistency checking, inference and decidability. The results of their work was an OWL translation of the EXPRESS files in a semantically rich product model they called OntoSTEP which can be easily integrated with OWL ontologies, additionally the creation of a Protegé plugin that extracts the beyond-geometry information of the product into its corresponding OntoSTEP representation.

Another approach that has been proposed to enrich STEP's product description is by including functional design knowledge [17]. The authors state that in order to complete the product data it is important to include the artifacts function during collaborative functional modeling. The approach extends their previous work on Behavior-driven Function-Environment-Structure (B-FES) but with an ontology-based scheme. The resulting functional design ontology B-FES/o aims at allowing various design agents the possibility to browse, search and integrate web services aimed at functional design along with the reuse of functional design knowledge.

The authors of [18] proposed an ontology based on STEP's AP 42 (Topological and Geometrical Representation) under the scope of the AIM@SHAPE [19] initiative. Although the full development and application of the ontology was not implemented, their work is relevant since the ontology is available and serves as a guideline on the mapping strategy they followed between EXPRESS classes and OW.

Although the differences between STEP and IGES are remarkable (file structure, data representation, product data support and applications, etc) the previous works denote the current ongoing efforts to extend the interoperability and information exploitation of CAD neutral files along with the tendency of semantically enrich the original models. Based on those evident needs along with the fact that little has been done towards IGES (and since it is still used and supported by CAD systems) this paper intends to provide a first approach at semantically representing the data and contents of IGES files.

# 3    IGES, a Neutral File Format for CAD System Integration

The Initial Graphics Exchange Specification (IGES) started as an American National Standards Institute (ANSI) Standard developed by the US National Bureau of Standards first created in 1980 and accepted as an ANSI standard later on 1981. It's creation aimed at providing CAD/CAM systems a specific information structure to represent and exchange of product definition data. The specifications provides the insights and details on the file structure along with elements such as language formats in order to represent "*geometric, topological and non-geometric product definition data*"[10].   The categories of Product Definition that the IGES standard supports are the following:

- *Administrative*: Product Identification and Structure
- *Design/Analysis*: Idealized Models
- *Basic Shape*: Geometric and Topological
- *Augmentation of Physical Characteristics*: Dimensions and Intrinsic Properties
- *Presentation Information.*

The importance of working with the IGES standard lies on the fact that the file does not only provide support for geometrical information (3D or 2D CAD models) but it also allows the user to retrieve product information stored within. The basic unit of the IGES file structure is the "entity" which can be divided into two groupings: geometric and non-geometric. The former contemplates entities that represent and describe the physical shape of the product (2D elements such as: Point, curve, arc, line as well as 3D elements such as: Sphere, Torus, Plane Surface, Ellipsoid, etc.), the latter considers entities that enrich and define the geometric entities (dimensions, units, annotations, associativity, etc.) Also it is important to note that IGES supports complementary product data for applications such as Finite Element Modeling (FEM), Architecture Engineering and Construction (AEC), Electrical Attributes along with Process Plant elements. The main structure of an IGES file will be briefly described in the following section.

## 3.1    IGES File Definition, Structure and Main Elements

According to the IGES specification [10], the file structure conforms of 5 sections:

1) Start Section (S)
2) Global Section (GS)
3) Directory Entry Section (DE)
4) Parameter Data Section (PD)
5) Terminate Section (TS)

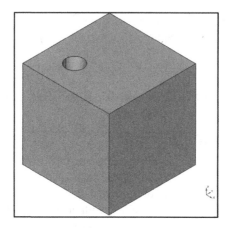

**Fig. 3.** Sample IGES 3D CAD model

An IGES file represents product data as an *"organized collection of entities"* [10] and so declaring an entity as the basic unit that is used to represent all the details and information of a product. As mentioned before each file comprises 5 Sections.

The Start Section aims at providing a "human readable" description of the file and the elements it contains but it is never used by any CAD system. The Global Section is the main section of the entire file since it contains vital information such as: model space scale and units, minimum resolution and maximum coordinate values, etc. The Directory Entry Section defines a fixed structure of 20 fields that describe the elements and corresponding attributes of all the entities (geometrical and non-geometrical) used in the IGES file, it is important to mention that such structure is iterated for every single entity. The Parameter Data Section contains the data of each entity listed in the DE Section. Since each entity has a varying number of parameters (for example a Color Definition uses 5 parameters to be described while a Relational B-Spline Curve entity uses 180 parameters) the PD section does have any defined structure as the DE Section does. The Terminate Section defines the amount of records each section uses in the file structure to avoid file integrity conflicts when read by a CAD system.

To have a better understanding of the IGES file structure, a sample IGES file is presented for explanation purposes. The file describes all related data of a 100-inch cube with a 20-inch diameter cylindrical thru-hole as shown in Figure 3. The complete file contains 683 lines so for brevity purposes Figures 4a, 4b and 4c show a sectioned view of the contents of the file to illustrate each one of the sections of the actual data contained within the file.

```
 1    Comment                                                                  S    1
 2    1H,,1H;,10HSolid Edge,12Hcubohole.igs,17H By Spatial Corp.,22HXPlus GENEG  1
 3    RIC/IGES 3.0,32,38, 6,308,15,7HUnknown,1.000,1,2HIN,1,1.000,15H20120424.G   2
 4    221533,3.9e-007,0.00,6HAuthor,5HTitle,11,0,15H20120424.221533;           G    3
 5         314       1      0      1      0      0      0      000010001D      1
 6         314       1      0      2      0      0      0            0D      2
 7         128       3      0      1      0      0      0      000010001D      3
 8         128       1      0      9      0      0      0            0D      4
 9         126      12      0      1      0      0      0      000010501D      5
10         126       1      0      3      0      0      0            0D      6
```

**Fig. 4a.** Start Section declared in line 1, GS declared on lines 2-4, DE starting at line 5

```
255       144     426      0      1      0      0      0      000000001D    251
256       144       1   -225      1      0      0      0            0D    252
257    314,75.29412508010864,75.29412508010864,75.29412508010864,10HMix    1P      1
258    edColor;                                                            1P      2
259    128,3,1,3,1,0,0,0,0,-1.,-1.,-1.,-1.,0.,0.,0.,0.,0.,0.,1.,1.,        3P      3
260    1.,0.33333333333333,0.33333333333333,1.,1.,0.33333333333333,       3P      4
261    0.33333333333333,1.,1.5748031496063,1.18110236220472,0.,           3P      5
262    1.5748031496063,0.39370078740158,0.,0.78740157480315,              3P      6
```

**Fig. 4b.** DE Section finalizing at line 256, PD Section starting at line 257

```
677    1.96850393700787,3.93700787401575,0.78740157480315,               245P    421
678    1.18110236220472,3.93700787401575,-7.85398163397448,              245P    422
679    -4.71238898038469;                                                245P    423
680    102,4,239,241,243,245;                                            247P    424
681    142,1,227,237,247,2;                                              249P    425
682    144,227,1,0,249;                                                  251P    426
683    S       1G      3D     252P     426                                  T      1
```

**Fig. 4c.** PD Section finalizing at line 682, TS declared in line 683

Figure 4a shows the first section of the sample IGES file, lines 2-4 represent the Global Section, which in turn holds a total of 26 elements that provide important information about the file and the elements within it. Elements such as: Native System ID (name of the CAD system that was used to create the original file), File name, Units name, model space scale, date and time of exchange file generation, name of author and author's organization, etc.

Identifying at first glance each element of the Global Section from a file that resembles what is depicted in Figure 4a does not imply expertise in CAD design or engineering knowledge but requires a perfect notion of the IGES documentation referring to the specific structures and rules of each Section. The same occurs on the following sections (DE and PS) since there's no more information than numbers on each line and without context it's hard to differentiate and understand the data presented. If the file is opened with any CAD software the user can look up specific elements such as units or the author's name, but it still, it is a time consuming task since there is no universal procedure to obtain such data that applies to all CAD systems.

## 4    Semantic Representation of IGES CAD Files

It is manifest that IGES observes a fixed and precise structure but yet the useful information it stores within (geometrical and non-geometrical) can't be identified straightforwardly. The need of having the full IGES Specification document at hand is imperative when analyzing the contents of a file without a CAD System. To address these complications in this paper the use of semantic representation is proposed to extend the IGES interoperability capabilities by providing a semantic structure to its data [20].

The idea is to extract all the data of an IGES file preserving as much as possible its original structure but expressing it according to the World Wide Web Consortium's (W3C) Resource Description Framework (RDF) standard model [21].

The semantic representation of IGES data focuses on creating an RDF version of all the contents and elements saved on each file. In order to do such modeling a lightweight ontology is proposed, it resembles the data structure described in the IGES documentation for their files but from a Semantic Web approach. By doing so the result of the instantiation of the ontology with the data from an IGES file extends the interoperability capabilities of the IGES files. The ontology provides a *"formal specification of a conceptualization"*[22].

The scope of the semantic representation of the IGES files focuses on:

- Represent the IGES file structure and elements using the RDF data model.
- Extract all the product information stored within any IGES file.
- Translate any IGES file to its semantic representation.
- Provide the user the possibility to explore and identify specific data from an IGES file without the need of a CAD system.

To test if the current approach provides enhanced functionalities versus an original IGES file, the following competency question served as the evaluation guidelines for the development of the ontology:

1. Can a semantic representation of the contents of an IGES file provide a user the ability to identify and extract specific information related to a product?
2. Can a user locate a specific file from a collection of IGES files based from their corresponding semantic representations?
3. Is it feasible to list all the information from a product stored within an IGES file without the use of any CAD system?

Derived from the competency questions enlisted the first thing was developing a semantic representation based on the RDF specification of the IGES file structure. All the vocabulary used on the RDF model is based on the terms and elements that the IGES documentation uses, that way if the user wants to get a deeper insight of the elements presented he/she can refer to the documentation and get a deeper understanding of what's presented in the resulting RDF model. Since RDF is based on the statement approach (subject-predicate-object) it is easier to identify the properties and elements of a sample IGES file product when declared as specific statements such as the ones presented in Table1.

**Table 1.** Sample elements based on a sample IGES product data file

| Num. | Subject | Objetct | Predicate |
|------|---------|---------|-----------|
| 1 | http://www.ontoIGES.test/slotrdf/ | hasSection | GlobalSection |
| 2 | http://www.ontoIGES.test/slotrdf/ | hasSection | DirectorySection |
| 3 | http://www.ontoIGES.test/slotrdf/DirectorySection/Entity=1/ | hasTypeNumber | 116 |
| 4 | http://www.ontoIGES.test/slotrdf/DirectorySection/Entity=1/ | hasLabel | Point |
| 5 | http://www.ontoIGES.test/slotrdf/GlobalSection | hasFileName | slot |
| 6 | http://www.ontoIGES.test/slotrdf/GlobalSection | hasNativeSystemID | slot.igs |
| 7 | http://www.ontoIGES.test/slotrdf/GlobalSection | hasUnitsName | IN |
| 8 | http://www.ontoIGES.test/slotrdf/GlobalSection | hasNameofAuthor | NVB |
| 9 | http://www.ontoIGES.test/slotrdf/GlobalSection | hasAuthorsOrganization | ITESM |
| 10 | http://www.ontoIGES.test/slotrdf/GlobalSection | hasDateandTimeofCreation | 20120424.192927 |

As mentioned before, one of the goals of the semantic representation of IGES files was to *"represent the IGES file structure..."*, the first two rows of Table 1 shows that the file structure of an IGES file can be represented as a statement. For instance the first row declares that the file *"slotrdf"* has a Section named "GlobalSection" while on the second row the statement declares that "slotrdf" has a Section named "DirectorySection". On the next rows it can be observed that the entity number 1 of the file has a TypeNumber "118" (row 3) and it has a Label of "Point". On the rest of the rows additional data from the Global Section of the file is represented, the Units Name along with the Author's Name and its Organization as well as the Date and Time when the file was created was successfully extracted and listed.

It is important to note that while Table 1 shows fragments of the contents of a file on the ontology all the sections and file structure was successfully represented. All the 26 elements from the Global Section and 20 elements from the Directory Section including the Parameter Section are covered. Table 2 shows an overview of all the elements that conform each section. The only sections that were not included where the Start and Terminate Section, that was because they don't provide significant information and they can confuse a user since their purpose is for file integrity verification for CAD systems.

All of the classes used for the ontology are based on the IGES file structure: Global Section, Directory Section and Parameter Section while the elements of each Section were used as the Object Properties. For each Object Property its corresponding Data type property was declared based on the IGES specification. For brevity purposes the details of each data type are not discussed here.

**Table 2.** Elements of the Global and Directory Section of all IGES files

| Element | Global Section | Directory Section |
|---|---|---|
| 1 | Parameter Delimiter Character. | Entity Type Number |
| 2 | Record Delimiter Character. | Parameter Data |
| 3 | Product ID from Sending System | Structure |
| 4 | File Name | Line font pattern |
| 5 | NativeSystem ID | Level |
| 6 | Preprocessor Version | View |
| 7 | Number of Binary Bits for Integer Representation | Transformation Matrix |
| 8 | Single Precision Magnitude | Label Display Associativity |
| 9 | Single Precision Significance | Status Number |
| 10 | Double Precision Magnitude | Sequence Number |
| 11 | Double Precision Significance | Entity Type Number |
| 12 | Product ID for Receiver | Line Weight Number |
| 13 | Model Space Scale | Color Number |
| 14 | Units Flag | Parameter Line Count Number |
| 15 | Units Name | Form Number |
| 16 | Maximum Number of Line Weights | Reserved 1 |
| 17 | Size of Maximum Line Width | Reserved 2 |
| 18 | Date and Time of Creation | Entity Label |
| 19 | Minimum User-Intended Resolution | Entity Subscript Number |
| 20 | Approximate Maximum Coordinate Value | Sequence Number 2 |
| 21 | Name of Author | |
| 22 | Author's Organization | |
| 23 | IGES Version Number | |
| 24 | Drafting Standard Code | |
| 25 | Model Creation or Last Change Date | |
| 26 | Application Protocol / Subset ID | |

To successfully extract and translate the contents of any IGES file a tool was developed. The operations performed by the tool are the following; listing of all the available IGES files stored on a target folder, once the user identifies the desired file and writes its name on the tool prompt, it extracts all the contents of the IGES file, then all of the data is instantiated according to the ontology and finally the output of such process is an RDF file named as the original IGES file. In the present approach the output files follow the RDF/XML serialization standard to improve the data exchange process with other systems and to ease the human reading/comprehension process.

To test the ability to locate a file based on its semantic representation there was the need to set up a triple store for the resulting RDF files in order to have the possibility to query the collection saved files. OpenLink Virtuoso server [23] was used for this purpose. In order for a user to consult from the dataset the user has to perform a SPARQL query. The SPARQL query capability and flexibility of the triple store allows the user to obtain specific information from the stored semantic representation of the IGES files. Some of the queries executed over the dataset (of about 100 translated IGES models) include: enlist all files that were drawn using the Inches Units (IN) (*UnitsName property*), list all the files created by a specific Author (*NameofAuthor* property), enlist all the files that were created by a Specific CAD system (*NativeSystemID property*) for instance AutoCAD, CATIA, SolidEdge, etc.

# 5    Concluding Remarks and Future Work

The presented work shows the first approach at creating a semantic representation of CAD models based on the IGES standard. The extraction of all the data stored on a native IGES file was successful as well as their translation into an RDF format. The resulting files were validated using the W3C's Validation Service in order to verify its RDF conformance. Also a small test was conducted with a series of colleagues that were presented first an original IGES file with 5 simple questions, then the corresponding semantic representation of the file was handed and the same questions were presented. The impressions obtained was that it resulted easier for them to identify the elements that were asked for on the questionnaire even though they had no background or previous knowledge regarding the IGES specification. This simple test served as a starting point to prove that users without any background or expertise could be able to find specific information from a semantic representation of an IGES file and that there could be no need for a CAD system to obtain such information.

There is more work to do in terms of perfecting the semantic representation of IGES files. Future work will focus on some aspects like; query capabilities to perform complex SPARQL queries over the current dataset, inclusion of diversity of the translated files (inclusion of 3D and 2D models, entity based queries), file size or modularity, inclusion of other ontologies to allow the reuse of the ontology, etc.

# References

1. Bordegoni, M., Rizzi, C.: Innovation in Product Design: From CAD to Virtual Prototyping. Springer, London (2011)
2. Zeid, I.: Mastering cad/cam. McGraw-Hill, Inc. (2004)
3. Rao, P.N.: CAD/CAM Principles and Applications. Tata McGraw-Hill Education (2004)
4. Kohler, C., et al.: A matrix representation of the CPM/PDD approach as a means for change impact analysis. In: International Design Conference, Dubrovnik, Croatia (2008)
5. Hanna, A.S., Swanson, J.: Risk allocation by law-cumulative impact of change orders. Journal of Professional Issues in Engineering Education and Practice, ASCE (2007)
6. Keller, R., Eckert, C.M., Clarkson, P.J.: Using an engineering change methodology to support conceptual design. Journal of Engineering Design 20(6) (2009)
7. Burati, J.L., Farrington, J.J., Ledbetter, W.B.: Causes of quality deviations in design and construction. Journal of Construction Engineering and Management (1992)
8. Radhakrishnan, P., Subramanyan, S., Raju, V.: CAD/CAM/CIM. New Age International (2008)
9. International Organization for Standardization. ISO 10303-11: Industrial automation systems and? integration – Product data representation and exchange – Part 1: Overview and fundamental principles (1994)
10. Initial Graphics Exchange Specification: IGES 5.3, N. Charleston, SC: U.S. Product Data Association, http://www.uspro.org/product-data-resources
11. Sutton, M.J.: Document management for the enterprise: principles, techniques, and applications. John Wiley & Sons, Inc. (1996)
12. Peltonen, H., Mannisto, T., Alho, K., Sulonen, R.: An engineering document management system. In: Proceedings of the ASME Winter Annual Meeting, pp. 6–9 (1993)

13. Kropsu-Vehkapera, H., Haapasalo, H., Harkonen, J., Silvola, R.: Product data management practices in high-tech companies. Industrial Management & Data Systems 109(6), 758–774 (2009)

14. Miller, E.: "What's PDM?" Computer-Aided Engineering Magazine (1997)

15. Sheth, A.: Changing focus on interoperability in information systems: from system, syntax, structure to semantics. In: Goodchild, M.F., et al. (eds.) Interoperating Geographic Information Systems. Kluwer, Dordecht (1999)

16. Krima, S., Barbau, R., Fiorentini, X., Rachuri, S., Sriram, R.: OntoSTEP: OWL-DL Ontology for STEP, National Institue of Standards and Technology, NISTIR 7561, Gaithersburg, MD 20899, USA (2009)

17. Zhang, W.Y., Lin, L.F., Tong, R.F., Li, X., Dong, J.X.: B-FES/o: an ontology-based scheme for functional modeling in design for semantic Web applications. In: Shen, W., James, A.E., Chao, K.-M., Younas, M., Lin, Z., Barthès, J.-P.A. (eds.) CSCWD (2), pp. 1146–1151. IEEE Computer Society (2005)

18. Andersen, O.A., Vasilakis, G.: Building an ontology of CAD model information. In: Geometric Modelling,Numerical Simulation, and Optimization: Applied Mathematics and SINTEF, pp. 11–40. Springer (2007)

19. Falcidieno, B., Spagnuolo, M., Alliez, P., Quak, E., Vavalis, E., Houstis, C.: Towards the Semantics of Digital Shapes: The AIM@ SHAPE Approach. In: EWIMT (2004)

20. Ray, S.R.: Interoperability standards in the semantic web. Journal of Computing and Information Science in Engineering (Transactions of the ASME) 2(1), 65–68 (2002)

21. Resource Description Framework (RDF), http://www.w3.org/RDF/

22. Gruber, T.R.: A translation approach to portable ontology specifications. Knowledge Acquisition 5(2), 199–220 (1993)

23. OpenLink Virtuoso,
http://virtuoso.openlinksw.com/dataspace/dav/wiki/Main

# Complexity of Verification of Fuzzy Multi-Agent Systems[*]

Michael I. Dekhtyar[1] and Mars K. Valiev[2]

[1] Dept. of CS, Tver St. Univ., Tver, Russia, 170000
Michael.Dekhtyar@tversu.ru
[2] Keldysh Inst. for Appl. Math., Moscow, Russia, 125047
valiev@keldysh.ru

**Abstract.** Some notions of fuzzy multi-agent systems are introduced. Agents of these systems are controlled by fuzzy logic programs. Complexity of verification of their dynamic properties are established. The properties are expressed as formulas of some variants of fuzzy temporal logic.

## 1 Introduction

The study of verification of temporal (dynamic) properties of program systems was initiated in [1]. One of the most successful approaches in this area is model checking (verification of formulas of different variants of temporal logic on models defined on transition systems). A wealth of results on model checking and its complexity is exposed in [2] and, in a more extent (including, in particular, results on probabilisic systems) in [3] (probabilistic transition systems correspond, in usual terminology, to Markov chains (MC) and decision processes (MDP)). Transition systems are very abstract: their states have no structure, and transitions are fixed in time. Multi-agent systems (MAS) in some sense generalize transition systems: states of their agents can be supplied by a structure, and transitions are controlled by some intelligent components of agents. The first results on verification of MAS (of different types) were obtained in [4–6]. Since then many extensions and generalizations of these results appeared, in particular, for probabilistic MAS (see f.e., [7–9]).

Probabilistic systems are used to model practical systems acting in uncertainty conditions. But often using fuzzy notions is more appropriate to model uncertainty. So, some fuzzy variants of MCs and MDP were defined in [10, 11] as variants of formalization of fuzzy dynamic control systems introduced in [12]. Here we introduce fuzzy MAS and study the complexity of the verification problem for them. Our approach here is similar to the approach we used for probabilistic MAS in [8, 9]. Namely, we propose an effective algorithm of simulation of any fuzzy MAS **A** by a fuzzy Markov system **M**. So, the solutions of various problems of verification of **A** are reduced to the solutions of the corresponding problems for **M** However, a difference from probabilistic case is that for probabilistic systems we can use known results [13, 14] on complexity of verification of usual MC and MDP while for fuzzy Markov systems such results were not known, and we had to establish them.

[*] This work was sponsored by the RFBR Grants 13-01-00643 and 13-01-00382.

## 2  Fuzzy Markov Decision Processes

Fuzzy MAS verification, as we propose it, is based on verification of finite fuzzy Markov systems. Fuzzy Markov systems can be formally defined in a number of ways (see [10, 11]). We follow the approach of Avrachenkov and Sanches [10] and sketch the definitions below.

A fuzzy Markov decision process (MDP) $\mathbf{M}$ is a controlled fuzzy Markov chain with a finite set of states $S = S_{\mathbf{M}}$. With every state $s \in S$, a finite set $Act_s$ of possible actions, which are available when the process is in state $s$, is associated. If the system is in a state $s \in S$ and an action $a \in Act_s$ is chosen, then the system executes a transition to a next state according to a given fuzzy transition distribution $p_{s,a} : S \to [0,1]$. Informally, $p_{s,a}(s')$ is the possibility to move from the state $s$ to the state $s'$ when the action $a$ is chosen in $s$.

To summarize, a fuzzy MDP $\mathbf{M}$ has the form $\langle S, \{Act_s | s \in S\}, \{p_{s,a} | s \in S, a \in Act_s\}\rangle$, where $S$ is a set of states, $Act_s$ is a set of actions, and $p_{s,a}$ is a distribution of transition possibilities. We choose the starting state of $\mathbf{M}$ as $s_0$.

The MDP $\mathbf{M}$ can be represented as a directed multigraph $G_M$ with the set of nodes $S$ and edges $(s, s')$ labeled by pairs of the form $\langle a, p_{s,a}(s')\rangle$, where $a \in Act_s$.

*Trajectories* of an MDP $\mathbf{M}$ are finite or infinite sequences of alternating states and actions $\tau = \langle s_1, a_1, s_2, a_2, \ldots\rangle$ such that for all $i$ $s_i \in S$, $a_i \in Act_{s_i}$ and for all $i$ there is an edge in $G_M$ from $s_i$ to $s_{i+1}$ labeled by $\langle a_i, p\rangle$ for some $p > 0$.

With each trajectory $\tau$ we associate a path $\pi_\tau = s_1, s_2, \ldots$ along the states of $G_M$. Given a path $\pi = s_1, s_2, \ldots$, we denote by $\pi^{(i)}$ the suffix of $\pi$ starting at $s_i$, i.e. $\pi^{(i)} = s_i, s_{i+1}, \ldots$.

The *possibility* $p(\tau)$ *of trajectory* $\tau$ is defined as the minimal possibility of the transitions along the trajectoty, i.e. $p(\tau) = \min\{p_{s_i,a}(s_{i+1}) | \langle s_i, a, s_{i+1}\rangle \in \tau\}$. *Possibility* $p(T)$ *of a set of trajectories* $T$ is defined as $\max\{p(\tau) | \tau \in T\}$.

A *decision policy* $u$ for an MDP $\mathbf{M}$ is a prescription for choosing actions at each point in time. Such a policy must select an action $a$ from the set $Act_s$ when the process is in state $s$, and it can base its selection on the history of the process up to that time. With each policy $u$, a set of trajectories $\mathcal{T}(u)$ is associated. $\mathcal{T}(u)$ includes all trajectories $\tau = \langle s_1, a_1, s_2, a_2, \ldots\rangle$, such that for all $i$ $u(s_1, a_1, s_2, a_2, \ldots, s_i) = a_i$.

Given a state $s \in S$, we denote as $T(s, u)$ the set of all trajectories of $\mathcal{T}(u)$ starting in $s$. One can view an MDP with a fixed policy as a fuzzy Markov chain (MC) on an infinite state space, namely on the set of all finite trajectories.

## 3  Fuzzy Popositional Temporal Logics

To specify dynamic properties of fuzzy MDPs and fuzzy MAS, we use temporal logics that correspond to the variants of temporal logics used for specification of the properties of regular MDPs and MCs (see, e.g. [3], ch. 9). We start with a definition of a fuzzy version $FCTL^*$ of the branching time logic $CTL^*$. This logic is similar to the probabilistic branching time logic $PCTL^*$ introduced in [15].

FCTL* (fuzzy computation tree logic star) is a branching-time temporal logic. Its formulas define properties of trees of paths of MDPs. Besides the standard propositional logic and temporal operators, it includes the possibilistic operator $[\varphi]_J$ where $\varphi$ is a path formula and $J$ is an interval of $[0,1]$. The path formula $\varphi$ imposes a condition on the set of paths, where $J = [a,b]$ indicates a lower bound $a$ and an upper bound $b$ on the possibility.

The syntax of $FCTL^*$ includes two types of formulas: *state formulas* and *path formulas*. Formulas of $FCTL^*$ are built from atomic propositions from a set $AP$ using Boolean and temporal operators and some fuzzy operators.

$FCTL^*$ state formulas are formed according to the following rules:

1. Any atomic proposition $x \in AP$ is a state formula.
2. If $f$ and $g$ are state formulas then $\neg f$ and $(f \wedge g)$ are state formulas.
3. If $f$ is a path formula and $J \subseteq [0,1]$ is an interval with rational bounds then $[f]_J$ is a state formula.

$FCTL^*$ path formulas are formed as follows:

1. All state formulas are path formulas.
2. If $f$ and $g$ are path formulas then $\neg f, (f \wedge g), X(f)$ and $(fUg)$ are path formulas.

A model $\mathbf{M}$ for $FCTL^*$ is a pair $\langle M, L \rangle$, where $M$ is a fuzzy MDP, and $L$ is a mapping from its state set $S$ to $2^{AP}$ which determines the meaning of the propositional variables on the states of $M$. Paths of $\mathbf{M}$ are paths (i.e. sequences of states) associated with trajectories of MDP $M$.

For a state $s$ of $M$ and a state fomula $f$ let $\mathbf{M}, s \models f$ mean "$f$ is satisfied on $s$". Analogously, $\mathbf{M}, \pi \models f$ denotes that the path formula $f$ is satisfied on the path $\pi$. As usual, whenever $\mathbf{M}$ is fixed, we omit it in these notations.

Formally, satisfaction is defined in the following inductive way (where $\pi$ is supposed to be of the form $(s_0, s_1, \ldots)$).

1. For a propositional variable $a$, $s \models a$ iff $s \in L(a)$.
2. The meaning of the Boolean connectives $\neg, \wedge$ for the state formulas and the path formulas is defined as usual.
3. Let $f$ be a state formula. Then $\pi \models X(f)$ iff $s_1 \models f$.
4. Let $f$ be a state formula. Then $\pi \models f$ iff $s_0 \models f$.
5. Let $f$ and $g$ be path formulas. Then $\pi \models (fUg)$ iff $\exists i. \pi^{(i)} \models g$ and $\forall j < i. \pi^{(j)} \models f$.
6. For a state $s$, a decision policy $u$ and a path formula $f$, let $T(s, u, f)$ denote the intersection of sets $T(s, u)$ and $T(s, f)$, where $T(s, u)$ is the set of all paths with the start state $s$, which are associated with trajectories of the Markov chain determined by $u$, and $T(s, f)$ is the set of all paths with the same start state which satisfy the formula $f$. Then the meaning of the formula $[f]_J$ is defined so: $s \models [f]_J$ iff for any decision policy $u$, $p(T(s, u, f)) \in J$.

We denote by $p_{min}(s, f)$ and $p_{max}(s, f)$ the minimal and maximal values of $p(T(s, u, f))$ among all decision policies $u$. Then, satisfiability of the formula $[f]_{[a,b]}$ on $s$ is reduced to two conditions: $a \leq p_{min}(s, f)$ and $p_{max}(s, f) \leq b$.

The logic $FCTL$, more restricted than $FCTL^*$, is obtained from $FCTL^*$ by defining path formulas through the only condition:

2'. If $f$ and $g$ are state formulas then $X(f)$ and $(fUg)$ are path formulas.

We also use another logic simpler than $FCTL^*$. This logic syntactically co-incides with the convenient propositional logic $LTL$ of linear time: its formulas are built from propositional variables by Boolean connectives and operators $X$ and $U$ as above in definition of path formulas of $FCTL^*$. So, formulas of this logic themselves do not contain any features to evaluate possibilities of formulas, however their interpretation on fuzzy MDP allows to speak about comparison of different decision policies $u$ with respect to values of $p(T(s, u, f))$. In particular, one can speak about the most optimistic and the most pessimistic policies allowing to reach a property of paths of $M$, expressed by a formula of $LTL$. Namely, for the most optimistic policy $u_{opt}$ $p(T(s_0, u_{opt}, f)) = p_{max}(s_0, f)$, and for the most pessimistic policy $u_{pes}$ $p(T(s_0, u_{pes}, f)) = p_{min}(s_0, f)$.

In the rest of the paper we consider two types of specifications of dynamic properties of fuzzy MDP: by formulas of the logic $FCTL^*$ (in particular, of $FCTL$) and by formulas of the logic $LTL$.

For specifications of the first type, the problem of verification of fuzzy MDPs is formulated as a problem of satisfiability of a $FCTL^*$−formula $f$ on a state $s_0$ of a fuzzy MDP $M$ (i.e. verifying that $M, s_0 \models f$.

For specifications of the second type, the possibilities of satisfiabilty of formulas depend on the decision policy used. Because there is a continuum of such policies, the problem in this case must be somehow restricted to special cases. The most interesting policies are policies $u_{pes}$ and $u_{opt}$ with extreme values of $p(T(s, u, f))$: if $p_{min}(s, f) > r$ then any policy reaches $f$ with possibility higher than $r$, and $p_{max}(s, f)$ is the highest possibility which can be reached in satisfying $f$. In the following section, we discuss some approaches to computing the values of $p_{min}(s, f)$ and $p_{max}(s, f)$. Note that in the probabilistic setting the corresponding functions are mutually expressible, and it is sufficient to compute one of them. For fuzzy MDP it is not true: computing $p_{min}(s, f)$ is more complicated than computing $p_{max}(s, f)$.

We also note that the algorithm for verification of $FCTL^*$ formulas uses the algorithms for computing $p_{min}(s, f)$ and $p_{max}(s, f)$ as a tool to evaluate meanings of subformulas of the form $[f]_J$. Of course, the algorithm for $FCTL^*$ can be also used for verification of formulas from $FCTL$, however for the latter logic, there exists a more efficient verification algorithm.

## 4    Complexity of Verification of Fuzzy MDP

The following theorem describes complexity of computing functions $p_{min}(s, f)$ and $p_{max}(s, f)$ for an $LTL$−formula $f$ and a state $s$ of a fuzzy MDP $M$.

**Theorem 1.** *i) There exists an algorithm which computes $p_{max}(s, f)$ and finds the corresponding policy $u_{opt}$ in the time polynomial in the size of $M$ and exponential in the size of $f$.*

*ii) There exists an algorithm which computes $p_{min}(s, f)$ and finds the corresponding policy $u_{pes}$ in the space polynomial in the size of $M$ and exponential in the size of $f$.*

The proof of this theorem, in general, follows [14], where similar results are proved for regular Markov processes. However there exist important differences in details. In particular, for regular MDPs the algorithm in part i) has double exponential time complexity with respect to the size of $f$, and a somewhat stronger variant of part ii) is an easy corollary of the variant of part i).

The proofs of both parts of the theorem are based on a construction of a nondeterministic Büchi automaton $A$ given a formula $f$, such that $A$ accepts exactly the paths of $M$ which satisfy $f$ (see [3, 13]). In the worst case, the size of $A$ can be exponential in the size of $f$. After this, a fuzzy Büchi automaton $B$ is constructed based on $M$ and $A$: a kind of product of $M$ and $A$. If $M$ contains a transition from $s$ to $s'$ with a label $a, p$ and $A$ contains a transition from a state $q$ to a state $q'$ with the label $s'$ then $B$ contains the transition from the state $(s, q)$ to the state $(s', q')$ with the label $(a, p, s')$. All states of $B$ with the second component being an accepting state of $A$ are chosen as accepting states for $B$.

After this, the values of $p_{min}(s, f)$ and $p_{max}(s, f)$ can be computed by solving some path searching problems in the diagram of $B$. Computing $p_{max}(s, f)$ can be done in polynomial time. Computing $p_{min}(s, f)$ is more complicated and goes over an exponential number of repeat-free paths in the diagram.

Theorem 1 can be used for constructing an algorithm for verification of formulas from $FCTL^*$. This algorithm recursively deconstructs the formula $f$ from inside to outside using parts i) and ii) of Theorem 1 for processing subformulas of the form $[f]_J$. Verification of formulas from $FCTL$ can be made with the same recursive scheme, but in this case it is sufficient to compute functions $p_{min}(s, f)$ and $p_{max}(s, f)$ for simple formulas of the form $Xf$ and $fUg$, where $f$ and $g$ are propositional variables. It can be made without transition from formulas to automata which allows to logarithmically lower the complexity of verification with respect to the size of $f$.

**Theorem 2.** *i) There exists an algorithm for verification of a formula $f$ from $FCTL^*$ on $M$ in space polynomial in the size of $M$ and the size of $f$.*

*ii) There exists an algorithm for verification of a formula $f$ from $FCTL$ on $M$ in time polynomial in the size of $M$ and exponential in the size of $f$.*

The main contribution to complexity in both parts of Theorem 2 is made by the computation of $p_{min}$ used to verify the lower bounds in formulas of the form $[f]_J$. One can propose some weaker variants of logics $FCTL^*$ and $FCTL$ (we can call them $FCTL_0^*$ and $FCTL_0$) which use only intervals [0,b]. For these logics the following theorem holds:

**Theorem 3.** *i) There exists an algorithm for verification of a formula $f$ from $FCTL_0^*$ on $M$ in time polynomial in the size of $M$ and exponential in the size of $f$.*

*ii) There exists an algorithm for verification of a formula $f$ from $FCTL_0$ on $M$ in time polynomial both in the size of $M$ and in the size of $f$.*

Theorems 1 and 2 show that algorithms for verifying fuzzy MDPs in the general case are of high complexity. The only case with the tractable verification problem we found is presented in Theorem 3(ii). It would be interesting to find out some other subclasses of fuzzy MDPs and temporary formulas which allow effective solutions of the verification problem.

## 5   Fuzzy MAS

We consider two classes of fuzzy MAS: FSMAS, which function sequentially, and FNMAS, which function nondeterministically. The former is a special case of the latter, but FSMAS are of special interest since they can be used as adequate models of many practical systems, and allow for a more efficient analysis of their behavior.

A FNMAS **A** has a finite set of interacting intelligent agents $A_i$ governed by some fuzzy logic programs. A finite set **C** of constants is connected with **A**. Moreover, two disjoint predicate signatures $\Sigma_R^A$ and $\Sigma_F^A$ are connected with each agent $A$ of the system. Atoms of the signature $\Sigma_R^A$ ($AR$-atoms) are of the form $q(t_1, \ldots, t_m)$ where $q \in \Sigma_R^A$ and $t_1, \ldots, t_m$ are constants or variables, and have a usual interpretation, i.e. ground atoms (facts) of this form can be only true or false. Atoms of the signature $\Sigma_F^A$ ($AF$-atoms) express inexact knowledge and are annotated atoms of the form $q(t_1, \ldots, t_m) : p$ where $q \in \Sigma_F^A$, and $p \in [0, 1]$. When this atom is ground, then $p$ is the degree of the confidence in this fact (or its possibility ). We call atoms of these two forms $A$-atoms. Each agent $A$ of the system has a finite internal database (IDB) $I_A$. $I_A$ consists of ground $A$-atoms. In addition to the IDB, the agent $A$ has a mailbox $MsgBox_A$, which contains messages received from other agents of the system before the current step. The current content of the IDB and the current content of the mailbox of the agent $A$ is its current local state $IM_A = (I_A, MsgBox_A)$.

Agents from **A** communicate with each other by transmission of messages of the form $msg(Sender, Receiver, Msg)$, where $Sender$ and $Receiver$ are agent names (source and addressee), and $Msg$ is a (transmitted) ground $Sender$-atom.

For each pair of agents $A, B$ from **A**, there is a communication channel $CH_{AB}$, into which messages sent by the agent $A$ to the agent $B$ fall. Then, they go from this channel into the mailbox $MsgBox_B$. The time in transit for each message is considered to be a fuzzy value assigned by a finite fuzzy discrete distribution. As $ps_{AB}(t)$ we denote the possibility that $B$ will receive the communication sent to it by agent $A$ exactly in $t$ steps after its departure ($t_0$ will denote the minimal number such that $ps_{AB}(t) = 0$ for all $t > t_0$ and for all agents $A$ and $B$ of the system).

The current state of the channel $CH_{AB}$ includes all the messages sent by the agent $A$ to the agent $B$ that have not yet reached $B$, with a statement specifying the duration of their staying in the channel. We denote the current state of the channel in the same way as the channel itself, that is, $CH_{AB} = \{(Msg, t) \mid$ *message $Msg$ from agent $A$ to agent $B$ is found in channel during $t$ steps*$\}$. We also use abbreviations $CH_{ij}$ and $p_{ij}$ for $CH_{A_i A_j}$ and $p_{A_i A_j}$, respectively.

With each agent $A$ we associate its base $ACT_A$ of parameterized actions of the type $(a(X_1, \ldots, X_m)$, $ADD_a(X_1, \ldots, X_m)$, $DEL_a(X_1, \ldots, X_m)$, $PUT_a(X_1, \ldots,$

$X_m$), $SEND_a(X_1, \ldots, X_m)$. Here, $a(X_1, \ldots, X_m)$ is the (parameterized) name of the action, $ADD_a(X_1, \ldots, X_m)$ and $DEL_a(X_1, \ldots, X_m)$ are sets of $A$-atoms. Arguments of atoms in these sets are either constants or parameters $X_1, \ldots, X_m$. These sets determine the changes in the IDB after execution of this action (this is clarified below in Section 7). The set $SEND_a(X_1, \ldots, X_m)$ includes messages of the type $msg(A, B, p(t_1, \ldots, t_k))$ sent to other agents. Let $c_1, \ldots, c_m$ be constants. We denote by $ADD_a(c_1, \ldots, c_m)$ the set of ground $AR$-facts obtained by the substitution of $c_1, \ldots, c_m$ for $X_1, \ldots, X_m$ into atoms from $ADD_a(X_1, \ldots, X_m)$. Sets $DEL_a(c_1, \ldots, c_m)$, $PUT_a(c_1, \ldots, c_m)$ and $SEND_a(c_1, \ldots, c_m)$ are defined in a similar way. We call the ground atoms of the form $a(c_1, \ldots, c_m)$ the ground action atoms (or simply ground actions).

The specific choice of the agent's actions to be executed in the given local state is determined by the pair $(FLP_A, Sel_A)$. Here, $FLP_A$ is a fuzzy logic program, which at each step determines for the current local state $IM_A$ a set $Perm_A$ of the annotated ground actions permissible for execution at this step ($Perm_A$ is defined more exactly below in the next section). $Sel_A$ is a polynomially computable operator, which nondeterministically eventually chooses some subset from $Perm_A$ for execution. The sequential FMAS are distinguished from the general case in that $Sel_A$ in this case is a polynomially computable deterministic operator.

## 6    Fuzzy Logic Programs

The fuzzy logic program $FLP_A$ of an agent $A$ consists of clauses of the form
$$H : p \leftarrow L_1, \ldots, L_n.$$
Here, $H$ is an action atom of the form $a(t_1, \ldots, t_m)$, where $t_1, \ldots, t_m$ are constants or variables, $p \in [0, 1]$, and literals $L_i$ may be

1) annotated action atoms,

2) $AR$-literals of the form $r(t_1, \ldots, t_k)$ or $\neg r(t_1, \ldots, t_k)$ where $r \in \Sigma_R^A$,

3) $AF$-atoms of the form $q(t_1, \ldots, t_k) : p$ where $q \in \Sigma_F^A$ and anotation $p \in [0, 1]$,

4) message literals of the form $msg(Sender, A, Msg)$, $\neg msg(Sender, A, Msg)$,

5) polynomially computable embedded predicates.

The program $FLP_A$, together with current local state $IM_A = (I_A, MsgBox_A)$ (i.e. the program $FLP_{A,IM_A} = LP_A \cup I_A \cup MsgBox_A$) determines a set $Perm_A$ ($= Sem(FLP_{A,IM_A})$) of annotated ground action atoms which represent candidates to be executed by $A$ at current step.

We define now semantics $Sem(P)$ for ground fuzzy logic programs $P$ of the kind introduced in this paper. Let us denote by $U$ the set of all ground (unannotated) atoms from $P$ (including both internal and action atoms). An interpretation $f$ associates with any atom $r(c_1, \ldots, c_k) \in U, r \in \Sigma_R^A$, its truth value $f(r(c_1, \ldots, c_k)) \in \{true, false\}$; with any atom $q(c_1, \ldots, c_m) \in U, r \in \Sigma_F^A$, it associates its possibility $f(q(c_1, \ldots, c_m)) \in [0, 1]$, and with any action atom $a(c_1, \ldots, c_m) \in U$ it associates its possibility $f(a(c_1, \ldots, c_m)) \in [0, 1]$.

An atom $r(c_1, \ldots, c_k) \in U$ is satisfied by interpretation $f$, if $f(r(c_1, \ldots, c_k)) = true$ and $\neg r(c_1, \ldots, c_k)$ is satisfied by $f$, if $f(r(c_1, \ldots, c_k)) = false$.

An annotated atom of the form $q(c_1, \ldots, c_k) : p$ is satisfied by the interpretation $f$, if $p \leq f(q(c_1, \ldots, c_k))$. An action atom $a(c_1, \ldots, c_m) : p$ is satisfied by the interpretation $f$, if $f(a(c_1, \ldots, c_m))$ is defined and $p \leq f(a(c_1, \ldots, c_m))$. Satisfiability of message literals of the form $msg(Sender, Msg)$ or $\neg msg(Sender, Msg)$ is defined in the standard way with respect to the current state of $MsgBox_A$. Satisfiability of embedded predicates is defined by their natural semantics.

A clause $a(c_1, \ldots, c_m) : p : -L_1, \ldots, L_n$ is satisfied by the interpretation $f$ (with respect to $MsgBox_A$), if inequality $f(a(c_1, \ldots, c_m)) \geq p$ holds when $L_i$ is satisfied by $f$ for all $i \in [1, n]$. The interpretation $f$ is a model of $P$ if all clauses of $P$ are satisfied by $f$. Let us define a partial order $\leq$ on the set of inerpretations as follows: $f_1 \leq f_2$ iff $f_1(q) \leq f_2(q)$ for each atom $q \in U$ (we suppose that $false < true$). A model $f$ of the program $P$ is a minimal model if $f_1 \leq f$ does not hold for any other model $f_1$ of $P$. The set of models of $P$ is closed under "minimization".

**Lemma 1.** *Let $f_1$ and $f_2$ be two models of the program $P$. Then the interpretation $f = min(f_1, f_2) = \{q : p \mid q \in U \wedge p = min(f_1(q), f_2(q))\}$ is a model of $P$.*

It follows from this lemma that there exists the minimal model of $P$. This model can be constructed by a standard procedure of fixpoint computation.

Since the heads of clauses of $FLP_A$ are action atoms only, any model of $FLP_{A,IM_A}$ includes all atoms of $IM_A$. Then, for ground $FLP_A$ the minimal model $f_{min}(FLP_{A,IM_A})$ can be computed by the following fixpoint computation.
**Step 0:** For all $a(c_1, \ldots, c_m) \in U$ let $f_0(a(c_1, \ldots, c_m)) = 0$.

    $\ldots$

**Step $i + 1$:** For all $a(c_1, \ldots, c_m) \in U$ let $f_{i+1}(a(c_1, \ldots, c_m))$ be the maximal element of the set $\{\{f_i(a(c_1, \ldots, c_m))\} \cup \{p \mid$ there is a clause $a(c_1, \ldots, c_m) : p : -L_1, \ldots, L_n \in FLP_A$ which is satisfied by the interpretation $f_i\}\}$.

Let $C_i$ be a subset of the clauses of $FLP_A$ which are satisfied by the interpretation $f_i$. It follows from the definition above that $C_i \subseteq C_{i+1}$. Therefore, for some $i, i \leq$ (number of clauses of $FLP_A$) an equality $f_i = f_{i+1}$ holds and we can set $f_{min}(FLP_{A,IM_A}) = f_i$.

**Theorem 4.** *For any fuzzy logic program $P$ (of the kind considered in this paper) there exists a minimal model $f_{min}(P)$ computable in polynomial time with respect to the size of the groundization $gr(P)$ of $P$.*

This way, we can define $Sem(P)$ as the set of annotated action atoms $\{a(c_1, \ldots, c_m) : p \mid p = f_{min}(P)(a(c_1, \ldots, c_m))\}$. We use often the notation $Perm$ instead of $Sem(P)$.

## 7   Global Behavior of FMAS

As is seen from the given definitions, FSMAS are similar, in a certain sense, to fuzzy Markov chains and FNMAS are similar to fuzzy Markov decision processes

([10]). We note that the main difference of FNMAS and FSMAS from Markov processes and chains is that transitions in FMAS are not defined explicitly, but are determined by some calculations. Additionally, states of FMAS have the structure of databases, which makes FMAS, in a sense, more expressive than fuzzy Markov chains or processes.

First, we define the operational semantcs of FNMAS, then we indicate changes in this definition required to obtain the semantics of FSMAS.

The global state $\mathbf{S}$ of a system $\mathbf{A}$ includes local states of the agents of the system and the states of all its channels. The set of all the global states $\mathbf{A}$ is denoted by $\mathbf{S_A}$.

The transition $\mathbf{S} \Rightarrow_{\mathbf{A}} \mathbf{S}'$ begins with emptying the mailboxes of all the agents. Then, the new contents of all the channels $CH_{ij}$ and the postboxes are formed: (1) the time counters of the messages found in the $CH_{ij}$ are increased by 1; (2) the pairs $(Msg, t)$ such that $t > t_0$ are removed from $CH_{ij}$; (3) for each pair $(Msg, t) \in CH_{ij}$ the fact $msg(A_i, A_j, Msg)$ is placed into the mailbox $MsgBox_j$ of the agent $A_j$ with the possibility $p_{ij}(t)$. Then, each agent $A_i$ forms a set $Perm_i = Sem(FLP_{i,IM_i})$ of all permissible, at the given step, annotated ground actions; and the operator $Sel_{A_i}$ chooses nondeterministically some subset $Selected_{A_i}$ from $Perm_i$. Let $SelAct_i$ denote the set $\{a \mid a : ps \in Selected_{A_i}\}$. After this, the fuzzy operation is applied to $SelAct_i$ choosing a fuzzy subset $Obl_i$ of it with possibility $\min\{ps \mid a : ps \in Perm_i, a \in Obl_i\}$. $Obl_i$ is the fuzzy set of actions to be executed by agent $A_i$. Finally, each agent $A_i$ performs actions from $Obl_i$ in the following way. It adds into each channel $CH_{ij}, (i \neq j)$ all the pairs $(Msg, 0)$, where $Msg$ is a ground instance of a message of the form $msg(A_i, A_j, p(t_1, \ldots, t_k))$ out of the set $SEND_a(c_1, \ldots, c_m)$ for some $a(c_1, \ldots, c_m)$ from $Obl_i$. The current state is updated as follows. Let $AddObl_i$ consist of all the $A$-atoms from all the sets $ADD_a(c_1, \ldots, c_l)$ such that a ground name $a(c_1, \ldots, c_l)$ from $Obl_i$ is unified with a parameterized name $a(X_1, \ldots, X_l)$. The sets $DelObl_i$ and $SendObl_i$ are defined similarly. Then all the facts belonging to $DelObl_i$ are deleted from the current state, and all the facts belonging to $AddObl_i$ are added to it.

The definition of the semantics for FSMAS practically coincides with the definition above; it is only required for FSMAS to take into account that for each agent $A$ the operator $Sel_A$ is deterministic and determines the set of executed actions unambiguously.

# 8  Simulation of FMAS by Fuzzy Markov Systems

We describe how FNMAS can be simulated by fuzzy Markov decision processes, after which we discuss how FSMAS can be simulated by Markov chains.

Let $\mathbf{A}$ be a FNMAS. We now define a fuzzy MDP $Mod_{\mathbf{A}}$ simulating $\mathbf{A}$.

The set of states of $Mod_A$ is defined as the set of global states of $\mathbf{A}$. Its actions are composite and are presented as tuples $Selected = (Selected_1, \ldots, Selected_n)$, where $Selected_i$ is a subset of the set of all annotated ground action atoms of the agent $A_i$. It remains to define possibility distrbutions $PS_{Selected}$ for any global state $S$ of the system $\mathbf{A}$ and action $Selected$. They are computed by the deterministic algorithm TransPossibility($Selected, S, S'$) that calculates the possibility of the transition from $S$ to another global state $S'$ of the system $\mathbf{A}$ under the condition that each agent $A_i$ chooses for execution the annotated actions from $Selected_i$.

**Algorithm.** TransPossibility($Selected, S, S'$)

1: **for all** $A_i, A_j \in \mathbf{A}$ $(i \neq j)$ **do**
2:     $M[i,j] := \{(m,t) | ((m,t) \in CH_{i,j})$ **and** $((m,t+1) \notin CH'_{i,j})\}$;
3:     $p_{i,j} := \min\{p_{i,j}(t) \mid (m,t) \in M[i,j]\}$;
4: **end for**
5: **for all** $A_j \in \mathbf{A}$ **do**
6:     $MsgBox_j := \emptyset$;
7:     **for all** $A_i \in \mathbf{A}$ $(i \neq j)$ **do**
8:         $MsgBox_j := MsgBox_j \cup \{msg(A_i, A_j, m) \mid \exists t((m,t) \in M[i,j])\}$;
9:     **end for**
10: **end for**
11: **for all** $A_i \in \mathbf{A}$ **do**
12:     $Perm_i := Sem(FLP_{A,IM_A})$
13:     **if** $Selected_i \not\subseteq Range(Sel_i(Perm_i))$ **then**
14:         **return** 0
15:     **end if**
16:     **for all** $A_i \in \mathbf{A}$ **do**
17:         $SelAct_i := \{a(c_1, \ldots, c_m) \mid a(c_1, \ldots, c_m) : p \in Selected_i\}$;
18:         $p_i := 0$;
19:         **for all** $Obl \subseteq SelAct_i$ **do**
20:             $AddObl := \bigcup\{ADD_a(c_1, \ldots, c_m) \mid a(c_1, \ldots, c_m) \in Obl\}$;
21:             $DelObl := \bigcup\{DEL_a(c_1, \ldots, c_m) \mid a(c_1, \ldots, c_m) \in Obl\}$;
22:             **if** $(I'_i := ((I_i \backslash DelObl) \cup AddObl)$ **and** $(\bigwedge_{m \neq i}\{ms \mid (ms, 0) \in CH'_{i,m}\} = \{ms \mid \exists a(c_1, \ldots, c_q) \in Obl(msg(A_i, A_m, ms) \in SEND_a(c_1, \ldots, c_q)\})$
              **then**
23:                 $p_i := \max\{p_i, \min\{p_a \mid a(c_1, \ldots, c_m) \in Obl$ **and** $a(c_1, \ldots, c_m) : p_a \in Selected_i\}\}$
24:             **end if**
25:         **end for**
26:     **end for**
27: **end for**
28: $p(S, S') := \min\{\{p_{i,j} \mid 1 \leq i, j \leq n, j \neq i\} \cup \{p_i \mid 1 \leq i \leq n\}\}$
29: **return** $p(S, S')$

In this algorithm, $M[i,j]$ in line 2 is the set of those messages from the channel $CH_{i,j}$ which are moved into $MsgBox_j$ under the transition from $S$ to $S'$. Then $p_{i,j}$ in line 3 is the possibility of the following event: *the set of messages received by $A_i$ from $A_j$ is equal to $M[i,j]$*. The value $p_i$ computed in lines 16 - 27 is the total possibility of obtaining new state $I'_i$ from $I_i$ under all possible choices of the executable actions set $Obl$.

**Theorem 5.** *Given two global states $S$ and $S'$ and a **M**-action Selected, algorithm TransPossibility(Selected, $S, S'$) computes the possibility $p_{Selected}(S, S')$ of the transition $S \Rightarrow S'$ under a **M**-action Selected of MDP $\mathbf{M_A}$ . The time complexity of the algorithm is bounded by $2^r pol(|\mathbf{A}| + |S| + |S'|)$, where $r$ is the maximal number of different ground actions of one agent of the system, pol is some polynomial which is independent of $\mathbf{M_A}$, and $|\mathbf{A}| + |S| + |S'|$ is the sum of the total size of MDP $\mathbf{A}$ and the sizes of both states $S$ and $S'$.*

When we consider FSMAS, parameter *Selected* is not required, and one can compute the possibility of the transition from $S$ to $S'$ directly (in this case we get a fuzzy Markov chain). It is enough to replace lines 13 - 15 in algorithm TransPossibility(*Selected, $S, S'$*) with the line (13') $Selected_i := Sel_i(Perm_i)$ and we get algorithm which computes the possibility $p(S, S')$ for FSMAS.

# 9  Verification of Dynamic Properties of FMAS

The results of Section 8 on simulation of fuzzy MAS by fuzzy Markov systems together with results of Section 4 on verification of dynamic properties of fuzzy Markov systems allow us to construct algorithms of verification of FMAS. But since states of MAS have structure of databases we can go somewhat further. Namely, for specification of dynamic properties of FMAS we can use first-order extensions of propositional logics used in Section 4 for fuzzy Markov systems.

Let $FO^{\mathbf{A}}$ denote the set of closed first-order formulas constructed from all $A$-atoms and message predicates for all $A \in \mathbf{A}$. Satisfiability of such formulas in global states is defined under the closed world assumption for all $A$-atoms (in particular, $AF$-literal $\neg q(c_1, \ldots, c_l) : ps$ is true on state $S$, if $q(c_1, \ldots, c_l) : ps$ is not in the local component $IDB_A$ of $S$). It can be checked in time polynomial of the size of the global state. Let $L$ be one of propositional logics $LTL, FCTL^*$ or $FCTL$, and $FO^{\mathbf{A}}$-$L$ denote the logic obtained from $L$ by permitting arbitrary formulas from $FO^{\mathbf{A}}$ instead of atomic propositions. Satisfiability of formulas of this logic in global states and trajectories of $\mathbf{A}$ is defined in a natural way. The states and trajectories of a simulated FMAS $\mathbf{A}$ and simulating Markov system $Mod_{\mathbf{A}}$ are the same. So, the notion of satisfiability of a formula from $FO^{\mathbf{A}}$-$L$ is transferred from $\mathbf{A}$ to $Mod_{\mathbf{A}}$, and in fact, they coincide.

So, now we formulate some of many results on the complexity of the verification problem for FMAS and FSMAS which follow from the discussion above.

**Theorem 6.** *i) The satisfiability of a LTL formula $f$ on a ground FSMAS $\mathbf{A}$ can be checked in a memory polynomial with respect to the sizes of $\mathbf{A}$ and $f$.*
*ii) The satisfiability of a LTL formula $f$ on a ground FNMAS $\mathbf{A}$ can be checked in a time exponential in the size of $\mathbf{A}$ and double exponential in the size of $f$.*

**Theorem 7.** *The satisfiability of a FCTL formula $f$ on a ground FSMAS or FNMAS $\mathbf{A}$ can be verified in a time exponential in the size $\mathbf{A}$ (for NPMAS with a higher basis of the exponent) and linear in the size of $f$.*

**Theorem 8.** *i) The satisfiability of a FCTL\* formula f on a ground FSMAS* **A** *can be verified in a time exponential in the size of* **A** *and linear in the size of f.*
*ii) The satiiability of a FCTL\* formula f on a ground FNMAS* **A** *can be verified in a time exponential in the size* **A** *and double exponential in the size of f.*

Groundization of non-ground MAS can exponentially increase size of the system. So, complexity of verification for non-ground systems in worst case is exponentially higher than for ground systems with respect to MAS size.

# 10   Example

As a small example we consider here a fuzzy MAS **SB** which simulates a simplified fuzzy version of alternative model of negotiation proposed by Rubinstein [16]. This model was adopted for probabilistic agents in [7]. In this model two agents *S(eller)* and *B(uyer)* take it in turns to make an action. The action can be either (i) put forward a proposal (offer), or (ii) accept the most recent proposal. We assume that negotiation takes place in a sequence of rounds. Agent $S$ begins, at round 0, by making a proposal $x^0$, which agent $B$ can either accept or reject. If the proposal is accepted, then the deal $x^0$ is implemented. Otherwise, the negotiation moves to another round, where agent $B$ makes a proposal (counter-offer) and agent $S$ chooses to either accept or reject it, and so on. $S$ will make proposals on even rounds and $B$ will make proposals on odd rounds. For an agent, the decision on the opponent's offer is a fuzzy one, which depends on the offered amount and the market situation. We consider two kinds of market situations: prices are going up (u) and prices are going down (d). Since our agents have no influence on the market situation, it is the source of nondeterminism in the negotiation process.

The value of agent's $a$ $i$-th offer is defined by functions $of_u^a(i)$ and $of_d^a(i)$, which depend on the market situation. For agent $S$ these functions are decreasing, and for agent $B$ they are increasing. For characterising the possibility of an agent's $a$ actions we introduce the so called Acceptance Possibility functions, $AP_u^a(x, i)$ and $AP_d^a(x, i)$, and Rejection Possibility functions $RP_u^a(x, t)$ and $RP_d^a(x, t)$ respectively, which return possibility values of the actions depending on the offer price $x^{(i)}$ and time (step number) $i$.

The internal database $I_a, a \in \{S, B\}$, during negotiations includes only one fact: $step(i)$ where $i$ is the number of current step of the agent $a$ (or the number of offers proposed by $a$). At the end of the negotiations, each agent adds a new fact $deal(x)$ into $I_a$, where $x$ is the price accepted by both agents. At the beginning of the negotiations, $I_a = \{step(0)\}, a \in \{S, B\}$.

Action base $ACT_a, a \in \{S, B\}$, consists of actions $deal(x)$, $accept_m(x)$, $re-ject_m(i)$, $m \in \{u, d\}$. Action $deal(x)$ puts the fact $deal(x)$ into $I_a$. Action $accept_m(x)$ sends to the counter-agent $\hat{a}$ the message $deal(x)$ and puts the same fact $deal(x)$ into $I_a$. Action $reject_m(i)$ sends to the counter-agent $\hat{a}$ the message with a new offer's price $of_m^a(i)$ and changes the number of steps from $i$ to $i+1$. In addition, $ACT_S$ includes action $start(x^0)$ which sends the message with initial seller price $x^0 = of_m^S(0)$ to $B$ and changes $S$'s step number to 1.

The agent's $a \in \{S, B\}$ fuzzy logic program $FLP_a$ consists of clauses of the following forms:
(1) $deal(x) : 1 \leftarrow msg(\hat{a}, deal(x))$.
(2S) $accept_m(x) : 1 \leftarrow msg(B, x), step(i), of_m^S(i) \leq x$.
(2B) $accept_m(x) : 1 \leftarrow msg(S, x), step(i), of_m^B(i) \geq x$.
(3) $accept_m(x) : AP_m^a(x, i) \leftarrow msg(\hat{a}, a, x), step(i)$.
(4) $reject_m(i) : RP_m^a(x, i) \leftarrow msg(\hat{a}, a, x), step(i)$.
In addition, $FLP_S$ includes the clause $start(x^0) : 1 \leftarrow step(0)$ which fires the action $start(x^0)$ to begin the negotiations.

The clause (1) fires when agent $a$ receives the message that $\hat{a}$ has accepted his last offer $x$. The clauses (2S) and (2B) assure that the agent $a$ accepts the last offer $x$ of $\hat{a}$ if his own next offer $of_m^a(i)$ will be worse than $x$. The clause (3) causes an acceptance of agent's $\hat{a}$ offer $x$ at step $i$ with the possibility degree $AP_m^a(x, i)$ and the clause (4) causes a rejection of the offer with the possibility degree $RP_m^a(x, i)$. We don't require that $AP_m^a(x, i) + RP_m^a(x, i) = 1$.

The nondeterministic operator $Sel_a$ chooses some subset $Obl$ from $Perm_a$ for execution as follows: if action $deal(x) : 1$ is included into $Perm_a$ then $Sel_a$ chooses this action, otherwise it "guesses" one of the two market situations $m \in \{u, d\}$ and selects the subset of appropriate actions, i.e. $Obl = Perm_a \cap \{accept_m(x) : 1, accept_m(x) : p, reject_m(i) : q\}$.

In the last case, there are following ways of executing the selected actions:
(1) if $accept_m(x) : 1 \in Obl$ then it always runs: sends message $msg(a, deal(x))$ to $\hat{a}$, otherwise,
(2) the action $accept_m(x)$ may run with possibility degree $p$;
(3) the action $reject_m(i)$ may run with possibility degree $q$;
(4) both actions may run with possibility degree $\min\{p, q\}$.
In case (4), agent $\hat{a}$ will receive two messages from $a$: $msg(a, deal(x))$ and $msg(a, of_m^a(i))$. But it will react on the first message only and will ignore the second one, i.e. $\hat{a}$ puts $deal(x)$ into $I_{\hat{a}}$ and stops.

We suppose that the communication channels $CH_{SB}$ and $CH_{BS}$ of MAS **SB** are reliable, i.e. a message sent by $a$ at the step $i$ will be received by $\hat{a}$ at the next step $(i + 1)$.

Now we fix values of the offer functions (Table 1), acceptance possibility functions (Table 2) and rejection possibility functions (Tables 3, 4) used by agents $S$ and $B$ during negotiations.[1] The sign '-' in these tables means that the appropriate value is irrelevent to the system behavior.

**Table 1.** Offer functions for $S$ and $B$

| $i$ | 0 | 1 | 2 | 3 | $i$ | 0 | 1 | 2 | 3 |
|---|---|---|---|---|---|---|---|---|---|
| $of_u^S(i)$ | 100 | 90 | 80 | 60 | $of_{su}^B(i)$ | 50 | 70 | 80 | 90 |
| $of_d^S(i)$ | 100 | 80 | 60 | 50 | $of_{sd}^B(i)$ | 40 | 50 | 60 | 80 |

---

[1] In [7] and [16] offer functions and acceptance probability functions are defined by some analitical formulas. Here, for simplicity, we specify our functions in a tabular form.

**Table 2.** Functions $AP_u^S(x,i)/AP_d^S(x,i)$ and $AP_u^B(x,i)/AP_d^B(x,i)$

| $x \setminus i$ | 1 | 2 | 3 | 4 | $x \setminus i$ | 0 | 1 | 2 | 3 |
|---|---|---|---|---|---|---|---|---|---|
| 90 | - | - | - | 1 / 1 | 100 | 0.1 / 0 | - | - | |
| 80 | - | - | 0.6 / 0.8 | 0.8 / 0.9 | 90 | - | 0.2 /0 | - | - |
| 70 | - | 0.6 / 0.7 | - | - | 80 | - | 0.4 / 0.2 | 0.3 / 0.1 | - |
| 60 | - | - | 0.5 / 0.6 | 0.5 / 0.6 | 60 | - | - | 0.5 / 0.4 | - |
| 50 | 0.1 / 0.2 | 0.2 / 0.3 | - | - | 50 | - | - | - | 1 / 0.9 |
| 40 | 0.05 / 0.1 | - | - | - | | | | | |

**Table 3.** Rejection possibility functions $RP_u^S(x,i)/RP_d^S(x,i)$

| $x \setminus i$ | 1 | 2 | 3 | 4 |
|---|---|---|---|---|
| 90 | - | - | - | 0.1 / 0 |
| 80 | - | - | 0.3 / 0.2 | 0.2 / 0.1 |
| 70 | - | 0.4 / 0.3 | - | - |
| 60 | - | - | 0.6 / 0.5 | 0.7/ 0.6 |
| 50 | 0.8 / 0.9 | 0.8 / 0.95 | - | - |
| 40 | 1 / 0.9 | - | - | - |

**Table 4.** Rejection possibility functions $RP_u^B(x,i)/RP_d^B(x,i)$

| $x \setminus i$ | 0 | 1 | 2 | 3 |
|---|---|---|---|---|
| 100 | 0.9 / 1 | - | - | |
| 90 | - | 0.8 / 0.9 | - | - |
| 80 | - | - | 0.7 / 0.8 | - |
| 60 | - | - | 0.5 / 0.4 | - |
| 50 | - | - | - | 0 / 0.1 |

Formally, as it was defined in section 7, a global state of MAS **SB** has the form $(I_S, I_B.CH_{SB}, CH_{BS})$. To simplify representations of states and trajectories we use $i$ to denote a database state of the form $\{step(i)\}$, $x$ to denote a communication channel state of the form $\{(x,0)\}$, $d(x)$ to denote fact $deal(x)$. For example, under these conventions, the global state $(\{step(2)\}, \{step(1)\}, \{(90,0)\}, \emptyset)$ is represented as $(2, 1, 90, \emptyset)$, and the state $(\{step(3)\}, \{step(2), deal(80)\}, \emptyset, \{(deal(80),0)\})$ as $(3, d(80), \emptyset, d(80))$. The initial state of **SB** is $(0, 0, \emptyset, \emptyset)$.

In Fig. 1 we show a part of the state space $\mathbf{S_{SB}}$ of MAS **SB** that includes all the trajectories representing negotiations finishing with the price of 80. On this diagram, agent $S$ acts in states $s_0, s_2, s_3, s_6, s_8$ and $s_{10}$, and agent $B$ acts in states $s_1, s_4, s_5$ and $s_9$. A label $m(p), m \in \{u, d\}$, of an edge $(s_k, s_j)$ means that the agent acting in $s_k$ guesses market situation $m$ and performs some of $m$-actions with the possibility degree $p$. For $S$ this action is $start(100)$ in state $s_0$ and $reject_m(i)$ in states $s_2, s_3, s_6$. In states $s_8$ and $s_{10}$, agent $S$ executes the action $deal(80)$ with possibility degree 1 (this action is not shown on Fig. 1). $B$ executes actions $reject_m(i)$ in states $s_1$ and $s_4$, and actions $accept_m(80)$ in states $s_5$ and $s_9$.

A decision policy for MAS **SB** is a function from the state space $\mathbf{S_{SB}}$ to $\{u, d\}$ which defines what kind of the market situation an acting agent choses in a

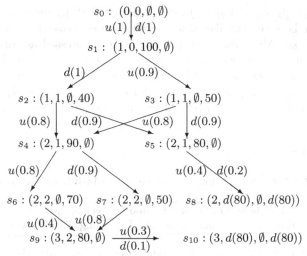

**Fig. 1.** State transitions diagram for the deal price 80

state. For example, the policy "always $u$" produces the following trajectory: $\tau = s_0, s_1, s_3, s_4, s_6, s_9, s_{10}$, which has the possibility degree $\min\{1, 0.9, 0.8, 0.8, 0.4, 0.3\} = 0.3$. Since for each state $s_k$ the choice of the market situation $m \in \{u, d\}$ uniquely defines the next state $s_j$, each decision policy can be defined by a word in the alphabet $\{u, d\}$.

Suppose that we are interested in what is the possibility degree that the negotiations terminate with the deal price 80? This question can be stated as the question about the possibility degree of *LTL*-formula $f = trueU deal(80)$. A direct analysis of the diagram in Fig. 1 allows us to obtain the following bounds on the possibility degree of $f$.

**Theorem 9.** *i) The decision policy $\pi_{opt} = uddu$ is the most optimistic policy for state $s_0$ and formula $f$. It has the maximal possibility degree $p_{max}(s_0, f) = 0.4$.*

*ii) The decision policy $\pi_{pes} = uduuud$ is the most pessimistic policy for state $s_0$ and formula $f$. It has the minimal possibility degree $p_{min}(S_0, f) = 0.1$.*

*Remark 1.* The decision policies proposed in this theorem are not unique. For example, the policy $\pi'_{opt} = uudu$ also is the most optimistic policy and the policy $\pi'_{pes} = uuudud$ is another most pessimistic policy.

*Remark 2.* Theorem 9 allows us to estimate some FCTL-formulas. E.g. $s_0 \models [f]_{[0.1, 0.4]}$ and $s_0 \not\models [f]_{[0.3, 0.4]}$.

## 11   Conclusion

In this paper we introduced the notion of fuzzy nondeterministic multi-agent systems (FNMAS) with agents controlled by fuzzy logic programs. FSMAS are a special case of NFMAS which function sequentially. It was shown that FNMAS can be effectively simulated by fuzzy MDP (FSMAS by fuzzy MC). Some complexity bounds were established for verification of dynamic properties of fuzzy MDP and fuzzy MC, when the properties are expressed as formulas of some variants of fuzzy temporal logic. Combining these results we obtain complexity bounds for verification of FNMAS and FSMAS. These bounds are rather high (with a few exceptions, exponential or hyperexponential). So, it will be interesting to find classes of fuzzy MAS with lower complexity of verification.

# References

1. Pnueli, A.: The temporal logic of programs. In: 18th IEEE Symp. on Foundations of Computer Science, pp. 46–57 (1977)
2. Clarke, E., Grumberg, O., Peled, D.: Model Checking. MIT Press (2000)
3. Baier, C., Katoen, J.: Principles of model checking. Kluwer Academic Publishers (2002)
4. Benerecetti, M., Giunchiglia, F.: Model checking-based analysis of multiagent systems. In: Rash, J.L., Rouff, C.A., Truszkowski, W., Gordon, D.F., Hinchey, M.G. (eds.) FAABS 2000. LNCS (LNAI), vol. 1871, pp. 1–15. Springer, Heidelberg (2001)
5. Wooldridge, M., Fisher, M., Huget, M.P., Parsons, S.: Model checking multi-agent systems with mable. In: Proc. of the First Intern. Conf. on Autonomous Agents and Multiagent Systems, pp. 952–959 (2002)
6. Dekhtyar, M., Dikovsky, A., Valiev, M.: Complexity of multi-agent systems behavior. In: Flesca, S., Greco, S., Leone, N., Ianni, G. (eds.) JELIA 2002. LNCS (LNAI), vol. 2424, pp. 125–136. Springer, Heidelberg (2002)
7. Ballarini, P., Fisher, M., Wooldridge, M.: Automated game analysis via probabilistic model checking: a case study. Electronic Notes in Theoretical Computer Science 149, 125–137 (2006)
8. Dekhtyar, M., Dikovsky, A., Valiev, M.: Temporal verification of probabilistic multi-agent systems. In: Avron, A., Dershowitz, N., Rabinovich, A. (eds.) Pillars of Computer Science. LNCS, vol. 4800, pp. 256–265. Springer, Heidelberg (2008)
9. Valiev, M., Dekhtyar, M.: Complexity of verification of nondeterministic probabilistic multiagent systems. Automatic Control and Computer Sciences 45, 390–396 (2011)
10. Avrachenkov, K., Sanches, E.: Fuzzy Markov chains and decision-making, pp. 143–159. Kluwer Academic Publishers (2002)
11. Buckley, J., Eslami, E.: An introduction to fuzzy logic and fuzzy sets. Physica-Verlag, Springer (2002)
12. Bellman, R., Zadeh, L.: Decision-making in a fuzzy environment. Management Science Series 17, 141–164 (1970)
13. Vardi, M., Wolper, P.: An automata-theoretic approach to automatic program verification (preliminary report). In: Logic in Computer Science, pp. 332–344 (1986)
14. Courcoubetis, C., Yannakakis, M.: The complexity of probabilistic verification. Journal of ACM 42, 857–907 (1995)
15. Aziz, A., Singhal, V., Balarin, F., Brayton, R.: It usually works: The temporal logic of stochastic systems. In: Wolper, P. (ed.) CAV 1995. LNCS, vol. 939, pp. 155–165. Springer, Heidelberg (1995)
16. Osborne, M.J., Rubinstein, A.: Bargaining and markets. Academic Press, London (1990)

# Using Activity Theory and Causal Diagrams for Designing MultiAgent Systems That Assist Human Activities

Héctor Ceballos, Juan Pablo García-Vázquez, and Ramón Brena

Tecnológico de Monterrey (ITESM), Intelligent Systems Research Chair
Campus Monterrey, Nuevo León, México
{ceballos,jpablo.garcia,ramon.brena}@itesm.mx

**Abstract.** In this paper, we propose to use the Activity Theory and causal diagrams for modelling human activities with the aim of facilitating the specification of an agent-based assistance system through the Prometheus methodology. As a case study, we consider the elder medication activity, a recurring, complex and context-rich activity that involves several individual and collective activities which may require assistance. From the data collected in a contextual study of the elder medication, we modeled the medical consultation and refill medicine activities. Our results demonstrate that causal diagrams allow to capture the dynamics of the modelled activity, introduce the assistance of intelligent agents, extract the multiple scenarios synthesized in the activity structure and translate them into Prometheus artifacts.

## 1 Introduction

Since the appearance of CommonKADS [1] and throughout the development of multiple multiagent systems methodologies [2–4], peoples' knowledge and their participation has been a key element in the system specifications. As a result, software agents have been proposed as intelligent assistants for human development activities with the purpose of learning from the expert and mimicking some limited functionality [5, 6]. In other approaches like Electronic Institutions [7], people are introduced in the decision loop through the use of User Agents that serve as an interface between them and other software agents in a regulated organization environment. This interaction typically required appropriate Human-Computer Interfaces for delivering information and capturing human feedback. But the most recent advances in pervasive computing are enabling many other alternative ways of perceiving human presence and activity [8].

For this reason, the development of multi-agent systems to assist human activities have become a tangible reality in whose design the human must be placed in the center again [9]. This assistance can take advantage of the vast Artificial Intelligence experience on the development of protocols for gathering information, negotiating, resolving conflicts, coordinating activities and allocating resources [10, 11].

F. Castro, A. Gelbukh, and M. González (Eds.): MICAI 2013, Part I, LNAI 8265, pp. 185–198, 2013.
© Springer-Verlag Berlin Heidelberg 2013

By modeling human activities, we can identify the conditions that must be enabled in order to facilitate their development. For instance, in [12] is proposed an ontology to model the context of the activities of daily living (ADL). The contextual information of the ADL is used by a multiagent-based component to support the activity or prevent an older adult from the a risk associated with the ADL. Other works propose to model a specific human activity. For instance in [13] authors model the human office activities and use multiagent systems to keep track of the state of their users so it can anticipate the users needs and proactively address them.

However, in these works exist a gap between the analysis of human activities and the specification of a Multiagent system that assist the activity. Therefore, in this paper we propose using activity theory to identify the contextual information of the activity and causal diagrams for modelling the dynamics of the activity, which facilitate the process of identification of the artifacts needed to build a multiagent system with the Prometheus methodology. To illustrate our proposal, we consider as a case study the elderly medication activity, since it is a recurrent, complex and context-rich activity, which involves several individual and collective activities, such as attending to medical consultations, taking prescribed medicines and refill medicines [14].

This paper is organized as follows. In section 2, we present the theories used for modelling human activities, some philosophical and modern approaches to causality, and a brief overview of the Prometeus methodology. In section 3 we present the findings of a contextual study of elder medication regarding doctor's visit activity, the modelling of this activity using Engeström's approach and present a methodology for translating it into an annotated causal diagram. In section 4, we present how agent-based assistance can be introduced in human activities and be codified in Prometheus artifacts. Finally, we present our conclusions and future work.

## 2   Background

### 2.1   Activity Theory

The activity theory (AT) is a multidisciplinary and philosophical framework that allows us to understand and study the different forms of the human activities as an individual and collective process [15]. There are three theoretical generations of AT [16]. The first generation is grounded on the concept of *mediation* proposed by Vygosky, which refers to a human performing an activity through a device or tool to achieve a particular objective. This approach considers that activity is an individual process. The second generation was represented by the ideas of Leonti'ev, who introduced the term of *labor division* to define an activity as collective or individual. In addition, Leonti'ev also defined a three-level scheme (activity-actions-operations) to describe a hierarchical structure of activity in which the *activity* is the basic unit of analysis. An Individual activity can be part of a collective activity that involves more than one person working on a same result or objective. Individual activities are composed of *actions*, that is

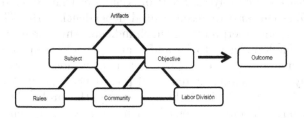

**Fig. 1.** Engeströms human activity system model

something that the person makes consciously to achieve a goal. Actions are comprised by *operations*, which describe how the person does the action.

The third generation of AT is represented by the ideas of Engeström, who consider the ideas of the first and second generation and adding new concepts, such as community, roles and rules to describe the *structure of human activity*. Engeström represent the human activity by a triangle (see Fig. 1) which is composed by the following concepts: a *subject* refers to the individual or sub-group chosen as the point of view in the analysis. The *object* refers to the raw material or a problem space at which the activity is directed and which is molded and transformed into the *results or outcome* with the help of *artifacts* that can be physical or symbolic. The *community* comprises multiple individuals and/or sub-groups that share the same general object and other elements such as *locations*. The *labor division* refers that every individual that participates in the activity has a role. Finally, the *rules* that refer to the explicit and implicit regulations, norms and conventions that represent actions and interactions within the activity system.

AT has been used in computer science to design computer applications, especially in the study of the incorporation of new technologies and computer human interfaces [15]. In addition, AT also has been used to model the context of human activities and to describe situations [17].

## 2.2 Causality

Since Aristotle, *Causality* has been used for explaining natural phenomena or processes in terms of changes [18]. Change is explained through causal relations between events, objects or states of affairs, where the second one (the effect) is a consequence of the first one (the cause), and the cause precedes invariably to the effect. In fact, Aristotle distinguished between four types of causes that intervene on a change: *material cause* (the physical matter used/consumed during change), *formal cause* (the form or plan used for transforming the matter), *efficient cause* (the agent performing the change) and *final cause* (the goal pursued by the agent).

Recently, Pearl revised Bayesian Networks claiming that directed arcs between random variables can also represent causal dependencies [19]. This is, the arc $V_1 \rightarrow V_2$ has a second interpretation which indicates that the event $V_1$ occurred previously or simultaneously to $V_2$ and that $V_2$ is a consequence of $V_1$. This assumption is different to the original statistical notion of correlation, which does not imply directionality or temporal precedence, and it is used by Pearl for developing the Do calculus, which estimates the probability of setting a condition $y$ through the intervention of $x$, denoted $P(y|do(x))$, based on previous observations of the phenomenon [20].

### 2.3   The Prometheus Methodology

Prometheus is an iterative methodology for designing, documenting and building intelligent agent system, which uses goals, beliefs, plans and events. The main difference of Prometheus with other multiagent methodologies is that it uses an iterative process over software engineering phases rather than a linear waterfall model [2].The Prometheus methodology consists of three phases:

- The *system specification phase* focuses on identifying the basic functions of the system, along with inputs (percepts), outputs (actions) and their processing. For instance, how precepts are to be handled and any important shared data sources to model the systems interaction with respect to its changing and dynamic environment.
- The subsequent *architectural design phase* determines which agents the system will contain and how they will interact.
- The *detailed design phase* describes the internals of each agent and the way in which it will achieve tasks within the overall system. The focus in on defining capabilities (modules within the agent), internal events, plans and detailed data structures.

The Prometheus methodology is supported by an open source tool called Prometheus Design Tool(PDT), which supports building agent based system[1].

## 3   The Elderly Medication Activity

Medication is an activity of daily living (ADL) critical for the elderly to be independent at home [14]. This activity is associated with the medical term *medication compliance* that is defined as *the extent to which a patient acts in accordance with the prescribed interval, and dose of a dosing regimen* [21]. During aging the older adults present cognitive and sensorial changes, such as visual acuity reduction or memory loss, then they face frequent problems associated with nonadherence, such as forgetting to take their medicines or forgetting the doctor appointment. To understand the elderly medication activity, a contextual study of medication was carried out [9]. The contextual study consisted of

---

[1] http://www.cs.rmit.edu.au/agents/pdt/

40-minute semi-structured and contextual interview based on Medication Management Instrument for Deficiencies in the Elderly (MedMaIDE), which is an assessment instrument for potential issues surrounding medication compliance and management in a home setting [14]. The participants were 17 elders ranging in age from 63 to 86 years old. Study results evidenced that some older adults are aware of some problems that they face to adhere to their medication, such as forget taking their medication or taking incorrect medicines and/or doses; therefore they create their own strategies to adhere to their medication, such as having a specific place to medicate, maintaining notes for indicating the purpose of taking the medicines and visiting periodically their doctor for refilling their medicines [9]. In this paper, we present the findings of the last strategy with the aim of modeling this activity using the Engreström's approach presented in section 2.1.

## 3.1   Findings on the Doctor Visit Activity

All older adults (17/17) comment that they visit monthly their doctor for their medical appraisal and refilling their medicines. Thirteen older adults (13/17) use the medical appointment card to remind the appointment date. For instance, the older adult (OA-02) said: "*I have a medical appointment card*" and the OA-03 comment: "*when I go to the hospital, I carry with me my card*". Whereas, other three older adults (3/17) use a calendar where they write a note to remind their doctor appointment. For instance, the OA-17 said: "*in my calendar I enclose with a circle the appointment date and write down doctor appointment*". Only one older adult (OA-01) require that a family member remind the doctor appointment, this older adult said: "*My daughter also goes to the hospital... we have the doctor appointment the same day... she calls me*". In addition, we identify that eleven older adults (11/17) require support of a family member to go to the hospital or pharmacy. For instance, the older adult (OA-03) said: "*I go to the hospital in taxi cab or my husband takes me... I do not know how to drive a car.*", and OA-16 said: "*my son takes me... but, depends of the date, if is friday my daughter does*".

**Activity Modelling.** From the findings, we deduce the elements of the activity. The *subject* is the older adult who visits his doctor. The *objective* of the activity is to be assessed with his health (medical appraisal). The activity *outcome* is get a prescription, supply the medicines and schedule the next doctor appointment. Several *artifacts* are used to perform the activity, such as the medical card and calendar. Additionally, we identify the *community* involved in the activity: family members, the doctor and doctor's assistant; who has a role in the activity, for example, the doctor who gives the prescription and the doctor assistant schedules the next appointment date; and finally, the *activity rules*, that indicate when to visit the doctor and how is the medicine provided. All these activity elements are shown in Fig. 2.

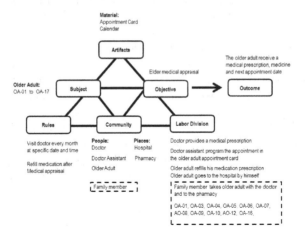

**Fig. 2.** Medical consultation activity elements

## 3.2   The Activity Causal Diagram

The activity structure proposed by Engeström identifies the main elements of the activity but it does not structure the dependencies between them or the valid sequences or alternatives that can be followed in the activity. In order to complement Engeströms approach we propose the use of causal diagrams for modelling the dynamics of the activity. In the first place we introduce the *Activitys Causal Structure* for identifying: the real-world elements that enable the execution of the activity (causes), the goal pursued by the subject (objective), and its observable consequences (outcomes).

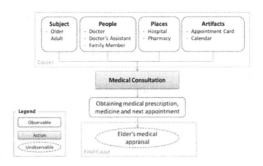

**Fig. 3.** The causal structure of the medical consultation activity

Fig. 3 illustrates the causal structure of the *Medical Consultation activity*, based on the activity structure given in Fig. 2. On one hand, the older adult, the artifacts (appointment card, calendar), and the community (family members, the doctor, the doctors assistant, hospital, pharmacy) are represented as *causes*. On the other, obtaining a new medical prescription, medicine and a new appointment (*the outcome*), can be observed immediately after the consultation, meanwhile the elders medical appraisal (*the objective*) is evidenced only through these outcomes. To this causal interpretation of the activity we incorporate the other two elements missing from the Engeström theory: rules and role division. Role division enumerates the list of actions performed by each agent, meanwhile rules constrain the way on which these actions must be performed. In order to order actions and represent the different ways the activity can be carried out, we express them as a set of subgraphs *cause → action → effect*. Then we chain them together by following this principle: An action $X_1$ precedes another action $X_2$ if exist some cause of $X_2$ that is a direct or indirect effect of $X_1$, expressed as Causes($X_2$) ∈ Anc (Effects($X_1$)). An arc connecting an effect $Z_1$ of $X_1$ to an action $X_3$ or a precondition $Z_2$ of $X_3$ is redundant if the graph already has a directed path from $Z_1$ to $Z_2$ or $X_3$. The resulting graph is *minimal* if it does not have *redundant* arcs and constitutes a Directed Acyclic Graph (DAG) if there are no cycles on it.

**Definition 1.** *An Activity Causal Diagram is represented by $D = \langle G,X,Z,I,F \rangle$, where $G$ is a minimal DAG which arcs denote causal dependencies between observable conditions (Z) and actions (X), and which have at least one causal path from the initial condition $I \in Z$ to every set of outcomes $F_i \in F$, being $F_i \subset (Z \setminus I)$.*

Fig. 4 shows the causal diagram of the *Medical Consultation activity*, constituted by the five actions described in the labor division of Fig. 2. It has six observable conditions or events ($Z_1$-$Z_6$) and five human actions ($X_1$-$X_5$). Despite actions do not have explicit preconditions and postconditions in the labor division description, these are expressed by using the elements of the activity structure (see Fig. 3). The initial condition is the appointment date ($Z_1$) and there are three possible outcomes of the activity: ($Z_4$, $Z_5$, $Z_6$), ($Z_4$, $Z_5$) and ($Z_4$). Given that the objective is not directly observable, this is not included in the causal diagram.

## 3.3   Semantic Annotations

In order to make explicit those dependencies between activitys elements we introduce the use of semantic descriptors over causal diagram nodes. Observable condition and action nodes are annotated with a conjunctive query, represented by a list of statements ⟨subject, predicate, object⟩ where the subject is a variable, the predicate is a label representing an attribute or relationship, and the object is another variable or constant; variables are denoted by a question mark prefix. Fig. 5 illustrates the annotation of two observable conditions ($Z_3$ and $Z_4$), and one action ($X_3$) from Fig. 4.

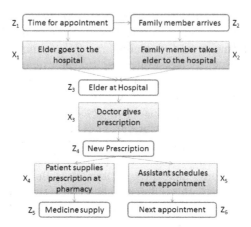

**Fig. 4.** The medical consultation causal diagram

Annotation variables refer to the elements of the activity structure (e.g. ?patient, ?hospital, ?prescription), and to the attributes of those elements (e.g. ?disease, ?medicine, ?frequency). Predicates describe relationships between activity entities (e.g. located_at, has_next_appointment), and properties of activity entities (e.g. on_date, prescribed_by). An observable condition can be annotated with multiple sets of annotations for indicating the different ways on which the event might occur. For instance, the new prescription might include medication (Ann($Z_{4.1}$)) or not(Ann($Z_{4.2}$)).

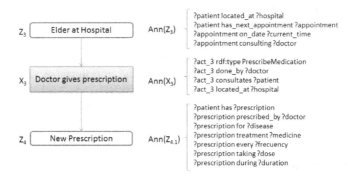

**Fig. 5.** Examples of semantic annotations

In action descriptions, actions execution is denoted by the variable ?act_i, the action is identified by a type (?act_i rdf:type ActionName), the agent performing/initiating the action is identified through the property done_by, and other attributes linking the action with its causes are also included (e.g. consultates ?patient, located_at ?hospital). Action and observable condition annotations are represented by $\text{Ann}(V_i)$, where $V_i$ represents an action $X_i$ or an observable $Z_i$, respectively. The set of variables used in $\text{Ann}(V_i)$ are denoted by $\text{Var}(\text{Ann}(V_i))$.

## 3.4  The Activity Binary Decision Diagram

The activity causal diagram in Fig. 6 codifies the different ways on which the *Medical Consultation activity* is carried out: unassisted (denoted by $X_1$) or assisted by a family member (denoted by $X_2$). Additionally, there exist three possible outcomes for the activity: getting a prescription, medicine and a new appointment ($Z_4$, $Z_5$, $Z_6$); getting a prescription, medicine and being discharged of further consultation ($Z_4$, $Z_5$); and finally, getting a prescription without medication and being discharged of consultation ($Z_4$).The resulting alternative plans are better illustrated by generating the Binary Decision Diagram (BDD) of the activity causal diagram [22].

Fig. 6 illustrates the BDD obtained from the Medical Consultation causal diagram. The Activity BDD is a compact representation of a decision tree that summarizes the valid sequences of actions (plans) that start in the initial condition and end with the achievement of the possible outcomes of the activity. In this BDD, a solid arrow outgoing from a node $X_i$ indicates that $X_i$ is executed as part of a valid plan, whereas a dotted arrow outgoing from $X_i$ indicates that the omission of $X_i$ is part of another valid plan. Actions are ordered in the BDD according to the partial order obtained from the precedence relations between nodes of the activity causal diagram that produces the minimal number of nodes. Valid plans identified by traversing the BDD are also listed in Fig. 6.

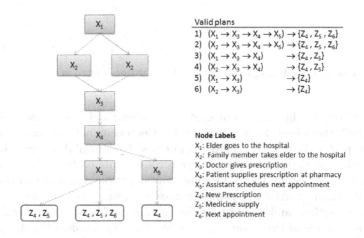

Valid plans
1) $(X_1 \rightarrow X_3 \rightarrow X_4 \rightarrow X_5) \rightarrow \{Z_4, Z_5, Z_6\}$
2) $(X_2 \rightarrow X_3 \rightarrow X_4 \rightarrow X_5) \rightarrow \{Z_4, Z_5, Z_6\}$
3) $(X_1 \rightarrow X_3 \rightarrow X_4)$ $\rightarrow \{Z_4, Z_5\}$
4) $(X_2 \rightarrow X_3 \rightarrow X_4)$ $\rightarrow \{Z_4, Z_5\}$
5) $(X_1 \rightarrow X_3)$ $\rightarrow \{Z_4\}$
6) $(X_2 \rightarrow X_3)$ $\rightarrow \{Z_4\}$

**Node Labels**
$X_1$: Elder goes to the hospital
$X_2$: Family member takes elder to the hospital
$X_3$: Doctor gives prescription
$X_4$: Patient supplies prescription at pharmacy
$X_5$: Assistant schedules next appointment
$Z_4$: New Prescription
$Z_5$: Medicine supply
$Z_6$: Next appointment

**Fig. 6.** The Medical Consultation BDD

# 4    Assisting Human Activities through Multiagent Systems

Causal diagrams can be used as a bridge between the analysis of human activities and the specification of a MultiAgent System that assist that activity. It allows introducing the assistance of intelligent agents and it can be used for making the system specification following the Prometheus Methodology.

## 4.1    Incorporating Intelligent Assistance to Human Activities

So far, the causal diagram only reflects human actions, which execution depends on the free will of each person and in consequence it cannot be controlled but modeled through observation. In order to assist the modeled human activity we can incorporate the participation of intelligent agents upon this structure. Depending on the functionality desired, an agent action can be added for: 1) *enabling* a condition $(X_E)$, or 2) *sensing* the effects of an action $(X_S)$. Fig. 7 shows how these two operations can be introduced around human actions. Note that the human action $X_1$ is replaced by an arc causes$(X_1) \rightarrow$ effects$(X_1)$, indicating that its effects might be observed with or without assistance.

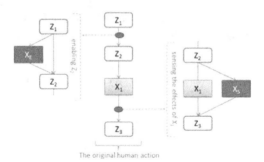

**Fig. 7.** Introducing agent actions for assisting human activities

Agent actions can be whether atomic or composite and are represented as $X_i'$ to distinguish them from human actions $X_i$. Composite actions can implement specialized protocols or be broken down into another causal diagram. These assistance actions are attributed to new agent roles identified by variables in their respective semantic annotations. Original human actions are removed from this extended diagram in order to obtain the *assisted-activity causal diagram*, which only contains actions and events that can be observed by software agents. Fig. 8 shows an example of two actions introduced for: 1) reminding the doctors appointment to the patient (atomic enabling action), and 2) keeping track of his GPS location for verifying if he attended the appointment (composite sensing action). Both actions are performed by an agent in charge of assisting to the patient $(Z_1')$ and use the patient cellphone as notification and tracking device.

In this example, $X_1'$ and $X_2'$ assist the human action $X_1$. Similarly, the medical consultation activity is assisted by another AssistantAgent that reminds to the family member when he has to take the patient to the doctors appointment, a HospitalAgent that connects to the clinical expedient database for getting patients prescription and next appointment, and a SmartHomeAgent that monitors changes on medicine dispenser levels.

## 4.2 Translating Causal Diagrams to Prometheus Artifacts

The translation from activity structures and causal diagrams to a Prometheus system specification is made in two phases: 1) stating the main system goals, and 2) expressing scenarios. In the first phase the main system goal is stated as assisting the ⟨human activity⟩ and it is decomposed in as many goals as documented activities we have: each activity objective constitutes a goal.

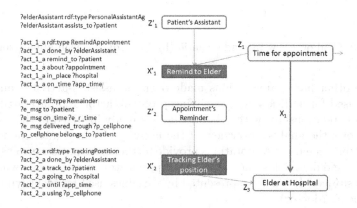

**Fig. 8.** An example of two actions for assisting medical consultation (with annotations)

In the second phase, since the activity structure and the causal diagram synthesizes several cases (one for each older person interviewed), the activity BDD is used for identifying all the possible scenarios in the activity. In our case study we modeled six scenarios: one for each valid plan (see Fig. 6). The assisted-activity causal diagram is used for delimiting the subgraph that represent each scenario. This subgraph is constituted by: a) the initial condition ($I$), b) outcome nodes considered in the plan ($F_i$), 3) the sequence of actions $X_i'$ that assist human actions $X_i$ in the selected plan, and 4) other observable conditions $Z_i$ and $Z_i'$ in the path from $I$ to $F_i$. Each node of the subgraph constitutes a step in the scenario and it is listed according to some partial order given by the causal diagram. Multiple partial orders indicate that there exist activities which can be performed in parallel without affecting the outcome achievement. Observable conditions $Z$

are classified as goal steps, atomic actions $X$ with effects on $Z$ are classified as *percept* steps (e.g. checking patients electronic expedient), atomic actions $X$ with effects on $Z$ (e.g. Remind appointment to Elder) are action steps, composite actions $X$ are represented as calls to another *scenario*, and steps introduced for awaiting for person actions are included as *other*. Fig. 9 illustrates the goal overview and the scenario for Medical Consultation activity when the patient goes by himself to the hospital.

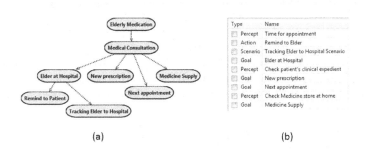

(a)                                    (b)

**Fig. 9.** Goal overview (a) and scenario (b) for medical consultation (alone)

On the other hand, annotations made over the assisted-activity causal diagram are used for additionally identifying protocol, actor and data artifacts, as well as their relationships with other artifacts already included in the scenarios. Fig. 10 shows the analysis overview of the activity obtained after modeling all other possible scenarios. Annotations provide further information such as actions parameters and data fields, indicated by the predicates on statements where they appear as subject. Roles are represented by variables used for identifying agents (e.g. ?patient, ?doctor).

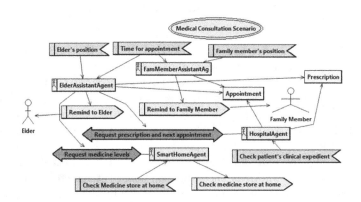

**Fig. 10.** Analysis overview for the medical consultation activity

Agent types included in the analysis overview are obtained from the community component of the activity structure, i.e. people participating in the activity (PersonalAssistantAg) and places enhanced with sensing capabilities and information systems (e.g. SmartHomeAg, HospitalAg).

## 5   Conclusion and Future Work

We motivated the use of the Activity Theory and causal diagrams for closing the gap between the analysis and the development of intelligent agent-based systems that assist daily living activities. For this purpose we introduced the activity causal diagram which structures the activity dynamics in such a way that enables extracting the different scenarios synthesized in the Engeström activity structure. Additionally, causal diagram's semantic annotations capture the relationships between activity elements and provide a formal language that can be used as the system ontology. Next we showed how intelligent agents assistance can be embedded in this causal diagram and be translated into artifacts of the Prometheus methodology.

We anticipate the implementation of a probabilistic decision making mechanism for converting the Causal Diagram into a Causal Bayesian Network where plan accuracy could be improved through parametric and structural Bayesian learning (IC* Algorithm [19]).

**Acknowledgments.** Authors thank Tecnologico de Monterrey for supporting this research through the Intelligent Systems Research Chair, and CONACYT for sponsoring both the postdoctoral fellowship C-290754 and the grant CB-2011-01-167460.

## References

1. Zhou, M., Ren, J., Qi, J., Niu, D., Li, G.: Commonkads methodology for developing power grid switching orders systems. In: Washio, T., Zhou, Z.-H., Huang, J.Z., Hu, X., Li, J., Xie, C., He, J., Zou, D., Li, K.-C., Freire, M.M. (eds.) PAKDD 2007. LNCS (LNAI), vol. 4819, pp. 87–98. Springer, Heidelberg (2007)
2. Padgham, L., Winikoff, M.: Prometheus: A methodology for developing intelligent agents. In: Giunchiglia, F., Odell, J.J., Weiss, G. (eds.) AOSE 2002. LNCS, vol. 2585, pp. 174–185. Springer, Heidelberg (2003)
3. Zambonelli, F., Jennings, N.R., Wooldridge, M.: Developing multiagent systems: The gaia methodology. ACM Trans. Softw. Eng. Methodol. 12, 317–370 (2003)
4. Bareiss, E.R.: Protos: A unified approach to concept representation, classification, and learning (ph.d. dissertation). Technical report, Austin, TX, USA (1988)
5. Tsang, Y.C.: Building software agents to assist teaching in distance learning environments. In: Proceedings of the Fifth IEEE International Conference on Advanced Learning Technologies, ICALT 2005, pp. 230–232. IEEE Computer Society, Washington, DC (2005)
6. Maes, P.: Agents that reduce work and information overload. Commun. ACM 37, 30–40 (1994)

7. Arcos, J., Esteva, M., Noriega, P., Rodriguez-Aguilar, J., Sierra, C.: Engineering open environments with electronic institutions. Engineering Applications of Artificial Intelligence, 191–204 (2005)
8. Chen, L., Nugent, C.: Ontology-based activity recognition in intelligent pervasive environments. International Journal of Web Information Systems 5, 410–430 (2009)
9. García-Vázquez, J.P., Rodríguez, M.D., Tentori, M.E., Saldaña, D., Andrade, Á.G., Espinoza, A.N.: An agent-based architecture for developing activity-aware systems for assisting elderly. j-jucs 16, 1500–1520 (2010)
10. Wu, J.: Contract net protocol for coordination in multi-agent system. In: Second International Symposium on Intelligent Information Technology Application, IITA 2008, vol. 2, pp. 1052–1058 (2008)
11. Gasparovic, B., Mezei, I.: Auction aggregation protocols for agent-based task assignment in multi-hop wireless sensor and robot networks. In: 2011 IEEE/ASME International Conference on Advanced Intelligent Mechatronics (AIM), pp. 247–252 (2011)
12. Saldaña-Jimenez, D., Rodríguez, M.D., García-Vázquez, J.-P., Espinoza, A.-N.: Elder: An ontology for enabling living independently of risks. In: Meersman, R., Herrero, P., Dillon, T. (eds.) OTM 2009 Workshops. LNCS, vol. 5872, pp. 622–627. Springer, Heidelberg (2009)
13. Myers, K.L., Yorke-Smith, N.: Proactive behavior of a personal assistive agent. In: Proceedings of the AAMAS Workshop on Metareasoning in Agent-Based Systems, Honolulu, HI, pp. 31–45 (2007)
14. Orwig, D., Brandt, N., Gruber-Baldini, A.L.: Medication management assessment for older adults in the community. The Gerontologist 46, 661–668 (2006)
15. Nardi, B.: Context and Consciousness: Activity Theory and Human-Computer Interaction. MIT Press (1996)
16. Engeström, Y., Miettinen, R., Punamäki, R.: Perspectives on Activity Theory. Learning in Doing: Social, Cognitive and Computational Perspectives. Cambridge University Press (1999)
17. Cassens, J., Kofod-Petersen, A.: Using activity theory to model context awareness: a qualitative case study. In: Proceedings of the Nineteenth International Florida Artificial Intelligence Research Society Conference, pp. 619–624 (2006)
18. Alvira, T., Clavell, L., Melendo, T.: Metafísica. Libros de Iniciación Filosófica. Universidad de Navarra, Ediciones (1982)
19. Pearl, J.: Causality. Models, Reasoning, and Inference. Cambridge University Press (2000)
20. Pearl, J., Robins, J.: Probabilistic evaluation of sequential plans for causal models with hidden variables. In: Besnard, P., Hanks, S. (eds.) Uncertainty in Artificial Intelligence, vol. 11, pp. 444–453 (1995)
21. Cramer, J.A., Roy, A., Burrell, A., Fairchild, C.J., Fuldeore, M.J., Ollendorf, D.A., Wong, P.K.: Medication compliance and persistence: Terminology and definitions. Value in Health 11, 44–47 (2008)
22. Akers, S.: Binary decision diagrams. IEEE Transactions on Computers C-27, 509–516 (1978)

# Challenges in Ontology Alignment and Solution to the Contradictory Evidence Problem

Maria Vargas-Vera[1] and Miklos Nagy[2]

[1] Facultad de Ingenieria y Ciencias
Universidad Adolfo Ibanez
Vinia del Mar, Chile
maria.vargas-vera@uai.cl
[2] The Open University, UK
m.nagy@open.ac.uk

**Abstract.** This paper introduces the main challenges when performing ontology mapping. These challenges vary from representational issues to conflicting information. For the latest category of challenges, namely conflicting information, we have designed a method to deal with the uncertainty on mappings. Then, our main contribution is the design and development of novel trust assessment formalism for handling contradicting evidence in the context of ontology mapping. The novelty of our proposed solution relays in the incorporation of the fuzzy voting model to the Dempster-Shafer theory. Finally, we present a case study where we show how our approach improves the ontology mapping problem.

## 1 Introduction

This section presents the main challenges for ontology mapping on the Semantic Web. These challenges are considered as roadblocks for developing real applications on the Semantic Web. Our proposed approach intends to resolve these challenges. Although, these challenges are just a subset of those that have been identified by the ontology mapping community ([1],[2]), in our view they are the most relevant ones that need to be addressed by any approach that intends to improve the quality of the mapping result. The identification of the challenges is based on the systems currently available at competitive level. So our key five challenges are as follows:

a). **Robustness across domains.** Most systems use multiple techniques such as heuristics, machine learning or Natural Language Processing (NLP) in order to transform the information in the ontologies into their internal representation. For example, ASMOV ([3]) uses domain specific background knowledge whereas RiMOM ([4]) applies pre-defined rules to assess similarities. Anchor-Flood ([5]) and TaxoMap ([6]) have been designed to exploit large textual descriptions of the ontology concepts, which is an assumption that cannot be satisfied across domains. These techniques have the problem that could impact domain independence negatively because they require a-priori knowledge from a designer. It is important to emphasize that ontology designers will always have the freedom to

F. Castro, A. Gelbukh, and M. González (Eds.): MICAI 2013, Part I, LNAI 8265, pp. 199–216, 2013.

model their domain according to their need. In the same way, database designers can come up with different models for the same problem. To overcome this problem, existing systems utilize various types of domain knowledge (heuristic rule or training data set).

b). **Uncertain reasoning.** Some ontology alignment systems provide limited reasoning support, in order to derive new information from the input ontologies. Unfortunately, not enough emphasis is placed on the reasoning part in spite of the fact that it has the potential to provide an added value to the systems. Furthermore, the uncertain reasoning possibility is completely missing from the existing systems.

c). **Managing conflicts.** Conflict detection is only provided as a post-processing functionality. However, conflicts that normally appear during the mapping process are not treated properly by the current solutions. Managing conflicting information does have the potential to improve the end results slightly or moderately depending on the domains. Conflicts can be a result of insufficient or contradicting information of different terms that are similar or even the same. We propose a conflict elimination approach using a fuzzy voting model. Based on our initial approach for eliminating conflicts ([7]), we propose different fuzzy variables, membership functions and a customized voting algorithm in order to provide more reliable results. The fuzzy voting model allows detecting and eliminating contradictory evidence, instead of discarding the whole scenario or combining them with contradictions. These contradictions can occur on any entities in the ontology e.g. classes, objects, data properties and instances.

d). **Mapping optimization.** Only two systems (RiMOM, TaxoMap) consider optimization of the mapping process, while other systems do not even consider it as a problem at this stage. This can be explained by the fact that most of the systems have not faced the problem of processing large-scale real world ontologies. While, it is true that optimization issues can be addressed later on, it is important that the mapping solutions are conceived with scalability options.

e). **Mapping visualization.** Each system presents the mapping result to the users, although little emphasis has been placed on how these results are presented. Most systems show the results as a list of mapping pairs, and only some employ two-dimensional graph-based visualization. Additionally, there is no way to examine how the system produced these results as only the end results are kept.

More details of each of the challenges is discussed in section 3. However, for the sake of space we only discuss a few challenges. The main contribution of this paper is that it proposes a conflict elimination method based on trust and fuzzy voting, before any conflicting belief is combined. We show that this idea works well and improves precision and recall in a ontology mapping system.

The paper is organized as follows: Section 2 presents the related work. Section 3 the main challenges in ontology mapping. Section 4 introduces our algorithm used in our solution; Section 5 shows a case of study and finally, section 6 describes future research directions and conclusions.

## 2  Related Work

We had reviewed the most relevant approaches to ontology alignment (also identified as state-of-the-art in [1]). In particular, our interest was on related work which considers uncertainty in the mapping process. Different approaches to eliminate contradictions for ontology mapping have been proposed by the ontology mapping community. These approaches can be classified into two distinct categories.

First group include solutions that consider uncertainty and fuzziness as an inherent nature of the ontology mapping and tries to describe it accordingly. Ferrara et al. (2008) model the whole ontology mapping problem as fuzzy where conflicts can occur therefore, their approach models the whole mapping process as an uncertain reasoning task, where the mapping results need to be validated at the end of the reasoning process. The reasoning is supported by fuzzy Description Logic approaches. As a consequence, their mapping validation algorithm interprets the output mapping pairs as fuzzy and tries to eliminate the inconsistencies from them [8].

Tang et al. (2006) formalise the ontology mapping problem as making decisions on mappings using Bayesian reasoning. Their system *RiMOM* [4] has participated in the OAEI competition as well. Their solution do consider two kinds of conflicts in the ontologies, namely the structure and naming conflicts. However, they use thesaurus and statistical techniques to eliminate them before combining the results. *RiMOM* approach produces ontology mapping using well-defined processing steps like *ontology pre-processing, strategy selection, strategy execution* and *alignment combination*. *RiMOM* has been very successful during OAEI competitions; however, its strategies have to be defined in advance together with their rules, which are selected during execution time. As a result, it is questionable how the system can be adapted to the Semantic Web environment, where domains can change dynamically. Furthermore, the assumption that ontologies with *similar features* are similar in reality might not be valid in all cases. Another weak point is that large ontologies cannot easily be loaded into the internal model and the approach does not consider optimisation for the mapping process. Nevertheless, the main idea is remarkable since it builds up its own structure and, hence, tries to interpret the ontology before processing it.

The second group, however, differ conceptually because they mainly utilise data mining and logic reasoning techniques in pre and post processing stages of the mapping.

For example, Liu et al. (2006), split the ontology mapping process into four different phases. Their approach first exploits the available labels in the ontologies then it compares the instances. After it recalls mappings from the previous mapping tasks and compares it with the structure of the ontologies. Their approach also tries to eliminate contradictions, using the previous experience and data mining techniques on the relations that are defined on the ontologies [9].

A similar solution has been proposed byJean-Mary et al. (2009); Jean- Mary & Kabuka (2008). The system ASMOV *Automated Semantic Mapping of Ontologies with Validation (ASMOV)* automates the ontology alignment process using a weighted average of measurements of similarity along four different features of ontologies, and performs semantic validation of resulting alignments. This system acknowledges that conflicting mappings are produced during the mapping process but they use an iterative post processing logic validation in order to filter out the conflicting mappings.

*Anchor-Flood* [5], is an ontology mapping tool conceived in the context of the *International Patent Classification (IPC)*. The mapping approach itself was designed to work as part of a *patent mining* system that assigns patent abstracts to existing IPC ontologies and it also uses a multi-phase approach to create the mapping results. These phases are *pre-processing, anchoring, neighbouring block collection* and *similarity measures*. Anchor-Flood also uses an internal representation form to which the ontologies are transformed before processing. The system is also reliant on the availability of individuals, which might not be always present in real life scenarios. There are also a number of weaknesses that are related to the fact that the approach is highly dependent on the correctness of the initial anchoring. Inconsistencies might not be eliminated and missed links might not be discovered it they do not fall into the context of already linked entities.

*TaxoMap* [6] is an approach that is based on the assumption that large-scale ontologies contain very extensive textual descriptions and well defined class structures but do not contain a large number of properties or individuals. The similarity assessment uses various *Natural Language Processing* techniques and frameworks like *TreeTagger* [10] and *structural heuristic-based* similarity algorithms like *Semantic Cotopy* [11]. In order to filter out inconsistent mappings, it uses a *refinement module*. End users have the possibility to define constraints and solutions using a logic-based language called *Mapping Refinement Pattern Language (MRPL)*. For example, this language allows the end users to express domain specific constraints that can remove a mapping pair on condition that the classes involved in the mapping do not have an equivalence relation in the source or target ontology. However, one weakness of the system is that it requires the fine-tuning of nine different threshold values, which is a challenge given the possible combinations and the possible impacts on the result set.

*Lily* [12] is a mapping approach which carries out the mapping in different phases. These phases are *pre-processing, match computing* and *post processing*. In the last phase, the system extracts the final mapping set based on the similarity assessments, and then it verifies that inconsistent mappings are indicated to the user, who can remove them manually. It is important to point out that the mapping approach recognises the fact that the interpretation of the ontologies involves dealing with uncertainty. However, the objective is only to reduce the amount of uncertainty instead of dealing or reasoning with it. As a result, the mapping process only reduces the negative effect of the matching uncertainty. Lily can also deal with large-scale ontology matching tasks thanks to its scalable ontology matching strategy.

# 3    Challenges in Ontology Alignment

## 3.1    Representation Problems and Uncertainty

The Semantic Web ([13]) was designed to achieve machine-processable interoperability through the semantic annotation of web content, which is based on distributed domain ontologies. This vision assumes that using Semantic Web resources, software agents are able to establish an understanding (at a certain level) of the data they process, and that they can then reason with this information. The purpose of such agents is to carry out various tasks on behalf of, or for, the users, like answering queries, searching for information or integrating data. Furthermore, data on the Semantic Web is described by ontologies, which typically consist of a number of classes, relations, individuals and axioms. These elements are expressed using a logical language. The W3C has proposed RDF(S) ([14]) and OWL ([15]) as Web ontology languages. However, OWL has three variants with different expressiveness. OWL Lite is the simplest and includes basic hierarchies that are most commonly used in current thesauri. OWL DL and OWL Full can be used for complex representational problems with or without complete reasoning support.

During 2009, W3C published a new recommendation called OWL 2, which redefines the core concepts in OWL and defines three profiles, namely: OWL 2 EL (large ontologies), OWL 2 QL (simple ontologies), and OWL 2 RL (complex ontologies). This profiles were defined in order to adjust the language expressiveness to the real world requirements of data integration and knowledge representation. In addition to the existing Web ontology languages, W3C has proposed other representations, such as SKOS ([16]), which is widely used for describing large thesauri or taxonomies on the Semantic Web. Euzenat (2002) pointed out early on that numerous questions need to be answered before semantic annotation becomes usable on the Web. One of the issues mentioned was entities in the domain can be represented differently in different ontologies, e.g., class labels as rdfs:label or properties of the class.

Consider the following excerpts: Fig. 1,2 from different Food and Agricultural Organization of the United Nations (fao) ontologies.Assuming that, we need to assess the similarity between entities of the two ontologies, in the fragment depicted in Fig.1 a class c 8375 is defined to represent Demospongiae sponges. In the class description only the ID is indicated, therefore, to determine the properties of the class one needs to extract the necessary information from the associated named individual. In Fig. 2 Demospongiae are represented as RDF individuals, where the individual properties are defined as data properties. One can note the difference in how the class labels are represented in Fig.1 through rdfs:label and in Fig.2 through hasNameScientific and hasNameLongEN tags.

Considering the correctness of both ontologies, they both comply with the OWL specifications; therefore, processing them individually with any logic reasoner would not lead to inconsistency problems. However, if one needs to create class and individual similarities between the two ontologies then several problems would occur. For example, when comparing the two ontologies a

```
    ...
<owl:Class rdf:ID="c_8375">
   <rdfs:subClassOf>
      <owl:Class rdf:ID="c_7033"/>
   </rdfs:subClassOf>
</owl:Class>
...
< c_8375 rdf:ID="i_8375">
   <aos:hasScopeNote xml:lang="EN">Isscaap group b-52
   </aos:hasScopeNote>
   <aos:hasScopeNote xml:lang="FR">Groupe b-52
   de la csitapa</aos:hasScopeNote>
   ...
   <rdfs:label xml:lang="en">Demospongiae</rdfs:label>
</c_8375>
...
```

**Fig. 1.** Ontology fragment from the AGROVOC ontology

```
    ...
<owl:Class rdf:about="#species">
<rdfs:subClassOf rdf:resource="#biological_entity"/>
<owl:disjointWith rdf:resource="#family"/>
<owl:disjointWith rdf:resource="#order"/>
<owl:disjointWith rdf:resource="#group"/>
</owl:Class>
...
<rdf:Description rdf:about="http://www.fao.org/
species_v1.0.owl#31005_17431">
<j.0:hasNameLongEN>Barrel sponge</j.0:hasNameLongEN>
<j.0:hasMeta>31005 </j.0:hasMeta>
<j.0:hasNameScientific> Demospongiae"</j.0:hasNameScientific>
</rdf:Description> ...
```

**Fig. 2.** Ontology fragment from the ASFA ontology

considerable amount of uncertainty arises over the classes and their properties. This uncertainty arises because, as a result of using different representations, certain elements will be missing for the comparison, e.g., we have a label in the fragment in Fig.1 that is missing from the fragment in Fig.2 but there is a hasNameLongEN tag in the fragment in Fig.2 that is missing in the fragment in Fig.1.Therefore, we argue that any process including ontology mapping that involves interpreting different ontologies in order to compare them will always involve dealing with uncertainties of some form.

## 3.2   Quality of Semantic Web Data

Data quality problems ( [17], [18]) in the context of database integration ([19]) emerged long before the Semantic Web concept was proposed. Gertz et al. (2004) investigated the important aspects of data quality and trust in the data itself in open and dynamic environments like the Web [20]. Their conclusions on how the sudden development of Internet-based applications and Web-based technologies brought data quality and trust issues into the spotlight also applies to the Semantic Web [20]. When individuals or organizations publish data on the Semantic Web, their reason for publishing the data may be dissimilar. For example, a library that makes available a list of books for search purposes and a publisher who actually sells books might emphasize different properties/aspects of the same book. Therefore, in scenarios where mapping and data exchange has to be made between two ontologies describing the aforementioned domain, incompleteness of data will always be an issue. Furthermore, given the distributed nature of the Semantic Web, data quality will always be an issue, because the applications should be able to process inaccurate, ill-defined and/or inconsistent data with minimal human expert input. Naturally, the required expert input at design time differs depending on the application domain because a simple search might include incomplete results; whereas querying integrated databases should not. The laborious nature of cleaning up data and its impact to data quality during any kind of data integration (data-warehouse or mediator based) is a well-known issue [21]. In this respect, various data syntax issues can be resolved using a standardized format for the application, e.g., defining a separation rule for compound terms like MScThesis, MSc Thesis. In the context of the Semantic Web, the major issue for any data integration solution is how to resolve semantic data quality issues without involving domain experts or any other user input. This is because it is unfeasible to foresee any ontology designer providing input for each source that is available on the Semantic Web. As such, the applications themselves need to be able to resolve these problems without involving too much domain expert knowledge and support, if any, during run-time. Additionally, applications should be able to independently analyze the ontology content and assess whether it can be used or not for a given purpose. Consider the example shown in Fig. 3, which is from the directories ontology.

As Fig. 3 shows, Windows Vista is defined as the subclass of the Operating systems class, however, the designer has indicated that it has a specific serial number, and therefore it should actually be considered as an individual. In short, the semantic data quality here is low, as the information is dubious, and therefore the Semantic Web application has to create its own hypotheses over the meaning of this data.

## 3.3   Efficient Ontology Mapping with Large-Scale Ontologies

Processing large-scale ontologies is a difficult and time-consuming task, using conventional approaches with limited resources. This has been discussed by Flahive et al. (2006), who propose to extract so called sub-ontologies using a

```
...
<owl:Class rdf:about="http://matching.com/3887.owl#
Windows_Vista">
<rdfs:label xml:lang="en"> Windows Vista Home
Edition </rdfs:label>
<j:hasSerialNumber>
 <rdfs:label >00043-683-036-658</rdfs:label>
</j:hasSerialNumber>
<rdfs:subClassOf>
 <owl:Class rdf:about="http://matching.com/3887.owl#
Operating_Systems">
 </owl:Class>
</rdfs:subClassOf>
</owl:Class>
...
```

**Fig. 3.** Ontology fragment from the Web directories ontology

distributed environment that can be used to process different parts of the mapping task in parallel [22]. For example, Li et al. (2010) report on a large-scale ontology summarization problem in the context of ontology visualization. The identified problems are similar because even displaying large ontologies for editing or review causes considerable difficulties for end users. A similar large-scale ontology extraction methodology has been proposed by Carlo et al. (2005) that is based on database view like definitions on the ontologies in order to manage the information overload in the context of ontology visualization [23]. Scalability issues can be considered as important because they can contribute to an acceptance or rejection of an approach once it reaches the end users. Consider for example an ontology mapping approach that can only work with small ontologies. While, the merits of the approach would be acknowledged, the applicability of the solution would be questioned when using real life large ontologies. Additionally, domains that continuously produce and maintain large lexical databases or general knowledge bases are good candidates for transforming their source into a more structured form like a web ontology.

Consider for example WordNet. Since the project started in 1985 WordNet has been used for a number of different purposes in information systems. It is popular a general background knowledge for ontology mapping systems because it contains around 150.000 synsets and their semantic relations. Other efforts to represent common sense knowledge as an ontology include the Cyc project, which consists of more than 300.000 terms and around 3.000.000 axioms. Another example is the Suggested Upper Merged Ontology (SUMO), which includes several domain ontologies. It contains around 20.000 concepts and 70.000 assertions. However, by far the largest semantic resource to date (to the best of our knowledge) in terms of individual number is DBpedia, with its 1.8 million entries, each linked to a Wikipedia article. Discovering correspondences between these large-scale semantic resources is an on-going effort, but only partial mappings have been established, i.e., SUMO-WordNet, due to the vast amount of human and computational effort involved in these tasks. The OAEI 2008 ([24]) also included a mapping track for large ontologies. This mapping track used three very large resources, namely WordNet, DBpedia and GTAA (Audiovisual Thesaurus in the Dutch language) [25]. These ontologies contain well over 100.000 entities and the numbers could reach millions when individuals are considered. Nevertheless, the idea of using only large-scale ontologies on the Semantic Web can be debated on the grounds that most organizations or individuals would rather develop small ontologies. However, from the scalability point of view it is indifferent if one needs to process a small number of large ontologies or a large number of small ontologies. Consider for example that in 2007 Swoogle [26] had already indexed more than 10.000 ontologies, which were available on the Web. The large number of concepts and properties that are implied by the scale or number of these ontologies poses several scalability problems from the reasoning point of view. Therefore, from the ontology mapping point of view there is a need to address various scalability issues. Specifically, scalability here has two aspects: first of all, the similarity assessments can be executed at the same time using distributed and parallel computation; secondly, the similarity combinations can be optimized.

# 4    Solution to Contradictory Evidences

The problem of trustworthiness in the context of ontology mapping can be represented in different ways. In general, trust issues on the Semantic Web are associated with the source of the information i.e. who said what and when and what credentials they had to say it. From this point of view the publisher of the ontology could greatly influence the outcome of the trust evaluation and the mapping process can prefer mappings that came from a more "trustful" source. However, we believe that in order to evaluate trust it is important to look into our processes that create the mappings between these ontologies. From the similarity point of view it is more important to see how the information in the ontologies are "conceived" by our algorithms than to assess a trust value based on the creator (university or private person) of these ontologies. For example, it is an important question to ask if our algorithms can exploit all the available information in the ontologies or just part of it.

The reason why we propose such trust evaluation is, because ontologies of the Semantic Web usually represent a particular domain and support a specific need. Therefore, even if two ontologies describe the same concepts and properties their relation to each other can differ depending on the conceptualisation of their creators, which is independent from the organisation where they belong. In our ontology mapping method, we propose that the trust in the provided similarity measures, which are assessed between the ontology entities depend on the actual understanding of the mapping entities. It is important to point out that similarity assessments are quite complex for ontology mapping, therefore the way they produce the similarity measure can differ from case to case. Imagine a situation where the similarity assessment involves consulting background knowledge to retrieve the synonyms of a particular entity. For the term "paper" one can use the meaning of the "scientific publication" or the "A4 sized paper sheet". As a consequence, the result will differ from case to case e.g. a similarity measure can be trusted in one case but not trustful in an another case during the same process. Our mapping algorithm that incorporates trust management into the process is described by Algorithm 1.

---

**Input**: Similarity belief matrices $S_{n \times m} = \{S_1, .., S_k\}$
**Output**: Mapping candidates

1  **for** $i=1$ **to** $n$ **do**
2      BeliefVectors BeliefVectors ← GetBeliefVectors($S[i, 1 - m]$) ;
3      Concepts ← GetBestBeliefs(BeliefVectors BeliefVectors) ;
4      Scenario ← CreateScenario(Concepts) ;
5      **for** $j=1$ **to** $size($Concepts$)$ **do**
6          | Scenario ← AddEvidences (Concepts) ;
7      **end**
8      **if** Evidences *are contradictory* **then**
9          **for** $count=1$ **to** $numberOf($Experts$)$ **do**
10             Voters ← CreateVoters($10$) ;
11             TrustValues ← VoteTrustMembership(Evidences) ;
12             ProbabilityDistribution ←
               CalculateTrustProbability(TrustValues) ;
13             Evidences ← SelectTrustedEvidences(ProbabilityDistribution) ;
14         **end**
15     **end**
16     Scenario ← CombineBeliefs(Evidences) ;
17     MappingList ← GetMappings(Scenario) ;
18 **end**

---

**Algorithm 1.** Belief combination with trust

The advantage of our proposed solution is that the evaluated trust is independent from the source ontologies themselves, and can change depending on the available information in the context.

DSSim's mapping Algorithm 1 receives the similarity matrices (both syntactic and semantic) as an input and produces the possible mappings as an output. The similarity matrices represent the assigned similarities between all concepts in ontology 1 and 2. Our mapping algorithm iterates, through all concepts in ontology 1, and selects the best possible candidate terms from ontology 2, which is represented as a vector of best beliefs(step 2). Once the best beliefs are selected, the algorithm gets the terms that corresponds to these beliefs and creates a mapping scenario. This scenario contains all possible mapping pairs between the selected term in ontology 1 and the possible terms from ontology 2(step 3 and 4). Once our mapping scenario is built, then, the algorithm starts adding evidence from the similarity matrices(step 6). These evidence might contradict because different similarity algorithms can assign different similarity measures for the same mapping candidates. If these evidence are contradictory, then the algorithm needs to evaluate, which measure i.e. mapping agents' belief we trust in this particular scenario (see step 8-15). The trust evaluation is invoked, which invalidates the evidence(agent beliefs) that cannot be trusted in this scenario. Once the conflict resolution routine is finished, the valid beliefs can be combined and the possible mapping candidates can be selected from the scenario.

The advantage of our proposed solution is that the evaluated trust is independent from the source ontologies themselves, and can change depending on the available information in the context.

## 5   OAEI Case Study

Experimental comparison of the conflict resolution has been carried out with the Ontology Mapping Evaluation Initiative data sets from 2007 and 2008. In this section the results of these experiments are presented.

The OAEI evaluation uses widely accepted measures for search systems called recall and precision. Both precision and recall have a fixed range between 0-1 (i.e. 0% and 100%).

**Definition 1.** *Precision shows how many correct mappings have been returned by the search engine or a mapping system.*

**Definition 2.** *Recall measures how many relevant mappings or search results have been returned from the possible set of correct responses.*

The first experiments have been carried out with the benchmark ontologies of the Ontology Alignment Evaluation Initiative(OAEI)[1], which is an international initiative that has been set up for evaluating ontology matching algorithms. The experiments were carried out to assess how trust management influences results of our proposed mapping algorithm. The main objective was to evaluate the impact of establishing trust before combining beliefs in similarities between concepts and properties in the ontology.

The benchmark tests are popular for evaluating systems in the ontology mapping community. The reason is that these tests were mainly generated from one reference ontology, discharging, transforming or replacing the content of the content and structure. Additionally, the size of the ontology is easily processable for any system, because the reference contained 33 named classes and 64 properties. Additionally, each test contains the reference alignment, which can be used to validate the generated results.

The benchmark tests can be grouped in to 3 different categories:

– Group 1xx: relatively simple tests such as comparing the reference with itself or with a totally different ontology.

---

[1] http://oaei.ontologymatching.org/

– Group 2xx: these tests are the most interesting ones for the evaluation. Different tests have been generated using the reference ontology and change it using a specific rule. For example, replacing class names with random strings, introducing different naming conventions, remove class hierarchy or reducing the expressiveness of the ontology from OWL FULL to OWL Lite.
– Group 3xx: four real ontologies of bibliographic references that were defined by different research institutions.

Due to the fact that the benchmark is the only test set in the OAEI tracks where the results are also available, we have first run our experiments where DSSim applies the fuzzy voting model for evaluating trust and one without it. Therefore, as a basic comparison we have modified the mapping algorithm (without trust), which does not evaluate trust before conflicting belief combination, just combine them using Dempster's combination rule. The recall and precision graphs for the algorithm with trust and without trust over the whole benchmarks are depicted in Fig. 4, 5. Experiments have proved that with establishing trust one can reach higher average precision and recall rate.

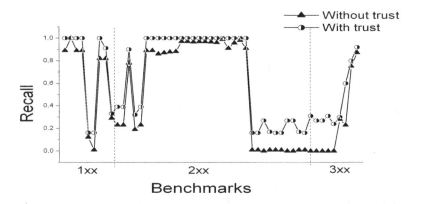

**Fig. 4.** Recall graph with and without applying fuzzy voting

Fig. 4 and 5 show the improvement in recall and precision that we have achieved by applying our trust model for combining contradictory evidence. From the precision point of view, the increased recall values have not impacted the results significantly, which is good because the objective is always the improvement of both recall and precision together.

We have measured the average improvement for the whole benchmark test set that contains 51 ontologies. Based on the experiments, the average recall has increased by 12% and the precision is by 16%. The relative high increase in precision compared to recall is attributed to the fact that in some cases the precision has been increased by 100% as a consequence of a small recall increase of 1%. This is perfectly normal because if the recall increases from 0 to 1% and the returned mappings are all correct (which is possible since the number of mappings are small) then the precision increases from 0 to 100%.

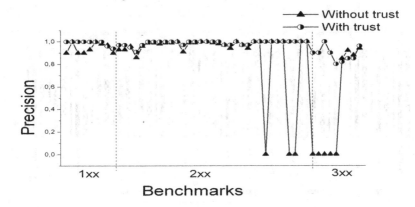

**Fig. 5.** Precision graph with and without applying fuzzy voting

Further the increase in recall and precision greatly varies from test to test. Surprisingly, the precision has decreased in some cases(5 out of 51). The maximum decrease in precision was 7% and maximum increase was 100%. The recall has never decreased in any of the tests and the minimum increase was 0.02% whereas the maximum increase was 37%.

In our ontology mapping solution there are number of mapping agents that carry out similarity assessments, hence create belief mass assignments for the evidence. Before the belief mass function is combined, each mapping agent need to calculate dynamically a trust value, which describes how confident the particular mapping agent is about the other mapping agents' assessment. This dynamic trust assessment is based on the fuzzy voting model, and depends on its own and other agents' belief mass function. In our ontology mapping framework, we assess trust between the mapping agents' beliefs and determine, which agents' belief cannot be trusted, rejecting the one, which is as the result of trust assessment become distrustful.

From the comparison point of view it is important to demonstrate that our mapping system compares well to other existing systems. Fig. 6 shows the 6 best performing systems out of 13 participants. Note that, we have ordered the systems based on their F-Value and the H-means because the H-mean unifies all results for the test and F-Value represents both precision and recall.

In the benchmark test DSSim has performed in the upper mid range compared to other systems. Depending on the group of tests our system compares differently to other solutions:

- Group 1xx: Our results are nearly identical to the other systems.
- Group 2xx: For the tests where syntactic similarity can determine the mapping outcome our system is comparable to other systems. However, where semantic similarity [27] is the only way to provide mappings our systems provides less mappings compared to the other systems in the best six.
- Group 3xx: Considering the F-value for this group only 3 systems SAMBO, RIMOM and Lily are ahead.

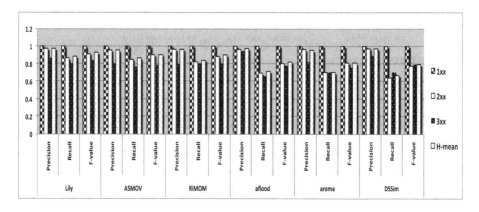

**Fig. 6.** Best performing systems in the benchmarks track based on H-mean and F-value

The weakness of our system is to provide good mappings, when only semantic similarity can be exploited is the direct consequence of our mapping architecture. At the moment, we are using four mapping agents where 3 carries our syntactic similarity comparisons and only 1 is specialised in semantics. However, it is worth to note that our approach seems to be stable compared to previous years performance. The precision and recall values were similar, in spite of the fact that more and more difficult tests have been introduced in 2008. As the DSSim architecture is easily expandable with adding more mapping agents, it is possible to enhance our semantic mapping performance in the future.

### 5.1 Directory

The directory track is a large and challenging track, because the tests were generated from existing Web directories i.e. real world ontologies. The size of the ontologies are relatively small, however, the number of tests are large. Further the generated ontologies do not have a deep class hierarchy and they do not contain any properties.

The specific characteristics of the dataset are:

- The root of the web directories has been included with a small number of classes for more than 4500 tests. Expert mappings for all the matching tasks.
- Each test contains only simple ontology relationships i.e. subclass
- The generated tests contain mistakes concerning the terminology in order to mimic the real world modelling scenario.

Fig. 7, 8 displays the result of the mapping with and without applying trust into the belief combination. In case of the directories, the measures without applying trust have been calculated based on the original results submitted to the OAEI organisers. During the OAEI evaluation DSSim has produced only one mapping file that included the trust assessment algorithm. Based on the results communicated by the organisers we have run the our mapping algorithm and compared the mapping file with the one that was submitted to OAEI. The library track shows large differences in some mappings (e.g. 50% better with applying trust), however, it is important to note that these large differences can be attributed to the fact that the ontologies contain only a couple of classes. In these cases, even improving the mapping with two new mapping pairs can result in a 50% increase in precision or recall. Therefore, the results should be interpreted considering this bias. Thanks to the large number of tests i.e. more than 4500 mapping tasks, it is possible to deduce an average improvement for both precision and recall. Considering recall, the average improvement was 8% and the precision increase was 11%.

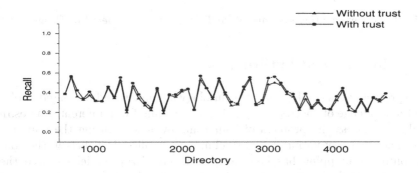

**Fig. 7.** Recall graph with and without applying fuzzy voting

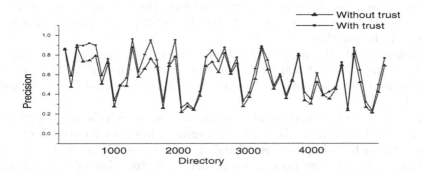

**Fig. 8.** Precision graph with and without applying fuzzy voting

In the directories track only 6 systems have participated the year 2008 (see Fig. 9). In terms of F-value DSSim has performed the best, however, the difference is marginal compared to the CIDER [28] or Lily [29] systems. The concepts in the directory ontologies mostly can be characterised as compound nouns e.g. "News_and_Media" and we need to process(split) them properly before consulting background knowledge in order to provide better mappings in the future.

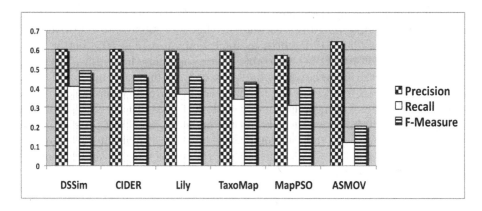

**Fig. 9.** All participating systems in the directories track ordered by F-value

## 6    Conclusions and Future Work

We have presented the challenges in the ontology alignment and presented a solution to the challenge of contradictory evidences coming from different sources.In particulat we adress the problem of conflicting evidences during the mapping process. Then, a fuzzy voting model to eliminate conflicts in beliefs in the context of ontology mapping has been proposed. The fuzzy model required the definition of what fuzzy trust means in the context of ontology mapping, and how the input and output variables of a fuzzy system needed to be defined to manage the contradictory beliefs. Through fuzzy trust, we have defined different trust levels, represented by linguistic variables. Recognising the importance of different trust levels is relevant, not just for ontology mapping but for the Semantic Web as a whole.

Experiments with the different OAEI tests were carried out. This experiments allow us to conclude that that by the addition to the combination rule, we had improved average recall up to 12% and the precision between 3-16% as depicted in Fig. 4 and Fig. 5.

Finally, we have described initial experimental results with the benchmarks of the Ontology Alignment Initiative, which demonstrates the effectiveness of our approach through the improved recall and precision rates. There are many areas of ongoing work, with our primary focus considering the effect of the changing number of voters and the impact on precision and recall or applying our algorithm in different application areas. In the future we also try to investigate how multilingual background knowledge can impact the mapping process for ontologies that are not in English.

# References

1. Shvaiko, P., Euzenat, J.: Ontology matching: State of the art and future challenges. IEEE Transactions on Knowledge and Data Engineering 25(1), 158–176 (2013)
2. Shvaiko, P., Euzenat, J.: Ten challenges for ontology matching. Technical Report DISI-08-042, University of Trento (2008)
3. Jean-Mary, Y.R., Shironoshita, E.P., Kabuka, M.R.: Ontology matching with semantic verification. Web Semantics: Science, Services and Agents on the World Wide Web 7(3), 235–251 (2009)
4. Tang, J., Li, J., Liang, B., Huang, X., Li, Y., Wang, K.: Using bayesian decision for ontology mapping. Web Semantics: Science. Services and Agents on the World Wide Web 4, 243–262 (2006)
5. Seddiqui, M.H., Aono, M.: An efficient and scalable algorithm for segmented alignment of ontologies of arbitrary size. Web Semantics: Science, Services and Agents on the World Wide Web 7(4), 344–356 (2009)
6. Hamdi, F., Niraula, B.S.N.B., Reynaud, C.: TaxoMap in the OAEI 2009 alignment contest. In: Proceedings of the 4th International Workshop on Ontology Matching (OM-2009). CEUR Workshop Proceedings, vol. 551 (2009)
7. Nagy, M., Vargas-Vera, M., Stolarski, P.: DSSim Results for OAEI 2008. In: Proceedings of the 3rd International Workshop on Ontology Matching (OM-2008) Collocated with the 7th International Semantic Web Conference (ISWC-2008), Karlsruhe, Germany. CEUR Workshop Proceedings, vol. 431, CEUR-WS.org (October 26, 2008)
8. Ferrara, A., Lorusso, D., Stamou, G., Stoilos, G., Tzouvaras, V., Venetis, T.: Resolution of conflicts among ontology mappings: a fuzzy approach. In: Proceedings of the 3rd International Workshop on Ontology Matching (2008)
9. Liu, X.J., Wang, Y.L., Wang, J.: Towards a semi-automatic ontology mapping - an approach using instance based learning and logic relation mining. In: Fifth Mexican International Conference (MICAI 2006) on Artificial Intelligence (2006)
10. Schmid, H.: Probabilistic Part-of-Speech Tagging Using Decision Trees. In: Proceedings of International Conference on New Methods in Language Processing, vol. 12, pp. 44–49 (1994)
11. Ehrig, M., Koschmider, A., Oberweis, A.: Measuring similarity between semantic business process models. In: Proceedings of the Fourth Asia-Pacific Conference on Conceptual Modelling, pp. 71–80. Australian Computer Society, Inc. (2007)
12. Wang, P., Xu, B.: Lily: Ontology Alignment Results for OAEI 2009. In: Proceedings of the 4th International Workshop on Ontology Matching (OM 2009). CEUR Workshop Proceedings, vol. 551 (2009)
13. Berners-Lee, T., Hendler, J., Lassila, O.: The Semantic Web. Scientific American 284(5), 34–43 (2001)
14. Beckett, D.: Rdf/xml syntax specification (2004)
15. McGuinness, D.L., van Harmelen, F.: Owl web ontology language
16. Miles, A., Bechhofer, S.: Skos simple knowledge organization system (2004)
17. Wang, R.Y., Kon, H.B., Madnick, S.E.: Data Quality Requirements Analysis and Modeling. In: Proceedings of the Ninth International Conference on Data Engineering, pp. 670–677 (1993)
18. Wand, Y., Wang, R.Y.: Anchoring data quality dimensions in ontological foundations. Communications of the ACM, 86–95 (1996)
19. Batini, C., Lenzerini, M., Navathe, S.B.: A comparative analysis of methodologies for database schema integration. ACM Computing Surveys 18(4), 323–364 (1986)

20. Gertz, M., Özsu, M.T., Saake, G., Sattler, K.U.: Report on the Dagstuhl Seminar: Data quality on the Web. SIGMOD Record 33(1), 127–132 (2004)
21. Rahm, E., Do, H.H.: Data cleaning: Problems and current approaches. IEEE Data Engineering Bulletin 23(4), 3–13 (2000)
22. Flahive, A., Apduhan, B.O., Rahayu, J.W., Taniar, D.: Large scale ontology tailoring and simulation in the Semantic Grid Environment. International Journal of Metadata, Semantics and Ontologies 1(4), 265–281 (2006)
23. Carlo, W., Tharam, D., Wenny, R., Elizabeth, C.: Large scale ontology visualisation using ontology extraction. International Journal of Web and Grid Services 1(1), 113–135 (2005)
24. Caracciolo, C., Euzenat, J., Hollink, L., Ichise, R., Isaac, A., Malaisé, V., Meilicke, C., Pane, J., Shvaiko, P., Stuckenschmidt, H., Šváb-Zamazal, O., Svátek, V.: First results of the Ontology Alignment Evaluation Initiative 2008. In: The 3rd International Workshop on Ontology Matching (2008)
25. Brugman, H., Malaisé, V., Gazendam, L.: A Web Based General Thesaurus Browser to Support Indexing of Television and Radio Programs. In: The 5th international conference on Language Resources and Evaluation (LREC 2006) (2006)
26. Ding, L., Finin, T., Joshi, A., Pan, R., Cost, R.S., Peng, Y., Reddivari, P., Doshi, V.C., Sachs, J.: Swoogle: A Search and Metadata Engine for the Semantic Web. In: Proceedings of the Thirteenth ACM Conference on Information and Knowledge Management (2004)
27. Nagy, M., Vargas-Vera, M., Motta, E.: Multi agent ontology mapping framework in the aqua question answering system. In: Gelbukh, A., de Albornoz, Á., Terashima-Marín, H. (eds.) MICAI 2005. LNCS (LNAI), vol. 3789, pp. 70–79. Springer, Heidelberg (2005)
28. Gracia, J., Mena, E.: Ontology matching with cider:evaluation report for the oaei 2008. In: Proceedings of the 3rd International Workshop on Ontology Matching (2008)
29. Wang, P., Xu, B.: Lily: Ontology alignment results for oaei 2008. In: Proceedings of the 3rd International Workshop on Ontology Matching (2008)

# Simple Window Selection Strategies for the Simplified Lesk Algorithm for Word Sense Disambiguation

Francisco Viveros-Jiménez[1], Alexander Gelbukh[1,2], and Grigori Sidorov[1,2]

[1] Centro de Investigación en Computación,
Instituto Politécnico Nacional, Mexico City, Mexico
[2] Institute for Modern Linguistic Research,
"Sholokhov" Moscow State University for Humanities, Moscow, Russia
pacovj@hotmail.com
www.gelbukh.com,www.g-sidorov.org

**Abstract.** The Simplified Lesk Algorithm (SLA) is frequently used for word sense disambiguation. It disambiguates by calculating the overlap of a set of dictionary definitions (senses) and the context words. The algorithm is simple and fast, but it has relatively low accuracy. We propose simple strategies for the context window selection that improve the performance of the SLA: (1) constructing the window only with words that have an overlap with some sense of the target word, (2) excluding the target word itself from matching, and (3) avoiding repetitions in the context window. This paper describes the corresponding experiments. Comparison with other more complex knowledge-based algorithms is presented.

## 1 Introduction

Words can have different meanings depending on the context. For example, in "John is playing the *bass*" and "John is eating a *bass*", the word *bass* has different meanings. Such meanings are represented as separate *senses* of words in explanatory dictionaries. Word sense disambiguation (WSD) is the task of automatically choosing an appropriate sense for a given word occurrence (*target word*) in a text (*document*) out of a set of senses listed in a given dictionary. WSD is useful in applications that deal with meaning of texts, like machine translation [3, 4, 15], wikification [9], etc.

Approaches to WSD can be classified into two large groups: knowledge-based systems and supervised learning systems. Approaches based on supervised learning have better performance, but they need large manually-tagged corpus, which is difficult to prepare. In contrast, knowledge-based approaches rely only on the information present in the dictionary selected for the task. In general, they are faster but have lower performance. Still, there are possibilities for their improvements. We discuss some of the possible improvements in this paper.

The Simplified Lesk Algorithm (SLA) [5] is a widely known knowledge-based algorithm for WSD. It is frequently used because of its simplicity and speed

F. Castro, A. Gelbukh, and M. González (Eds.): MICAI 2013, Part I, LNAI 8265, pp. 217–227, 2013.

[8, 19]. Given a word, the algorithm chooses the sense that has the greatest overlap between its dictionary definition and the context (see Algorithm 1) [8]. Usually, the context (*context window*) is a local context, like the current sentence or $N$ words in the text around the target word. Auxiliary words (*stop words*) are ignored, because they carry no lexical meaning. The SLA's main drawback is its low recall: it cannot provide an answer for many words, because there are no overlaps or several senses have the same overlap score.

---

**Algorithm 1.** The Simplified Lesk Algorithm (SLA)

---

1  **foreach** *target word W of the document* **do**
2  │   $i = 1$
3  │   **while** $i < N$ *(the context window size)* **do**
4  │   │   **foreach** *direction* $\in$ {left, right} **do**
5  │   │   │   $w$ = the word at distance $i$ from $W$ in *direction*
6  │   │   │   // Count the overlaps
7  │   │   │   **if** *w is not a stop word* **then**
8  │   │   │   │   **foreach** *sense s of W* **do**
9  │   │   │   │   │   **foreach** *word u in s (i.e., in definition of the sense s)* **do**
10 │   │   │   │   │   │   **if** $u = w$ **then**
11 │   │   │   │   │   │   │   $overlap(s) = overlap(s) + 1$

12 │   │   $i = i + 1$
13 │   **if** arg max $overlap(s)$ *is unique* **then**
14 │   │   Select the sense $s$ for $W$
15 │   **else**
16 │   │   Fail to make a decision for $W$ (or use a back-off algorithm to provide it)

---

In this paper, we propose three simple strategies that significantly improve the performance of the SLA while preserving its simplicity and speed. The proposed strategies are: (1) constructing the window only with words that have an overlap with some sense of the target word, (2) excluding the target word itself from matching, and (3) avoiding repetitions of words in the window, i.e., count the words only once.

Our motivation in this paper is to study the impact of these strategies on a simple classical algorithm, the SLA. Better understanding of such simple building blocks is very useful for the development of more complex systems [7]. Besides, we apply the same strategies to other methods obtaining better results. Our implementation for the SLA and several other knowledge-based algorithms is publicly available at http://fviveros.gelbukh.com (Java source code and data).

## 2   Experimental Setup

As usual, we use precision (P) and recall (R) for measuring performance of algorithms. In WSD, they are calculated as follows:

$$P = \frac{\text{correct answers}}{\text{total answers}} \qquad R = \frac{\text{correct answers}}{\text{total target words}} \qquad F1 = \frac{2PR}{P+R}$$

where an *answer* is a target word for which the algorithm made some decision (line 14 of Algorithm 1), and a *correct answer* is an answer that coincides with the one provided by human annotators as the gold standard [11].

All experiments were carried out using Senseval 2 [13] and Senseval 3 [17] test sets as the gold standard. We used WordNet 3.0 [10] (the current version of the WordNet) glosses and samples as sense definitions. Note that Senseval test sets are labeled with previous version of the WordNet. Thus, the results can vary depending on the version of the WordNet used. We used the Stanford POS tagger [18] for tagging the definitions of the senses.

## 3   Discussion about the Use of Back-Off Algorithms

WSD algorithms are often used together with some back-off algorithm for providing an answer when the main algorithm fails to make a decision (line 16 of Algorithm 1). But what happens if the back-off algorithm is actually better than the main algorithm? When this happens, the lower the coverage of the main algorithm is, the more final decisions will be made by the back-off algorithm; consequently, the better the performance observed for the combined algorithm will be. So, it is better that the main algorithm does not participate in decision making. This sounds really unnatural.

The SLA is frequently used with the Most Frequent Sense (MFS) heuristic as the back-off algorithm. The MFS consists of selecting the sense that is most frequent in a given corpus. It has good performance mainly due to the skewed distribution of the frequencies of the senses. The MFS outperforms SLA, so when MFS data is available, practical applications should use the MFS heuristic directly without any need for the SLA.

However, the MFS is a supervised method: it needs the frequencies of the individual senses from a hand-tagged corpus, which is not easily available, especially for less studied languages. There exist methods for unsupervised learning of the MFS data [7], but they do not provide the same quality as a hand-tagged corpus.

Both its supervised nature and the "the worse the better" effect that it produces make the MFS an unsuitable option as the back-off algorithm for our study. The proper behavior of the SLA (an unsupervised algorithm) can be analyzed correctly only without a back-off algorithm of a different nature (supervised). On the other hand, practical applications that use some knowledge-based algorithm (without the MFS) can also use unsupervised back-off algorithms, like random sense selection: when the algorithm cannot make a choice, a random sense is selected. We report the results obtained both without back-off algorithms and, for the sake of completeness, with the two mentioned back-off algorithms (the random sense and the MFS). Note that if we use a back-off algorithm, then $P = R = F1$, so we just report $P$.

## 4  Influence of Size of the Context Window on the SLA

The SLA has better performance when using larger window sizes, as can be seen in Table 1. The *MFS* and *Rnd* columns contain the $P$ values observed when the most frequent sense and the random sense were used as the back-off algorithms. It can be observed that the SLA recall increases when $N$ grows, because the larger window increases the number of overlaps. It has the best recall for the window equal to the whole document (for the Senseval 2 data). This means that the words useful for the SLA are present in the document, but they are not visible in a small window. In our experiments, the average number of significant words in test documents was 740. Table 2 contains an example of words that have overlaps in small and large windows.

**Table 1.** SLA performance for various window sizes ($N$)

| Window size | Senseval 2 | | | | | Senseval 3 | | | | |
|---|---|---|---|---|---|---|---|---|---|---|
| | F1 | P | R | MFS | Rnd | F1 | P | R | MFS | Rnd |
| 0 | 0 | 0 | 0 | **67.1** | 40.4 | 0 | 0 | 0 | **66.1** | 35.0 |
| 1 | 4.2 | 47.2 | 2.2 | 66.9 | 42.2 | 5.8 | 29.6 | 3.2 | 63.9 | 35.0 |
| 2 | 8.0 | 48.0 | 4.4 | 66.9 | 43.6 | 9.9 | 29.7 | 5.9 | 62.8 | 35.3 |
| 4 | 11.9 | 44.8 | 6.9 | 66.4 | 42.6 | 14.4 | 28.8 | 9.6 | 60.4 | 35.8 |
| 16 | 25.4 | 42.5 | 18.1 | 62.5 | 46.7 | 21.9 | 27.2 | 18.3 | 51.2 | 36.7 |
| 64 | 35.5 | 42.5 | 30.4 | 56.4 | 46.9 | 27.6 | 30.0 | 25.4 | 43.3 | 36.8 |
| 256 | 41.7 | 43.8 | 39.7 | 50.7 | 47.4 | 31.2 | 29.9 | 32.6 | 39.6 | 36.7 |
| Document | 44.1 | 45.1 | 43.1 | 47.9 | 46.9 | 33.2 | 34.0 | 32.4 | 38.4 | 36.5 |

**Table 2.** Example of overlapping words for the window of 4 words and for the window equal to the whole document

| Correct answer | 4-word window | Whole document |
|---|---|---|
| $art_1$ | – | $art_N$, $work_N$ |
| $bell_1$ | $sound_N$ | $sound_N$, $ringing_N$, $make_V$ |
| $service_3$ | – | $sunday_N$, $rule_N$, $worship_N$, $service_N$, $follow_V$ |
| $teach_1$ | – | $knowledge_N$, $French_J$ |
| $child_2$ | – | $human_J$, $child_N$, $college_N$, $kid_N$ |

## 5  Composition of the Context Window

Another important consideration for the SLA is the "quality" of the words selected as the context window. For illustrating this, let us measure the frequency of words in the dictionary definitions. We use the dictionary version of the inverse document frequency measure ($IDF_D$), similar to the IDF calculated for a corpus [5]. The $IDF_D$ is calculated using the following equation:

$$IDF_D(w) = -\log \frac{|\{g : w \in g\}|}{G} \tag{1}$$

where $G$ is the total number of glosses in the dictionary and $|\{g : w \in g\}|$ is the number of glosses where the lemma $w$ appears. In this manner, the words that appear very often in the dictionary (general words) such as *be*, *have* or *not* have low $IDF_D$ values.

Table 3 contains a list with the five words that have the greatest overlap scores for the context window of 4 words and for the window equal to the whole document. As expected, the SLA often uses general words for making decisions. When we use the whole document as the window, the usage of these words in the algorithm is greatly increased. We can observe that more specific words like *cell*, *bell* and *gene* have less importance for the algorithm in comparison with the general words like *be*, *make* and *use*.

**Table 3.** Top five words with overlaps between the window and the answer (definition of the sense chosen by the SLA)

| 4 words window | | | | | |
|---|---|---|---|---|---|
| Senseval 2 | | | Senseval 3 | | |
| Lemma | $IDF_D$ | Answers | Lemma | $IDF_D$ | Answers |
| $not_R$ | 3.2 | 35 | $be_V$ | 1.5 | 379 |
| $other_J$ | 4.4 | 12 | $have_V$ | 2.4 | 25 |
| $gene_N$ | 7.0 | 10 | $man_N$ | 5.0 | 13 |
| $bell_N$ | 7.3 | 10 | $do_V$ | 4.3 | 12 |
| $cell_N$ | 5.5 | 7 | $time_N$ | 4.5 | 11 |
| Whole document window | | | | | |
| Senseval 2 | | | Senseval 3 | | |
| Lemma | $IDF_D$ | Answers | Lemma | $IDF_D$ | Answers |
| $not_R$ | 3.2 | 546 | $be_V$ | 1.5 | 1481 |
| $be_V$ | 1.5 | 298 | $have_V$ | 2.4 | 322 |
| $make_V$ | 3.3 | 206 | $make_V$ | 3.3 | 223 |
| $new_J$ | 5.0 | 164 | $do_V$ | 4.3 | 169 |
| $use_V$ | 3.0 | 147 | $house_N$ | 5.6 | 123 |

The overlap count of these general words increases almost exponentially for larger windows as presented in Table 4. It can be observed that few context words produce large overlap count values when using larger window sizes. We believe that this is the reason for decreasing of the SLA precision. However, we made experiments that showed that simply removing these general words does not improve the performance.

**Table 4.** Average number of words and average overlap count observed in Senseval 2 (left) and Senseval 3 (right) test sets using various window sizes

| Window size | Senseval 2 | | Senseval 3 | |
|---|---|---|---|---|
| | Words | Overlap count | Words | Overlap Count |
| 4 | 1.0 | 1.1 | 1.1 | 1.15 |
| 16 | 1.2 | 1.3 | 1.4 | 1.9 |
| 64 | 1.5 | 2.5 | 1.9 | 5.3 |
| 256 | 2.5 | 6.5 | 2.8 | 18.3 |
| Whole document | 3.7 | 17.4 | 3.6 | 45.5 |

# 6  Using the First $N$ Overlapping Words as the Context Window

In previous sections we analyzed the possibility of using large context windows, even the whole document, that increases the performance of the SLA. Still, there are even better strategies for the context window selection.

The SLA does not really use all words from the document. In fact, it uses an average of 4 words as shown in Table 4. So we propose using only these "useful" words as the context window instead of the whole document. In this way, we filter out all words that do not have an overlap with some sense of the target word, but we limit the number of words to the $N$ "nearest" words only. Algorithm 2 describes the proposed window selection strategy.

---

**Algorithm 2.** Window selection algorithm that considers the first $N$ words with overlaps

---

1  Set $i = 1$;
2  **while** $sizeOf(Win) < N$ *and there are unchecked words in the document* **do**
3  $\quad$ Look for a word $W_p$ at $i$ positions to the (RIGHT and LEFT) of the target word $W$;
4  $\quad$ **if** $W_p$ *exists in some sense of* $W$ *and* $sizeOf(Win) < N$ **then**
5  $\quad\quad$ Add $W_p$ to $Win$;
6  $\quad$ Set $i = i + 1$;

---

The proposed window will contain the first $N$ words that produce an overlap with some sense of the target word. The window words will be extracted from the context closest to the target word, but they do not have to be very close to it in token offsets. If the SLA does not find these words, then the context window can contain less than 4 words. We leave the question of the optimal size of $N$ for future work. Note that the complexity of the disambiguation of a word with the SLA increases from $O(PN)$ to $O((PN)^2)$, where $N$ is the window size and $P$ is the polysemy of the target word, but this increment is quite acceptable.

The strategy of using 4 words that have overlaps as the context window gives better performance to the SLA than using the whole document as the window, as shown in Table 5, where "4 words" is the original selection method for 4 words, "Document" is the whole document as the context window, "4 O" corresponds to the strategy of selection of only words that have overlaps (4 words, in this case), "T" means that the target word is excluded, and "D" stands for counting duplicates only once (for description of the last two strategies, see Section 7).

**Table 5.** Performance of various strategies of the context window selection. Where "4 words" is the standard selection of 4 words, "Document" is the whole document as the context window, "4 O" corresponds to the strategy of selection of only words that have overlaps, "T" means that the target word is excluded, and "D" stands for counting duplicates only once.

| Window selection | Senseval 2 | | | | | Senseval 3 | | | | |
|---|---|---|---|---|---|---|---|---|---|---|
| | F1 | P | R | MFS | Rnd | F1 | P | R | MFS | Rnd |
| 4 words | 11.9 | 44.8 | 6.9 | 66.4 | 42.6 | 14.4 | 28.8 | 9.6 | 60.4 | 35.8 |
| Document | 44.1 | 45.1 | 43.1 | 47.9 | 46.9 | 33.2 | 34.0 | 32.4 | 38.4 | 36.5 |
| 4 O | 44.0 | 45.1 | 43.1 | 51.4 | 46.4 | 34.0 | 34.9 | 33.2 | 44.0 | 37.2 |
| 4 O T | 47.3 | 48.5 | 46.1 | 55.5 | 49.9 | 34.0 | 34.9 | 33.1 | 44.3 | 37.8 |
| 4 O D | 47.6 | 48.7 | 46.6 | 56.6 | 50.3 | 35.7 | 36.6 | 34.8 | 46.6 | 37.8 |
| 4 O T D | **47.8** | **48.9** | **46.6** | 56.7 | 50.8 | **35.8** | **36.7** | **34.9** | 46.8 | 39.7 |

## 7 Excluding the Target Word and Duplicates from the Context Window

The SLA sometimes can find the target word itself in the context window. This happens when the target word is included in the window and in some dictionary definitions as well. For example, senses 3, 4, and 5 of the word $bell_N$ contain the word $bell_N$ itself: "(3) *The sound of a **bell** being struck*; (4) *(nautical) Each of the eight half-hour units of nautical time signaled by strokes of a ship's **bell**...*; (5) *The shape of a **bell**;*". In this manner, there are false overlaps. Removing the target word increases the performance of the SLA, as shown in Table 5.

On the other hand, repetitions of words in the context window are also bad for the SLA, because the repeated words are often general words with low $IDF_D$ values, i.e., frequent words in the dictionary. Therefore, if we consider repetitions, then the general words would have higher frequencies and more influence on the SLA's disambiguation process. Considering the overlapping words only once (i.e., ignoring their frequencies) improves the SLA performance, as can be seen in Table 5.

## 8 Comparison with Other Knowledge-Based Algorithms

We also made a comparison of the SLA (with the proposed improvements) with various knowledge-based WSD algorithms such as Graph Indegree [16], Conceptual Density [2], the original Lesk Algorithm [6] and the SLA with lexical chaining window [19]. These algorithms were configured as follows: (1) they use the current sentence as the context window, (2) their individual parameters (if any) are set to the optimal values specified in the corresponding paper, (3) *depth* = 4 was used for the depth-first search conducted over the WordNet taxonomy used in the Conceptual Density algorithm as recommended in [12], and (4) back-off algorithms are not used. The observed performance of these WSD algorithms can vary as compared with the previously reported results due to the use of WordNet 3.0 and differences in the context window sizes.

Table 6 shows the performance of all these algorithms. The results are statistically significant because we applied the Mann Whitney U test with a 95% confidence level and it confirms that the answer set of the proposed SLA is different from the answer sets of the other algorithms. The following observations can be made:

- The recall of the modified SLA became significantly better as compared with the original SLA. In general, the obtained recall is comparable or in some cases better than the results obtained by other methods that have higher complexity and use additional resources like WordNet taxonomy.
- The modified SLA has the precision similar to other knowledge-based algorithms. The Conceptual Density algorithm has the best precision.
- The original Lesk Algorithm has good results, but it is well known that it has very high complexity, which makes it unviable in practical applications.

**Table 6.** Comparison of knowledge-based algorithms. WN means use of WordNet taxonomy; in the Compl. column: P stands for polysemy, N for window size, M for the depth of the search tree.

| | Compl. | WN | Senseval 2 | | | Senseval 3 | | |
|---|---|---|---|---|---|---|---|---|
| | | | P | R | F1 | P | R | F1 |
| Graph Indegree [16] | $O(NP^4)$ | yes | 57.6 | 57.3 | 57.4 | 53.4 | 52.9 | 53.5 |
| **Modified SLA** | $O((PN)^2)$ | no | 48.9 | 46.6 | 47.8 | 36.7 | 34.9 | 35.7 |
| Complete Lesk Alg. [6] | $O(P^N)$ | no | 48.2 | 46.1 | 47.1 | 39.8 | 37.6 | 38.6 |
| Conceptual Density [2] | $O(NP^M)$ | yes | 59.2 | 19.4 | 29.3 | 57.2 | 18.1 | 27.4 |
| SLA, lexical chaining [19] | $O((PN)^2)$ | yes | 35.2 | 19.2 | 24.9 | 23.0 | 12.4 | 16.1 |
| Original SLA | $O(NP)$ | no | 44.5 | 13.5 | 20.7 | 29.1 | 14.7 | 19.5 |

## 9   Analysis of Changes in SLA Results

We observed several changes of the SLA results after applying the proposed window selection strategies. These can be summarized as follows:

- Total number of overlaps is reduced from the order of 100,000 overlaps to roughly 10,000 on both test sets, i.e, ten times.
- The proposed window selection strategies cause a reduction of the number of addressed senses (senses with *overlap* > 0), as presented in Table 7.
- The proposed window selection strategies reduce the usage of general words and increase the usage of words with higher $IDF_D$ (Figure 1).

Note that the improved SLA can be a good sense filter. It discards about half of the senses with the precision of at least 75%, as shown in Table 7. If we use the SLA as a sense filter, then we choose only senses with the *overlap* ≥ 1 as the sense inventory for other WSD algorithms.

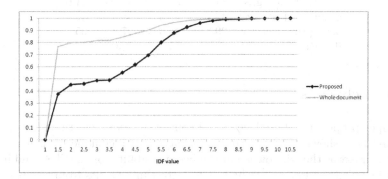

**Fig. 1.** Cumulative distribution of $IDF_D$ of the words producing overlaps for Senseval 3

**Table 7.** Polysemy reduction percentage and probability of having the correct answer among the remaining senses for some window selection strategies

| Window selection | Senseval 2 | | Senseval 3 | |
|---|---|---|---|---|
| | Reduction | P(correct) | Reduction | P(correct) |
| Whole document | 15 | 93 | 11 | 92 |
| 4 O | 50 | 77 | 45 | 71 |
| 4 O T | 59 | 74 | 56 | 65 |
| 4 O D | 44 | 83 | 36 | 81 |
| 4 O T D | 54 | 79 | 49 | 75 |

## 10   Integration with Other WSD Algorithms

We also checked if the proposed window selection procedure is aplicable to other WSD algorithms and with the Lesk similarity measure [1]. Table 8 shows the performance changes observed when using our window selection procedure. The following observations can be obtained from this table:

- Our window selection procedure is applicable to other overlap based methods. However, Graph InDegree method did not consistently perform better when using our window selection procedure. We will test the compatibility of our window selection filters with some other classical an state-of-the-art WSD systems in near future.
- Our window selection procedure is compatible with the Lesk similarity measure. This measure was the best out of the six in [14]. However, we will perform a compatibility analysis with the other five measures in future research.

**Table 8.** F1 measure observed when using our window selection procedure with some other WSD algorithms and with Lesk similarity measure

|  | Senseval 2 | | Senseval 3 | |
| --- | --- | --- | --- | --- |
|  | 4 words | 4 O T D | 4 words | 4 O T D |
| Graph InDegree | 57.4 | 58.7 | 53.5 | 51.0 |
| Complete Lesk alg. | 47.1 | 49.5 | 38.6 | 42.0 |
| Conceptual Density | 29.3 | 43.0 | 27.4 | 35.8 |
| SLA with Lesk sim. | 48.3 | 55.2 | 43.0 | 50.8 |

# 11   Conclusions

This paper proposes and analyzes novel context window selection strategies for the SLA. It is shown that the commonly accepted technique of using a small nearest context as the window is not the best possibility for the SLA, and in general for knowledge based algorithms. The algorithm benefits from words present in the document that are outside of the nearest context. It is shown that the performance of the algorithm can be significantly improved using the following strategies: (1) considering only the words that have an overlap with some sense of the target word, (2) excluding the target word itself from the context window, and, (3) considering repeated words (duplicates) only once, i.e., ignoring frequencies. These modifications lead to performance improvements. The performance observed for the SLA with the proposed window selection is also applicable to other knowledge-based approaches such as Graph-based WSD, Conceptual Density, etc. Note that these approaches are more complex and use additional resources such as WordNet taxonomy.

**Acknowledgements.** Work done under partial support of Mexican Government (CONACYT, SNI), Instituto Politécnico Nacional, Mexico (projects SIP-IPN 20131441, 20131702; COFAA-IPN, PIFI-IPN), Mexico City Government (ICYT-DF project PICCO10-120), and European Commission (project 269180). The authors thank Prof. Dr. Anton Zimmerling (MSUH) for the valuable discussions during the development of this work.

# References

1. Banerjee, S., Pedersen, T.: An adapted lesk algorithm for word sense disambiguation using WordNet. In: Gelbukh, A. (ed.) CICLing 2002. LNCS, vol. 2276, pp. 136–145. Springer, Heidelberg (2002)
2. Buscaldi, D., Rosso, P., Masulli, F.: Finding predominant word senses in untagged text. In: Workshop Senseval-3, Proc. of ACL, ACL 2004, pp. 77–82. Association for Computational Linguistics (2004)
3. Carpuat, M., Shen, Y., Yu, X., Wu, D.: Toward integrating word sense and entity disambiguation into statistical machine translation. In: Proc. of IWSLT, IWSLT 2006, pp. 37–44 (2006)

4. Chan, Y.S., Ng, H.T.: Word sense disambiguation improves statistical machine translation. In: Proc. of ACL, ACL 2007, pp. 33–40 (2007)
5. Kilgarriff, A., Rosenzweig, J.: Framework and results for english SENSEVAL. Computers and the Humanities 34(1-2), 15–48 (2000)
6. Lesk, M.: Automatic sense disambiguation using machine readable dictionaries: how to tell a pine cone from an ice cream cone. In: Proc. of SIGDOC, SIGDOC 1986, pp. 24–26. ACM, New York (1986)
7. McCarthy, D., Koeling, R., Weeds, J., Carroll, J.: Finding predominant word senses in untagged text. In: Proc. of ACL, ACL 2004, pp. 280–287. Association for Computational Linguistics, Stroudsburg (2004)
8. Mihalcea, R.: Knowledge-based methods for WSD. In: Word Sense Disambiguation: Algorithms and Applications, Text, Speech and Language Technology, pp. 107–132. Springer, Dordrecht (2006)
9. Mihalcea, R., Csomai, A.: Wikify!: linking documents to encyclopedic knowledge. In: Proc. of CIKM, CIKM 2007, pp. 233–242. ACM, New York (2007)
10. Miller, G.A.: WordNet: A lexical database for English. Communications of the ACM 38, 39–41 (1995)
11. Navigli, R.: Word sense disambiguation: A survey. ACM Comput. Surv. 41, 10:1–10:69 (2009)
12. Navigli, R., Lapata, M.: An experimental study of graph connectivity for unsupervised word sense disambiguation. IEEE Trans. Pattern Anal. Mach. Intell. 32(4), 678–692 (2010)
13. Palmer, M., Fellbaum, C., Cotton, S., Delfs, L., Dang, H.T.: English tasks: All-words and verb lexical sample (2001)
14. Patwardhan, S., Banerjee, S., Pedersen, T.: Using measures of semantic relatedness for word sense disambiguation. In: Gelbukh, A. (ed.) CICLing 2003. LNCS, vol. 2588, pp. 241–257. Springer, Heidelberg (2003)
15. Pinto, D., Vilario, D., Balderas, C., Tovar, M., Beltran, B.: Evaluating n-gram models for a bilingual word sense disambiguation task. Computación y Sistemas 15(2) (2011)
16. Sinha, R., Mihalcea, R.: Unsupervised graph-based word sense disambiguation using measures of word semantic similarity. In: Proc. of ICSC, ICSC 2007, pp. 363–369 (2007)
17. Snyder, B., Palmer, M.: The English all-words task (2004)
18. Toutanova, K., Manning, C.D.: Enriching the knowledge sources used in a maximum entropy part-of-speech tagger. In: Proc. of EMNLP, EMNLP 2000, pp. 63–70. ACL, PA (2000)
19. Vasilescu, F., Langlais, P., Lapalme, G.: Evaluating variants of the lesk approach for disambiguating words. In: Proc. of LREC, LREC 2004, pp. 633–636. Lisbon, Portugal (May 2004)

# Disambiguating Wikipedia Articles on the Basis of plWordNet Lexico-semantic Relations

Maciej Piasecki, Michał Kaliński, and Agnieszka Indyka-Piasecka

Institute of Informatics, Wrocław University of Technology, Poland
maciej.piasecki@pwr.wroc.pl

**Abstract.** A method for mapping Wikipedia articles (treated as a large informal resource describing concepts) to wordnet synsets (relation-based word meaning descriptions) is proposed. In contrast to previous approaches, the method focuses mainly on wordnet relation structure as the main means for meaning description. The description is supplemented by knowledge automatically extracted from a corpus in the form of Measure of Semantic Relatedness. Several different ways of building synset meaning descriptions are analysed. We noticed that the problem is similar to wordnet-to-wordnet mapping, as both resources utilise relation structure to describe meanings and provide partition into lexical meanings. A set of inter-resource semantic relations was introduced as a basis for the manual evaluation of the mapping algorithms. Several algorithms were tested on polysemous and monosemous articles from Polish Wikipedia.

## 1  Introduction

Large ontologies that provide formalised description of concepts, and large wordnets, like Princeton WordNet (henceforth PWN)[1] [3], that describe lexical meanings, are of great importance for the natural language processing. A crucial feature is linking an ontology with a wordnet by concept-to-sense mapping. However, the construction of such large scale resources is a very complex process, as well as a high quality mapping. The mapping must be built manually, as concepts are abstract objects and they have no prior connection to lexical meanings[2].

Publicly available, large scale resources, e.g. Wikipedia[3], can be an alternative, since it describes concepts with short text articles, and includes links between concepts and implicit links between concepts and lexical meanings. By comparing Wikipedia articles with wordnet synsets one can try to establish links between concepts and lexical meanings in an explicit way.

---

[1] A wordnet is *lexico-semantic network* which follows the basis assumptions of Princeton WordNet [3]. Every wordnet includes synsets – sets of near-synonyms – linked by lexico-semantic relations. Synsets represent distinct lexical meanings. WordNet became a commonly used language resource in the natural language processing.

[2] English words and expressions are used to name concepts in ontologies, but formally they are only labels and cannot be fully trusted, because as their usage can be slightly incompatible with lexical meanings described in a wordnet.

[3] http://en.wikipedia.org and http://pl.wikipedia.org

F. Castro, A. Gelbukh, and M. González (Eds.): MICAI 2013, Part I, LNAI 8265, pp. 228–239, 2013.
© Springer-Verlag Berlin Heidelberg 2013

Our goal is to develop a method for the automated mapping of Wikipedia articles onto wordnet synsets. This idea is not new, see Sec. 2, however most previous works were done for the mapping Wikipedia to PWN and are based on similarity between two texts. Wikipedia articles are compared with glosses (short text descriptions of the synset meaning) provided in PWN for all synsets by computing text similarity. In many wordnet glosses are written only for some synsets or are not present at all, e.g. plWordNet includes only short comments for selected synset. Lexical meanings are described by lexico-semantic relations in wordnets. Moreover, the construction of PWN is based on the assumption that "synsets represent lexicalised concepts", relations linking synsets are called "conceptual relations" and synsets are larger and tend to be more descriptive than in the case of plWordNet. Thus, first, we need to find a source of information that can be used instead of text glosses. Secondly, the encyclopaedic structure must be mapped to a linguistic lexical semantic network, i.e. articles describing concepts must be mapped onto synsets characterising lexical meanings with the help of lexico-semantic relations.

Each Wikipedia article can be perceived as a description of its headword meaning. However, meanings identified for a word in Wikipedia can be different than meanings described for this word in a wordnet. The coverage of word senses can be also different between Wikipedia and a wordnet, e.g. the 'confusion' meaning of Polish *chaos* is not described in Wikipedia, Wikipedia mathematical *chaos* is not described in plWordNet, while *chaos* as substance type is shared by both. Both problems must be solved in mapping.

In Sec. 2 we present a short overview of the mapping methods developed for a specific case of English Wikipedia and PWN. Next we discuss possible knowledge sources that can be a basis for the mapping in Sec. 3. In Sec. 4 a mapping algorithm is presented. The application of several algorithm variants to a test sample and the manual evaluation of the results is presented in Sec. 5.

## 2 Related Works

The computation of similarity between Wikipedia article text content and a wordnet gloss written for a synset is a starting point for the vast majority of the proposed methods. Ruiz-Casado et al. [12] use vector model to compute text similarity to link Wikipedia articles with PWN synsets. Pozetto and Navgli [10] in order to find the best match of an article and a synset first construct for articles and synset "disambiguation context" – a bag of words including words associated with the given article or synset. Next, they calculate text overlap for different article-synset pairs and selects the synset that maximises probability of representing the same set as the article.

In [7] the authors extend the model by transforming flat disambiguation contexts into subgraphs of the wordnet graph by taking into account all wordnet senses of the Wikipedia headword and associated synsets (a structure used in wordnet-based Word Sense Disambiguation). Sense selection is done on the basis of the length of the graph paths linking it to the words from the disambiguation context of the Wikipedia article. The Wikipedia link structure is processed only during the construction of the disambiguation contexts.

Fernando & Stevenson [4] first generate a small set of candidate articles for each noun synset. The candidates are selected by two criteria: words in WordNet synset against Wikipedia article title matching and information retrieval system to search the full text of the article for these words. Then, from the set of candidate articles for each noun synset the best matching article is identified. The standard TF-IDF weighting for text similarity and distinct metric for title similarity are used. The similarity is computed mainly on glosses. At the last stage of the process, the mappings are refined by removing all mappings with more then one synset mapped to the same Wikipedia article, so only 1-to-1 mapping are accepted. The article is confirmed to be a good match only if bi-directional links between this article and another mapped article exist.

Niemann and Gurevych [8] explore the wordnet relation graph in the mapping algorithm. The Wikipedia graph of links is not so precisely defined and can be built on the basis, e.g., links between articles, categories and infobox attributes. Thus its shape and link types are significantly different from the wordnet graph. Niemann and Gurevych do not attempt to compare graph locations of an article and a synset. Instead they used the wordnet graph to describe meanings of articles and synset by subgraphs of the wordnet graph $G = (V, E)$, where $V$ are synsets and $E$ and lexico-semantic relation links. Next, the subgraphs are used to compare the meanings of Wikipedia articles and wordnet synsets. Both are described by the *activation patterns* in $G$ obtained as a result of the Page Rank algorithm.

First, the bag of word representation is built for articles and synsets. Next, for each article and synset, the initial vector of activated synset-nodes is calculated. Synsets whose elements occur in the bag of words for the given article or synset described receive non-zero activation values. Next, a personalised Page Rank [1] is run to propagate activations. The final article activation pattern is compared with the final activation patterns for each preselected synset by $\chi^2$ measure.

Most existing approaches depend heavily on text similarity between articles and wordnet glosses. Different wordnet relations and relation structures are used in a limited way. The majority of works are focused on PWN, while there are small, but significant differences between PWN and some other wordnets.

## 3    Data Sources

Most approaches to Wikipedia-to-wordnet mapping were developed for PWN. In PWN every synset is described by a gloss. However, not all wordnets do have glosses due to two main reasons. Writing glosses is time consuming and demanding while glosses are not really necessary for the meaning description in a wordnet – lexico-semantic relations are the basic means. plWordNet [6] – a very large wordnet for Polish – is an example of such a wordnet. Moreover, the basic building blocks of plWordNet are *lexical units* (word and sense number pairs), that are grouped into synsets only if they share lexico-semantic relations [9]. In plWordNet relations linking synsets are directly derived from lexico-semantic relations linking lexical units. There are also many relations defined only on the level of lexical units. plWordNet does not have glosses for synsets, but there are short comments for selected lexical units, cf the statistics below. Moreover, plWordNet has a rich set of relations and a high density of relation links per a lexical unit [6]. This is the main means for describing word senses.

Following [10], we represent Wikipedia articles and wordnet synsets by *disambiguation contexts*, i.e. collections of words (a particular word can occur several times) built on the basis of words associated with the given article or synset. However, due to the lack of glosses, we prepared two variants of the description for both articles and synsets: *simple* and *enhanced*, presented below. The variants differ in the number of different knowledge sources used to build the disambiguation contexts and hence in size and the richness of the contexts. In the *enhanced variant* we try to enrich the contexts in order to substitute the gloss-based information. We assumed that disambiguation contexts for both sides, Wikipedia and plWordNet, should be of similar size and description power to facilitate their comparison.

**Simple Variant** of disambiguation contexts (SV):

- Wikipedia *article* disambiguation context includes:
    - *bracket words* – syntactic head elements of the expressions enclosed in brackets in the article headwords,
    - *categories* – head elements of the category names, that describe the given article and words included in the brackets in those category names,
    - *links* – words from the titles of the outgoing links from the given article.
- plWordNet *synset s* disambiguation context includes:
    - *synonyms* – all words included in *s*,
    - direct *hypernyms* – words from synsets that are direct hypernyms of *s*,
    - direct *hyponyms* – words from synsets linked by hyponymy with *s*,
    - direct *meronyms* – as above,
    - *co-hyponyms* – words from synsets that share with *s* a direct hypernym (co-hyponyms of headwords occur often in their Wikipedia articles).

The article headword (article title) is not included in the disambiguation context, since only synsets including it are considered as the mapping targets by the algorithm, cf Sec. 4.

Bracket words are short expressions, typically one or two word long that are included in the round brackets and attached directly to the headword, e.g. *Broda* 'beard' (*zarost* 'facial hair') or *Szczep* 'graft' (*ogrodnictwo* 'gardening'). The bracket words are used to semantically disambiguate or classify the headword. Wikipedia categories should classify the article content. However, categories are written by different authors, according to different patterns, and their semantic relation to the article content and the head word can be very different, e.g. *Skałki Karkonoszy* 'rocks of Karkonosze (Giant Mountains), *Single wydane w roku 1954* 'Singles published in the year 1954' or *Szwajcarskie filmy historyczne* 'Swiss historical movies'.

Many categories are multi-word expressions, but we need lexical units (including multi-word) to match elements of disambiguation context on the wordnet side. We had to extract semantic heads, that express the main semantic class, from the categories, e.g. for the above categories: *skałka* 'rock', *singiel* 'single' and *film* 'movie' (or *film historyczny* 'historical movie'). This was done by a simple, but effective heuristics applied also to bracket expressions. Bracket expressions and categories are morpho-syntactically tagged and the first noun in the plural number and nominative case is extracted as its head.

**Enhanced Variant** (EV) of disambiguation contexts:

- Wikipedia *article* disambiguation context includes:
  - all words from the **Simple Variant** plus
  - *content words* – nouns from the first paragraph of the article.
- disambiguation context for a plWordNet *synset s* includes:
  - all words from the **Simple Variant** plus
  - a set of co-hyponyms extended to the set of *cousins* according to the path-pattern ($m$ hyponymy links up, $n$ hypernymy links down): $(2, 1)$ and $(2, 2)$,
  - indirect hypernyms and hyponyms up to 3 links (synset members),
  - *other relations*: inter-register synonymy, inhabitant, type, instance, holonymy, femininity, cf [6],
  - all words from the *comments* (i.e. draft glosses, mostly very short) to lexical units and the synset.
  - the *most semantically related words* due to a Measure of Semantic Relatedness.
    * based on the position in *k-MLists* for $s$ members,
    * and those words that are shared between *k-MLists* for $s$ members and words from $s$ simple context.

A Wikipedia article usually starts with a kind of definition in the first paragraph, but the following paragraphs are more semantically diversified. Thus, we added to the disambiguation context only nouns extracted from the first paragraph.

In the case of wordnet, firstly we extended the set of relations used to construct the disambiguation context with relations similar to synonymy, hypernymy or hyponymy, cf [9,6]. Secondly, we looked for other possible knowledge sources. The set of relations was expanded with indirect relations (homogeneous relation paths). Indirect hypernyms introduce generalisation to the description, and indirect hyponyms are more specific words that can occur in Wikipedia definitions. A path pattern: $(m, n)$ matches a path going $m$ hypernymy links up the hierarchy and than $n$ hyponymy links down. For a synset $s$, the patterns $(2, 1)$ and $(2, 2)$ cover all *cousins* linked to $s$. The set of close cousins describes a narrow semantic field, and its element are also likely to occur in the Wikipedia definitions. The whole set of words extracted from the wordnet relations describes semantically the sense represented by a synset and its members, i.e. words included in the synset that are often polysemous.

plWordNet does not include proper glosses, but there are short working comments written by linguists for selected lexical units and synsets. In the test sample only around 55% synsets have a comment (for a synset or its member). The comments were morpho-syntactically tagged and next all nouns were extracted.

The *Measure of Semantic Relatedness* (MSR) assigns a numerical value to a word pair in such a way that the value describes how closely semantically related the given two words are. MSR is built on the basis of the analysis of word distributions in a corpus. A good MSR should return higher values for words linked by lexico-semantic relations – synonyms should be assigned the highest values. An MSR was constructed on the basis of a general Polish corpus including 1.8 billion tokens[4]. In MSR construction we followed the method presented in [9]. About 70 000 nouns included in plWordNet 2.0 were described by their basic morpho-lexico-syntactic relations to adjectives, nouns and verbs.

For a given word $w$, the top $k$ words most related to $w$ (i.e. with the highest MSR values) that are returned by the MSR – henceforth called *k-MList* – include words associated with $w$ with a variety of relations, weakly related (in some context only), as well as non-related, i.e. errors, e.g. for the word *skałka* ('a rock', 'a small rock' or 'a piece of rock') the applied MSR returns: *skała* 'rock' 0.239, *urwisko* 'precipice'0.201, *klif* 'cliff' 0.199, *głaz* 'rock, boulder' 0.197, *pagórek* 'hill' 0.192, *ostaniec* 'inselberg' 0.188, *urwisek* 'a small rascal' (an error, an infrequent word) 0.184, *turnia* 'crag' 0.181, *wąwóz* 'ravine' 0.162, *wzgórze* 'hill' 0.158, *wydma* 'dune' 0.158, *wychodnia* 'outcrop' 0.153, *piarg* 'scree' 0.152 . . .

The MSR describes words not lexical units and does not differentiate between different word meanings. Very often only one or two most prominent meanings dominate the list. A *k-MList* associates words used in similar contexts and shows the context of use of the described word. We assumed that *k-MLists* can substitute absent synset glosses to some extent. The most accurate associations are on the top of every *k-MList*. In order to provide good description for less frequent words too, for each synset member $w$ we took only the $k = 5$ first positions from *k-MLists*. Next we added all words shared between the *k=20-MLists* of $w$ and *k=20-MLists* of the words from the synset simple disambiguation context.

## 4    Mapping Algorithm

The algorithm inspired by [10] is based on the idea of collecting votes for the association of article – synset pairs. Each word shared between the disambiguation contexts (DCs) of an article and a synset is a vote for linking these two. The strength of this vote is simply the joint number of occurrences of the given word. We assume that knowledge sources are carefully selected, independent and most of them are based on meta-data, so every word use is very meaningful.

for each Wikipedia head word $w$

1. let $syn(w) = \{S : w \in S\}$
2. let $art(w)$ = set of all Wikipedia articles with $w$ as a head word.
3. $map(w) = argmax_{S \in syn(w)} p(S|w)$, where

$$p(S|w) = \frac{score(w, S) + 1}{\sum_{w' \in art(w)} \sum_{S' \in syn(w)} score(w', S') + 1}$$

---

[4] The corpus includes several available Polish corpora, cf [9] and texts collected from Internet.

The *score* measures how much two DCs are related. We considered two types of the measure. The first is a modified version of the one proposed in [10]:

$$score_s(w, S) =$$

$$\sum_{x \in (DC(S) \cup DC(w))} \min \left( \frac{c(x, DC(S))}{cmax(x, WdnKS(S, x))}, \frac{c(x, DC(w))}{cmax(x, WikiKS(w, x))} \right)$$

where $DC()$ returns a disambiguation context for a headword/synset, $c(x, Y)$ returns the number of occurrences of $x$ in the collection $Y$, $cmax(x, Z)$ returns the maximal number of occurrences of $x$ across the set of knowledge sources delivered as the second parameter, and $WdnKS(S, x)$ and $WikiKS(W, x)$ are sets of knowledge sources including $x$ in the context for synset/headword.

DCs are collections and multiple occurrences of a word $x$, coming from different knowledge sources and increase the $x$ weight. The frequencies are used directly as weights. The $cmax()$ is being used for normalisation.

In the case of MSR, corpus frequencies can be biased and an MSR generated directly on the basis of the word frequencies expresses mostly much worse accuracy than an MSR based on the frequencies filtered and transformed into weighted features. We assumed that not all knowledge sources are equally informative for the mapping task. Thus, we introduced the second type of the $score_w$ measure in which DC words are weighted. The weights are based on the correlation between different knowledge sources according to words occurrences shared between them. As knowledge sources classify articles and synsets, and we expect that there is a corresponding synset for most articles, and that the knowledge source that represents higher correlation is more informative for the mapping. The weights are calculated in a following way:

- $x$ is a word pair from the knowledge source $X$, e.g. a set of direct hypernyms used in synset DCs, or a set of words extracted from the Wikipedia categories
- $c(x, X)$ is the frequency of $x$ in the knowledge source $X$.

For two knowledge sources $X$ and $Y$ we analyse how much information they deliver about each other with the help of Mutual Information:

- $p(x, X) = \frac{c(x,X)}{|X \cup Y|}$
- $p(x, Y) = \frac{c(x,Y)}{|X \cup Y|}$
- $p(x, x) = \frac{min(c(x,X), c(x,Y))}{|X,Y|}$
- $weight(X, Y) = I(P(x), P(y)) = \sum_{x \in X \cup Y} p(x, x) log \frac{p(x,x)}{p(x,X)p(x,Y)}$

Next, knowledge source weights are used to assign weights to DC words:

$$lw(x, w, S) = \max_{\substack{X \in WikiKS(w,x), \\ Y \in WdnKS(S,x)}} weight(X, Y)$$

Finally, the *score* function is modified with weights defined for words:

$$score_w(S, w) =$$

$$\sum_{x \in (DC(S) \cup DC(w))} lw(x, w, S) \min \left( \frac{c(x, DC(S))}{cmax(x, WdnKS(S,x))}, \frac{c(x, DC(w))}{cmax(x, WikiKS(w,x))} \right)$$

Ponzetto and Navigli [10] assumed that a monosemous headword $w$, i.e. occurring only once in Wikipedia, can be directly mapped to the only synset that includes $w$. However, as we tested on a sample of the monosemous headwords, this assumption is not true, see the next section.

Both variants of the algorithm abstain if there is no single synset with the best value of $p(S|w)$, as there is no basis to choose one synset among several with the same probability.

## 5  Experiments and Results

Wikipedia mapping is typically evaluated by comparing it with manual mapping done for a sample, e.g. [8,4]. However, manual annotation of a statistically significant sample would take substantial time: for each article several synsets have to be considered. Instead, we decided to manually evaluate the generated results of the mapping. First, we have drawn a large representative sample of polysemous 1064 Wikipedia articles. 690 of them have corresponding synsets in plWordNet 1.6 (the version used in our experiments). plWordNet includes very little number of Proper Names (PNs) that are described only in specific cases. Thus, we tried to filter all PNs from the sample obtaining finally 399 headwords. PN headwords were recognised by a heuristic:

- an article includes geo-coordinates in its infobox,
- or a bracket expression which begins with big letter and includes one of the predefined about 30 words recognised as signalling PN headword.

Different criteria were proposed for Wikipedia mapping evaluation in literature. In [10] mappings are simply evaluated as "correct" (505 from 1000 possible) and incorrect. In a similar way: "The annotation task was to label each sense pair either as alignment or not." in [8]. According to such definitions, there are no intermediate classes. In [4] three types of relations between 200 synsets and articles were manually annotated: *matching article* 63% ( the same concept as the synset), *related article* (two subcategories: *part-of related* 5.5% – a synset corresponds to a part of an article, *other related* 18%).

What is the proper set of relation types? Both Wikipedia and wordnet describe meanings and in both meanings are linked by relations (lexico-semantic in wordnet, links, categories and infoboxes in Wikipedia). In both meanings can be partitioned in different ways for a given word. Thus, we can notice that Wikipedia mapping task is similar to wordnet-to-wordnet mapping. A manual analysis of the sample showed that the relation between Wikipedia articles and synsets resemble inter-lingual relations used for mapping wordnets. As a result, we adapted for the evaluation a set of inter-lingual wordnet relations [13,11]:

- $s$ – inter-resource *synonymy* – links a Wikipedia article with a synset such that the article describes exactly the same lexical meaning as the synset,
- $h$ – inter-resource *hyponymy* – a Wikipedia article describes a more specific sense than the synset linked to it,
- $H$ – inter-resource *hypernymy* – a Wikipedia article is more general then a synset, typically, the article describes several meanings in its content and one of them corresponds to the linked synset, a quite frequent situation,
- $m$ – inter-resource *meronymy* – an article describes a sense that is in meronymy relation (e.g. a part of) with the linked synset,
- $o$ – inter-resource *holonymy* – the reverse situation, the synset sense is a meronym of the article sense,
- $p$ – inter-resource *partial synonymy* – an article and a synset overlap semantically, there is a shared part of their meanings, but they have also separate parts, none of the two senses is completely included in the other,
- $c$ – inter-resource *cousins* – an article and a synset are not directly linked, but they share a hypernym (potentially indirect) in the wordnet structure,
- $f$ – inter-resource *fuzzynymy* – an article and a synset cannot be linked by any of the above relations, but an annotator sees a strong semantic association between the two, they must be in the same narrow semantic domain,
- $e$ – *error* – linked but not semantically associated.

Consider an instance of *I-hyponymy*: for *Aspirant* 'warrant officer' (*stopień strażacki* 'a rank in fire department') in plWordNet there is a general sense {aspirant 2}, a hyponym of {podoficer 1 'non-commissioned officer'}; I-hypernymy: *Bezpiecznik* 'in general: fuse, safety binding, safety catch, safety valve, etc.' linked to {bezpiecznik 2} a hyponym of {urządzenie mechaniczne 1 'mechanical device'}; I-meronymy: *Secesja (architektura)* 'Art Nouveau in architecture' linked to {secesja 2} a hyponym of {kierunek w sztuce 1 'artistic movement'}.

All experiments were performed on the selected test sample. The calculation of the MI-based weights for the knowledge resources was performed on a separate randomly selected sample of articles (the computation for the whole Wikipedia would be costly). We tested all four possible combinations of:

- the two DC variants: *simple* (DC-S) and *enhanced* (DC-E),
- and the two scoring functions: *simple* (Sim) and *weighted* (W).

The baseline algorithm selects randomly one synset for each test article from those including the headword. All five algorithms were applied to the same test sample, and the generated results were evaluated by two annotators according to the link types defined above. The results are shown in Tables 1 and 2 below.

Table 1 presents manual classification of the generated links. The links were first evaluated independently by two evaluators. Next, they discussed differences in their decisions. After this phase only 52 difference from 1649 evaluating decisions in total remained. The remaining disagreements were finally solved by the

**Table 1.** Relations assigned by evaluators (in %) to the generated links

|          | Baseline | Sim&DC-S | W&DC-S | Sim&DC-E | W&DC-E |
|----------|---------|----------|--------|----------|--------|
| Coverage | 100.00  | 47.36    | 52.63  | 64.66    | **71.67** |
| s [%]    | 22.81   | **68.78** | 64.76 | 56.97    | 55.59  |
| h [%]    | 5.26    | 3.7      | 3.8    | **6.97** | 5.94   |
| H [%]    | 2.01    | **2.11** | 1.9    | 1.55     | 1.04   |
| m [%]    | **1.00** | 0.52    | 0.47   | 0        | 0.34   |
| o [%]    | 0.00    | **0.52** | 0.47   | 0.38     | 0.34   |
| p [%]    | 4.01    | 2.11     | 1.9    | 3.87     | **4.89** |
| c [%]    | 0.75    | 0.52     | 0.47   | **0.77** | 0.69   |
| f [%]    | **5.76** | 4.23    | 3.8    | 3.1      | 2.09   |
| e [%]    | **58.40** | 17.46  | 22.3   | 26.35    | 29     |

third super-evaluator. *Coverage* is the percentage of the Wikipedia articles that were mapped to a synset. The baseline achieved 100%, as exactly one synset was randomly selected for every article. Other algorithms abstained for a number of articles. As we could expect, enhanced DCs (DC-E), with more words per context, improve the coverage by a richer description. However, the percentage of I-synonymy links is smaller, but mainly due to the higher error, as the ratio to other relations is stable. Larger contexts can generate more accidental links. The unsupervised weight estimation appeared to be too fuzzy to select the most descriptive words.

In order to analyse the frequencies in Table 1, we applied well-known measures of precision, recall (in relation to the whole test sample) and F-measure, see Table2. The relations were grouped into three classes: $S$ only synonymy, $H$ – synonymy plus hypo/hypernymy and $W$ all relations (weak association).

All algorithms outperformed baseline, even in the case of recall (correctly mapped / size of the test sample). The precision of the baseline is too low. The same situation is with F-measure and F-measure calculated for the precision and coverage (FC in Table2).

Weighted score ($W$ in Table2) produced slightly worse results than simple score ($Sim$). This can be caused by specific words that select correct senses but occur in the knowledge sources of the lower weights. Enhanced DCs result in lower precision but also in higher recall and much higher coverage.

The obtained precision is lower than reported for PWN, but this can be caused by two factors. First, synsets do not included glosses and their DCs do not describe their senses well enough. This observation was confirmed by our preliminary experiments with Word Sense Disambiguation algorithm based on the plWordNet data. Second, our criteria for inter-resource relations seem to be stricter than those used in literature.

Manual inspection of a sample of monosemous Wikipedia articles mapped to their corresponding synsets showed that almost half of the mappings is incorrect, which is contrary to common assumption in literature. Many articles describe senses absent in plWordNet 1.6. We identified a threshold over the sum

**Table 2.** Coverage, precision and recall (in %) of the mapping Wikipedia on a wordnet

| | Baseline | Sim&DC-S | W&DC-S | Sim&DC-E | W&DC-E |
|---|---|---|---|---|---|
| Coverage | 100.00 | 47.36 | 52.63 | 64.66 | **71.67** |
| PrecS | 22.81 | **68.78** | 64.76 | 56.97 | 55.59 |
| PrecH: | 34.09 | **76.71** | 72.38 | 69.37 | 67.48 |
| PrecW: | 41.60 | **82.53** | 77.61 | 73.64 | 70.97 |
| RecallS | 22.81 | 32.58 | 34.08 | 36.84 | **39.84** |
| RecallH | 34.09 | 36.34 | 38.09 | 44.86 | **48.37** |
| RecallW | 41.60 | 39.09 | 40.85 | 47.61 | **50.87** |
| FS | 22.81 | 44.21 | 44.65 | 44.74 | **46.38** |
| FH | 34.09 | 49.31 | 49.91 | 54.48 | **56.34** |
| FW | 41.60 | 53.05 | 53.52 | 57.83 | **59.26** |
| FCS | 37.14 | 56.09 | 58.06 | 60.57 | **62.61** |
| FCH | 50.84 | 58.56 | 60.94 | 66.93 | **69.51** |
| FCW | 58.76 | 60.18 | 62.72 | 68.85 | **71.31** |

of frequencies of the DC words equal to 15.0 that improves precision by filtering out incorrect mappings. *W&DC-E* algorithm was run with the threshold added. The coverage decreased to 43.35%, but the precision was significantly increased: *PrecS*=62.42%, *PrecH*=75.14% and *PrecW*=78.61%. The recall was decreased, but to a smaller degree than the coverage: *RecallS*=27.06%, *RecallH*=32.58% and *RecallW*=34.08%. Thus, for some test sample articles there are no matching synsets and a kind of filtering procedure should be built into the mapping.

## 6    Conclusions

We presented a method for mapping Wikipedia articles on plWordNet synsets not on the basis of the content of the linked elements, but primarily on the basis of the semantic relations describing them. As plWordNet does not include glosses, but only short comments for a limited number of synsets, the proposed method cannot follow a typical blueprint for the Wikipedia mapping task, in which text-to-text similarity is fundamental.

We showed that a rich relation structure in plWordNet allows for building synset representation that is rich enough to achieve good accuracy in the mapping task. Even better results were obtained in expanding synset descriptions with the help of the Measure of Semantic Relatedness. The method can be applied to other wordnets without glosses or lexical semantic networks.

The evaluation was based on the observed analogy between Wikipedia mapping and wordnet to wordnet mapping. A set of inter-resource semantic relations was proposed as better charactersing different relations between Wikipedia articles and wordnet synset. The evaluation was performed by two annotators who achieved very good inter-annotator agreement.

Only the local link structure is considered in the method for building representations for articles and synsets. In further research we want to explore the possibility of comparing relation subgraphs as descriptions for the meaning of articles and synsets. The lack of improvement in the weighted scoring shows that a more local version of the weighting algorithm is required.

# References

1. Agirre, E., Soroa, A.: Personalizing Page Rank for word sense disambiguation. In: Proceedings of the 12th Conference of the European Chapter of the ACL (EACL 2009), pp. 33–41. Association for Computational Linguistics, Athens (2009)
2. Calzolari, N., Choukri, K., Declerck, T., Dogan, M.U., Maegaard, B., Mariani, J., Odijk, J., Piperidis, S. (eds.): Proceedings of the Eighth International Conference on Language Resources and Evaluation (LREC 2012). ELRA, Istanbul (2012)
3. Fellbaum, C. (ed.): WordNet – An Electronic Lexical Database. The MIT Press (1998)
4. Fernando, S., Stevenson, M.: Mapping wordnet synsets to wikipedia articles. In: Calzolari, et al. (eds.) [2]
5. Isahara, H., Kanzaki, K. (eds.): JapTAL 2012. LNCS, vol. 7614. Springer, Heidelberg (2012)
6. Maziarz, M., Piasecki, M., Szpakowicz, S.: Approaching plWordNet 2.0. In: Fellbaum, C., Vossen, P. (eds.) Proceedings of 6th International Global Wordnet Conference, pp. 189–196. The Global WordNet Association, Matsue (2012)
7. Navigli, R., Ponzetto, S.: BabelNet: The automatic construction, evaluation and application of a wide-coverage multilingual semantic network. Artificial Intelligence 193, 217–250 (2012)
8. Niemann, E., Gurevych, I.: The people's web meets linguistic knowledge: Automatic sense alignment of Wikipedia and WordNet. In: Proc. of the International Conference on Computational Semantics (IWCS), pp. 205–214. Oxford (2011)
9. Piasecki, M., Szpakowicz, S., Broda, B.: A Wordnet from the Ground Up. Oficyna Wydawnicza Politechniki Wrocławskiej (2009), http://www.site.uottawa.ca/~szpak/pub/A_Wordnet_from_the_Ground_Up.pdf
10. Ponzetto, S.P., Navigli, R.: Knowledge-rich word sense disambiguation rivaling supervised systems. In: Proceedings of the 48th Annual Meeting of the Association for Computational Linguistics, pp. 1522–1531. Association for Computational Linguistics, Uppsala (2010)
11. Rudnicka, E., Maziarz, M., Piasecki, M., Szpakowicz, S.: A strategy of mapping Polish Wordnet onto Princeton Wordnet. In: Proceedings of COLING 2012: Posters, pp. 1039–1048. The COLING 2012 Organizing Committee, Mumbai (2012)
12. Ruiz-Casado, M., Alfonseca, E., Castells, P.: Automatic Assignment of Wikipedia Encyclopedic Entries to WordNet Synsets. In: Szczepaniak, P.S., Kacprzyk, J., Niewiadomski, A. (eds.) AWIC 2005. LNCS (LNAI), vol. 3528, pp. 380–386. Springer, Heidelberg (2005)
13. Vossen, P.: EuroWordNet General Document Version 3. Tech. rep., Univ. of Amsterdam (2002)

# Recognising Compositionality of Multi-Word Expressions in the Wordnet Oriented Perspective

Paweł Kędzia, Maciej Piasecki, Marek Maziarz, and Michał Marcińczuk

Institute of Informatics, Wrocław University of Technology, Poland
{pawel.kedzia,maciej.piasecki,marek.maziarz,michal.marcinczuk}@pwr.wroc.pl

**Abstract.** A method for the recognition of the compositionality of Multi Word Expressions (MWEs) is proposed. First, we study associations between MWEs and the structure of wordnet lexico-semantic relations. A simple method of splitting plWordNet's MWEs into compositional and non-compositional on the basis of the hypernymy structure is discussed. However, our main goal is to build a classifier for the recognition of compositional MWEs. We assume prior MWE detection. Several experiments with different classification algorithms were performed for the purposes of this task, namely Naive Bayes classifier, Multinomial logistic regression model with a ridge estimator and Decision Table classifier. A heterogeneous set of features is based on: t-score measure for word co-occurrences, Measure of Semantic Relatedness and lexico-syntactic structure of MWEs. MWE compositionality classification is analysed as a knowledge source for automated wordnet expansion.

## 1 Introduction

Multi-word Expressions (henceforth MWEs), are characterised in [30] as "lexical items that can be decomposed into single words and display idiosyncratic features". Depending on the extent of MWE idiosyncrasy, MWEs can be divided into several classes along the opposition *compositional* and *non-compositional*. Following [12], the compositionality is a degree to which MWE meaning can be explained by a function of the meanings of the MWE constituents and the way in which they are combined. Compositionality can be also perceived as a degree of predictability of MWE in its meaning and its structure knowing the MWE constituents. MWE syntactic idiosyncrasy is also treated as a marker of its non-compositionality. Following this definition it can be said, that a MWE is compositional when the composition of the semantic representations of its constituents determines the semantic representation of the whole MWE. A non-compositional MWE is an expression which is more metaphorical and its meaning cannot be predicated on the basis of the semantics of all MWE elements.

One word and multi-word lexemes (i.e. MWEs) are described in every wordnet by the lexico-semantic relations. Knowledge about the compositionality of a given MWE can be very helpful in identifying particular instances of lexico-semantic relations in which the given MWE participates, e.g. one can expect that

F. Castro, A. Gelbukh, and M. González (Eds.): MICAI 2013, Part I, LNAI 8265, pp. 240–251, 2013.

the head of a compositional MWE is linked to the whole MWE by hypernymy. Thus, the knowledge of MWE compositionality could be especially helpful for automated methods of wordnet expansion.

In the work presented here, we wanted to explore both issues. Hypernymy/hyponymy is of the greatest importance for the wordnet structure. So, firstly, we investigated a hypothesis that compositional MWEs are hyponyms (more specific) of their syntactic heads[1]. Assuming that the hypothesis is true, compositional MWEs can be located in preselected places of the wordnet hypernymy structure. Secondly, our goal was to develop a method for recognising compositional MWEs on the basis of their distributions in a large corpus. We aimed at achieving accuracy to utilise enough high information about the MWE compositionality in finding its place in the wordnet.

## 2 Related Work

Various degrees of MWE compositionality have been proposed in literature. Two classes: compositional and non-compositional is the simplest solution, e.g. [27]. However greater number of classes are also proposed. For instance, during the DiSCo 2011 Workshop[2] two measures of the compositionality level were used: *coarse-grained* and *fine-grained* scoring. The coarse-grained scoring defines three levels of compositionality: *low, medium* and *high* – compositional. The fine-grained scoring represents MWE compositionality by numerical values from the range: $[0, 100]$. Low-compositional MWEs are located in $[0, 25]$, medium corresponds to $[38, 62]$, high ones are in $[75, 100]$. All other MWEs were removed from the coarse-grained data test set. The authors of [29] used six-levels compositionality scale: 1 means that MWE is non-compositional ("No word in the expression has any relation to the actual meaning of the expression") and 6 represent fully compositional MWEs. In [13,18,22], only three levels of compositionality are used: *low, medium,* and *high*. The distinction between compositional and non-compositional MWEs is identical to coarse-grained scoring of DiSCo'2011. In [23], a *compositionality level* $(D)$ is measured by multiplying the semantic distance between the MWE and each of its constituents. The $D$ score is computed as the square root of the product using the following formula: $D(M) = \sqrt{\prod_{i=1}^{n} SD(M, w_i)}$, where $M$ is a MWE, $w_i$ is its constituent and $SD$ is a semantic distance function. The $SD$ value depends on the number of connections between MWE, its constituents and the semantic fields in the lexicon. $SD$ and $D$ range between $[0, 1]$. $D$ is equal to 1 for strongly compositional MWE and 0 for non-compositional MWE.

Regardless the number of the compositionality levels, there are many approaches to the recognition of the MWE compositionality. In [1] corpus-based and WordNet-based semantic similarity measures were used to analyse MWE

---

[1] A head is defined here as the main syntactic constituent of a MWE which expresses syntactic properties of the whole MWE and can replace the whole MWE, as far as only the syntactic properties are considered.

[2] Distributional Semantics and Compositionality Workshop at ACL/HLT 2011.

compositionality. Concerning the former a modified Lin's approach [16] was applied (LSA method and cosine measure), for the latter: Resnik distance [25] and Hirst and St-Onge distance [10] were used. Similarity between the MWE head and the whole MWE was analysed for noun-noun and verb-particle MWEs. In the case of noun-noun MWE the best correlation between LSA and WordNet based similarity measures was achieved for LSA and Resnik (the correlation 0.108), and in the case of verb-particle for LSA and HSO (the correlation 0.225). A hypothesis that the pairs with a high value of $LSA(mwe, word_i)$ have $MWE$ being a hyponym of $word_i$ was tested, and appeared to be true only for rare MWEs. Korkontzelos and Suresh [12] proposed unsupervised approach to compare MWE meaning with its semantic head on the basis of Distributional Semantics. The meaning representation was extracted form a tagged and parsed corpus, cf [11]. The authors focused on complex nominal units, proper names and adjective-noun structures. In [18] the authors take into account only bigrams (two-element MWEs, often: a head and its modifier) and divide MWEs into three groups. They follow McCarthy work [20] on measuring similarity between a phrasal verb and main verb (e.g. *blow up* and *blow*) in which the similarity was an indicator of compositionality. Pedersen [22] studies many distributional similarity measures (e.g. t-score, Jaccard, Dice and PMI) to determine MWE compositionality. The best results were obtained for the context window of 10 words. Only two-element MWEs were processed as in [18]. MWE compositionality level was analysed in relation to the coarse grained and fine grained scales. Concerning the former, first a pair $(MWE, MWE_{head})$ was assigned a value from the range $[0, 100]$. Next, these values were mapped onto the coarse grained scale consisting of three compositionality levels, cf [18]. The best results are reported in [22] for t-score measure in coarse grained scale, where the higher value of t-score signals higher value of compositionality. A different approach to recognition of non-compositionality is presented in [8]. The authors propose knowledge-free, training-free and language-independent *Multiword Explanation Distance* (MED) to recognise MWE compositionality. MED in several configurations was compared with PMI and was evaluated in Named Entity extraction task with $F1 = 0.83$. Salehi and Cook [27] shows how MWE translation to other language can be helpful for the compositionality detection. Their approach can be used for any MWE and any language. They applied binary classification of compositionality and used *Panlex*[3] to translate MWEs and their constituents. The authors argue that compositional MWEs are more likely to be word-for-word translated than non-compositional.

## 3     Compositionality and the Hypernymy Structure

A higher number of the compositionality levels can improve description precision, but as there was no Polish lexical resource describing MWE compositionality and a larger number of classes can decrease inter-annotator agreement we decided to

---

[3] Multilingual dictionary, available at http://panlex.org/

apply a relatively simple binary division of MWEs into: *compositional* and *non-compositional*. The notion of compositionality is vague and needs clarification [28, p. 82]. According to [17] the meaning of a *composite expression*[4] is *a function* of the meanings of its constituents. It is said that the final meaning is *determined by* the meaning of its parts and also by the mode of composition, that is by the way the constituent parts are put together [21, p. 12]. Svensson distinguishes few aspects (dichotomies) of the term [28]: transparency/opacity, analysability/un-analysability, literal/figurative meaning, partial/full compositionality. Thus, (1) a compositional expression (unit) must be transparent, i.e., it should be possible to find out complex the meaning out of meanings of the constituent units; (2) compositionality means analysability – the complex expression should be decomposable into meanings of constituent units, (3) composite expressions are used in their literal meaning, so they are non-figurative expressions, (4) partial compositionality means that only some constituent units determine the final meaning, while others do not. Taking into account the properties of the compositional expressions identified in the literature, we call a lexical unit *compositional* if it meets jointly the following criteria:

- meaning of a complex lexical unit $X$ is composed of meanings of its constituents,
- meaning of a complex lexical unit $X$ need not be limited to meanings of its constituent lexical elements and may contain some additional, surplus features (coming for instance from the *mode of composition*),
- this encore cannot have metaphorical or metonimical character,
- if the final meaning is determined by only one of its constituents such lexical unit is not compositional,
- partial compositionality is non-compositionality.

Otherwise the lexical unit would be called non-compositional.

### 3.1   plWNCompNoncomp Algorithm

We noticed that a synset which includes a compositional noun MWE is often linked by the *hyponymy*, *inter-register synonymy* or *instance of* (for definitions see [19]) relations to a synset including the syntactic head of this MWE. Thus we have formulated a hypothesis: compositional MWEs are hyponyms of their syntactic heads or are related to their syntactic heads by *inter-register synonymy* and *instance of* relation. Next, we implemented a simple wordnet-based classifier of the MWE compositionality (see Algorithm 1) to verify how far we can go with it. The classifier divides plWordNet [24] MWEs into: compositional and non-compositional. It is shown in Sec. 3.3.

---

[4] A composite expression encompasses also a multi-word lexical unit.

**Algorithm 1.** Wordnet-based classification of MWEs

1: **Input:** plWN **and** MWE
2: **Output:** Decision about compositionality
3:
4: **if** ∃ MWE **in** plWN **and** MWE is not artificial **then**
5:     $H = Head(MWE)$
6:     **if** ∃ synset $S$ with lemma $L = H$ **and** $Rel(L, H) = synonymy$ **then**
7:         **return** $MWE$ is **compositional**
8:     **else**
9:         **if** ∃ $hyponym$ $S$ with lemma $L = H$ **then**
10:             **return** $MWE$ is **compositional**
11:         **else**
12:             **if** ∃ synset $S$ with lemma $L = H$ **and** $Rel(L, H) = instance\_of$ **then**
13:                 **return** $MWE$ is **compositional**
14:             **else**
15:                 **return** $MWE$ is **non-compositional**
16:             **end if**
17:         **end if**
18:     **end if**
19: **else**
20:     Cannot classify MWE
21: **end if**

## 3.2 Data Set and Annotation

First, we extracted from plWordNet all two-element noun MWEs and made the list of the most frequent of them in a huge Polish test corpus (*Kgr7*) [5] of around 1.8 billion tokens. MWEs representing artificial lexical units (i.e. expressions, not proper lexical units cf [24]) were excluded. Next we applied plWNCompNoncomp algorithm to the extracted MWEs obtaining 9508 compositional MWEs and 4035 non-compositional MWES.

A sample of 1564 MWEs was selected from the most frequent ones according to *Kgr7* corpus. Only the most frequent MWEs were considered because of the classification methods based on corpus distribution that are presented in Sec. 4. We used plWNCompNoncomp classifier in order to have similar numbers of compositional and non-compositional MWEs. Next two annotators manually assigned MWEs to both classes following the formulated annotation guidelines. The results are presented in Tab. 1. Cohen's Kappa is equal to 0.6 that means by [15] that the agreement is moderate (from 0.61 is substantial agreement), according to Cicchetti [6] and Fleiss [7], the agreement is good. In spite of the good agreement we asked a senior linguist to decide in contradictory cases. As a result we obtained 705 compositional and 859 non-compositional. Examples of annotator decisions are presented in Tab. 2. The columns A1, A2, A3 are

---

[5] Kgr7 corpus contains many documents from *Korpus IPI PAN*, Polish Wikipedia, *Korpus Rzeczypospolitej*[26] and texts extracted from Internet; Kgr7 was used in plWordNet development, cf [3].

decisions of two annotators and the supervisor (A3). For example, MWE *bułka tarta* is classified as non-compositional by the first annotator, as compositional by the second and the final decision of supervisor is compositional. In case of *dom kultury* MWE, A1 classified it as non-compositional, A2 as compositional and the final decision is non-compositional.

**Table 1.** Decisions about MWE compositionality: A1, A2 - first and second annotator

|  | A1 - Compositional | A1 - Non-compositional |
|---|---|---|
| **A2 - Compositional** | 586 | 153 |
| **A2 - Non-compositional** | 162 | 663 |
| **Cohen's Kappa** | 0.6 | |

**Table 2.** Examples of decisions about compositionality of MWE

| MWE | A1 | A2 | A3 Supervisor |
|---|---|---|---|
| bułka tarta (crumbs) | non-comp. | comp. | **comp.** |
| chłonny rynek (eady market) | comp. | non-comp. | **comp.** |
| dom kultury (culture house) | non-comp. | comp. | **non-comp.** |
| fałszywy ślad (false trail) | comp. | non-comp. | **non-comp.** |
| aparat fotograficzny (photo camera) | **comp.** | **comp.** | — |
| blada twarz (paleface) | **non-comp.** | **non-comp.** | — |

For the need of processing and recognition of MWE occurrences in text, plWordNet MWEs have been divided into about 100 structural classes [2,14]. A lexico-morpho-syntactic constraint is defined for each class. The constraints describe the key lexical and syntactic properties (e.g. the number, order of the MWE constituents and morpho-syntactic dependencies among them). Moreover, MWE classes are divided into two groups cf. [2,14]: *fix* of fixed order of constituents and *flex* in which the linear order of constituents is not constrained – their distribution in our dataset is presented in Tab. 3. We can notice that non-compositional MWEs tend to belong to the Fix classes. It seems that the lack of compositionality is expressed in Polish by the lack of flexibility in word order, while Polish is weakly constrained word order language.

### 3.3 Evaluation of Hypernymy Based Algorithm

plWNCompNoncomp classifier for MWEs (Sec. 3.1) was evaluated on the annotated MWE test sample. It should be emphasised that the algorithm works on MWE lemmas and heads. It does not disambiguate their senses. MWE heads were identified due to the MWE structural classes. The evaluation results are presented in Tab. 4.

The algorithm achieved high precision for true negatives and high recall for compositional MWEs. For non-compositional MWEs the recall is relatively low: 0.62 and $F_1$ measure is equal to 0.72. For compositional MWEs, $F_1$ is lower (0.67)

**Table 3.** Cardinality of MWEs with division on Fix and Flex classes

| Fix/Flex Class | Compositional | Non-compositional | All |
|---|---|---|---|
| Fix (number of MWEs): | 525 | 541 | 1066 |
| Flex (number of MWEs): | 334 | 164 | 498 |
| Fix (% of MWEs): | 0.61 | 0.77 | 0.68 |
| Flex (% of MWEs): | 0.39 | 0.23 | 0.32 |

**Table 4.** Precision, recall and accuracy of the plWNCompNoncomp algorithm

| | Compositional | Non-compositional |
|---|---|---|
| Precision | 0.57 | 0.86 |
| Recall | 0.83 | 0.62 |
| F-Measure | 0.67 | 0.72 |
| Accuracy | 0.7 | |

that is caused by the low precision for true positives (0.57). The basic rule of the algorithm causes over-generation, but anyway a hyponymy link between MWE and its head seems to be a positive signal in favour of the MWE compositionality.

There are some cases when a MWE is not described by *hyponymy*, *inter-register synonymy* or *instance of* relations but it is still intrinsically compositional, e.g. a synset *{zysk ekonomiczny 1}*[6] (*economic profit*) includes MWE classified by the algorithm as non-compositional because there is no synset including its head *zysk* (*profit*) and connected with it by one of the expected relations. However *zysk ekonomiczny* is compositional, and has 7 hypernyms: *{wartość ekonomiczna 1}* (*economic value*), *{wartość 1}* (*value*), *{pojęcie matematyczne 1}* (*mathematic concept*), *{pojęcie 2}* (*concept*), *{wytwór umysłu 2}* (*product of a mind*), *{wytwór 1}* (*product*), *{rezultat 1}* (*result*).

However, the compositionality of polysemous MWEs very often cannot be judged unless we consider their particular senses, e.g. *język angielski* (*English language*) can mean a written/spoken language – compositional in this sense – or as a school activity – non-compositional.

## 4    Corpus-Based MWE Classification

plWNCompNoncomp process MWE from plWordNet has limited precision. We need to look for additional knowledge sources in the corpus in order to better classify both plWordNet MWEs and new MWEs.

### 4.1    MSR and t-score Approach

First we reimplemented Pedersen's approach based on t-score measure [22] and tested it on the MWE test sample (Sec. 3.2) and *Kgr7* corpus. T-score values

---

[6] A synset includes lexical units, here understood as pairs: lemma plus sense number.

were calculated for co-occurrences of MWE syntactic heads and whole MWEs in *Kgr7* using window size $\langle 0, 10 \rangle$ that covers also most of the discontinuous MWEs. However, contrary to [22], we did not find correlation between t-score values and MWE compositionality, cf Fig. 1 were t-score values are presented on x-axis for compositional – the value 1 on y-axis, and non-compositional – the value 0 MWEs. Above the threshold $\geq 3000$ we can find only non-compositional MWEs, but their total number is around 30.

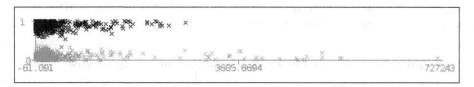

**Fig. 1.** T-score values in compositional and non-compositional class

Next, we tried to use a Measure of Semantic Relatedness (MSR) for MWE heads and the whole MWEs to identify compositional MWEs. We assumed that MSR values were significantly higher for compositional MWEs. MSR was extracted from *Kgr7* and calculated for all noun one-word and multi-word lemmas described in plWordNet 1.8. Lemma occurrences were described by lexico-morpho-syntactic features, cf [24], and a MSR based on PMI and cosine measure was computed with the help of *SuperMatrix* system [4]. We compared MSR values for head-MWE pairs for compositional and non-compositional MWEs, but the similarity values did not provide enough clear distinction cf Fig. 2. However, we found that almost only non-compositional MWEs occur below the threshold equal to 0.044. This observation is illustrated by precision, recall, accuracy and $F_1$ measure presented in Tab. 5 We took the weighted average values of precision (**0.698**), recall (**0.701**) and $F_1$ measure (**0.695**) as our baseline in classification process.

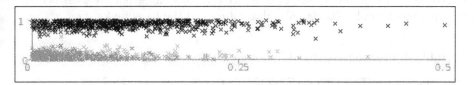

**Fig. 2.** MSR values in compositional and non-compositional class

**Table 5.** Precision, recall and accuracy with MSR threshold $= 0.044$ – baseline

|  | Compositional | Non-compositional |
|---|---|---|
| **Precision** | 0.65 | 0.736 |
| **Recall** | 0.815 | 0.562 |
| **F-Measure** | 0.72 | 0.636 |
| **Accuracy** | 0.69 | |

## 4.2    Combination of Features

In a similar way to [29] we decided to build a classifier based on a combination of features. We used three classifiers: Naive Bayes (NB), Multinomial logistic regression (LR) and Decision Tables (DT) from Weka [9], evaluated according to the ten-fold stratified cross-validation scheme.

First, we analysed combinations of two features based on t-score and MSR. Results obtained with the three classifiers (NB, LR, DT) and the two features used separately and together are presented in Tab. 6. Neither single MSR and t-score nor combination of both features did not outperform the baseline.

**Table 6.** Precision, recall, F-measure for MSR and t-score features

| Feature(s): | M | | | T | | | M+T | | |
|---|---|---|---|---|---|---|---|---|---|
| Classifier: | **NB** | **LR** | **DT** | **NB** | **LR** | **DT** | **NB** | **LR** | **DT** |
| **Precision** | 0.674 | 0.684 | 0.69 | 0.543 | 052 | 0.586 | 0.639 | 0.69 | 0.687 |
| **Recall** | 0.652 | 0.681 | 0.686 | 0.529 | 0.522 | 0.585 | 0.66 | 0.688 | 0.685 |
| **F-Measure** | 0.644 | 0.68 | 0.68 | 0.432 | 0.442 | 0.586 | 0.647 | 0.688 | 0.683 |

In addition to the two features based on corpus distribution, we introduced the third one based on the MWE structure analysis. The structural class can be also predicted on the basis of MWE behaviour in the corpus. Results are presented in Tab. 7. Three variants of the structural feature were tested: **C1** is structural class of MWE with information encoded in it (including fix/flex distinction), **C2** – only MWE word order is represented by values: *fix* and *flex* and **C3** is morpho-syntactic class of MWE without information about word ordering. Boldfaced cells in F-Measure row mean that the baseline of $F_1$ was achieved. Our results confirm the claim form [29] that MWE classification based on the merged features express better performance than any single feature classifier. In our experiments, only NB classifier did not exceed the baseline for $F_1$.

**Table 7.** Precision, recall and F-measure for different feature configurations

| Features: | M+T+C1+C3 | | | M+C3 | | | M+C2+C3 | | |
|---|---|---|---|---|---|---|---|---|---|
| Classifier: | **NB** | **LR** | **DT** | **NB** | **LR** | **DT** | **NB** | **LR** | **DT** |
| **Precision** | 0.667 | 0.706 | 0.724 | 0.696 | 0.691 | 0.725 | 0.669 | 0.683 | 0.725 |
| **Recall** | 0.658 | 0.705 | 0.724 | 0.68 | 0.688 | 0.725 | 0.663 | 0.68 | 0.725 |
| **F-Measure** | 0.651 | **0.705** | **0.723** | 0.676 | 0.688 | **0.724** | 0.661 | 0.68 | **0.724** |

## 4.3    Features and Instance Selection

As the next step, we performed feature selection with different configuration of evaluator and search method. The best results were shown in Tab. 8.

**Table 8.** Feature selection in MWE classification task

| Evaluator | Search method | Features | Classifier | P | R | F1 |
|---|---|---|---|---|---|---|
| CfsSubstEval | BestFirst | M + C1 | NB | 0.702 | 0.687 | 0.683 |
| | | | LR | 0.695 | 0.692 | 0.692 |
| | | | DT | 0.723 | 0.722 | **0.722** |
| ClassifierSubsetEval (Decision Table) | BestFirst | M + T + C1 | NB | 0.677 | 0.66 | 0.647 |
| | | | LR | 0.7 | 0.699 | 0.699 |
| | | | DT | 0.724 | 0.724 | **0.723** |
| ClassifierSubstEval (Decision table) | GeneticSearch | M + T + C3 | NB | 0.664 | 0.648 | 0.634 |
| | | | LR | 0.703 | 0.701 | 0.701 |
| | | | DT | 0.723 | 0.723 | **0.723** |

In the last experiment we reduced the number of training examples with the help of SMOTE method (Synthetic Minority Over-sampling Technique [5]), but we kept the whole set of features. see Tab. 9.

**Table 9.** SMOTE for whole set of features: M, T, C1, C2, C3

| Classifier | Precision | Recall | F-Measure |
|---|---|---|---|
| NB | 0.697 | 0.697 | 0.697 |
| LR | 0.719 | 0.727 | 0.709 |
| DT | 0.741 | 0.748 | 0.741 |

# 5 Conclusions and Future Works

We found the vast majority of compositional MWE in the Polish wordnet are linked by hyponymy, inter-register synonymy or instance of relations with their syntactic heads. So, compositionality of a MWE can be very helpful in placing it in the wordnet structure, but potential MWE compositionality must be first checked. On the basis of plWordNet data a set of the most frequent compositional and non-compositional MWEs was automatically extracted and next corrected by a linguist. Using this Polish test data set we verified results in recognition of compositional MWEs by re-implementation of Pedersen's method [22] with the help of t-score measure. This approach does not seem to work for Polish. However, we showed also that a combination of several features that can be extracted from a corpus as an input to the selected classifiers provides good results in recognition of compositional MWEs. Besides t-score the features included a Measure of Semantic Relatedness (MSR) and information about MWE syntactic structure. Thus we combined three levels of knowledge about MWE: co-occurrences (t-score), various context dependencies (MSR) and MWE syntax.

# References

1. Baldwin, T., Bannard, C., Tanaka, T., Widdows, D.: An empirical model of multiword expression decomposability. In: Proc. of the ACL 2003 Workshop on Multiword Expressions: Analysis, Acquisition and Treatment, MWE 2003, vol. 18, pp. 89–96. ACL (2003)
2. Broda, B., Derwojedowa, M., Piasecki, M.: Recognition of Structured Collocations in An Inflective Language. Systems Science 34(4), 27–36 (2008); the previous version was published in the Proceedings of AAIA 2008, Wisla Poland
3. Broda, B., Maziarz, M., Piasecki, M.: Tools for plWordNet Development. Presentation and Perspectives. In: Calzolari, N., et al. (eds.) Proceedings of the Eight International Conference on Language Resources and Evaluation (LREC 2012), pp. 3647–3652. ELRA, Istanbul (2012)
4. Broda, B., Piasecki, M.: SuperMatrix: a general tool for lexical semantic knowledge acquisition. In: Proc. of IMCSIT – 3rd International Symposium Advances in Artificial Intelligence and Applications (AAIA 2008), pp. 345–352 (2008)
5. Chawla, N.V., Bowyer, K.W., Hall, L.O., Kegelmeyer, W.P.: Smote: Synthetic minority over-sampling technique. Journal of Artificial Intelligence Research 16, 321–357 (2002)
6. Cicchetti, D.V., Volkmar, F., Sparrow, S.S., Cohen, D., Fermanian, J., Rourke, B.P.: Assessing the reliability of clinical scales when the data have both nominal and ordinal features: proposed guidelines for neuropsychological assessments. J. Clin. Exp. Neuropsychol. 14(5), 673–686 (1992)
7. Fleiss, J.L.: Statistical Methods for Rates and Proportions. Wiley series in probability and mathematical statistics. John Wiley & Sons, New York (1981)
8. Gurrutxaga, A., Alegria, I.: Measuring the compositionality of nv expressions in basque by means of distributional similarity techniques. In: Calzolari, N., et al. (eds.) Proceedings of the Eight International Conference on Language Resources and Evaluation (LREC 2012). ELRA, Istanbul (2012)
9. Hall, M., Frank, E., Holmes, G., Pfahringer, B., Reutemann, P., Witten, I.H.: The weka data mining software: an update. SIGKDD Explor. Newsl. 11(1), 10–18 (2009)
10. Hirst, G., St-Onge, D.: Lexical chains as representations of context for the detection and correction of malapropisms (1997)
11. Korkontzelos, I., Klapaftis, I., Man, S.: Graph connectivity measures for unsupervised parameter tuning of graph-based sense induction systems (2009)
12. Korkontzelos, I., Manandhar, S.: Detecting compositionality in multi-word expressions. In: Proceedings of the ACL-IJCNLP 2009 Conference Short Papers, ACLShort 2009, pp. 65–68. ACL (2009)
13. Krčmář, L., Ježek, K., Pecina, P.: Determining compositionality of word expressions using word space models. In: Proceedings of the 9th Workshop on Multiword Expressions, pp. 42–50. Association for Computational Linguistics, Atlanta (2013)
14. Kurc, R., Piasecki, M., Broda, B.: Constraint based description of polish multiword expressions. In: Proceedings of the Eight International Conference on Language Resources and Evaluation (LREC 2012). ELRA, Istanbul (2012)
15. Landis, J.R., Koch, G.G.: The Measurement of Observer Agreement for Categorical Data. Biometrics 33(1), 159–174 (1977)
16. Lin, D.: An information-theoretic definition of similarity. In: Proceedings of the Fifteenth International Conference on Machine Learning, ICML, pp. 296–304. Morgan Kaufmann Publishers Inc., San Francisco (1998)

17. Lyons, J.: Linguistic Semantics. Cambridge University Press (1995)
18. Maldonado-Guerra, A., Emms, M.: Measuring the compositionality of collocations via word co-occurrence vectors: Shared task system description. In: Proceedings of the Workshop on Distributional Semantics and Compositionality, pp. 48–53. ACL, Portland (2011)
19. Maziarz, M., Piasecki, M., Szpakowicz, S.: Approaching plWordNet 2.0. In: Fellbaum, C., Vossen, P. (eds.) Proceedings of 6th International Global Wordnet Conference, pp. 189–196. The Global WordNet Association, Matsue (2012)
20. McCarthy, D., Keller, B., Carroll, J.: Detecting a continuum of compositionality in phrasal verbs. In: Proc. of the ACL 2003 Workshop on Multiword Expressions: Analysis, Acquisition and Treatment, vol. 18, pp. 73–80. ACL (2003)
21. Pagin, P.: Is compositionality compatible with holism? Mind & Language 12, 11–33 (1997)
22. Pedersen, T.: Identifying collocations to measure compositionality: shared task system description. In: Proceedings of the Workshop on Distributional Semantics and Compositionality, DiSCo 2011, pp. 33–37. ACL, Stroudsburg (2011)
23. Piao, S.S., Rayson, P., Mudraya, O., Wilson, A., Garside, R.: Measuring mwe compositionality using semantic annotation. In: Proceedings of the Workshop on Multiword Expressions: Identifying and Exploiting Underlying Properties, pp. 2–11. ACL, Sydney (2006)
24. Piasecki, M., Szpakowicz, S., Broda, B.: A Wordnet from the Ground Up. Oficyna Wydawnicza Politechniki Wrocławskiej (2009)
25. Resnik, P.: Using information content to evaluate semantic similarity in a taxonomy. In: Proceedings of the 14th International Joint Conference on Artificial Intelligence, pp. 448–453 (1995)
26. Korpus rzeczpospolitej (1993-2002),
    http://www.cs.put.poznan.pl/dweiss/rzeczpospolita
27. Salehi, B., Cook, P.: Predicting the compositionality of multiword expressions using translations in multiple languages. In: *SEM, Proc. of the Main Conference and the Shared Task: Semantic Textual Similarity, vol. 1, pp. 266–275. ACL (2013)
28. Svensson, M.H.: A very complex criterion of fixedness: Non-compositionality, ch. 5, pp. 81–93. John Benjamins Publishing Company (2008)
29. Venkatapathy, S., Joshi, A.K.: Measuring the relative compositionality of verb-noun (v-n) collocations by integrating features. In: Proceedings of the Conference on Human Language Technology and Empirical Methods in Natural Language Processing, HLT 2005, pp. 899–906. ACL (2005)
30. Vincze, V., Nagy, T.I., Berend, G.: Detecting noun compounds and light verb constructions: a contrastive study. In: Workshop on Multiword Expressions: from Parsing and Generation to the Real World, MWE 2011, pp. 116–121. ACL (2011)

# Automatic Processing of Linguistic Data as a Feedback for Linguistic Theory

Vladislav Kuboň, Markéta Lopatková, and Jiří Mírovský

Charles University in Prague
Faculty of Mathematics and Physics
Institute of Formal and Applied Linguistics
{vk,lopatkova,mirovsky}@ufal.mff.cuni.cz

**Abstract.** The paper describes a method of identifying a set of interesting constructions in a syntactically annotated corpus of Czech – the Prague Dependency Treebank – by application of an automatic procedure of analysis by reduction to the trees in the treebank. The procedure clearly reveals certain linguistic phenomena that go beyond 'dependency nature' (and thus generally pose a problem for dependency-based formalisms). Moreover, it provides a feedback indicating that the annotation of a particular phenomenon might be inconsistent.

The paper contains discussion and analysis of individual phenomena, as well as the quantification of results of the automatic procedure on a subset of the treebank. The results show that a vast majority of sentences from the subset used in these experiments can be analyzed automatically and it confirms that most of the problematic phenomena belong to the language periphery.

## 1 Introduction

Gathering various kinds of linguistic resources has become one of the major activities of many linguists during the past twenty years.

One of the factors which substantially influence the quality of linguistic resources, is the annotation consistency. The annotation consistency is very difficult to maintain especially for large data resources. In the process of annotation, the annotators have to make a huge number of small decisions related especially to borderline phenomena or to phenomena from the language periphery. A series of such decisions may lead to an annotation which, when viewed from the outside, may look unnatural or inconsistent.

In this paper we try to tackle the problem of annotation correctness and consistency of a large scale linguistic resource with very detailed syntactic annotation. This resource, the Prague Dependency Treebank (PDT) [1], actually provided a feedback for the theory it has been based upon, namely the Functional Generative Description [2]. This interesting fact has been described esp. in [3]. Our investigation takes this problem one step further – it identifies phenomena which have been annotated in a problematic way. It provides the feedback to the annotation, not to the underlying theory directly (although some of the findings may have consequences for the theory itself).

F. Castro, A. Gelbukh, and M. González (Eds.): MICAI 2013, Part I, LNAI 8265, pp. 252–264, 2013.
© Springer-Verlag Berlin Heidelberg 2013

In our experiments we concentrate on the crucial relation for all dependency-based theories, the relation of dependency itself. We are going to define it through analysis by reduction (introduced in Section 2), a stepwise simplification of a sentence preserving its correctness [4, 5]. We want to gain better insight into the problem by means of the application of a semi-automatic procedure (requiring, of course, a subsequent manual checking) on a relatively large subset of PDT data. The results are presented in Section 4. In this way we can verify the concept against real data and, at the same time, shed more light on the way how individual linguistic phenomena are annotated.

## 1.1   The Background

In the world of dependency representation, there are three essential (and substantially different) syntactic relationships, namely 1. *dependencies* (the relationship between a governing and a modifying sentence member, as e.g. a verb and its object, or a noun and its attribute), 2. *'multiplication'* of two or more sentence members or clauses (esp. coordination), and 3. *word order* (i.e., the linear sequence of words in a sentence).[1] In this paper we are concentrating on the phenomenon 1. and 3, i.e., on the relationships of dependency and word order. These two basic syntactic relationships (dependency and word order) are relatively complex especially in languages with a higher degree of word order freedom.

Within dependency linguistics, these relationships have been previously studied especially within the Meaning-Text Theory: the approaches aiming at the determination of dependency relations and their formal description are summed up esp. in [7]. An alternative formal description of dependency syntax can be found in [8]. Our approach is based on the Czech linguistic tradition represented mainly in [2].

The second notion important for our experiments is the notion of an *analysis by reduction*. This notion helps to define the dependency relations: if, in the course of a stepwise reduction of a sentence, one of the words creating possible governor-modifier pair can be deleted without changing the distribution properties of the pair (i.e., the ability to appear in the same syntactic context) then it is considered as a modifying one (dependent on the latter one). This is applicable to endocentric constructions (as, e.g. *small table, Go home!*); for exocentric constructions (as *Peter met Mary*), the principle of analogy on the part-of-speech level is applied. Roughly speaking, as a sentence containing an intransitive verb is correct (*e.g., Peter sleeps*), an object is considered as dependent on a (transitive) verb as well; similarly for other types of objects as well as for a subject (as subject-less verbs exist in Czech, e.g., *Prší* '(It) rains'), see [2, 4].

The reason for exploiting the analysis by reduction is obvious: it allows for examining dependencies and word order independently. The method of AR has been described in detail in [4, 5], its formal modeling by means of restarting automata can be found in [9–11]. A brief description of its basic principles follows in Section 2.

---

[1] [6] considers linear order vs. structural order and also divides the structural relationships between connexion (now dependency) and junction (coordination).

## 2   Methodology – Analysis by Reduction

Let us now describe the main ideas behind the method used for sentence analysis. *Analysis by reduction (AR)* is based on a stepwise simplification of an analyzed sentence. It defines possible sequences of reductions (deletions) in the sentence – each step of AR is represented by *deleting* at least one word of the input sentence; in specific cases, deleting is accompanied by a *shift* of a word form to another word order position.

Let us stress the basic constraints imposed on the analysis by reduction, namely:

(i) the obvious constraint on preserving individual word forms, their morphological characteristics and/or their surface dependency relations;
(ii) the constraint on preserving the correctness (a grammatically correct sentence must remain correct after its simplification);
(iii) the application of the shift operation is limited to cases where it is enforced by the correctness preserving principle of AR.

Note that the possible order(s) of reductions reflect dependency relations between individual sentence members, as it is described in [5, 11]. The basic principles of AR can be illustrated on the following Czech sentence (1).

**Example**

(1)   *Marie   se   rozhodla   nepřijít.*
    Marie – *refl* – decided – not to come
    'Marie has decided not to come.'

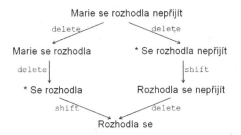

**Fig. 1.** Scheme of AR for sentence (1)

The analysis by reduction can be summarized in the scheme in Fig. 1. The sentence can be simplified in two ways:

(i) Either by simple deletion of the dependent infinitive verb *nepřijít* 'not to come' (see the left branch of the scheme).
(ii) Or by deleting the subject *Marie*[2] (the right part of the scheme). However, this simplification results in an incorrect word order variant starting with a clitic

---

[2] Note that Czech is a pro-drop (null-subject) language; thus it is possible to reduce a sentence subject (if present at all) at any moment and the sentence remains correct (if some word order constraint is not violated).

$se^3 \rightarrow_{shift}$ *Se rozhodla nepřijít*. Thus the word order has to be adjusted (by applying a shift) in order to preserve the syntactic correctness of the sentence: $\rightarrow_{shift}$ *Rozhodla se nepřijít*. '(She) decided not to come'.

Now, we can proceed in a similar way until we get the minimal correct simplified sentence *Rozhodla se*. 'She decided.'

We can notice that the order of reductions reflects the dependency relations in the corresponding dependency tree. Informally, the words are 'cut from the bottom of the tree'; i.e., a governing node must be preserved in a simplified sentence until all its dependent words are deleted, see [4]. In other words, AR corresponds to the dependency tree for sentence (1).

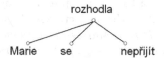

**Fig. 2.** Dependency tree of sentence (1); PDT-like (surface) syntactic annotation

**Projectivity.** The phenomenon of (non-)projectivity is one of very interesting and problematic language phenomena [14].[4] As a supplementary result, we are going to quantify how many sentences can be completely processed by a simple analysis by reduction (analysis by reduction with delete operation only). For this reason, we allow only for projective reductions. In other words, dependent word in a distant position cannot be deleted (with the only exception of limited technical non-projectivities caused, e.g., by prepositions).

The constraint allowing only projective reductions makes it possible to describe a core projective word order. It shows that – even within projective constructions – certain constraints on word order exist, esp. in connection with the position of clitics.

Let us demonstrate the processing of non-projective reductions on the following example (2) (based on [15], modified).

**Example**

(2)  *Petr   se   Marii   rozhodl   tu knihu   nekoupit.*
Petr – *refl* – to Mary – decided – the book – not to buy
'Petr has decided not to buy the book to Mary.'

The word *Marii* 'Mary' (indirect object of the verb *nekoupit* 'not to buy') cannot be reduced because it is 'separated' from its governing verb by the main predicate

---

[3] Czech has strict grammatical rules for clitics – roughly speaking, they are usually located on the sentence second (Wackernagel's) position, see esp. [12, 13]

[4] Informally, projective constructions meet the following constraint: having two words $n_{gov}$ and $n_{dep}$, the second one being dependent on the first one – then all words between these two words must also (transitively) depend on $n_{gov}$.

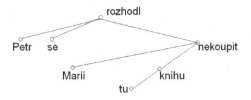

**Fig. 3.** Dependency tree of sentence (2)

*rozhodl* 'decided' (i.e., by the root of the dependency tree) and thus the relation *Marii – nekoupit* 'to Mary – not to buy' is represented by a non-projective edge in the dependency tree. Thus within the projective AR, a shift must be performed to make the reduction possible: *Petr se Marii rozhodl tu knihu nekoupit.* →$_{shift}$ *Petr se rozhodl Marii tu knihu nekoupit.* →$_{delete}$ *Petr se rozhodl tu knihu nekoupit.*

## 3   Semi-automatic Application of AR on the PDT Data

### 3.1   Data

For humans, especially for native speakers of a particular natural language, it is easy to apply the analysis by reduction, at least when simple sentences are concerned. However, this application exploits the fact that the human understands the sentence and that (s)he is naturally able to reduce the sentence step by step. When we are aiming at applying AR automatically, we have to 'substitute' (at least to some extent) the understanding using the syntactically annotated data (with subsequent manual correctness checking).

For our experiments we make use of the data from the Prague Dependency Treebank 2.0 (PDT, see [1]).[5] The syntactic structure – given by dependency trees (a single tree for a single sentence) – actually guided the process of AR.

The PDT contains very detailed annotation of almost 49,500 Czech sentences. The annotation is performed at multiple layers, out of which the analytical layer – describing (surface) syntactic structure employing so called analytical functions – is the most relevant for our experiments; we are taking into account only training data (38,727 sentences) (leaving the test set for evaluation in the future).

Investigating individual linguistic phenomena is easier if only simple sentences are taken into account. In the initial phase of our experiments, we concentrate on sentences which do not contain phenomena of obviously non-dependent character (esp. coordination, apposition, and parentheses). We also focus only on sentences with a single *finite verb* (and thus typically consisting of a single clause only). Note that even these sentences can have quite complex structure, including non-projectivities, see ex. (2).

For obtaining a suitable set of test sentences for AR as well as for searching the data, we exploit a PML-TQ search tool, which has been primarily designed

---

[5] http://ufal.mff.cuni.cz/pdt2.0/

for processing the PDT data. PML-TQ is a query language and search engine designed for querying annotated linguistic data [16], based on the TrEd toolkit [17]. TrEd with the PML-TQ extension allows users to formulate complex queries on richly annotated linguistic data.

This tool makes it possible to extract a subset of the corpus containing sentences with desired properties (we want to filter out sentences with too many phenomena), namely the sentence length limited to 10-25 tokens; no coordination and apposition nodes; no parentheses; just one finite verb; and no numerals.

Out of the 38,727 sentences of the training data of PDT, only 2,453 sentences remained after the application of this preprocessing filter. Although this number constitutes only 6.33% of the training set, it is still too big for manual inspection and it clearly shows the necessity of a semi-automatic method of applying AR to the data.

## 3.2   The Automatic Procedure

The automatization of the analysis by reduction requires a very careful approach. It is necessary to guarantee the correctness of the analyzed sentences in each step of the AR. The process is oriented bottom-up, it starts with the leaves of the dependency tree and it removes all dependent nodes stepwise, preserving one very important word-order condition, namely the condition that the neighboring nodes must always be removed first, followed by those which are connected by projective edges. The second very important condition is the *preservation of non-projectivity*. A node cannot be reduced if this reduction would result in some non-projective edge becoming projective, see sentence (2).

Let us now describe how individual linguistic phenomena are handled by the automatized AR.

**Arguments, Adjuncts and Attributes.** These categories are actually the simplest ones because they are the most regular ones. This group includes all nodes marked by analytical functions for attributes (Atr), adverbials (Adv), objects (Obj) and subjects (Sb). All these types of nodes can be reduced automatically, they represent the most natural dependency relationships.

**Prepositions.** This part of speech actually represents one of the most obvious examples of a phenomenon which is not naturally of a dependency nature. Prepositions typically serve as a kind of a morpho-syntactic feature of a noun (similarly as, e.g. a morphological case). However, many dependency-based theories and treebanks (including PDT) prefer to represent prepositions as governing nodes for the whole prepositional groups.

For our procedure it means that if a node is governed by a preposition (analytical function AuxP), it is necessary to reduce both nodes at once, in a single step. This has an important consequence: prepositions (AuxP) are also ignored when projectivity is tested – i.e., if the only source of a non-projective edge is a preposition, the sentence is treated as projective (this is justified by rather technical annotation of prepositions in PDT).

A special category of multiword prepositions is handled in a similar way – all words depending on the preposition (with the AuxP analytical function) are being ignored by AR until the governing preposition is being reduced – at this moment all the dependent words of the preposition are being reduced as well. For example, in the sentence *Byl zrušen s výjimkou programu.* 'It was cancelled with the exception of the program.' it is necessary to delete both the noun *programu* 'program' and the multiword preposition *s výjimkou* 'with (the) exception of' in one step. The sentence will then be reduced to *Byl zrušen.* '(It) was cancelled.'

**Comparison.** The constructions *čím – tím* (as in, e.g., *čím starší, tím lepší* 'the older the better') constitutes a very special case, which goes beyond the dependency nature of AR. For the time being, we skip sentences with this construction in our experiments.

Other types of comparisons, as, e.g., *než* 'than' (analytical function AuxC), *jako* 'as' (AuxY or AuxC combined with ellipsis marked ExD), do not cause any problems, they are always reduced together with their last child. Let us demonstrate this reduction on the sentence

**Example**

(3)  *Míra  nezaměstnanosti by    se    měla    vyvíjet    protikladně,*
     rate – unemployment – *cond* – *refl* – should – develop – opposite –
     *než    ve    standardní ekonomice.*
     than – in – standard – economy
     'The unemployment rate should develop in the opposite manner than in a standard economy.'

After deleting the adjective *standardní* 'standard', the stepwise reduction deletes within a single step of AR:
  – the noun *ekonomice* 'economy' (analytical function ExD)
  – together with the governing preposition *ve* 'in' (AuxP), and
  – the comma 'AuxX' (a node depending on *než* 'than' (AuxC) node;
  – further, the conjunction *než* 'than' (AuxC) is reduced.
Thus the reduced sentence *Míra nezaměstnanosti by se měla vyvíjet protikladně.* 'The unemployment rate should develop in the opposite manner.' is obtained. The reduction process may then continue further.

**Clitics.** Clitics have a relatively strictly defined position in grammatical Czech sentences – they must typically be located on a sentence second (Wackernagel's position) and thus they constitute a serious obstacle for our automatic procedure – they are reduced only together with their governing word, and, on top of that, no reduction may be performed which would leave a clitic on the sentence first position and thus make the reduced sentence ungrammatical.

Let us use the partially reduced sentence from the previous subsection as an example. It can be further reduced in several steps into → *Míra by se měla.* 'The rate should.' and no further, because reducing the subject *Míra* 'rate' would leave the clitics *by* and *se* in the sentence first position.

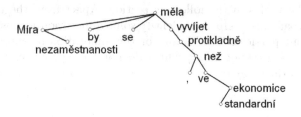

**Fig. 4.** Dependency tree of sentence (3)

**Particles.** Particles (AuxY) are in principle being reduced in a standard way (similarly as e.g. adverbials), it is only necessary to make sure that their reduction will not result in word order constraint violation. However, there is a special set of particles which constitute an exception – *coby, jako, jakoby, jakožto* 'as, like, as if' are being reduced together with their parent, similarly as in the case of comparison.

**Emphasizing Expressions.** If the word order permits it, emphasizing particles (AuxZ) can be reduced in the same way as, e.g., adverbials. If a prepositional group is involved in the emphasizing expression, it is reduced as a single unit. When checking the word order constraint, the nodes marked by AuxY (particles) are being ignored.

**Punctuation and Graphical Symbols.** Reduction of these symbols (AuxX, AuxG) can be applied when the governing word is being reduced, if the word order constraint permits it. Some problematic issues are caused by inconsistent treatment of expressions containing dashes or apostrophes (as, e.g., names like *Marie-Anne, Koh-i-noor, B-konto, Preud'homme* etc.) – these expressions clearly constitute a single unit, but they are not understood as such in some cases at the analytical layer of the treebank.

**Conjunctions.** A (subordinating) conjunction (AuxC) is reduced together with its last daughter node (which is not an emphasizing word (AuxZ), graphical symbol (AuxG) or punctuation itself (AuxX); if present, all these nodes are reduced, too). This simple rule may be used also due to the fact that sentences containing coordinations were left out from our sample set of sentences, their reduction may be more complicated when sentences with coordinations are included into the sample set in the future.

**Full Stop.** Sentence ending punctuation (AuxK) is always reduced as a final step of AR.

Note that in some cases, we do not insist on a complete reduction (with only the predicate left at the end). Even with the set of test sentences mentioned above and the uncomplete reductions, the automatic AR gives us interesting results – see the tables in the following section. Apart from the numerical results, this approach also helped to identify some annotation inconsistencies (for example the four particles listed above or the annotation of names containing special characters) or phenomena which do not have dependency nature and their annotation thus may cause technical problems (prepositions, some types of comparison, etc.).

# 4   Analysis of the Results of the Automatic Procedure

## 4.1   Quantitative Analysis of the Results

Let us now quantify and analyze the results of the automatic AR applied on the test sentences from the PDT. First of all, Table 1 provides numbers of sentences where specific problematic phenomena appear (from the complete set of the training data from PDT, i.e., from 38,727 sentences).

**Table 1.** Numbers of sentences with specific syntactic phenomena in PDT

|        | phenomenon |
|-------:|------------|
| 12,345 | sentences containing clitic(s); |
|        | out of which 3,244 non-projective |
| 850 | with the comparison or complement (AuxY or AuxC) introduced by *coby, jako, jakoby, jakožto*; |
|        | out of which 451 non-projective |
| 895 | with the comparison expressed by *než* (AuxC); |
|        | out of which 323 non-projective |
| 844 | with the comparison with ellipsis (ExD); |
|        | out of which 302 non-projective |
| 32 | with the comparison expressed by *čím – tím*; |
|        | out of which 17 non-projective |

Let us mention the reasons why we consider these phenomena problematic from the point of view of AR. First, clitics have a strictly specified position in a Czech sentence; thus they may cause a complex word order (including number of non-projective edges, see examples (1) and (2)). Second, a comparison (frequently accompanied by ellipses) has also complex and non-dependency character, as shown in example (3).

Let us now look at the results of simple (projective) reductions as described in the previous sections. The first column of Table 2 describes the number of nodes (= word forms) to which sentences were reduced; the second column gives the number of corresponding sentences and the third column gives their proportion with respect to the whole test set of 2,453 sentences.

We can see that our 'careful' automatic model of the simple AR (projective AR without shifts) can process almost 67% of the test set (plus 15.6% sentences are reduced into simple structures with 2 or 3 nodes). Note that (out of 2,453 test

**Table 2.** PDT – number of resulting nodes for analyzed sentences

| nodes | sentences | % | cumulative coverage |
|---|---|---|---|
| 1 | 1,640 | 66.86 | |
| 2 | 29 | 1.18 | 68.04 |
| 3 | 354 | 14.43 | 82.47 |
| 4 | 235 | 9.58 | 92.05 |
| 5 | 113 | 4.61 | 96.66 |
| 6 | 44 | 1.79 | 98.45 |
| 7 | 21 | 0.86 | 99.31 |
| 8 | 10 | 0.41 | 99.72 |
| 9 | 5 | 0.20 | 99.92 |
| 10 | 2 | 0.08 | 100.00 |

sentences), 282 sentences were non-projective (and thus cannot be fully reduced in the course of projective AR).

The results presented in Table 2 actually support the claim that the automatic procedure works surprisingly well given the complexity of the task. It is able to reduce more than 92% of input sentences to trees with 4 or less nodes. On top of that, it fails to reduce the tree (by a failure we understand the reduction to 7 or more nodes) in 1.6% of cases only.

## 4.2 Manual Analysis of the Results

After a manual analysis of the sentences that were reduced automatically to two nodes (29 in total), we can see that 23 sentences contain a clitic (dependent on the predicate), which prevents the full reduction; or an auxiliary verb (6 cases); or punctuation (1 case) (both auxiliary verbs and punctuation are represented as separate nodes in PDT). Further, 5 sentences which start with subordinating conjunction complete the list (as, e.g., → *Že rozeznáte* 'That (you) recognize'). The results for sentences that were reduced to 3 and 4 nodes, respectively, are shown in Table 3.

**Table 3.** PDT – the analysis of sentences reduced to 2, 3 and 4 nodes

| resulting in 1 node | resulting in 2 nodes | | phenomenon | | resulting in 3 nodes | | resulting in 4 nodes | |
|---|---|---|---|---|---|---|---|---|
| 1,640 | | 29 | # sentences | | | 354 | | 235 |
| – | 23 / | 0 | 1 clitic | / 2 clitics | 307 / | 3 | 149 / | 10 |
| 0 | 6 / | 1 | aux. verb | / punctuation | 74 / | 0 | 30 / | 2 |
| – | | – | 1 non-proj. | / 2 non-proj. | 37 / | – | 82 / | 2 |
| 0 | | 5 | others | | | 0 | | 0 |

In order to illustrate the most complicated cases, let us look at one sentence from the 'bottom' part of Table 2.

**Example**

(4)  *V ČR   se    využívá   v   menším   rozsahu   než    v zemích.*
    In CR– *refl* – is used – in – smaller – extent – than – in countries
    'In the Czech Republic it is used in a smaller extent than in countries.'

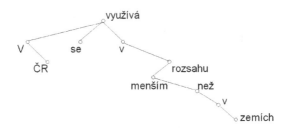

**Fig. 5.** Dependency tree for sentence (4)

In this case, 10 nodes remain as a result of the simple AR: The prepositional group *V ČR* 'In the Czech Republic' must be preserved in order to preserve correct position of the reflexive particle (clitic) *se*; further, the non-projective edge *menším–než* 'smaller–than' in the comparison ('separated' by the governing node *rozsahu* 'extent') stops the process of AR. So, as we can see, the sentence contains a complicated interplay of three phenomena – nonprojectivity, clitic and comparison, and thus constitutes a substantial challenge to the AR.

Let us now summarize the results from the point of view of language phenomena. Our experiments with the automatic AR have revealed that for the phenomena belonging to the language core (as, e.g., arguments, adjuncts and attributes) the AR works very smoothly (at this point it is important to remind that coordinations, appositions and parentheses were filtered out for this phase of our experiments). A vast majority of problems or irregularities is caused by the phenomena from language periphery (where, in many cases, the relations are not dependency-based and the syntactic structure is unclear).

The experiments also gave a feedback to the annotation of PDT – it has revealed that certain particles (with the analytical function of AuxY) which introduce comparison (lemmas *coby, jako, jakoby, jakožto* 'as, like, as if') behave in a completely different way than other nodes with the same analytical function. From the point of view of AR they have similar properties as the conjunctions *než* 'than', *jako* 'as' (which are annotated as AuxC). It is not clear why they have been annotated in this way and whether there are any reasons for this annotation, especially when the annotation manual of PDT does not give any answer to this question [18].

# Conclusion and Perspectives

In this paper we have tried to achieve a deeper insight into the phenomenon of dependency and its annotation. The investigation has been performed by means of a semi-automatic analysis of a subset of a large corpus. This analysis proved the consistency of the annotation of the majority of sentences from the selected subset of PDT on the one hand, on the other hand it also helped to identify problematic constructions and syntactic phenomena.

In the future we would like to continue the research by examining more complex sentences containing linguistic phenomena that have been left out in this initial experiment. The most natural phenomenon which causes serious problems to all dependency theories and which definitely requires further investigation, is coordination. It would also be interesting to develop a (semi-)automatic method for an optimal application of the shift operation that would allow for projectivization of processed sentences and their full reduction.

**Acknowledgments.** The research reported in this paper has been supported by the Czech Science Foundation GA CR, grant No. GA P202/10/1333 and partially grant No. GA P406/2010/0875. This work has been using language resources stored and/or distributed by the LINDAT-Clarin project of MŠMT (project LM2010013).

# References

1. Hajič, J., Panevová, J., Hajičová, E., Sgall, P., Pajas, P., Štěpánek, J., Havelka, J., Mikulová, M., Žabokrtský, Z., Ševčíková-Razímová, M.: Prague Dependency Treebank 2.0. LDC, Philadelphia (2006)
2. Sgall, P., Hajičová, E., Panevová, J.: The Meaning of the Sentence in Its Semantic and Pragmatic Aspects. Reidel, Dordrecht (1986)
3. Hajičová, E.: Corpus annotation as a test of a linguistic theory: The case of Prague Dependency Treebank, pp. 15–24. Franco Angeli, Milano (2007)
4. Lopatková, M., Plátek, M., Kuboň, V.: Modeling Syntax of Free Word-Order Languages: Dependency Analysis by Reduction. In: Matoušek, V., Mautner, P., Pavelka, T. (eds.) TSD 2005. LNCS (LNAI), vol. 3658, pp. 140–147. Springer, Heidelberg (2005)
5. Lopatková, M., Plátek, M., Sgall, P.: Towards a Formal Model for Functional Generative Description: Analysis by Reduction and Restarting Automata. The Prague Bulletin of Mathematical Linguistics 87, 7–26 (2007)
6. Tesnière, L.: Eléments de syntaxe structurale. Librairie C. Klincksieck, Paris (1959)
7. Mel'čuk, I.A.: Dependency in language. In: Proceedings of DepLing 2011, Barcelona, pp. 1–16 (2011)
8. Gerdes, K., Kahane, S.: Defining dependencies (and constituents). In: Proceedings of DepLing 2011, Barcelona, pp. 17–27 (2011)
9. Jančar, P., Mráz, F., Plátek, M., Vogel, J.: On monotonic automata with a restart operation. Journal of Automata, Languages and Combinatorics 4, 287–311 (1999)
10. Otto, F.: Restarting Automata. In: Reichel, H. (ed.) FCT 1995. LNCS, vol. 965, pp. 269–303. Springer, Heidelberg (1995)

11. Plátek, M., Mráz, F., Lopatková, M.: (In)Dependencies in Functional Generative Description by Restarting Automata. In: Proceedings of NCMA 2010, Wien, Austria, Österreichische Computer Gesellschaft. books@ocg.at, vol. 263, pp. 155–170 (2010)

12. Avgustinova, T., Oliva, K.: On the Nature of the Wackernagel Position in Czech. In: Formale Slavistik, pp. 25–47. Vervuert Verlag, Frankfurt am Main (1997)

13. Hana, J.: Czech Clitics in Higher Order Grammar. PhD thesis, The Ohio State University (2007)

14. Hajičová, E., Havelka, J., Sgall, P., Veselá, K., Zeman, D.: Issues of Projectivity in the Prague Dependency Treebank. The Prague Bulletin of Mathematical Linguistics 81, 5–22 (2004)

15. Holan, T., Kuboň, V., Oliva, K., Plátek, M.: On Complexity of Word Order. Les grammaires de dépendance – Traitement automatique des langues (TAL) 41, 273–300 (2000)

16. Pajas, P., Štěpánek, J.: System for Querying Syntactically Annotated Corpora. In: Proceedings of the ACL-IJCNLP 2009 Software Demonstrations, pp. 33–36. ACL, Singapore (2009)

17. Pajas, P., Štěpánek, J.: Recent Advances in a Feature-Rich Framework for Treebank Annotation. In: Proceedings of CoLING 2008, vol. 2, pp. 673–680. The Coling 2008 Organizing Committee, Manchester (2008)

18. Mikulová, M., Bémová, A., Hajič, J., Hajičová, E., Havelka, J., Kolářová, V., Kučová, L., Lopatková, M., Pajas, P., Panevová, J., Razímová, M., Sgall, P., Štěpánek, J., Urešová, Z., Veselá, K., Žabokrtský, Z.: Annotation on the tectogrammatical level in the Prague Dependency Treebank. Annotation manual. Technical Report 30, Prague, Czech Rep. (2006)

# Interval Semi-supervised LDA: Classifying Needles in a Haystack

Svetlana Bodrunova, Sergei Koltsov, Olessia Koltsova,
Sergey Nikolenko, and Anastasia Shimorina

Laboratory for Internet Studies (LINIS),
National Research University Higher School of Economics,
ul. Soyuza Pechatnikov, d. 16, 190008 St. Petersburg, Russia

**Abstract.** An important text mining problem is to find, in a large collection of texts, documents related to specific topics and then discern further structure among the found texts. This problem is especially important for social sciences, where the purpose is to find the most representative documents for subsequent qualitative interpretation. To solve this problem, we propose an interval semi-supervised LDA approach, in which certain predefined sets of keywords (that define the topics researchers are interested in) are restricted to specific intervals of topic assignments. We present a case study on a Russian LiveJournal dataset aimed at ethnicity discourse analysis.

**Keywords:** topic modeling, latent Dirichlet allocation, text mining.

## 1 Introduction

Many applications in social sciences are related to text mining. Researchers often aim to understand how a certain large body of text behaves: what topics interest the authors of this body, how these topics develop and interact, what are the key words that define these topics in the discourse and so on. Topic modeling approaches, usually based on some version of the LDA (latent Dirichlet allocation) model [1], are very important in this regard. Often, the actually interesting part of the dataset is relatively small, although it is still too large to be processed by hand and, moreover, it is unclear how to separate the interesting part from the rest of the dataset. Such an "interesting" part may be, for instance, represented by certain topics that are defined, but not limited to, certain relevant keywords (so that a simple search for these keywords would yield only a subset of the interesting part). In this short paper, we propose a method for identifying documents relevant to a specific set of topics that also extracts its topical structure based on a semi-supervised version of the LDA model. The paper is organized as follows. In Section 2, we briefly review the basic LDA model and survey related work concerning various extensions of the LDA model. In Section 3 we introduce two extensions: semi-supervised LDA that sets a single topic for each predefined set of key words and interval semi-supervised LDA that maps a set of keywords to an interval of topics. In Section 4, we present a case study of mining ethnical

F. Castro, A. Gelbukh, and M. González (Eds.): MICAI 2013, Part I, LNAI 8265, pp. 265–274, 2013.

discourse from a dataset of Russian LiveJournal blogs and show the advantages of the proposed approach; Section 5 concludes the paper.

## 2    The LDA Model and Extensions

### 2.1    LDA

The basic latent Dirichlet allocation (LDA) model [1,2] is depicted on Fig. 1a. In this model, a collection of $D$ documents is assumed to contain $T$ topics expressed with $W$ different words. Each document $d \in D$ is modeled as a discrete distribution $\theta^{(d)}$ over the set of topics: $p(z_w = j) = \theta^{(d)}$, where $z$ is a discrete variable that defines the topic for each word $w \in d$. Each topic, in turn, corresponds to a multinomial distribution over the words, $p(w \mid z_w = j) = \phi_w^{(j)}$. The model also introduces Dirichlet priors $\alpha$ for the distribution over documents (topic vectors) $\theta$, $\theta \sim \mathrm{Dir}(\alpha)$, and $\beta$ for the distribution over the topical word distributions, $\phi \sim \mathrm{Dir}(\beta)$. The inference problem in LDA is to find hidden topic variables $z$, a vector spanning all instances of all words in the dataset. There are two approaches to inference in the LDA model: variational approximations and MCMC sampling which in this case is convenient to frame as Gibbs sampling. In this work, we use Gibbs sampling because it generalizes easily to semi-supervised LDA considered below. In the LDA model, Gibbs sampling after easy transformations [2] reduces to the so-called *collapsed Gibbs sampling*, where $z_w$ are iteratively resampled with distributions

$$p(z_w = t \mid \mathbf{z}_{-w}, \mathbf{w}, \alpha, \beta) \propto$$

$$\propto q(z_w, t, \mathbf{z}_{-w}, \mathbf{w}, \alpha, \beta) = \frac{n_{-w,t}^{(d)} + \alpha}{\sum_{t' \in T} \left( n_{-w,t'}^{(d)} + \alpha \right)} \frac{n_{-w,t}^{(w)} + \beta}{\sum_{w' \in W} \left( n_{-w,t}^{(w')} + \beta \right)},$$

where $n_{-w,t}^{(d)}$ is the number of times topic $t$ occurs in document $d$ and $n_{-w,t}^{(w)}$ is the number of times word $w$ is generated by topic $t$, not counting the current value $z_w$.

### 2.2    Related Work: LDA Extensions

Over the recent years, the basic LDA model has been subject to many extensions; each of them presenting either a variational of a Gibbs sampling algorithm for a model that builds upon LDA to incorporate some additional information or additional presumed dependencies. Among the most important extensions we can list the following:

- *correlated topic models* (CTM) improve upon the fact that in the base LDA model, topic distributions are independent and uncorrelated, but, of course, some topics are closer to each other and share words with each other; CTM use logistic normal distribution instead of Dirichlet to model correlations between topics [3];

- *Markov topic models* use Markov random fields to model the interactions between topics in different parts of the dataset (different text corpora), connecting a number of different hyperparameters $\beta_i$ in a Markov random field that lets one subject these hyperparameters to a wide class of prior constraints [4];
- *relational topic models* construct a hierarchical model that reflects the structure of a document network as a graph [5];
- the *Topics over Time* model applies when documents have timestamps of their creation (e.g., news articles); it represents the time when topics arise in continuous time with a beta distribution [6];
- *dynamic topic models* represent the temporal evolution of topics through the evolution of their hyperparameters $\alpha$ and $\beta$, either with a state-based discrete model [7] or with a Brownian motion in continuous time [8];
- *supervised LDA* assigns each document with an additional response variable that can be observed; this variable depends on the distribution of topics in the document and can represent, e.g., user response in a recommender system [9];
- *DiscLDA* assumes that each document is assigned with a categorical label and attempts to utilize LDA for mining topic classes related to this classification problem [10];
- the *Author-Topic model* incorporates information about the author of a document, assuming that texts from the same author will be more likely to concentrate on the same topics and will be more likely to share common words [11, 12];
- finally, a lot of work has been done on nonparametric LDA variants based on Dirichlet processes that we will not go into in this paper; for the most important nonparametric approaches to LDA see [13–17] and references therein.

The extension that appears to be closest to the one proposed in this work is the *Topic-in-Set knowledge* model and its extension with Dirichlet forest priors [18,19]. In [19], words are assigned with "$z$-labels"; a $z$-label represents the topic this specific word should fall into; in this work, we build upon and extend this model.

## 3    Semi-supervised LDA and Interval Semi-supervised LDA

### 3.1    Semi-supervised LDA

In real life text mining applications, it often happens that the entire dataset $D$ deals with a large number of different unrelated topics, while the researcher is actually interested only in a small subset of these topics. In this case, a direct application of the LDA model has important disadvantages. Relevant topics may have too small a presence in the dataset to be detected directly, and one would need a very large number of topics to capture them in an unsupervised fashion.

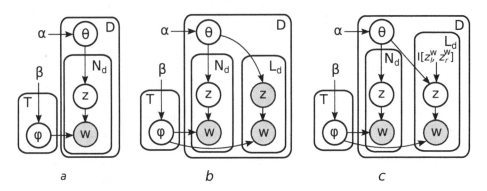

**Fig. 1.** Probabilistic models: (*a*) LDA; (*b*) semi-supervised LDA; (*c*) interval semi-supervised LDA

For a large number of topics, however, the LDA model often has too many local maxima, giving unstable results with many degenerate topics.

To find relevant subsets of topics in the dataset, we propose to use a semi-supervised approach to LDA, fixing the values of $z$ for certain key words related to the topics in question; similar approaches have been considered in [18, 19]. The resulting graphical model is shown on Fig. 1b. For words $w \in W_{\text{sup}}$ from a predefined set $W_{\text{sup}}$, the values of $z$ are known and remain fixed to $\tilde{z}_w$ throughout the Gibbs sampling process:

$$p(z_w = t \mid \boldsymbol{z}_{-w}, \boldsymbol{w}, \alpha, \beta) \propto \begin{cases} [t = \tilde{z}_w], & w \in W_{\text{sup}}, \\ q(z_w, t, \boldsymbol{z}_{-w}, \boldsymbol{w}, \alpha, \beta) & \text{otherwise}. \end{cases}$$

Otherwise, the Gibbs sampler works as in the basic LDA model; this yields an efficient inference algorithm that does not incur additional computational costs.

## 3.2   Interval Semi-supervised LDA

One disadvantage of the semi-supervised LDA approach is that it assigns only a single topic to each set of keywords, while in fact there may be more than one topics about them. For instance, in our case study (see Section 4) there are several topics related to Ukraine and Ukrainians in the Russian blogosphere, and artificially drawing them all together with the semi-supervised LDA model would have undesirable consequences: some "Ukrainian" topics would be cut off from the supervised topic and left without Ukrainian keywords because it is more likely for the model to cut off a few words even if they fit well than bring together two very different sets of words under a single topic.

Therefore, we propose to map each set of key words to *several* topics; it is convenient to choose a contiguous interval, hence *interval semi-supervised LDA* (ISLDA). Each key word $w \in W_{\text{sup}}$ is thus mapped to an interval $[z_l^w, z_r^w]$, and the probability distribution is restricted to that interval; the graphical model is shown on Fig. 1c, where $I[z_l^w, z_r^w]$ denotes the indicator function: $I[z_l^w, z_r^w](z) = 1$ iff $z \in [z_l^w, z_r^w]$. In the Gibbs sampling algorithm, we simply need to set the probabilities of all topics outside $[z_l^w, z_r^w]$ to zero and renormalize the distribution inside:

$$p(z_w = t \mid \mathbf{z}_{-w}, \mathbf{w}, \alpha, \beta) \propto \begin{cases} I[z_l^w, z_r^w](t) \frac{q(z_w, t, \mathbf{z}_{-w}, \mathbf{w}, \alpha, \beta)}{\sum_{z_l^w \leq t' \leq z_r^w} q(z_w, t', \mathbf{z}_{-w}, \mathbf{w}, \alpha, \beta)}, & w \in W_{\text{sup}}, \\ q(z_w, t, \mathbf{z}_{-w}, \mathbf{w}, \alpha, \beta) & \text{otherwise.} \end{cases}$$

Note that in other applications it may be desirable to assign intersecting subsets of topics to different words, say in a context when some words are more general or have homonyms with other meanings; this is easy to do in the proposed model by assigning a specific subset of topics $Z^w$ to each key word, not necessarily a contiguous interval. The Gibbs sampling algorithm does not change:

$$p(z_w = t \mid \mathbf{z}_{-w}, \mathbf{w}, \alpha, \beta) \propto \begin{cases} I[Z^w](t) \frac{q(z_w, t, \mathbf{z}_{-w}, \mathbf{w}, \alpha, \beta)}{\sum_{t' \in Z^w} q(z_w, t', \mathbf{z}_{-w}, \mathbf{w}, \alpha, \beta)}, & w \in W_{\text{sup}}, \\ q(z_w, t, \mathbf{z}_{-w}, \mathbf{w}, \alpha, \beta) & \text{otherwise.} \end{cases}$$

## 4 Mining Ethical Discourse

### 4.1 Case Study: Project Description

We have applied the method outlined above to a sociological project intended to study ethnical discourse in the Russian blogosphere. The project aims to analyze ethnically-marked discourse, in particular, find: (1) topics of discussion connected to ethnicity and their qualitative discursive interpretation; (2) ethnically-marked social milieus or spaces; (3) ethnically-marked social problems; (4) "just dangerous" ethnicities that would be surrounded by pejorative / stereotyped / fear-marked discourse without any particular reason for it evident from data mining. This study stems from constructivist research on inequalities in socio-economical development vs. ethnical diversity, ethnicities as social borders, and ethnicities as sources of moral panic [20–22]; our project goes in line with current research in mediated representations of ethnicity and ethnic-marked discourse [23–26].

The major issues in mediated representation of ethnicity may be conceptualized as criminalization of ethnicity, sensibilization of cultural difference and enhancing cultural stereotypes, problematization of immigration, reinforcement of negativism in image of ethnicities, unequal coverage of ethnic groups, labeling and boundary marking, and flawed connections of ethnicity with other major areas of social cleavages, e.g. religion. The approach needs to be both quantitative and qualitative; we need to be able to automatically mine existing topics from a large dataset and then qualitatively interpret these results. This led us to topic modeling, and ultimately to developing ISLDA for this project. Thus, the second aim of the project is methodological, as we realize that ethnic vocabulary may not show up as the most important words in the topics, and discursive significance of less frequent ethnonyms (like Tajik or Vietnamese) will be very low. As for the most frequent ethnonyms (in case of the Russian blogosphere, they include American, Ukranian, or German), our hypothesis was that they may provide varying numbers of discussion topics in the blogosphere, from 0 (no clear topics evident) up to 4 or 5 major topics, which are not always spotted by regular LDA.

## 4.2   Case Study Results and Discussion

In this section, we present qualitative results of the case study itself and compare LDA with ISLDA. In this case study, the dataset consisted of four months of LiveJournal posts written by 2000 top bloggers. In total, there were 235,407 documents in the dataset, and the dictionary, after cleaning stopwords and low frequency words, contained 192,614 words with about 53.5 million total instances of these words. We have performed experiments with different numbers of topics (50, 100, 200, and 400) for both regular LDA and Interval Semi-Supervised LDA.

Comparing regular LDA results for 100 and 400 topics, it is clear that ethnic topics need to be dug up at 400 rather than 100 topics. The share of ethnic topics was approximately the same: 9 out of 100 (9%) and 34 out of 400 (8.5%), but in terms of quality, the first iteration gives "too thick" topics like Great Patriotic war, Muslim, CEE countries, "big chess play" (great world powers and their roles in local conflicts), Russian vs. Western values, US/UK celebrities and East in travel (Japan, India, China and Korea). This does not provide us with any particular hints on how various ethnicities are treated in the blogosphere.

The 400-topic LDA iteration looks much more informative, providing topics of three kinds: event-oriented (e.g., death of Kim Jong-il or boycotting Russian TV channel NTV in Lithuania), current affairs oriented (e.g., armed conflicts in Libya and Syria or protests in Kazakh city Zhanaozen), and long-term topics. The latter may be divided into "neutral" descriptions of country/historic realities (Japan, China, British Commonwealth countries, ancient Indians etc.), long-term conflict topics (e.g., the Arab-Israeli conflict, Serb-Albanian conflict and the Kosovo problem), and two types of "problematized" topics: internal problems of a given country/nation (e.g., the U.S.) and "Russia vs. another country/region" topics (Poland, Chechnya, Ukraine). There are several topics of particular interest for the ethnic case study: a topic on Tajiks, two opposing topics on Russian nationalism ("patriotic" and "negative"), and a Tatar topic. Several ethnicities, e.g., Americans, Germans, Russians, and Arabs, were subject of more than one topic.

In ISLDA results, the 100-topic modeling covered the same ethnic topics as regular LDA, but Ukrainian ethnonyms produced a new result discussed below. 400-topic ISLDA gave a result much better than regular LDA. For ex-Soviet ethnicities (Tajik and Georgian), one of two pre-assigned topics clearly showed a problematized context. For Tajiks, it was illegal migration: the word collection also showed the writers from opposing opinion camps (Belkovsky, Kholmogorov, Krylov) and vocabulary characteristic of opinion media texts. For Georgians, the context of the Georgian-Ossetian conflict of 2008 clearly showed up, enriched by current events like election issues in South Ossetia. French and Ukrainian, both assigned 4 topics, showed good results. France had all topics more or less clearly connected to distinctive topics: a Mediterranean topic, Patriotic wars in Russia (with France and Germany), the current conflict in Lybia and general history of Europe. Here, we see that topics related to current affairs are easily de-aligned from long-term topics.

In general, we have found that ISLDA results have significant advantages over regular LDA. Most importantly, ISLDA finds *new important topics* related to the chosen semi-supervised subjects. As an example, Table 1 shows topics from our runs with 100 and 400 topics related to Ukraine. In every case, there is a strong topic related to Ukrainian politics, but then differences begin. In the 100 topic case (Figs. 1a and 1c), ISLDA distinguishes a Ukrainian nationalist topic (very important for our study) that was lost on LDA. With 400 topics (Figs. 1b and 1d), LDA finds virtually the same topics, while ISLDA finds three new important topics: scandals related to Russian natural gas transmitted through Ukraine, a topic devoted to Crimea, and again the nationalist topic (this time with a Western Ukrainian spin). The same pattern appears for other ethnical subjects in the dataset: ISLDA produces more informative topics on the specified subjects.

As for numerical evaluation of modeling results, we have computed the held-out perplexity on two test sets of 1000 documents each; i.e., we estimated the value of

$$p(\mathbf{w} \mid D) = \int p(\mathbf{w} \mid \Phi, \alpha\mathbf{m})p(\Phi, \alpha\mathbf{m} \mid D)d\alpha d\Phi$$

for each held-out document $\mathbf{w}$ and then normalized the result as

$$\text{perplexity}(D_{\text{test}}) = \exp\left(-\frac{\sum_{\mathbf{w} \in D_{\text{test}}} \log p(\mathbf{w})}{\sum_{\mathbf{w} \in D_{\text{test}}} N_d}\right).$$

To compute $p(\mathbf{w} \mid D)$, we used the left-to-right algorithm proposed and recommended in [27, 28]. The test sets were separate datasets of blog posts from the same set of authors and around the same time as the main dataset; the first test set $D_{\text{test}}$ contained general posts while the second, $D_{\text{test}}^{\text{key}}$, was comprised of posts that contain at least one of the key words used in ISLDA. Perplexity results are shown in Table 2; it is clear that perplexity virtually does not suffer in ISLDA, and there is no difference in the perplexity between the keyword-containing test set and the general test set. This indicates that ISLDA merely brings the relevant topics to the surface of the model and does not in general interfere with the model's predictive power.

For further sociological studies directed at specific issues, we recommend to use ISLDA with the number of preassigned topics (interval sizes) chosen *a priori* larger than the possible number of relevant topics: in our experiments, we saw that extra slots are simply filled up with some unrelated topics and do not deteriorate the quality of relevant topics. However, the results begin to deteriorate if more than about 10% of all topics (e.g., 40 out of 400) are assigned to the semi-supervised part; one always needs to have sufficient "free space" to fill with other topics. This provides a certain tension that may be resolved with further study (see below).

**Table 1.** A comparison of LDA topics related to Ukraine: (a) LDA, 100 topics; (b) LDA, 400 topics; (c) ISLDA, 100 topics; (d) ISLDA, 400 topics

| | | | | | | | |
|---|---|---|---|---|---|---|---|
| (a) | Ukraine 0.043 | Ukraine 0.049 | | | | | |
| | Ukrainian 0.029 | Ukrainian 0.017 | | | | | |
| | Polish 0.012 | Timoshenko 0.015 | | | | | |
| | Belorussian 0.011 | Yanukovich 0.015 | | | | | |
| | Poland 0.011 | Victor 0.012 | | | | | |
| | Belarus 0.010 | president 0.012 | | | | | |
| (b) | Ukraine 0.098 | Ukraine 0.054 | dragon 0.026 | | | | |
| | Ukrainian 0.068 | Timoshenko 0.019 | Kiev 0.022 | | | | |
| | Belorussian 0.020 | Yanukovich 0.018 | Bali 0.012 | | | | |
| | Belarus 0.018 | Ukrainian 0.016 | house 0.010 | | | | |
| | Kiev 0.018 | president 0.015 | place 0.006 | | | | |
| | Kievan 0.012 | Victor 0.013 | work 0.006 | | | | |
| (c) | Ukraine 0.065 | Ukraine 0.062 | Ukrainian 0.040 | Crimea 0.046 | | | |
| | gas 0.030 | Timoshenko 0.023 | Ukraine 0.036 | Crimean 0.015 | | | |
| | Europe 0.026 | Ukrainian 0.022 | Polish 0.021 | Sevastopol 0.015 | | | |
| | Russia 0.019 | Yanukovich 0.018 | Poland 0.017 | Simferopol 0.008 | | | |
| | Ukrainian 0.018 | Kiev 0.015 | year 0.009 | Yalta 0.008 | | | |
| | Belorussian 0.018 | Victor 0.014 | L'vov 0.006 | source 0.007 | | | |
| | Belarus 0.017 | president 0.013 | Western 0.005 | Orjonikidze 0.005 | | | |
| | European 0.015 | party 0.013 | cossack 0.005 | . sea 0.005 | | | |
| (d) | Ukraine 0.065 | Ukraine 0.062 | Ukrainian 0.040 | Crimea 0.046 | | | |
| | gas 0.030 | Timoshenko 0.023 | Ukraine 0.036 | Crimean 0.015 | | | |
| | Europe 0.026 | Ukrainian 0.022 | Polish 0.021 | Sevastopol 0.015 | | | |
| | Russia 0.019 | Yanukovich 0.018 | Poland 0.017 | Simferopol 0.008 | | | |
| | Ukrainian 0.018 | Kiev 0.015 | year 0.009 | Yalta 0.008 | | | |
| | Belorussian 0.018 | Victor 0.014 | L'vov 0.006 | source 0.007 | | | |
| | Belarus 0.017 | president 0.013 | Western 0.005 | Orjonikidze 0.005 | | | |
| | European 0.015 | party 0.013 | cossack 0.005 | sea 0.005 | | | |

**Table 2.** Held-out perplexity results

| # of topics | Perplexity, LDA | | Perplexity, ISLDA | |
|---|---|---|---|---|
| | $D_{\text{test}}$ | $D_{\text{test}}^{\text{key}}$ | $D_{\text{test}}$ | $D_{\text{test}}^{\text{key}}$ |
| 100 | 12.7483 | 12.7483 | 12.7542 | 12.7542 |
| 200 | 12.7457 | 12.7457 | 12.7485 | 12.7486 |
| 400 | 12.6171 | 12.6172 | 12.6216 | 12.6216 |

# 5  Conclusion

In this work, we have introduced the Interval Semi-Supervised LDA model (ISLDA) as a tool for a more detailed analysis of a specific set of topics inside a larger dataset and have showed an inference algorithm for this model based on collapsed Gibbs sampling. With this tool, we have described a case study in ethnical discourse analysis on a dataset comprised of the Russian LiveJournal blogs. We show that topics relevant to the subject of study do indeed improve in the ISLDA analysis and recommend ISLDA for further use in sociological studies of the blogosphere.

For further work, note that the approach outlined above requires the user to specify how many topics are assigned to each keyword. We have mentioned that there is a tradeoff between possibly losing interesting topics and breaking the model up by assigning too many topics in the semi-supervised part; in the current model, we can only advise to experiment until a suitable number of semi-supervised topics is found. Therefore, we propose an interesting open problem: develop a nonparametric model that chooses the number of topics in each semi-supervised cluster of topics separately and also chooses separately the rest of the topics in the model.

**Acknowledgements.** This work was done at the Laboratory for Internet Studies, National Research University Higher School of Economics (NRU HSE), Russia, and partially supported by the Basic Research Program of NRU HSE. The work of Sergey Nikolenko was also supported by the Russian Foundation for Basic Research grant 12-01-00450-a and the Russian Presidential Grant Programme for Young Ph.D.'s, grant no. MK-6628.2012.1.

# References

1. Blei, D.M., Ng, A.Y., Jordan, M.I.: Latent Dirichlet allocation. Journal of Machine Learning Research 3(4-5), 993–1022 (2003)
2. Griffiths, T., Steyvers, M.: Finding scientific topics. Proceedings of the National Academy of Sciences 101 (suppl. 1), 5228–5335 (2004)
3. Blei, D.M., Lafferty, J.D.: Correlated topic models. Advances in Neural Information Processing Systems 18 (2006)
4. Li, S.Z.: Markov Random Field Modeling in Image Analysis. Advances in Pattern Recognition. Springer (2009)
5. Chang, J., Blei, D.M.: Hierarchical relational models for document networks. Annals of Applied Statistics 4(1), 124–150 (2010)
6. Wang, X., McCallum, A.: Topics over time: a non-Markov continuous-time model of topical trends. In: Proceedings of the 12th ACM SIGKDD International Conference on Knowledge Discovery and Data Mining, pp. 424–433. ACM, New York (2006)
7. Blei, D.M., Lafferty, J.D.: Dynamic topic models. In: Proceedings of the 23rd International Conference on Machine Learning, pp. 113–120. ACM, New York (2006)
8. Wang, C., Blei, D.M., Heckerman, D.: Continuous time dynamic topic models. In: Proceedings of the 24th Conference on Uncertainty in Artificial Intelligence (2008)

9. Blei, D.M., McAuliffe, J.D.: Supervised topic models. Advances in Neural Information Processing Systems 22 (2007)

10. Lacoste-Julien, S., Sha, F., Jordan, M.I.: DiscLDA: Discriminative learning for dimensionality reduction and classification. In: Advances in Neural Information Processing Systems, vol. 20 (2008)

11. Rosen-Zvi, M., Griffiths, T., Steyvers, M., Smyth, P.: The author-topic model for authors and documents. In: Proceedings of the 20th Conference on Uncertainty in Artificial Intelligence, pp. 487–494. AUAI Press, Arlington (2004)

12. Rosen-Zvi, M., Chemudugunta, C., Griffiths, T., Smyth, P., Steyvers, M.: Learning author-topic models from text corpora. ACM Trans. Inf. Syst. 28, 1–38 (2010)

13. Teh, Y.W., Jordan, M.I., Beal, M.J., Blei, D.M.: Hierarchical Dirichlet processes. Journal of the American Statistical Association 101(476), 1566–1581 (2004)

14. Blei, D.M., Jordan, M.I., Griffiths, T.L., Tennenbaum, J.B.: Hierarchical topic models and the nested chinese restaurant process. Advances in Neural Information Processing Systems 13 (2004)

15. Teh, Y.W., Jordan, M.I., Beal, M.J., Blei, D.M.: Sharing clusters among related groups: Hierarchical Dirichlet processes. Advances in Neural Information Processing Systems 17, 1385–1392 (2005)

16. Williamson, S., Wang, C., Heller, K.A., Blei, D.M.: The IBP compound Dirichlet process and its application to focused topic modeling. In: Proceedings of the 27th International Conference on Machine Learning, pp. 1151–1158 (2010)

17. Chen, X., Zhou, M., Carin, L.: The contextual focused topic model. In: Proceedings of the 18th ACM SIGKDD International Conference on Knowledge Discovery and Data Mining, pp. 96–104. ACM, New York (2012)

18. Andrzejewski, D., Zhu, X., Craven, M.: Incorporating domain knowledge into topic modeling via Dirichlet forest priors. In: Proc. 26th Annual International Conference on Machine Learning, ICML 2009, pp. 25–32. ACM, New York (2009)

19. Andrzejewski, D., Zhu, X.: Latent Dirichlet allocation with topic-in-set knowledge. In: Proc. NAACL HLT 2009 Workshop on Semi-Supervised Learning for Natural Language Processing, SemiSupLearn 2009, pp. 43–48. Association for Computational Linguistics, Stroudsburg (2009)

20. Barth, F.: Introduction. In: Barth, F. (ed.) Ethnic Groups and Boundaries: The Social Organization of Culture Difference, pp. 9–38. George Allen and Unwin, London (1969)

21. Hechter, M.: Internal colonialism: the Celtic fringe in British national development, pp. 1536–1966. Routledge & Kegan Paul, London (1975)

22. Hall, S.: Ethnicity: Identity and difference. Radical America 23(4), 9–22 (1991)

23. Voltmer, K.: The Media in Transitional Democracies. Polity, Cambridge (2013)

24. Nyamnjoh, F.B.: Africa's Media, Democracy and the Politics of Belonging. Zed Books, London (2005)

25. ter Wal, J. (ed.): Racism and cultural diversity in the mass media: An overview of research and examples of good practice in the EU member states, 1995-2000, pp. 1995–2000. European Monitoring Centre on Racism and Xenofobia, Vienna (2002)

26. Downing, J.D.H., Husbands, C.: Representing Race: Racisms, Ethnicity and the Media. Sage, London (2005)

27. Wallach, H.M., Murray, I., Salakhutdinov, R., Mimno, D.: Evaluation methods for topic models. In: Proceedings of the 26th International Conference on Machine Learning, pp. 1105–1112. ACM, New York (2009)

28. Wallach, H.M.: Structured topic models for language. PhD thesis, University of Cambridge (2008)

# A Reverse Dictionary Based on Semantic Analysis Using WordNet

Oscar Méndez, Hiram Calvo, and Marco A. Moreno-Armendáriz

Centro de Investigación en Computación - Instituto Politécnico Nacional
Av. Juan de Dios Bátiz, 07738, Distrito Federal, México
`omendez_a12@sagitario.cic.ipn.mx`

**Abstract.** In this research we present a new approach for reverse dictionary creation, one purely semantic. We focus on a semantic analysis of input phrases using semantic similarity measures to represent words as vectors in a semantic space previously created assisted by WordNet. Then, applying algebraic analysis we select a sample of candidate words which passes through a filtering process and a ranking phase. Finally, a predefined number of output target words are displayed. A test set of 50 input concepts was created in order to evaluate our system, comparing our experimental results against OneLook Reverse Dictionary to demonstrate that our system provides better results over current available implementations.

**Keywords:** reverse dictionary, semantic analysis, search by concept, vector space model.

## 1 Introduction

Over the years, people have used dictionaries for two well-defined purposes. Both of them are reflected on the dictionary's definition that is a collection of words listed alphabetically in a specific language, which contains their usage informations, definitions, etymologies, phonetics, pronunciations, and other linguistic features; or a collection of words in one language with their equivalents in another, also known as a lexicon. When these different ideas come together we understand why this resource hasn't lost importance and continue to be widely used around the world.

As part of the technological evolution the world has experienced during the last years, dictionaries are now available in electronic format. This resource has different advantages over the traditional printed dictionary, being the most important the easy access that it allows users and the very fast response time. Lexicographers constantly improve this resource, in order to assist language users, by increasing the number of words defined in the dictionary and adding lots more information associated with each one of them. Its performance is simple, just mapping words to their definitions, i.e. it does a lookup based on the correct spelling of the input word to find the definition.

F. Castro, A. Gelbukh, and M. González (Eds.): MICAI 2013, Part I, LNAI 8265, pp. 275–285, 2013.

This traditional approach is really helpful mostly for readers and language students, but isn't good enough taking into account the perspective of people who produce language. We all have experienced the problem of being unable to express a word that represents an idea in our mind although we are conscious of related terms, a partial description, even the definition. This may be due to a lack of knowledge in the word's meaning or a recall problem. People mainly affected by this problem are writers, speakers, students, scientists, advertising professionals, among others. For them, traditional dictionary searches are often unsuccessful because these kind of search demands an exact input, while a language producer tends to require a reverse search where the input are a group of words forming a formal definition or just a series of related terms, and the output is a target word.

The need for a different search access mode in a dictionary led to the creation of a reverse dictionary. Its basic objective is to retrieve a target word when a group of words which appear in its definition are entered. In other words, given a phrase describing a desired concept or idea, the reverse dictionary provides words whose definitions match the entered phrase. The chances of giving an exact definition of a concept is very difficult so synonym words or related words could also be considered during the search.

In this research we developed a new method to generate a reverse dictionary based on a large lexical English database known as WordNet and the implementation of different semantic similarity measures which help us in the generation of a semantic space.

## 2    State of the Art

Only three printed reverse dictionaries exist for English language. The reason is probably the complexity of its elaboration, especially the fact of choosing the proper form to distribute the information. The Bernstein's Reverse Dictionary [4] was the first of its kind, in this book, the definitions of 13,390 words were reduced to their most brief form and then ordered alphabetically.

With the availability of dictionaries in electronic format, the interest for a reverse lookup application has been growing during the last years. Unlike printed versions, several attempts have been made in the creation of the reverse lookup method seeking for the best performance.

In the reverse electronic dictionary presented in [7], synonyms were used to expand search capabilities. They create a dictionary database with words numerically encoded for quick and easy access; adding also synonym group numeric codes in order to extend the searching process. In every search the numeric codes of the input words are found and stored. Then, main entry words having the numeric codes of the input words within their definitions are located and displayed as output candidates.

The magnitude of this natural language application is appreciated when dictionaries for different languages are constructed like [5]. For this Japanese reverse dictionary three different databases were created, using traditional IR concepts. Each database stored all dictionary words (EDR, 1995) with their definitions as vectors, reflecting the term frequencies in each definition, with standard similarity metrics values (tf-idf, tf, binary values) as its elements. The reverse lookup method is separated in two stages. First, they parse the input concept with a morphological analyzer and create its vector, and then compare to the definition vectors to obtain the closest matching concept in the dictionary. To calculate the similarity between vectors they used cosine measure.

A different reverse lookup method was created in [8]. Their algorithm for French language does a reverse search using two main mechanisms. The first one extracts sets of words, from their lexical database of French words, which delimit the search space. For example, in the definition 'a person who sells food' the algorithm extracts all the sets of persons. The second mechanism computes a semantic distance between each candidate word in the extracted sets and the input definition to rank the output words. This latter value is based on the distances in the semantic graph, generated by their database, between hypernyms and hyponyms of the words being analyzed.

Another proposal was based on the notion of association: every idea, concept or word is connected [14]. Given a concept (system input) and following the links (associations) between input members, a target word would be reached. They proposed a huge semantic network composed of nodes (words and concepts) and links (associations), with either being able to activate the other.

In [15] the reverse lookup method depends on an association matrix composed of target words and their access keys (definition elements, related concepts). Two different sources were selected as corpus for the databases: WordNet and Wikipedia. The one based on WordNet used as target words the words defined in the dictionary and as access keys their definitions. The corpus based on Wikipedia used the page's raw text as target words (after a filtering process) and the words co-occurrences within a given window of specific size as access keys. Finally for every input phrase, their members are identified and the reverse search results in a list of words whose vectors contain the same input terms.

The most recent reverse dictionary application we found is shown in [12]. To construct their database they created for every relevant term $t$ in the dictionary its Reverse Mapping Set (RMS) which requires finding all words in whose definition relevant term $t$ appears. For every input phrase a stemming process is required, then a comparison is made between the input and the RMS looking for the words whose definitions contain the input members; this generates a group of candidates that pass through a ranking phase based on similarity values computed using a similarity measure implemented on WordNet and a parser.

The systems presented above share different methodological features. All of them consider not only the terms extracted from the user input phrase, but also terms similar or related to them (synonyms, hyponyms, hyperyms) and also needed a previous dictionary processing in order to form their databases. The reverse search done by [7] [14] [15] and [12] at some point of its procedure does a comparison between the user input phrase to every definition in their databases looking for definitions containing the same words as the user input phrase, while [8] and [5] based their reverse search on the highest similarity values measuring graph distances and cosine respectively. All of this demonstrates a tendency during reverse lookup algorithms creation until now.

Our proposal presents a new approach for reverse dictionary creation, one purely semantic. We focus on a semantic analysis of input phrases using semantic similarity measures to represent words as vectors in a semantic space previously created assisted by WordNet. Then, applying algebraic analysis we select a sample of candidate words which passes through a filtering process and a ranking phase. Finally, a predefined number of output target words are displayed. It's important to mention that this project considers only nouns as word members of the semantic space, this part of speech restriction is due to the form in which vectors are constructed and the fact that it's only possible to calculate semantic similarity or semantic relatedness with words that belong to the same part of speech. Besides, it is well known that in natural language, concepts are expressed mostly as noun phrases [13].

## 3   WordNet as a Resource for Semantic Analysis

WordNet is a large lexical database for English and other languages. It groups words into sets of synonyms called synsets and describes relations between them. Lexical relations hold between word forms and semantic relations hold between word meanings.

The structure of word strings in WordNet specifies a specific sense of a specific word as shown below; this is used to avoid word sense disambiguation problems:

$$word\#pos\#sense$$

where pos is the part of speech of the word and its sense is represented by an integer number.

WordNet has a hierarchical semantic organization of its words, also called by computer scientists as "inheritance system" because of the inherited information that specific items (hyponyms) get from their superordinates. There are two forms to construe the hierarchical principle. The first one considers all nouns are contained in a single hierarchy. The second one proposes the partition of the nouns with a set of semantic primes representing the most generic concepts and unique beginners of different hierarchies [11]. To create WordNet's semantic space this project makes use of the second form and 25 top concepts were defined as semantic primes to represent the dimensions of word vectors.

The top concepts, with its specific sense, that were chosen are:

activity#n#1, animal#n#1 artifact#n#1, attribute#n#2, body#n#1, cognition#n#1, communication#n#2, event#n#1, feeling#n#1, food#n#1, group#n#1, location#n#1, motive#n#1, natural_object#n#1, natural_phenomenon#n#1, human_ being#n#1, plant#n#2, possession#n#2, process#n#6, quantity#n#1, relation#n#1, shape#n#2, state#n#1, substance#n#1, time#n#5

This is also the order given to the top concepts during the vector representation of words mentioned further on.

WordNet also includes the implementation of similarity and relatedness measures. A semantic relatedness measure uses all WordNet's relations for its calculation meanwhile a semantic similarity measure only uses the hyponymy relation. Three measures were considered for database construction: Jiang and Conrath (JCN) [9], Lin [10] and the Lesk algorithm (Lesk) [2]. The first two are similarity measures which have demonstrated to have a good performance among other measures that use WordNet as their knowledge source [6]; the last one is an adaptation of the original Lesk relatedness measure that take advantage of WordNet's resources [1].

Jiang and Conrath: this measure combines the edge-based notion with the information content approach. It calculates the conditional probability of encountering an instance of a child-synset given an instance of a parent synset, specifically their lowest super-ordinate (lso). The formula is expressed in 1.

$$dist_{JCN}(c_1, c_2) = 2\log(p(lso(c_1, c_2))) - (\log(p(c_1)) + \log(p(c_2))) \tag{1}$$

Lin: based on his similarity theorem: "The similarity between A and B is measured by the ratio between the amount of information needed to state the commonality of A and B and the information needed to fully describe what A and B are." It uses the same elements of JCN measure but in a different way. The formula is expressed in 2.

$$sim_{LIN}(c_1, c_2) = \frac{2\log p(lso(c_1, c_2))}{\log p(c_1) + \log p(c_2)} \tag{2}$$

Lesk: the original algorithm measures the relatedness between two words by the overlap between their corresponding definitions as provided by a dictionary. Basically the steps are:

1. Retrieve from an electronic dictionary all sense definitions of the words to be measured.
2. Determine the definition overlap for all possible sense combinations.
3. Choose senses that lead to highest overlap.

In WordNet an extended gloss overlap measure is available, which combines the advantages of gloss overlaps with the structure of a concept hierarchy to create an extended view of relatedness between synsets [1].

## 4    Semantic Space Construction

In this section we describe the construction process of the semantic space that contains the numeric representation of all WordNet's nouns as vectors of 25 dimensions determined by the top concepts mentioned before. For every noun we create its vector measuring semantic similarity between the word and each top concept, then it is stored in the semantic space. After reading and creating the vectors for every noun, the process ends. This procedure is detailed in Figure 1.

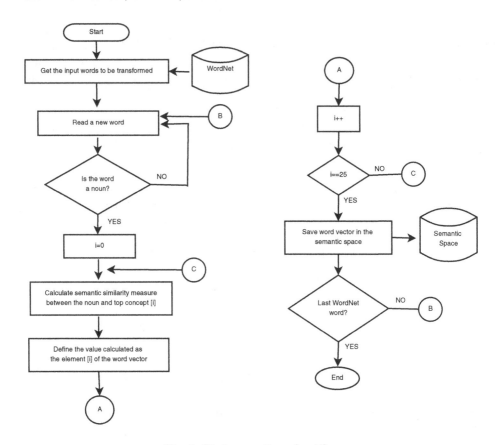

**Fig. 1.** Vector creation algorithm

The process was repeated for each of the different measures mentioned above, resulting on a semantic space with JCN measured vectors, another with Lin measured vectors, and the last one with Lesk measured vectors.

With the databases created, a normalization procedure was performed. For all word vectors maximum values of each dimensions were obtained in order to subsequently divide all word vectors dimensions by each respective maximum value previously obtained. Finally we have word vectors inside the semantic space with this form:

Genius → 0.05748, 0.04058, 0.09603, 0.06138, 0.06117, 0.04774, 0.07306, 0.02822, 0.06301, 0.07750, 0.05024, 0.05693, 0.03530, 0.12316, 0.01008, 0.01046, 0.00898, 0.05117, 0.03144, 0.05603, 0.04203, 0.07932, 0.03364, 0.02163, 0.07081

## 5    Search-by-Concept Process

A reverse dictionary receives a definition as input and gets a word that represents that concept as output. The search-by-concept dictionary proposed in this project is based on this principle.

The system input consists of a concept formed of $n$ nouns. Once the input is defined, the system looks for the word vectors of their $n$ components in the database and calculates their average. This gives as a result a new vector that should be located in the semantic space representing the word that combines all the characteristics given on the input concept. Regardless of whether the new vector already exists in the semantic space representing a word, a sample of twelve neighbor vectors is taken. This sample selection considers two parameters:

1. The euclidean distance value between vectors need to be:

   (a) For JCN less than 0.1
   (b) For Lin less than 0.8
   (c) For LSK less than 0.1

   These threshold values were determined after numerous testing. For vectors with euclidean distances bigger than the values mentioned above, the words they represented tend to have no relationship with the input concepts.

2. The product of the semantic similarity measure between each member of the input and the word represented by the neighbor vector is calculated; the top $n$ words with the highest values are chosen to form the system output.

# 6    Results

Before showing some results, a complete example for JCN semantic space is shown below:

```
Input concept - gym_shoe#n#1 athletic_contest#n#1 race#n#2

gym_shoe#n#1 ->
0.05383, 0.03492, 0.11093, 0.05720, 0.05738, 0.04458, 0.06833, 0.02628,
0.05933, 0.07286, 0.04694, 0.05249, 0.03347, 0.11451, 0.00944, 0.00927,
0.00782, 0.04819, 0.02938, 0.05237, 0.03932, 0.07490, 0.03153, 0.02020,
0.06700

athletic_contest#n#1 ->
0.08950, 0.03136, 0.07729, 0.07229, 0.05214, 0.06832, 0.08528, 0.04630,
0.07227, 0.07297, 0.05879, 0.04805, 0.04601, 0.10280, 0.00946, 0.00849,
0.00708, 0.05869, 0.02943, 0.06550, 0.04902, 0.09036, 0.02934, 0.02281,
0.08023

race#n#2 ->
0.09333, 0.03214, 0.07960, 0.07480, 0.05331, 0.07113, 0.08805, 0.04859,
0.07433, 0.07472, 0.06073, 0.04942, 0.04732, 0.10539, 0.00970, 0.00866,
0.00724, 0.06035, 0.03020, 0.06766, 0.05061, 0.09279, 0.03003, 0.02350,
0.08229
```

```
Average vector ->
0.07888, 0.03280, 0.08927, 0.06809, 0.05427, 0.06134, 0.08055, 0.04039,
0.06864, 0.07351, 0.05548, 0.04998, 0.04226, 0.10756, 0.00953, 0.00880,
0.00738, 0.05574, 0.02967, 0.06184, 0.04631, 0.08601, 0.03030, 0.02217,
0.07650
```

After the search-by-concept process these are the results:

The seven output words with highest ranking are shown in Table 1. The most relevant result is **meet\#n\#1**. The proximity of its vector's dimensions values with the ones of the average vector previously calculated is notable.

```
meet#n#1 ->
0.08617, 0.03065, 0.07523, 0.07008, 0.05108, 0.06587, 0.08282, 0.04433,
0.07043, 0.07140, 0.05706, 0.04682, 0.04483, 0.10047, 0.00925, 0.00833,
0.00693, 0.05719, 0.02873, 0.06359, 0.04762, 0.08818, 0.02873, 0.02220,
0.07838
```

**Table 1.** System output for concept: gym_shoe#n#1 athletic_contest#n#1 race#n#2

| Product of semantic similarity values | Euclidean distance | Word | Gloss |
|---|---|---|---|
| 0.02642 | 0.02015 | meet#n#1 | a meeting at which a number of athletic contests are held |
| 0.00580 | 0.02755 | Olympic_Games#n#1 | the modern revival of the ancient games held once every 4 years in a selected country |
| 0.00426 | 0.02755 | horse_race#n#1 | a contest of speed between horses |
| 0.00426 | 0.02755 | footrace#n#1 | a race run on foot |
| 0.00387 | 0.05936 | game#n#2 | a single play of a sport or other contest |
| 0.00325 | 0.03846 | track_meet#n#1 | a track and field competition between two or more teams |
| 0.00293 | 0.04428 | race#n#1 | any competition |

This process is done with the three different semantic spaces for every input concept. Table 2 and Table 3 show the reverse search of three different concepts with the two highest ranked output words from our system and the two highest ranked output words from an existing reverse dictionary [3] (OneLook Reverse Dictionary Online) respectively for comparison terms.

**Table 2.** Reverse search for three different concepts - System output

| Concept | | System results | |
|---|---|---|---|
| nature evolution life | JCN | growth#n#2 | A progression from simpler to more complex forms. |
| | | chemical_reaction#n#1 | (Chemistry) a process in which one or more substances are changed into others. |
| | Lesk | oxidative_phosphorylation#n#1 | An enzymatic process in cell metabolism that synthesizes ATP from ADP. |
| | | blooming#n#1 | The organic process of bearing flowers. |
| | Lin | growth#n#2 | A progression from simpler to more complex forms. |
| | | heat_sink#n#1 | A metal conductor specially designed to conduct (and radiate) heat. |
| antenna screen broadcast | JCN | serial#n#1 | A serialized set of programs. |
| | | wide_screen#n#1 | A projection screen that is much wider than it is high. |
| | Lesk | rerun#n#1 | A program that is broadcast again. |
| | | receiver#n#1 | Set that receives radio or tv signals. |
| | Lin | electrical_device#n#1 | A device that produces or is powered by electricity. |
| | | surface#n#1 | The outer boundary of an artifact or a material layer constituting or resembling such a boundary. |
| thunderbolt cloud water | JCN | atmospheric_electricity#n#1 | Electrical discharges in the atmosphere. |
| | | precipitation#n#3 | The falling to earth of any form of water. |
| | Lesk | atmospheric_electricity#n#1 | Electrical discharges in the atmosphere. |
| | | cumulus#n#1 | A globular cloud. |
| | Lin | atmospheric_electricity#n#1 | Electrical discharges in the atmosphere. |
| | | atmospheric_phenomenon#n#1 | A physical phenomenon associated with the atmosphere. |

**Table 3.** Reverse search for three different concepts - OneLook Reverse Dictionary output

| Concept | OneLook Reverse Dictionary results |
|---|---|
| nature evolution life | natural Huxley |
| antenna screen broadcast | set-top box tv-antenna |
| thunderbolt cloud water | thunder cloud |

**Table 4.** Evaluation

| Output source | Aspect 1 | Aspect 2 | |
|---|---|---|---|
| Our system | 94% | JCN | 42% |
| | | Lin | 6% |
| | | Lesk | 32% |
| OneLook Reverse Dictionary | 74% | 20% | |

At first sight, the results of our system seem to be correct answers for each concept, but in which way could we measure the quality of our results? We create a test set with 50 different concepts and for each concept we show the two highest ranked output words from our system and the two highest ranked output words from OneLook Reverse Dictionary, as in Table 2 and Table 3. A group of 10 people evaluated the test set under the following considerations:

1. Indicate if the output words converges with their associative reasoning.
2. Indicate which one of the sources gave the best results. And in case our system output was selected, specify the source of semantic space.

We resume the evaluation information in Table 4. Analyzing its content, it is clear that the performance of our system is better than OneLook Reverse Dictionary. Not only in the proximity with human associative reasoning capacity, it also gave the best results during the reverse search; where the concepts obtained from JCN semantic space demonstrate to combine better the characteristics of meaning of the input phrases.

# 7    Conclusions

In this paper, we described a new method for reverse dictionary construction with a semantic approach. We proposed the creation of three different semantic spaces, each one containing vectors created from different sources of semantic similarity measures. Also we described the different parts that constitute our reverse search together with an example. Our experimental results show that our system provides better results over current available implementations, including an improved system output providing also the gloss of every output word. This is very helpful in terms of evaluation because the user doesn't have to waste time looking for a definition in order to verify the quality of the output.

As future work we propose the creation of two new semantic spaces based on different resources, a distributional thesaurus and latent Dirichlet allocation(LDA). A distributional thesaurus is a thesaurus generated automatically from a corpus by finding words which occur in similar contexts to each other. Meanwhile LDA is a generative probabilistic model for collections of discrete data. This enables an analysis of reverse search from different approaches to determine which one is the closest to human associative reasoning. A supervised approach (WordNet), semi-supervised approach (distributional thesaurus) and unsupervised approach (LDA).

**Acknowledgements.** The authors wish to thank to Instituto Politécnico Nacional (SIP-IPN grants 20130018 and 20130086, COFAA-IPN and PIFI-IPN) and the government of Mexico (SNI and CONACYT) for providing the necessary support to carry out this research work.

# References

1. Banerjee, S., Pedersen, T.: An adapted lesk algorithm for word sense disambiguation using wordnet. In: Gelbukh, A. (ed.) CICLing 2002. LNCS, vol. 2276, pp. 136–145. Springer, Heidelberg (2002)
2. Banerjee, S., Pedersen, T.: Extended gloss overlaps as a measure of semantic relatedness. IJCAI 3, 805–810 (2003)
3. Beeferman, D.: Onelook Reverse Dictionary (2013),
   http://www.onelook.com/reverse-dictionary.shtml (accessed January-2013)
4. Bernstein, T., Wagner, J.: Bernstein's reverse dictionary. Quadrangle/New York Times Book Co. (1975)
5. Bilac, S., Watanabe, W., Hashimoto, T., Tokunaga, T., Tanaka, H.: Dictionary search based on the target word description. In: Proc. of the Tenth Annual Meeting of The Association for NLP (NLP 2004), pp. 556–559 (2004)
6. Budanitsky, A., Hirst, G.: Evaluating wordnet-based measures of lexical semantic relatedness. Computational Linguistics 32(1), 13–47 (2006)
7. Crawford, V., Hollow, T., Crawford, J.: Reverse electronic dictionary using synonyms to expand search capabilities. Patent, 07 1997; US 5649221 (1997)
8. Dutoit, D., Nugues, P.: A lexical database and an algorithm to find words from definitions (2002)
9. Jiang, J.J., Conrath, D.W.: Semantic similarity based on corpus statistics and lexical taxonomy. arXiv preprint cmp-lg/9709008 (1997)
10. Lin, D.: An information-theoretic definition of similarity. In: ICML, vol. 98, pp. 296–304 (1998)
11. Miller, G.A.: Nouns in wordnet: a lexical inheritance system. International Journal of Lexicography 3(4), 245–264 (1990)
12. Shaw, R., Datta, A., VanderMeer, D., Dutta, K.: Building a scalable database-driven reverse dictionary. IEEE Transactions on Knowledge and Data Engineering 25(3), 528–540 (2013)
13. Sowa, J.F.: Conceptual structures: Information processing in mind and machine (1984)
14. Zock, M., Bilac, S.: Word lookup on the basis of associations: from an idea to a roadmap. In: Proceedings of the Workshop on Enhancing and Using Electronic Dictionaries, ElectricDict 2004, pp. 29–35. Association for Computational Linguistics, Stroudsburg (2004)
15. Zock, M., Schwab, D.: Lexical access based on underspecified input. In: Proceedings of the workshop on Cognitive Aspects of the Lexicon, pp. 9–17. Association for Computational Linguistics (2008)

# Applying Rogerian Psychologist in Human-Computer Interaction: A Case Study

Tomáš Nestorovič[1] and Václav Matoušek[2]

[1] New Technologies for the Information Society
[2] Department of Computer Science and Engineering,
University of West Bohemia in Pilsen, Univerzitni 8, 30614 Pilsen, Czech Republic
{nestorov,matousek}@kiv.zcu.cz

**Abstract.** This paper concerns a design, application, and testing of a Rogerian psychologist strategy for information elicitation in dialogue management. Our results show that keeping the initiative in dialogue at users' side as long as they know what to say improves information exchange rate by 37.5 %. We also discuss applicability and implications for other domains.

**Keywords:** dialogue systems, dialogue management, knowledge elicitation, artificial intelligence.

## 1    Introduction

Human-machine dialogue management focuses on finding machine's best response given an interaction history with the user. Ranging from simple finite state machines to Markov decision networks, there is a wide collection of methods to implement a dialogue management. Our approach, however, follows the BDI architecture (Beliefs, Desires, Intentions) [1]. When designing the conversation agent we focused on its knowledge elicitation (i.e. Intentions in terms of BDI). The usual approach to solve a task with a user is to formulate an open-ended prompt, and if it does not manage to gain enough information to meet the objective of the task, then ask for missing information, one piece at a time [2, 3]. In terms of initiative distribution, this corresponds with applying the *user-initiative* and *system-initiative* strategies, respectively. However, as users generally adopt the interaction style suggested by the system [4], then once applying the system-initiative guidance, the task is constrained to a linear progress. Thus we focused on avoiding this side-effect by modifying the above outlined interaction pattern.

## 2    Rogerian Psychologist Strategy

Our modification to the outlined interaction style therefore accounts for the user keeping the initiative as long as s/he knows what to say. More particularly we involve a *Rogerian psychologist* into our model whose goal is to gain more information by "encouraging the user to keep on talking" (in terms of Rogerian therapy, clients are

F. Castro, A. Gelbukh, and M. González (Eds.): MICAI 2013, Part I, LNAI 8265, pp. 286–293, 2013.

better helped if they are encouraged to focus on their current subjective understanding rather than on some unconscious motive or someone else's interpretation of a situation) [5]. One of the well known implementations of this approach is Weizenbaum's Elisa [6], a general chatting robot for leading a conversation in an uninformed way, i.e. without properly modeling information state of what is being discussed and continuing the conversation only using simple rule-driven or context-free sentences (e.g. user's "I visited my friend yesterday" can be continued by system's "That sounds interesting, tell me more about it"). The Rogerian psychologist is also one of strategies humans use in common conversation. For instance, Wallis, Das, and O'Dea observed a phone call agent to use it when attempting to gain more information from a client during a car booking [7]. It therefore is a familiar approach for humans which they can respond to. The problem we can spot now is to find conditions under which it could be used in dialogue management.

The most obvious applicability of this strategy is in cases in which the user has provided some information that is, however, useless in the scope of a given task or domain (formally, if we have extracted some useless semantics, or simply know the user was not silent, respectively). Of course, this strategy cannot be over-used – a conversational agent must always make a trade-off between being reactive and proactive, i.e. giving the user chance to provide relevant information, and taking over the initiative. Therefore, the Rogerian psychologist strategy can be applied in dialogues that can be evaluated as well progressing. In our case, we approach this by checking that user's last response contributed to the current task satisfaction (i.e. if the user knew what to say last, there is a chance s/he will know what to say now as well), and by tracking the recognition score (if user's responses are less certain, it is more safe to interact directly than recovering from errors in the dialogue). Another constraint is to cases in which the agent expects (misses) multiple pieces of information (if only one piece is expected, it may be more efficient to ask for it directly). Finally, this strategy can be applied in cases in which user's intentions are unknown (i.e. after the open-ended initial prompt) or ambiguous (later in the dialogue when recognizing user's subintentions). Table 1 summarizes the criteria along with conditions for the other two strategies our information elicitation model accommodates, and Fig. 1 shows the strategy in the context of generating agent's prompts. Let us also note that apart of general context-free sentences the model can handle domain specific alternatives as well (i.e. analogous to Elisa's rule-driven ones, e.g. "Please try to detail the *train* [to find departure of; further; a bit more;…]").

**Table 1.** Modified information elicitation model strategies and selection criteria

| System-initiative strategy | User-initiative strategy | Rogerian psychologist |
|---|---|---|
| • dialogue quality estimation | • dialogue quality estimation | • dialogue quality estimation |
| • correction of information elicited using higher initiative strategy | • correction of information elicited using higher initiative strategy | • user's intention is unknown |
| | | • user's subintention is ambiguous |
| • information to gain is of large range | • high recognition score | • level of perplexity is high |
| • low recognition score | • user's intention is unknown | • user's previous response contributed to the intention solved |
| | • acceptable recognition score | • acceptable recognition score |

```
1  Procedure SelectBestStrategy ( ) {
2     Let R denote user's response when discussing intention I.
3     Evaluate how well each strategy fits current state of a dialogue and choose strategy S that fits it
      best.
4     If S is the Rogerian psychologist strategy {
5        If ¬A & B & ¬C & D & E (see legend below) {
6           If dialogue stagnates (system generates the same prompt as in its previous turn) {
7              If R supplied some information that supports getting I solved {
8                 User has satisfied one of future expectations – ground with "Uhu.", "Ok.", or "I see."
9              } else {
10                Response R did not bring any information into I – remain silent.
11             }
12          } else {
13             System is about to generate a different utterance than in its previous turn because the
               expectation has been met – randomly choose one of sentences available to the Rogerian
               psychologist (e.g. "Please say me more.")
14          }
15       } else {
16          Rogerian psychologist strategy cannot be applied. Do not drop it, just override it by
            another strategy in this turn (thus temporarily assign S a different value).
17       }
18    }
19    Generate response in accordance with the strategy S.
20 }
```

**Fig. 1.** Agent's utterance generating procedure with the Rogerian psychologist approach at Lines 5–17; $A$ = agent's focus has changed, $B$ = user's intention is known, $C$ = user's first turn response expected, $D$ = agent produces a dialogue move that the Rogerian psychologist *can* be applied to (e.g. it *cannot* be applied to a *Yes-No-Question* move), $E$ = two or more pieces of information expected (missed)

## 3    Experiment, Results, and Discussion

To verify the applicability of the Rogerian psychologist in human-computer interaction, we designed a timetable domain and conducted an experiment focused on determining if the strategy improves or impairs the information exchange rate. For this purpose, six users carried out the three tasks in Fig. 2 with the agent with the Rogerian psychologist strategy enabled, and six different users carried out the same three tasks with having it forbidden. Before a session, each user read through on-line instructions on how to use the system and then called it by phone. During each session the tasks were performed sequentially and users were obliged to write down information obtained from the system. Each of the interactions supplied us a set of automatic measurements of how well a particular dialogue proceeded (Table 2). These data included: *Timeouts* (the number of times the user did not say anything within a given time frame), *Misrecognitions* (the number of misrecognized pieces of information), *Turns* (the number of turns required in user's interaction), *Psychologist's Turns*, and *Time* (the number of seconds user's interaction lasted).

**Table 2.** Session measures: $TO$ = Timeouts, $MR$ = Misrecognitions, $TR$ = Turns, $TM$ = Time in seconds, $PT$ = Psychologist's turns, $Q_{\{1,...,6\}}$ = Response to Question$_{\{1,...,6\}}$, $US$ = User Satisfaction = $\sum_{(i)} Q_i$

| # | TO | MR | TR | TM | PT | $Q_1$ | $Q_2$ | $Q_3$ | $Q_4$ | $Q_5$ | $Q_6$ | US |
|---|----|----|----|----|----|----|----|----|----|----|----|----|
| U01 | 1 | 2 | 13 | 196 | 2 | 5 | 3 | 4 | 4 | 4 | 5 | 25 |
| U02 | 3 | 4 | 17 | 276 | 1 | 3 | 3 | 3 | 4 | 3 | 2 | 18 |
| U03 | 1 | 0 | 8 | 107 | 2 | 5 | 4 | 5 | 5 | 5 | 5 | 29 |
| U04 | 3 | 2 | 23 | 359 | 1 | 2 | 1 | 1 | 4 | 2 | 2 | 12 |
| U05 | 3 | 5 | 17 | 262 | 1 | 2 | 2 | 2 | 4 | 3 | 2 | 15 |
| U06 | 2 | 3 | 17 | 223 | 3 | 3 | 3 | 3 | 4 | 3 | 3 | 19 |
| U07 | 3 | 7 | 21 | 314 | 0 | 1 | 2 | 2 | 4 | 3 | 2 | 14 |
| U08 | 0 | 4 | 17 | 193 | 0 | 3 | 3 | 4 | 4 | 3 | 3 | 20 |
| U09 | 0 | 1 | 10 | 132 | 0 | 5 | 4 | 4 | 5 | 4 | 5 | 27 |
| U10 | 3 | 4 | 17 | 281 | 0 | 3 | 3 | 2 | 4 | 3 | 2 | 17 |
| U11 | 1 | 1 | 12 | 167 | 0 | 4 | 3 | 4 | 5 | 4 | 4 | 24 |
| U12 | 4 | 5 | 20 | 337 | 0 | 2 | 2 | 2 | 3 | 3 | 2 | 14 |

When finished with their tasks, users were given a survey focused on telling us what they reckon about the interaction (Fig. 3). We wanted to know their overall feeling (Question 1) broken down into five narrowed questions about the speed of the interaction (Question 2), opinion on clarity of system's prompts (Question 3), system's response latency (Question 4), the way the system managed the dialogue (Question 5), and users' attitude to eventual future use of the system (Question 6). Responses ranged over five predefined values (representing that the user *does not agree, rather does not agree, does not know, rather agrees*, and *agrees*) mapped to integers 1...5 (with 5 representing full agreement). Based on these questions, we computed *User Satisfaction* as a sum of each question score (i.e. with range from 6 to 30).

*Task 1.* Try to find the **cheapest** connection (bus, train, and/or airplane) that goes **to Utrecht** at **11 o'clock**. If you cannot find an exact match, try to find the one with the closest departure time. Please write down the exact departure time of the connection you found.

*Task 2.* For connections of your choice from Task 1, try to find their **total travel time**. You might need to use your math skills to find out. Please write down the exact time you have found.

*Task 3.* Try to buy a **ticket** for **you**. Remember you are on buying the **cheapest** one. Please write down the total price you have been told by the system.

**Fig. 2.** Task scenario

To reveal how the *User Satisfaction* depends on the above metrics, we employed the PARADISE framework [8] for spoken dialogues evaluation. The PARADISE framework quantifies the relative importance of independent evaluation metrics to performance, and is used to derive a performance function in the form

$$User\ Satisfaction\ =\ \textstyle\sum_{(i)} w_i \cdot N\ (\ measure_i\ ).$$

To compute the unknown coefficients (i.e. weights $w_i$), we used a multiple linear regression. These coefficients describe the contribution of the measures for the variance in *User Satisfaction*. The $N(x)$ is a Z-score normalization function to guarantee that the measures enter the linear regression as relative values. Thus, the normalization is present here to overcome the different scales (e.g. the *Time* is measured in seconds while the *Misrecognitions* is counted in terms of number of observations). The normalization function is computed as

$$N(x)\ =\ (\ x\ -\ \bar{x}\ )\ /\ \sigma_x$$

where $\bar{x}$ and $\sigma_x$ are the means and standard deviation for the $x$ variable, respectively. However, before applying the PARADISE framework, we excluded the *Time* measure as it highly correlates with the *Turns* measure ($corr > 0.95$). The application of the PARADISE framework shows that the most significant contributors to the *User Satisfaction* are *Timeouts* ($p < 0.045$) and *Misrecognitions* ($p < 0.003$). Hence, the formula that best explains the *User Satisfaction* is

$$User\ Satisfaction\ =\ \begin{array}{l} -0.53 \cdot N\ (\ Timeouts\ ) \\ -0.64 \cdot N\ (\ Misrecognitions\ ). \end{array}$$

This implies that the Rogerian psychologist strategy does not affect the *User's Satisfaction* ($p > 0.89$), i.e. users are not annoyed (surprised) by the system exceptional utterances and can handle them the same way as they would if heard from another person.

By comparing the number of turns that participants in the two groups required to solve the tasks, we can find an improvement of 5.2 %. This result is caused due to the Rogerian psychologist acting as a "prolonged user-initiative strategy" – participants in the group with the strategy turned on took advantage of being able to provide more pieces of information at a time. Nonetheless, although the improvement may be seen marginal, let us consider the following two aspects. First, the whole dialogue is involved, i.e. including agent's prompts that the psychologist cannot be applied to (e.g. *Validation* moves implicitly expect only yes-no answer). If we focused only on prompts the strategy can be applied to (i.e. no matter if the agent really applied it), we get an improvement of 37.5 % (compared to one-by-one way of querying).

*Question 1.* Do you think it was easy to obtain the information we requested you?

*Question 2.* Was the pace of interaction appropriate? Were you able to follow the information said by the system?

*Question 3.* Did you know what you could say at each point of the dialogue?

*Question 4.* Do you reckon the speed of system's reactions was appropriate?

*Question 5.* Did the system work the way you expected it to during the dialogue?

*Question 6.* Based on your current experience, do you think you would use the system regularly to access schedules or book tickets, e.g., when away from home?

**Fig. 3.** Task scenario

**Table 3.** Dialogue between the system (S) and a user (U). Errors introduced during user's utterance processing (ASR + Parser) are italicized. The *RPS* column indicates applicability of the Rogerian psychologist strategy: *Yes/No* = RPS was/was not used, "–" = RPS cannot be applied to the current turn.

| Agent | Utterance | RPS |
|---|---|---|
| $S_1$ | Welcome in the Simple Timetable System. How can I help you? | – |
| $U_1$ | I need to get to Utrecht. | – |
| $S_2$ | Please say me more. | Yes |
| $U_2$ | I need a cheap connection about eleven. *(Input: Cheap)* | – |
| $S_3$ | Which transportation means do you prefer? | No |
| $U_3$ | Cheap, so bus or train? | |
| $S_4$ | What time approximately would you like to depart? | No |
| $U_4$ | About eleven. | – |
| $S_5$ | I understood you want from Delft to Utrecht by the cheapest bus or train departing at eleven. Please confirm this or say your correct request. | – |
| $U_5$ | Yes. | – |
| $S_6$ | The next cheapest bus from Delft to Utrecht leaves at 3:30pm, train at 1pm, and bus at 1:30pm. Can I help you any further? Do you want to order a ticket now? | – |
| $U_6$ | What are the prices? | – |
| $S_7$ | The ticket for bus departing at 3:30pm from Delft to Utrecht costs 10 coins, train at 1pm 11 coins, and bus at 1:30pm 11 coins. Can I help you any further? Do you want to order a ticket now? | – |
| $U_7$ | No. When does the train arrive? | – |
| $S_8$ | The train departing from Delft at 1pm arrives in Utrecht at 2pm. Can I help you any further? Do you want to order a ticket now? | – |
| $U_8$ | And the early bus? *(Input: Bus)* | – |
| $S_9$ | The bus departing from Delft at 3:30pm arrives in Utrecht at 4pm, and 1:30pm at 2pm. Can I help you any further? Do you want to order a ticket now? | – |
| $U_9$ | Yes. | – |
| $S_{10}$ | Ticket ordering. Uhu. | Yes |
| $U_{10}$ | [ Timeout. ] | – |
| $S_{11}$ | How many persons will be traveling? | No |
| $U_{11}$ | One. | – |
| $S_{12}$ | Do you have any discounts? | No |
| $U_{12}$ | No. | – |
| $S_{13}$ | Do you want to order a full prized bus ticket for one person leaving Delft at 1:30pm, arriving Utrecht at 2pm? The total price is 11 coins. | – |
| $U_{13}$ | Yes. | – |
| $S_{14}$ | Thank you for your order. How can I help you? | – |

Second, let us also note that we deal here with a blind adaptability approach without any interaction habits-model of a particular user. While some systems make use of domain-dependent features to predict agent's utterance that best corresponds with user's behavior [9, 10], we would like to stick in our future work to domain-independent features as Hjalmarsson demonstrates in her work by making an extended use of the PARADISE framework [11].

Finally, the timetable domain is relatively a simple one and more complex domain with more pieces of information to discuss with the user would be valuable. However, with a more complex domain there is also the ASR performance point of view and it can be argued that for complex domains with high variability input (i.e. utterances which possibly can carry lot of different information) the ASR may fail to recognize confidently as it is exposed to too wide portion of a language. This holds especially for the context-free sentences (e.g. "Please say me more"), however, the ASR effectiveness can be recovered by supplying context-aware alternatives (e.g. the already mentioned "Please try to detail the *train*") which would narrow the amount of possible information and keep the language reasonably constrained. Last but not least, the context-aware sentences prevent the Rogerian style of interaction to draw a lot of irrelevant information by suggesting what the user should talk about, yet without pushing him to say something narrowed.

## 4    Conclusion

This paper concerned a BDI agent-based management for task-oriented dialogues, particularly focusing on agent's information elicitation. We showed an extended elicitation model aimed at increasing the information exchange rate. Omitting the above plotted issue regarding the ASR efficiency, the current state of the Rogerian psychologist strategy tends to shorten a dialogue. The three-task scenario in which users were interacting with the system to gain some information showed more accurately the difference between the common state-of-the-art way of interaction and interaction with handing the initiative back to the user. Keeping the initiative at users' side as long as they knew what to say resulted in 37.5 percent information exchange rate improvement (or five percents if considering whole dialogues) – a result saying that this way of information elicitation is 37.5 percent more efficient than the common unrepeated open-ended querying performed by the user-initiative strategy.

**Acknowledgment.** This work was supported by grant No. SGS-2013-029, "Advanced Computing and Information Systems".

## References

1. Rao, A., Georgeff, M.: BDI agents: From Theory to Practice. In: 1st International Conference on Multi-Agent Systems, pp. 312–319. MIT Press (1995)
2. Bohus, D., Rudnicky, A.: The RavenClaw Dialog Management Framework: Architecture and Systems. J. Computer Speech and Language 23, 332–361 (2009)

3. Turunen, M., Hakulinen, J., Häihä, K., Salonen, E., Kainulainen, A., Prusi, P.: An Architecture and Applications for Speech-based Accessibility Systems. IBM Systems Journal 44, 485–504 (2005)
4. Gustafson, J., Bell, L.: Speech Technology on Trial: Experiences from the System. J. Natural Language Engineering: Special Issue on Best Practice in Spoken Dialogue Systems 3, 273–286 (2003)
5. Rogers, C.: Client Centered Therapy: Current Practice, Implications and Theory. Houghton Mifflin, Boston (1951)
6. Weizenbaum, J.: ELIZA – A Computer Program for the Study of Natural Language Communication Between Man and Machine. J. Communications of the Association for Computing Machinery 9, 36–45 (1966)
7. Wallis, P., Mitchard, H., Das, J., O'Dea, D.: Dialogue Modeling for a Conversational Agent. In: Stumptner, M., Corbett, D.R., Brooks, M. (eds.) Canadian AI 2001. LNCS (LNAI), vol. 2256, pp. 532–544. Springer, Heidelberg (2001)
8. Walker, M., Litman, D., Kamm, C., Abella, A.: Evaluating Spoken Dialogue Agents with PARADISE: Two Case Studies. J. Computer Speech and Language 22, 317–347 (1998)
9. Komatani, K., Ueno, S., Kawahara, T., Okun, H.: User Modeling in Spoken Dialogue Systems for Flexible Guidance Generation. In: Eurospeech, pp. 745–748 (2003)
10. Chu-Carroll, J.: MIMIC: An Adaptive Mixed-initiative Spoken Dialogue System for Information Queries. In: 6th ACL Conference on Applied Natural Language Processing, pp. 97–104 (2000)
11. Hjalmarsson, A.: Towards User Modeling in Conversational Dialogue Systems: A Qualitative Study of the Dynamics of Dialogue Parameters. In: Interspeech, pp. 869–872 (2005)

# HuLaPos 2.0 – Decoding Morphology

László János Laki[1,2], György Orosz[1,2], and Attila Novák[1,2]

[1] MTA-PPKE Hungarian Language Technology Research Group
[2] Pázmány Péter Catholic University, Faculty of Information Technology and Bionics,
50/a Práter Street, 1083 Budapest, Hungary
{laki.laszlo,orosz.gyorgy,novak.attila}@itk.ppke.hu

**Abstract.** In this paper, a language-independent morphological annotation tool is presented that is based on the Moses SMT toolkit. Taking Hungarian as an example, we demonstrate that the algorithm performs very well for morphologically rich languages. In order to reach a very high, more than 98%, annotation accuracy, the presented system uses a trie-based suffix guesser, which enables the tool to handle words unseen in the training data effectively. The system yields state-of-the-art performance among language-independent tools for morphological annotation of Hungarian. For PoS tagging, it even outperforms the best hybrid tagger, which includes a language-specific morphological analyzer.

**Keywords:** PoS tagging, lemmatization, SMT, decoder, suffix guesser.

## 1 Introduction

Automatic morphological annotation, which consists of Part-of-speech (PoS) tagging and lemmatization, is a crucial task of natural language processing. Accuracy of morphological annotation can significantly affect the performance of a natural language processing chain. Although existing implementations have relatively high token accuracy, even relatively small differences in the accuracy of morphological annotation can lead to great quality differences at higher levels of linguistic processing. This motivates researchers to create better and better algorithms. Morphological annotation can be regarded as a translation problem, which inspired us to apply an SMT decoder to this task.

In this paper, we present a language-independent morphological annotation tool that is based on the Moses SMT toolkit [8]. Its ability to handle rich language models and the beam-search-based stack decoding algorithm implemented in the Moses decoder make it a promising tool to apply to this task.

The structure of our paper is as follows. We first present the special problems that make morphological annotation of agglutinating languages difficult. This is followed by an overview of the characteristics of the Moses SMT decoder and that of related work. Then a baseline Moses-based annotation system is presented, which is enhanced by adapting the models and optimizing the parameters used in the system to the task of generating morphological annotation for a morphologically rich language. The performance of the optimized system is compared to that of other morphological annotation tools, including the state-of-the-art PurePos system.

F. Castro, A. Gelbukh, and M. González (Eds.): MICAI 2013, Part I, LNAI 8265, pp. 294–305, 2013.
© Springer-Verlag Berlin Heidelberg 2013

# 2  Motivation and Background

## 2.1  Complete Morphological Disambiguation for Agglutinating Languages

Complete morphological disambiguation means to determine the morphosyntactic tag (part-of-speech plus additional inflectional features) and the lemma of each word in a sentence simultaneously. There are several tools that perform PoS tagging or lemmatization only, but only few are capable of doing complete morphological disambiguation.

What makes tagging of agglutinative languages like Hungarian, Turkish or Finnish more difficult than that of a morphologically less complicated language like English or French is data sparseness. On the one hand, while an open class English word has about 4–6 different word forms, it has several hundred or thousand different productively suffixed forms in agglutinating languages. This also means that there are more than a thousand of PoS tags for Hungarian, because all different possible inflected forms correspond to at least one different morphosyntactic tag. In contrast, the tagset contains only a few dozen tags for English. On the other hand, there is a big difference in the number of different word forms in a given corpus, which relates to the tagset size as well. If we compare Hungarian with English, we find that if we would like to reach a given level of vocabulary coverage for a text consisting of a given number of word tokens, a 8-10 times bigger training corpus is needed for Hungarian than for English [12].

The identification of the correct lemma is not trivial either, especially for the unseen words. For example, in Hungarian, there is a group of verbs the lemmas of which end in an -ik suffix (e.g. *törik* 'break intrans.'). Other verbs do not have this ending (e.g. *tör* 'break trans.'). Massive lemma ambiguities follow from the fact that the two paradigms are identical with the single exception of the third person singular present tense indicative form (the lemma), and that there are identical productive suffixes (e.g. -z vs. -zik) that produce derived verbs from the same root belonging either to the *ik*-less paradigm or the one with the -ik suffix [13].

## 2.2  SMT Decoding – Theoretical Background

The goal of machine translation is to implement a mapping between two languages, be those languages natural or artificial ones. A statistical machine translation (SMT) system learns the needed transformation rules from a bilingual parallel corpus applying an unsupervised learning algorithm.

If $F$ is a sentence in the source language, its optimal translation, $\hat{E}$ can be identified as

$$\hat{E} = argmax_{E}\ p(E|F) = argmax_{E}\ p(F|E)p(E) \tag{1}$$

where $\hat{E}$ maximizes a combination of the language model $p(E)$ and the translation model $p(F|E)$ scores [7].

This decoding model is isomorphic with noisy-channel models of PoS tagging where $p(E)$ is the tag transmission probability model and $p(F|E)$ is the output (or lexical) probability model. The main difference between the model implemented in the SMT decoder and that in an HMM-based PoS tagger is the way these probabilities are estimated. The main reasons that motivated us to use an SMT framework, in particular the open-source Moses toolkit [8], to the task of morphological annotation were the following:

1. The Moses training chain is fast to create a translation model (i.e. a lexical probability model) from a given word aligned corpus. Furthermore, in contrast to usual HMM decoders, the translation model may contain long phrases, which allows the system to tag long sequences of words as one unit.
2. The language model (i.e. the tag transmission probability model) is trained with a modified Kneser-Ney smoothing [6], which has a state-of-the-art performance in the creation of language models.
3. The decoder (tagger) uses an efficient beam search algorithm applying stack decoding. The advantage of this decoding technique is that it is able to do the translation in an arbitrary order (in contrast to e.g. the strict left-to-right decoding applied in an HMM tagger).
4. It is easy to integrate a morphological guesser or pre-annotation into the decoding process.

## 3   Related Work

The first statistical PoS tagger for Hungarian was created by Oravecz and Dienes [12]. They used an adapted version of the HMM-based TnT tagger [1] for the morphological disambiguation of Hungarian.

Halácsy et al. reimplemented TnT creating a PoS tagger called HunPos [5]. In HunPos, like in TnT, a trie-based suffix guesser is used to handle unknown words. A morphological table including a list of possible tags for each word in the input can be used to decrease the search space of the decoding algorithm. This can improve accuracy significantly when tagging a morphologically rich language, like Hungarian. The customized version of TnT used by Oravecz and Dienes also included the possibility to optionally load a morphological table. The tools mentioned above perform only tagging, not lemmatization.

Orosz and Novák [13] presented an open source, HMM based, hybrid morphological annotation tool called PurePos. Unlike HunPos or TnT, PurePos has a complete integration of a morphological analyzer (HUMor [10]), that is used to find the correct lemma candidates and PoS tags for out-of-vocabulary (OOV) words.

In contrast to the trie guesser, the morphological analyzer returns only the morphologically appropriate and possible annotations. In addition, in contrast to a morphological-table-based solution, it can analyze any word form covered by the morphological description loaded, which may be a cyclic and thus infinite set of words. The main disadvantage of using morphological analyzer is that this solution is limited only to supported languages and annotation schemes. Otherwise the PurePos system – omitting the morphological analyzer – is able to operate language-independently, but in that case, it loses its advantage.

Beside the HMM-based taggers, there is an annotation tool for Hungarian using a maximum entropy model: Magyarlanc [15], which is an NLP toolkit that was developed for IR systems. It contains an adaptation of the Stanford tagger for Hungarian, a tokenizer and a lemmatizer as well. In this system, the morphdb.hu [14] morphological analyzer was integrated, which uses a special variant of the MSD coding system [3] (different from the Humor scheme integrated into PurePos).

The main advantage of our system to the ones above is that it operates in a completely language- and tagset-independent manner. Moreover, previous tagger implementations have limited possibilities concerning the selection of decoding order and the units of translation. HMM-based taggers are restricted to left-to-right processing. When assigning an analysis to a word, the system can only rely on the analysis of its left-hand-side neighbors. The system performs a search for the best global analysis at the end of the sentence. The maximum-entropy-based algorithm implemented in e.g. Magyarlanc begins the analysis with the least ambiguous words, and then goes on with analysis of more ambiguous words. Analyses of nearest neighbors are relied on in the process.

In contrast, the decoder in the tagger described in this paper is in theory able to use arbitrarily long terms as separate translation units, and word analysis can take into account not only left-hand-side, but also right-hand-side neighbors. In addition, the language model used for implementing the tag-transition model – thanks to the improved Kneser-Ney smoothing – proved more effective than the trigram-model used by the HMM-based systems above.

Mora and Sánchez [4] were the first who used an SMT decoder as a PoS tagger. The system was used for morphological disambiguation for English (not including lemmatization). A word-frequency-based model and an exception list of 11 word ending patterns were used to manage OOV words. Their paper concluded that the best results for English language could be achieved with setting both the translation phrase length limit and the order of the language model to three.

An SMT-decoder-based tagger for Hungarian is described by Laki [9] applying the methods of Mora and Sanchez. Parameters and models used by Mora and Sánchez for English produced well below state-of-the-art results for Hungarian, which, due to its agglutinating nature, requires much more advanced techniques to handle the much more frequent OOV words.

In this work, we describe a language- and tag-set-independent morphological annotation system that includes ingredients from the previous SMT-decoder-based and HMM-based solutions, which performs better at the task of morphological annotation of Hungarian than the existing language-independent systems, and it is competitive with even the hybrid PurePos version, which uses a language-specific morphological analyzer.

## 4    Data and Baseline

### 4.1    Corpus

In our work, we used Szeged Corpus 2 [2], which is the only large-scale freely available completely annotated corpus for Hungarian. Szeged Corpus 2 was created by the Language Technology Group of the University of Szeged and contains morphological annotation using the MSD-coding system. The corpus contains manually checked and corrected annotation.

We performed some filtering on the corpus. First, sentences where multi-word phrases (named entities) were annotated as a single token were filtered out. If we would like to process these phrases in a manner that is compatible with the corpus, a NER system would need to be integrated in the system as a preprocessing step, which would make it difficult to measure the quality of the morphological disambiguation tool alone. Moreover, in the MSD-coding system used in Szeged Corpus 2, erroneous words (typos) have special tags, which were used by the annotators to mark wrongly spelled and foreign words. We also filtered out sentences that contain this type of tags. Finally, the filtered corpus has 64 395 segments (sentences) which contain 1 042 546 tokens. These cover 112 100 different word-form types.

To make our system comparable to the state-of-the-art PurePos system, which includes an integrated morphological analyzer, the evaluation was also performed on a modified version of the Szeged Corpus, in which the morphosyntactic annotation was converted to the HUMor annotation scheme used by the morphological analyzer integrated into PurePos.

### 4.2    Evaluation

To evaluate the performance of our systems, we calculated the accuracy of PoS tagging and lemmatization separately as well as the accuracy of the full morphological annotation including both lemmas and morphosyntactic tags. We calculated accuracies both at word and sentence level. We optimized the system for the accuracy of full word level morphological analysis.

The corpus was divided into 10%-10%-80% development, test and training sets. System parameters were tuned on the development set and final testing was performed on the test set.

### 4.3    Baseline

In the following section, we describe how the system was developed, adding and changing components and optimizing parameters to improve its performance to a state-of-the art level for Hungarian morphological analysis. We implemented a system along the lines described in [9].

**The Baseline System.** Paper [9] included several different setups, of which we used the one that included complete morphological annotation and PoS tagging as a baseline for this work. This system has the following properties:

1. The complete Moses chain was used to train that system, which means that the Giza++ tool [11] was used to align surface word forms with their analyses consisting of a lemma and a tag.
2. The system translates from surface word forms to lemma#PoS pairs, and this is the format of the training parallel corpus. Note that this formalism does not provide any generalizing power to the system.
3. The weakest point of this system is the way it handles OOV words not seen in the training corpus (this is a rather frequent event in the case of an agglutinating language). The decoder simply copies unseen words to the output. The lemma is then considered identical to the word form itself, and simply the most frequent tag (nominative singular noun) is assigned to it. Note that unseen words always block both higher-order translation model and language model matches.

The baseline entry in Table 1 shows the results of the system described in [9].

# 5   Improvements

In this section, we describe step-by-step improvements to the baseline system. The performance of each version of the tool was evaluated on the development set. The results are shown in Table 1.

**Table 1.** Evaluation of various configurations on the development set

| System Test | Token accuracy | | | Sentence accuracy | |
|---|---|---|---|---|---|
| | tag | lemma | morph | tag | morph |
| Baseline | 86.521% | 89.674% | 86.365% | 16.571% | 16.246% |
| MONO+GENLEM+4SFX-5-5 | 94.958% | 96.393% | 93.530% | 45.652% | 35.405% |
| MONO+GENLEM+4SFX-7-3 | 95.000% | 96.405% | 93.563% | 46.024% | 35.653% |
| +PRO+NUM | 95.803% | 96.433% | 94.323% | 50.907% | 38.971% |
| +GUESS | 99.570% | 96.817% | 96.418% | 92.435% | 52.829% |
| +OPEN+S-INI=HuLaPos2 | **99.566%** | **97.242%** | **96.837%** | **92.358%** | **57.402%** |

## 5.1   Using Monotone Alignment

Determining word alignment in parallel sentences is the most important step in the training of a statistical machine translation system. In the case of translation between natural languages, this is a hard task, which is usually solved using unsupervised machine learning algorithms, like the ones implemented in Giza++. By contrast, word alignment for morphological disambiguation is trivial: there must be a one-to-one monotone mapping between tokens and their analyses. Using a Giza++ alignment both takes a long time to generate and can only impair the quality of the system. Therefore, in all the setups described below, a monotone alignment was used instead of using Giza++.

## 5.2   Generalized Lemmatization

As it was discussed in chapter 4.3, the baseline system directly translates surface word forms to lemma#PoS pairs, and it does not contain any model to generalize either lemmatization or tag assignment to unseen words, which leads to severe data sparseness problem for the simple baseline model. This approach also leads to a huge target dictionary: there are 106 586 different items in it. A different representation is needed that has both generalizing power and can decrease the complexity of the model.

For suffixing languages like Hungarian, lemmas can be easily represented as a tuple that describes the transformation to be performed on the word form to get the lemma: $\langle cut, paste \rangle$, where $cut$ is how many characters are to be cut from the end of the string, and $paste$ is the string to be joined to the end of the result of the cut operation. For example in the case of the Hungarian word form *palotában* 'in the palace', the lemma of which is *palota* 'palace', the generalized representation of the lemma is "4#a" which means that the last four characters of the surface form are to be removed and an *a* character is to be attached. This representation reduces the size of the target dictionary size to 3571, which is closer for the size of the PoS tag set (1141 items).

## 5.3   Basic Handling of OOV Words

One of the PoS tagger configurations described in [9] (but not the system that we used as a baseline here) uses a simple suffix-based model to handle the tagging of OOV items. All hapaxes in the training corpus were replaced by a string of the form unk_#abcd, where abcd is the last four characters of the word. The same coding was used for OOV words in the text to be annotated. This method is compatible with the generalized lemmatization described above and provides a limited power of generalization to the system.

The entry MONO+GENLEM+4SFX-5-5 in Table 1 shows the results of the system using monotone alignment, the generalized lemmatizer and the four-character-suffix-based OOV handling with the default phrase length and laguage order settings, which is 5 for both values. The accuracy of lemmatization was greatly improved, which also resulted in an increased morpheme precision compared to the baseline system.

## 5.4   Optimizing Phrase Extraction

As it was discussed in section 2.2, the main advantage of the Moses decoder is that it is able to translate longer phrases as one unit. The maximum length of phrases used in translation and the order of language models influence the quality of the system. The optimal setting was determined empirically: the MONO+GENLEM+4SFX system was tested using different length settings. The results measured on the development set are shown in table 2.

**Table 2.** Determining the optimal phrase length and language model parameters

| LM order | max phrase length | | | | | |
|---|---|---|---|---|---|---|
| | 3-gram | 4-gram | 5-gram | 6-gram | 7-gram | 8-gram |
| 3-gram | 96.3499% | 96.3486% | 96.3480% | 96.3518% | **96.3518%** | 96.3499% |
| 4-gram | 96.3092% | 96.3131% | 96.3131% | 96.3150% | 96.3144% | 96.3118% |
| 5-gram | 96.3182% | 96.3202% | 96.3208% | 96.3234% | 96.3221% | 96.3208% |
| 6-gram | 96.3234% | 96.3234% | 96.3247% | 96.3266% | 96.3247% | 96.3241% |
| 7-gram | 96.3221% | 96.3221% | 96.3234% | 96.3247% | 96.3247% | 96.3234% |

The optimal setting for the maximum phrase length turned out to be 7, while that for the order of the language model was 3. Results for this model are shown in Table 1 as MONO+GENLEM+4SFX-7-3. All further models discussed below were trained using the same phrase length and language model parameters.

It should be mentioned that in the case of higher order language models, the accuracy of lemmatization slightly increases, but the precision of PoS tagging shows significant reduction at the same time.

When performing an error analysis of the MONO+GENLEM+4SFX-7-3 system, a few major errors were found. To improve performance, we had to handle the capitalization of lemmas of OOV words and the translation of open-class items, such as numbers.

### 5.5   Handling Proper Names

The main problem with proper names is that they are often OOV words, moreover the replaced form created by the 4SFX method often remained OOV because the system had not seen a word ending similarly in the training corpus. In that case, the original algorithm tagged the proper name as a common noun, which is the most probable tag. To solve this problem, the original 4SFX method was modified to distinguish capitalized words from lower-case ones, and the default tag for capitalized words was modified to be proper noun instead of common noun.

### 5.6   Handling Numbers

The baseline algorithm never annotates OOV open class items, like numbers, correctly. Numbers written in digits were thus replaced with a generic tag in the training corpus and in the input text using a simple regular expression. Since lemmatization is based on the actual word form and not on the generic tag, this method, while it solves the tagging problem of numbers, does not interfere with proper lemmatization.

As results for the entry called +PRO+NUM in Table 1 show, these simple modifications resulted in a significant improvement of tagging and full annotation accuracies.

## 5.7   Improved Handling of OOV Words

In order to increase the accuracy of the system further, we introduced a better algorithm to handle OOV words replacing the 4SFX method, because to use the most probable tag (common noun) for all unknown words is obviously not an optimal solution. To improve tagging and lemmatization of OOV words, a morphological guesser was integrated, which is similar to the one implemented in PurePos. The guesser learns [lemma transformation, tag] pairs (TTP) for the given suffixes from rare words in the training data. A reverse trie of suffixes is built, in which each node can have a weighted list containing the corresponding TTPs.

The guesser was integrated into the decoder in the following manner. The Moses decoder is able to read a set of predefined translations from the input, which can be used to handle words not seen in the training corpus. In this setup, hapaxes are left intact in the training corpus, while OOV words are pre-translated in the input. This is an optimal solution because the guesser can assign PoS tags and lemmas based on a smoothed interpolated model of various suffix lengths. Moreover, this solution does not force the system to default to a unigram language model when encountering an OOV word.

**Table 3.** Determining the optimal guesser training frequency threshold

| frequency threshold | Token accuracy | | | Sentence accuracy | |
|:---:|---|---|---|---|---|
| | tag | lemma | morph | tag | morph |
| < 2 | 99.570% | 96.817% | **96.418%** | 92.435% | 52.829% |
| < 3 | 99.575% | 96.712% | 96.314% | 92.497% | 51.511% |
| < 4 | 99.575% | 96.598% | 96.200% | 92.513% | 50.612% |
| < 5 | 99.580% | 96.521% | 96.127% | 92.590% | 49.853% |
| < 6 | 99.580% | 96.436% | 96.044% | 92.606% | 49.171% |
| < 7 | 99.580% | 96.358% | 95.965% | 92.606% | 48.504% |
| < 8 | 99.580% | 96.302% | 95.909% | 92.621% | 48.086% |

The guesser is to be used for handling rare unseen words, therefore it should be trained on rare words. But how rare should the words in the training set be exactly? We determined this experimentally, and as can be seen in Table 3, the threshold value for which we obtained the best annotation accuracy was 2, i.e. the guesser should be trained on hapaxes. Using a higher threshold slightly improves the accuracy of tagging, but overall annotation accuracy is impaired due to a more pronounced decrease in lemmatization quality.

The performance of this configuration is shown as the entry called +GUESS in Table 1.

## 5.8    Further Improvements

Examining errors made by the system, we identified further possibilities for improvement.

**Distinction of Numbers, Identifiers and Percentages.** In the MSD coding system, various open word classes have different PoS tags, so the scheme handling numerals was extended to other categories like identifiers, percentages, Roman numerals and indices.

**Lemma Capitalization of Sentence-Initial Words.** To improve the accuracy of lemmatization, a special handling of sentence-initial words was introduced that uses the most frequent case form of the lemma for these words.

The entry called called +OPEN+S-INI=HuLaPos2 in Table 1, shows the results for this configuration.

## 6    Comparison with Other Systems

We compared the performance of the best configuration, HuLaPos2, with that of the state-of-the-art tool called PurePos. As it was mentioned in section 3, PurePos can optionally use an integrated morphological analyzer, which uses the HUMor tagset.

Table 4 shows the comparison of the performance of HuLaPos2 with that of PurePos not using the integrated morphological analyzer trained and tested on the same MSD coded version of Szeged Corpus 2. HuLaPos2 outperforms PurePos in all evaluation metrics both at the token and the sentence level. The token-level morphological accuracy was 2.074% better, which corresponds to a 39.603% relative error rate reduction.

**Table 4.** Comparison of results on the MSD-tagged version of Szeged Corpus 2

| System | Token accuracy | | | Sentence accuracy | |
|---|---|---|---|---|---|
| | tag | lemma | morph | tag | morph |
| HuLaPos2 | 99.566% | 97.242% | 96.837% | 92.358% | 57.402% |
| PurePos_MSD | 96.742% | 96.348% | 94.763% | 58.968% | 44.784% |

HuLaPos2 was also trained on a modified version of the Szeged Corpus 2, which uses HUMor tags. This makes it possible to compare our system with the language-dependent hybrid version of the state-of-the-art PurePos tool. HuLaPos2 was compared with PurePos with and without the integrated morphological analyzer on the Humor-tagged version of the corpus. HuLaPos2 performs better at tagging, with a 17.264% relative error rate reduction compared to PurePos with the integrated MA. Its lemmatization and thus its overall annotation accuracy, on the other hand, is lower than that of PurePos+MA, while it is better than that of PurePos not using a MA. Most lemmatization errors are due to incorrect lemmatization of verbs the lemma of which can end either in *-ik* or in no suffix. Since it is a purely lexical property of these verbs, and lexical information is unavailable for OOV words, the system can only select the right lemma by chance.

**Table 5.** Comparison of results on the HUMor-tagged version of Szeged Corpus 2

| System | Token accuracy | | | Sentence accuracy | |
|---|---|---|---|---|---|
| | tag | lemma | morph | tag | morph |
| HuLaPos2 | 99.181% | 98.230% | 97.621% | 87.910% | 70.188% |
| PurePos | 96.499% | 96.270% | 94.534% | 57.206% | 43.618% |
| PurePos+MA | 98.959% | 99.532% | 98.774% | 85.194% | 82.916% |

## 7   Conclusion

In this paper, we described a language-independent morphological annotation tool that performs PoS tagging and lemmatization simultaneously based on the Moses framework. The presented system employs a trie-based suffix guesser, which effectively handles the problem of OOV words, typical of morphologically rich languages like Hungarian. The performance of the system was compared to the state-of-the-art language-dependent and -independent systems for annotating Hungarian. Our method outperforms the language-independent system in all measures. Furthermore, the accuracy of PoS tagging is better and the accuracy of lemmatization is comparable to that of the language-dependent system, which uses an integrated morphological analyzer.

**Acknowledgment.** This research was partially supported by the project grants TÁMOP–4.2.1./B–11/2-KMR-2011-0002 and TÁMOP–4.2.2./B–10/1-2010-0014.

## References

1. Brants, T.: Tnt - a Statistical Part-of-Speech Tagger. In: Proceedings of the Sixth Applied Natural Language Processing (ANLP 2000), Seattle, WA (2000)
2. Csendes, D., Csirik, J.A., Gyimóthy, T.: The Szeged Corpus: A POS Tagged and Syntactically Annotated Hungarian Natural Language Corpus. In: Sojka, P., Kopeček, I., Pala, K. (eds.) TSD 2004. LNCS (LNAI), vol. 3206, pp. 41–47. Springer, Heidelberg (2004)
3. Erjavec, T.: MULTEXT-East Version 3: Multilingual Morphosyntactic Specifications, Lexicons and Corpora. In: Fourth International Conference on Language Resources and Evaluation, LREC 2004, pp. 1535–1538. ELRA (2004)
4. Gascó i Mora, G., Sánchez Peiró, J.A.: Part-of-Speech tagging based on machine translation techniques. In: Martí, J., Benedí, J.M., Mendonça, A.M., Serrat, J. (eds.) IbPRIA 2007. LNCS, vol. 4477, pp. 257–264. Springer, Heidelberg (2007)

5. Halácsy, P., Kornai, A., Oravecz, C., Trón, V., Varga, D.: Using a morphological analyzer in high precision POS tagging of Hungarian. In: Proceedings of LREC 2006, pp. 2245–2248 (2006)
6. James, F.: Modified Kneser-Ney smoothing of n-gram models. Tech. rep. (2000)
7. Jurafsky, D., Martin, J.H.: Speech and Language Processing: An Introduction to Natural Language Processing, Computational Linguistics and Speech Recognition, 2nd edn. Prentice Hall series in artificial intelligence. Prentice Hall, Pearson Education International, Englewood Cliffs, NJ (2009)
8. Koehn, P., Hoang, H., Birch, A., Callison-Burch, C., Federico, M., Bertoldi, N., Cowan, B., Shen, W., Moran, C., Zens, R., Dyer, C., Bojar, O., Constantin, A., Herbst, E.: Moses: Open Source Toolkit for Statistical Machine Translation. In: Proceedings of the ACL 2007 Demo and Poster Sessions, pp. 177–180. Association for Computational Linguistics, Prague (2007)
9. Laki, L.: Investigating the Possibilities of Using SMT for Text Annotation. In: Simões, A., Queirós, R., da Cruz, D. (eds.) 1st Symposium on Languages, Applications and Technologies. Open Access Series in Informatics (OASIcs), vol. 21, pp. 267–283. Schloss Dagstuhl–Leibniz-Zentrum Informatik, Dagstuhl (2012)
10. Novák, A.: What is good Humor like? In: I. Magyar Számítógés Nyelvészeti Konferencia, pp. 138–144. SZTE, Szeged (2003)
11. Och, F.J., Ney, H.: Improved statistical alignment models. In: Proceedings of the 38h Annual Meeting on Association for Computational Linguistics, Hongkong, China, pp. 440–447 (2000)
12. Oravecz, C., Dienes, P.: Efficient stochastic Part-of-Speech tagging for Hungarian. In: Proc. of the Third LREC, pp. 710–717. ELRA (2002)
13. Orosz, G., Novák, A.: PurePos – an open source morphological disambiguator. In: Sharp, B., Zock, M. (eds.) Proceedings of the 9th International Workshop on Natural Language Processing and Cognitive Science, Wroclaw, pp. 53–63 (2012)
14. Trón, V., Halácsy, P., Rebrus, P., András Rung, P.V., Simon, E.: Morphdb.hu: Hungarian lexical database and morphological grammar. In: LREC, pp. 1670–1673 (2006)
15. Zsibrita, J., Vincze, V., Farkas, R.: Ismeretlen kifejezések és a szófaji egyértelműsítés. In: VII. Magyar Számítgépes Nyelvészeti Konferencia, Szegedi Tudományegyetem, Szeged, pp. 275–283 (2010)

# Hybrid Text Segmentation
# for Hungarian Clinical Records

György Orosz[1,2], Attila Novák[1,2], and Gábor Prószéky[1,2]

[1] Pázmány Péter Catholic University, Faculty of Information Technology and Bionics
50/a Práter street, 1083 Budapest, Hungary
[2] MTA-PPKE Hungarian Language Technology Research Group
50/a Práter street, 1083 Budapest, Hungary
{oroszgy,novak.attila,proszeky}@itk.ppke.hu

**Abstract.** Nowadays clinical documents are getting widely available to researchers who are aiming to develop resources and tools that may help clinicians in their work. While several attempts exist for English medical text processing, there are only few for other languages. Moreover, word and sentence segmentation tasks are commonly treated as simple engineering issues. In this study, we introduce the difficulties that arise during the segmentation of Hungarian clinical records, and describe a complex method that results in a normalized and segmented text. Our approach is a hybrid combination of a rule-based and an unsupervised statistical solution. The presented system is compared with other algorithms that are available and commonly used. These fail to segment clinical text (all of them reach $F$-scores below 75%), while our method scores above 90%. This means that only the hybrid tool described in this study can be used for the segmentation of Hungarian clinical texts in practical applications.

**Keywords:** text segmentation, clinical records, sentence boundary detection, log-likelihood ratios.

## 1  Introduction

Hospitals produce a large amount of clinical records, containing valuable information about patients: these documents might be utilized to help doctors in making better diagnoses, but they are generally used only for archiving and documentation purposes. To be able to extract information from such textual data, they should be properly parsed and processed, thus proper text segmentation[1] methods are needed. However, although performing well on the general domain, existing preprocessing algorithms have diverse problems in the case of Hungarian medical records. These difficulties arise because documents produced in the clinical environment are very noisy. The typical sources of errors are the following: *a)* typing errors (i.e. mistyped tokens, nonexistent strings of falsely concatenated words), *b)* nonstandard usage of Hungarian. While errors of the

---

[1] While the term *text segmentation* is widely used for diverse tasks, in our work it is used as the process of dividing text into word tokens and sentences.

F. Castro, A. Gelbukh, and M. González (Eds.): MICAI 2013, Part I, LNAI 8265, pp. 306–317, 2013.
© Springer-Verlag Berlin Heidelberg 2013

first type can generally be corrected with a rule-based tool, others need advanced methods.

For English, there are many solutions that deal with such noisy data, but for Hungarian, only a few attempts have been made. [24,25]. Studies reporting about processing clinical texts generally do not include a description of the segmentation part. Furthermore, the existence of a reliable segmentation tool is essential, since error propagation in a text-processing chain is an important problem. This is even more notable in the case of clinical records, where noise is generally present at various levels of processing.

In this study, a hybrid approach to normalization and segmentation of Hungarian clinical records is presented. The method consists of three phases: first, a rule-based clean-up step is performed; then tokens are partially segmented; finally, sentence boundaries are determined. It is shown below how these processing units are built upon one another. Then key elements of the sentence boundary detection (SBD) algorithm are described. The presented system is evaluated against a gold standard corpus, and is compared with other tools as well.

## 2   Related Work

### 2.1   Previous Work on Text Segmentation

The task of text segmentation is often composed of subtasks: normalization of noisy text (when necessary), segmentation of words, and sentence boundary detection. The latter may involve the identification of abbreviations as well. Furthermore, there are attempts (e.g. [32]), where text segmentation and normalization are treated as a unified tagging problem, and there are some that handle the problem with rule-based solutions (such as [13,8]).

Although segmentation of tokens is generally treated as a simple engineering problem[2] that aims to split punctuation marks from word forms, SBD is a much more researched topic. As Read et al. summarize [19], sentence segmentation approaches fall into three classes: 1) rule-based methods, that employ domain- or language-specific knowledge (such as abbreviations); 2) supervised machine learning approaches, which, since they are trained on a manually annotated corpus, may perform poorly on other domains; 3) unsupervised learning methods, which extract their knowledge from raw unannotated data.

Riley [21] presents an application of decision-tree learners for disambiguating full stops, utilizing mainly lexical features, such as word length and case, and probabilities of a word being sentence-initial or sentence-final. The SATZ system [16] is a framework which makes it possible to employ machine learning algorithms that are based on not just contextual clues but PoS features as well. The utilization of the maximum entropy learning approach for SBD was introduced by Reynar and Ratnaparkhi [20]. Later, Gillick presented [7] a similar approach

---

[2] In the case of alphabetic writing systems.

for English that relies on support vector machines resulting in a state-of-the-art performance.

In [13], Mikheev utilizes a small set of rules that are able to detect sentence boundaries (SB) with a high accuracy. In another system presented by him [12], the rule-based tokenizer described above is integrated into a PoS-tagging framework, which allows to assign labels to punctuation marks as well: these can be labeled as a sentence boundary, an abbreviation or both. Punkt [9] is a tool presented by Kiss and Strunk, that employs only unsupervised machine learning techniques: the scaled log-likelihood ratio method is used for deciding whether a *(word, period)* pair is a collocation or not.

There are some freely available systems specific to Hungarian: Huntoken [8] is an open source tool that is mainly based on Mikheev's rule-based system; and `magyarlanc` [33], which is a full natural language processing chain that contains an adapted version of MorphAdorner's tokenizer [10] and sentence splitter.

### 2.2  Processing Medical Text

For Hungarian clinical records, Siklósi et al. [24] presented a baseline system to correct spelling errors found in clinical documents. Their algorithm tries to fix a subset of possible spelling errors, relying on various types of language models. An improved version of their system was introduced recently [25], but sentence boundary detection is still not touched in it.

Tokenization and SBD is currently not a hot area in natural language processing, but there are some attempts at dealing with the segmentation of medical texts. Sentence segmentation methods, employed by clinical text processing systems, fall into two classes: many of them apply rule-based settings (e.g. [31]), while others employ supervised machine learning algorithms (such as [1,3,22,27,29]). Tools falling into the latter category mainly use maximum entropy or CRF learners, thus a handcrafted training material is essential. This corpus is either a domain-specific one or derived from the general domain. In practice, training data from a related domain yields better performance, while others [28] argue that the domain of the training corpus is not critical.

## 3  Resources and Metrics

### 3.1  Clinical Records

Our aim was to develop a high-performance text segmentation algorithm for Hungarian clinical records, since the resulting outcome is intended to be used by shallow parsing tools, which may be parts of a greater text processing system. To ensure the high quality of the processed data, input texts had to be normalized and a gold standard corpus was created for testing purposes. The normalization process had to deal with the following errors[3]:

---

[3] Text normalization is performed using regular expressions, which are not detailed here.

1. doubly converted characters, such as '&gt;',
2. typewriter problems (e.g. '1' and '0' is written as 'l' and 'o'),
3. dates and date intervals that were in various formats with or without necessary whitespaces (e.g. '2009.11.11', '06.01.08'),
4. missing whitespaces between tokens that usually introduced various types of errors:
   (a) measurements were erroneously attached to quantities (e.g. '0.12mg'),
   (b) lack of whitespace around punctuation marks (e.g. 'töröközegek.Fundus:ép.'),
5. various formulation of numerical expressions.

In order to investigate possible pitfalls of the algorithm being developed, the gold standard data set was split into two sets of equal sizes: a development and a test set, containing 1320 and 1310 lines respectively. The first part was used to identify typical problems in the corpus and to develop the segmentation methods, while the second part was used to verify our results. The comparison of clinical texts and a corpus of general Hungarian (Szeged Corpus [4]) reveals the following differences :

1. 2.68% of tokens found in clinical corpus sample are abbreviations while the same ratio for general Hungarian is only 0.23%;
2. sentences taken from the Szeged Corpus almost always end in a sentence final punctuation mark (98.96%), while these are totally missing from clinical statements in 48.28% of the cases;
3. sentence-initial capitalization is a general rule in Hungarian (99.58% of the sentences are formulated properly in the Szeged Corpus), but its usage is not common in the case of clinicians (12.81% of the sentences start with a word that is not capitalized);
4. the amount of numerical data is significant in medical records (13.50% of sentences consist exclusively of measurement data and abbreviations), while text taken from the general domain rarely contains statements that are full of measurements.

These special properties together make the creation of a specialized text segmentation algorithm for clinical texts necessary.

### 3.2   Metrics Used for Comparison

There are no metrics that are commonly used across text segmentation tasks. Researchers specializing in machine learning approaches prefer to calculate precision, recall and $F$-measure, while others, basically having a background in speech recognition, prefer to use NIST and Word Error Rate. Recently, Read et al. have reviewed [19] the current state-of-the-art in sentence boundary detection, and have proposed a unified metric that makes it possible to compare the performance of different approaches. Their method allows for the detection of sentence boundaries after any kind of character: characters can be labeled as sentence-finals or non sentence-finals, and thus accuracy is used for comparison.

In our work, the latter unified metric was generalized in order to be employed for the unified segmentation problem: viewing the text as a sequence of characters and empty strings between each character, the task can be treated as a classification problem, where all entities (characters and empty string between them) are labeled with the following tags:

$\langle \mathbf{T} \rangle$ – if the entity is a token boundary,
$\langle \mathbf{S} \rangle$ – if it is a sentence boundary,
$\langle \mathbf{None} \rangle$ – if the entity is neither.

The usage of this classification scheme enables us to use accuracy as a measure. Moreover, one can calculate precision, recall and $F$-measure as well.

In our work, we use accuracy as described above, to monitor the progress of the whole segmentation task. Since it is important to measure the two subtasks separately, precision and recall values are calculated for both word tokenization and SBD. Precision becomes more important than recall during the automatic sentence segmentation of clinical documents: an erroneously split sentence may cause information loss, while statements might still be extracted from multi-sentence text. Thus $F_{0.5}$ measure is employed for SBD, while word tokenization is evaluated against the balanced $F_1$ measure.

## 4   The Proposed Method

Tasks not examined previously need a baseline method that can be used for comparison. In our case, the method detailed below is compared with others. This algorithm was found to perform well with unambiguous boundaries, thus it was kept as a base of the proposed tool. Further extensions to the algorithm are detailed in section 4.2, which made it possible to deal with more complicated cases.

### 4.1   Baseline Word Tokenization and Sentence Segmentation

The baseline rule-based algorithm is composed of two parts. The first performs the word tokenization (BWT), while the second marks the sentence boundaries (BSBD). One principle that was kept in mind for the word segmentation process was not to detach periods from the ends of the words. It was necessary since BWT did not intend to recognize abbreviations: this task was left to the sentence segmentation process. The tokenization algorithm is not detailed here, since it performs tasks generally implemented in standard tokenizers.

The subsequent system in the processing chain is BSBD: to avoid information loss (as described in section 3.2.), it is minimizing the possibility of making false-positive errors. Sentences are only split if there is a high confidence of success. These cases are when:

1. a period or exclamation mark directly follows another punctuation mark token[4];
2. a line starts with a full date, and is followed by other words (The last white-space character before the date is marked as SB.);
3. a line begins with the name of an examination followed by a semicolon and a sequence of measurements.

Pipelining these algorithms yields 100% precision and 73.38% recall for the token segmentation task[5], while the corresponding values for the sentence boundary detection are 98.48% and 42.60% respectively. The latter values mean that less than half of the sentence boundaries are discovered, which obviously needs to be improved. An analysis of errors produced by the whole process showed that the whole tokenization process has difficulties only with separating sentence final periods. A detailed examination suggests that an improvement in sentence boundary detection can result in higher recall scores for word tokenization as well. Because of these, hereunder we only concentrate on improving the BSBD module.

### 4.2   Improvements on Sentence Boundary Detection

Usually, there are two kinds of indicators for sentence boundaries: the first is when a period ($\bullet$) is attached to a word: in this case a sentence boundary is found for sure only if the token is not an abbreviation; the second is when a word starts with a capital letter and it is neither part of a proper name nor of an acronym. Unfortunately, these indicators are not directly applicable in our case, since medical abbreviations are diverse and clinicians usually introduce new ones that are not part of the standard. Furthermore, Latin words and abbreviations are sometimes capitalized by mistake and there are subclauses that start with capitalized words. Moreover, as shown above, several sentence boundaries lack both of these indicators.

However, these features can still be used in SBD. A full list of abbreviations is not necessary: it is enough to find evidence for the separateness of a word and the attached period to be able to mark a sentence boundary. We found that the utilization of the scaled log-likelihood ratio method worked well in similar scenarios [9], thus its possible adaptation was examined.

The algorithm was first introduced in [6]: it was used for identifying collocations. Later it was adapted for the sentence segmentation task by Kiss and Strunk [9]. Their idea was to handle abbreviations as collocations of words and periods. In practice, this is formulated via a null hypothesis (1) and an alternative one (2).

$$H_0 : P(\bullet|w) = p = P(\bullet|\neg w) \tag{1}$$

$$H_A : P(\bullet|w) = p_1 \neq p_2 = P(\bullet|\neg w) \tag{2}$$

---

[4] Question marks are not considered as sentence-final punctuation marks, since they generally indicate a questionable finding in clinical texts.

[5] The values that are presented in this section were measured on the development set.

$$log\lambda = -2log\frac{L(H_0)}{L(H_A)} \tag{3}$$

(1) expresses the independence of a *(word, •)* pair, while (2) formulates that their co-occurrence is not just by chance. Based on these hypotheses $log\lambda$ is calculated (3), which is asymptotically $\chi^2$ distributed, thus it could be applied as a statistical test [6]. Kiss and Strunk found that pure $log\lambda$ performs poorly[6] in abbreviation detection scenarios, and thus they introduced scaling factors [9]. In that way, their approach loses the asymptotic relation to $\chi^2$ and becomes a filtering algorithm.

Since our aim is to find those candidates that co-occur only by chance, the scaled log-likelihood ratio method was used with inverse score ($iscore = 1/log\lambda$). Several experiments were performed on the development set that showed that the scaling factors described below give the best performance.

Our case contrasts to [9]: counts and count ratios did not indicate properly whether a token and the period is related in a clinical record, since frequencies of abbreviation types are relatively low. As the original work proposes, good indicators of abbreviations is their lengths *(len)*: shorter tokens tend to be abbreviations, while longer ones do not. Formulating this observation, a function is required that penalizes words that only have a few characters, while increasing the scores of others. Having a medical abbreviation list of almost 200 elements[7] we found that that more than 90% of the abbreviations are shorter than three characters. This fact encouraged us to set the first scaling factor as in (4). This enhancement is not just able to boost the score of a pair but it can also decrease it as well.

$$S_{length}(iscore) = iscore \cdot \exp{(len/3 - 1)} \tag{4}$$

Recently, HuMor [17,18] – a morphological analyzer (MA) for Hungarian – was extended with the content of a medical dictionary [14]. Therefore this new version of the tool could be used to enhance the sentence segmentation algorithm. HuMor is able to analyze possible abbreviations and full words as well, thus its output is utilized by an indicator function (5). Since the output of a MA is very strong evidence, a scaling component based on it needs larger weights compared to others. This led us to formulate (6).

$$indicator_{morph}(word) = \begin{cases} 1 & \text{if } word \text{ has an analysis of a known full word} \\ -1 & \text{if } word \text{ has an analysis of a known abbreviation} \\ 0 & \text{otherwise} \end{cases}$$

$$\tag{5}$$

$$S_{morph}(iscore) = iscore \cdot \exp{(indicator_{morph} \cdot len^2)} \tag{6}$$

Another indicator was discovered during the analysis of the data: a hyphen is generally not present in abbreviations but rather occurs in full words. This led

---

[6] In terms of precision.

[7] The list is gathered with an automatic algorithm that uses word shape properties and frequencies, then the most frequent elements are manually verified and corrected.

us to the third factor (7) where $indicator_{hyphen}$ is 1 only if the word contains a hyphen, otherwise it is 0.

$$S_{hyphen}(iscore) = iscore \cdot \exp\left(indicator_{hyphen} \cdot len\right) \qquad (7)$$

Scaled *iscore* is calculated for all *(word, •)* pairs that are not followed by another punctuation mark. If this value is higher than 1.5, the period is regarded as a sentence boundary and it is detached. Investigating the performance of the method described above, it was pipelined after the BSBD module producing 77.14% recall and 97.10% precision.

In order to utilize the second source of information (word capitalization), another component was introduced. It deals with words that begin with capital letters . Good SB candidates of these are the ones that do not follow a non sentence terminating[8] punctuation, and are not part of a named entity. Sequences of capitalized words are omitted and the rest is processed with HuMor: words known to be common are marked as the beginning of a sentence. In our case common words are those that do not have a proper noun analysis. Chaining only this component with BSBD results in 65.46% of recall and 96.37% of precision.

## 5   Evaluation

Our hybrid algorithm was developed using the development set, thus it is evaluated against the rest of the data.

**Table 1.** Accuracy of the input text and the baseline segmented one

|                       | Accuracy |
| --------------------- | -------- |
| Preprocessed          | 97.55%   |
| Segmented (baseline)  | 99.11%   |

Accuracy values in Table 1 can be used as good bases for the comparison of the overall segmentation task, but one must note that this metric is not well balanced. Its values are relatively high even for the preprocessed text, thus the increase in accuracy needs to be measured. Relative error rate reduction scores are provided in Table 2, which are calculated over the baseline method. We investigated each part of the sentence segmentation algorithm and examined their collaboration as well. The unsupervised SBD algorithm is marked with $LLR^9$, while the second is indicated by the term *CAP*.

A more detailed analysis of the SBD task is made by comparing precision, recall and $F_{0.5}$ values (see Table 3.). Each component significantly increases the recall, while precision is just barely decreased.

---

[8] Sentence terminating punctuation marks are the period and the exclamation mark for this task.

[9] Referring to the term log-likelihood ratio.

**Table 2.** Error rate reduction over the accuracy of the baseline method

|         | Error rate reduction |
|---------|----------------------|
| LLR     | 58.62%               |
| CAP     | 9.25%                |
| LLR+CAP | 65.50%               |

**Table 3.** Evaluation of the proposed sentence segmentation algorithm compared with the baseline

|          | Precision | Recall | $F_{0.5}$ |
|----------|-----------|--------|-----------|
| Baseline | 96.57%    | 50.26% | 81.54%    |
| LLR      | 95.19%    | 78.19% | 91.22%    |
| CAP      | 94.60%    | 71.56% | 88.88%    |
| LLR+CAP  | 93.28%    | 86.73% | 91.89%    |

The combined hybrid algorithm[10] brings significant improvement over the well-established baseline, but a comparison with other available tools is also presented. Freely available tools for segmenting Hungarian texts are magyarlanc and Huntoken. The latter can be slightly configured by providing a set of abbreviations, thus two versions of Huntoken are compared. One which employs the built-in set of general Hungarian abbreviations (*HTG*), and another one that extends the previous list with medical ones described in section 4.2 (*HTM*). Punct [9] and OpenNLP [2] – a popular implementation of the maximum entropy SBD method [20] – were involved in the comparison as well. Since the latter tool employs a supervised learning algorithm, Szeged Corpus is used as a training material.

**Table 4.** Comparision of the proposed hybrid SBD method with competing ones

|               | Precision | Recall | $F_{0.5}$ |
|---------------|-----------|--------|-----------|
| magyarlanc    | 72.59%    | 77.68% | 73.55%    |
| HTG           | 44.73%    | 49.23% | 45.56%    |
| HTM           | 43.19%    | 42.09% | 42.97%    |
| Punkt         | 58.78%    | 45.66% | 55.59%    |
| OpenNLP       | 52.10%    | 96.30% | 57.37%    |
| Hybrid system | 93.28%    | 86.73% | 91.89%    |

Values in Table 4 show that general segmentation methods failed on sentences of Hungarian clinical records. It is interesting that the maxent approach has high recall, but boundaries marked by it are false positives in almost half of the cases. Rules provided by magyarlanc seem to be robust, but the overall performance inhibits its application for clinical texts. Others do not just provide low recalls, but their precision values are around 50%, which is too low for practical purposes.

Our approach mainly focuses on the sentence segmentation task, but an improvement of word tokenization is expected as well. Better recognition of words

---

[10] It is the composition of the BWT, BSBD, LLR and CAP components.

**Table 5.** Comparing tokenization performance of the new tool with the baseline one

|  | Precision | Recall | $F_1$ |
|---|---|---|---|
| Baseline | 99.74% | 74.94% | 85.58% |
| Hybrid system | 98.54% | 95.32% | 96.90% |

that are not abbreviations results in a higher recall (see Table 5), while it does not significantly decrease precision.

# 6   Conclusion

We presented a hybrid approach that consists of several rule-based algorithms and an unsupervised machine learning algorithm to tokenization and sentence boundary detection. Owing to the special properties of Hungarian clinical texts, emphasis was laid on the direct detection of sentence boundaries. The method performs word tokenization first, partially segmenting tokens. Attached periods are left untouched in order to help the subsequent sentence segmentation process. The SBD method described above is based mainly on the calculation of $log\lambda$, which was adapted to the task in order to improve the overall performance of our tool. A unique property of the algorithm presented is that it is able to incorporate the knowledge of a morphological analyzer as well, increasing the recall of sentence segmentation.

The segmentation method successfully deals with several sorts of imperfect sentence boundaries. As described in section 5, the given algorithm performs better in terms of precision and recall than competing ones. Only magyarlanc reached an $F_{0.5}$-score above 60%, which is still too low for practical applications. The method presented in this study achieved a 92% of $F_{0.5}$-score, which allows the tool to be used in the Hungarian clinical domain.

**Acknowledgement.** We would like to thank Borbála Siklósi and Nóra Wenszky for their comments on preliminary versions of this paper. This work was partially supported by TÁMOP – 4.2.1.B – 11/2/KMR-2011-0002 and TÁMOP – 4.2.2/B – 10/1–2010–0014.

# References

1. Apostolova, E., Channin, D.S., Demner-Fushman, D., Furst, J., Lytinen, S., Raicu, D.: Automatic segmentation of clinical texts. In: Annual International Conference of the IEEE Engineering in Medicine and Biology Society, EMBC 2009, pp. 5905–5908. IEEE (2009)
2. Baldridge, J., Morton, T., Bierner, G.: The OpenNLP maximum entropy package (2002)
3. Paul, S., Cho, R.K., Taira, Kangarloo, H.: Text boundary detection of medical reports. In: Proceedings of the AMIA Symposium, p. 998. American Medical Informatics Association (2002)

4. Csendes, D., Csirik, J., Gyimóthy, T.: The Szeged Corpus: A POS tagged and syntactically annotated Hungarian natural language corpus. In: Proceedings of the 5th International Workshop on Linguistically Interpreted Corpora, pp. 19–23 (2004)
5. Dridan, R., Oepen, S.: Tokenization: returning to a long solved problem a survey, contrastive experiment, recommendations, and toolkit. In: Proceedings of the 50th Annual Meeting of the Association for Computational Linguistics, pp. 378–382. Association for Computational Linguistics (2012)
6. Dunning, T.: Accurate methods for the statistics of surprise and coincidence. Computational linguistics 19(1), 61–74 (1993)
7. Gillick, D.: Sentence boundary detection and the problem with the US. In: Proceedings of Human Language Technologies: The 2009 Annual Conference of the North American Chapter of the Association for Computational Linguistics, Companion Volume: Short Papers, pp. 241–244. Association for Computational Linguistics (2009)
8. Halácsy, P., Kornai, A., Németh, L., Rung, A., Szakadát, I., Trón, V.: Creating open language resources for Hungarian. In: Proceedings of Language Resources and Evaluation Conference (2004)
9. Kiss, T., Strunk, J.: Unsupervised multilingual sentence boundary detection. Computational Linguistics 32(4), 485–525 (2006)
10. Kumar, A.: Monk project: Architecture overview. In: Proceedings of JCDL 2009 Workshop: Integrating Digital Library Content with Computational Tools and Services (2009)
11. Meystre, S.M., Savova, G.K., Kipper-Schuler, K.C., Hurdle, J.F.: Extracting information from textual documents in the electronic health record: a review of recent research. In: Yearbook of Medical Informatics, pp. 128–144 (2008)
12. Mikheev, A.: Tagging sentence boundaries. In: Proceedings of the 1st North American chapter of the Association for Computational Linguistics Conference, pp. 264–271. Association for Computational Linguistics (2000)
13. Mikheev, A.: Periods, capitalized words, etc. Computational Linguistics 28(3), 289–318 (2002)
14. Orosz, G., Novák, A., Prószéky, G.: Magyar nyelvű klinikai rekordok morfológiai egyértelműsítése. In: IX. Magyar Számítógépes Nyelvészeti Konferencia, Szeged, pp. 159–169. Szegedi Tudományegyetem (2013)
15. Palmer, D.D., Hearst, M.A.: Adaptive sentence boundary disambiguation. In: Proceedings of the fourth conference on Applied natural language processing, pp. 78–83. Association for Computational Linguistics (1994)
16. Palmer, D.D., Hearst, M.A.: Adaptive multilingual sentence boundary disambiguation. Computational Linguistics 23(2), 241–267 (1997)
17. Prószéky, G.: Industrial applications of unification morphology. In: Proceedings of the Fourth Conference on Applied Natural Language Processing, Morristown, NJ, USA, p. 213 (1994)
18. Prószéky, G., Novák, A.: Computational Morphologies for Small Uralic Languages. In: Inquiries into Words, Constraints and Contexts, Stanford, California, pp. 150–157 (2005)
19. Read, J., Dridan, R., Oepen, S., Solberg, L.J.: Sentence Boundary Detection: A Long Solved Problem? In: 24th International Conference on Computational Linguistics (Coling 2012), India (2012)
20. Reynar, J.C., Ratnaparkhi, A.: A maximum entropy approach to identifying sentence boundaries. In: Proceedings of the Fifth Conference on Applied Natural Language Processing, pp. 16–19. Association for Computational Linguistics (1997)

21. Riley, M.D.: Some applications of tree-based modelling to speech and language. In: Proceedings of the Workshop on Speech and Natural Language, pp. 339–352. Association for Computational Linguistics (1989)

22. Savova, G.K., Masanz, J.J., Ogren, P.V., Zheng, J., Sohn, S., Schuler, K.K., Chute, C.G.: Mayo clinical text analysis and knowledge extraction system (ctakes): architecture, component evaluation and applications. Journal of the American Medical Informatics Association 17(5), 507–513 (2010)

23. Schmid, H.: Unsupervised learning of period disambiguation for tokenisation. Technical report (2000)

24. Siklósi, B., Orosz, G., Novák, A., Prószéky, G.: Automatic structuring and correction suggestion system for hungarian clinical records. In: De Pauw, G., De Schryver, G.M., Forcada, M.L., Tyers, F.M. (eds.) 8th SaLTMiL Workshop on Creation and Use of Basic Lexical Resources for Lessresourced Languages, pp. 29–34 (2012)

25. Siklósi, B., Novák, A., Prószéky, G.: Context-aware correction of spelling errors in hungarian medical documents. In: Dediu, A.-H., Martín-Vide, C., Mitkov, R., Truthe, B. (eds.) SLSP 2013. LNCS, vol. 7978, pp. 248–259. Springer, Heidelberg (2013)

26. Stevenson, M., Gaizauskas, R.: Experiments on sentence boundary detection. In: Proceedings of the Sixth Conference on Applied Natural Language Processing, pp. 84–89. Association for Computational Linguistics (2000)

27. Taira, R.K., Soderland, S.G., Jakobovits, R.M.: Automatic structuring of radiology free-text reports. Radiographics 21(1), 237–245 (2001)

28. Tomanek, K., Wermter, J., Hahn, U.: A reappraisal of sentence and token splitting for life sciences documents. Studies in Health Technology and Informatics 129(pt. 1), 524–528 (2006)

29. Tomanek, K., Wermter, J., Hahn, U.: Sentence and token splitting based on conditional random fields. In: Proceedings of the 10th Conference of the Pacific Association for Computational Linguistics, pp. 49–57 (2007)

30. Wrenn, J.O., Stetson, P.D., Johnson, S.B.: An unsupervised machine learning approach to segmentation of clinician-entered free text. In: AMIA Annu. Symp. Proc., pp. 811–815 (2007)

31. Xu, H., Stenner, S.P., Doan, S., Johnson, K.B., Waitman, L.R., Denny, J.C.: Medex: a medication information extraction system for clinical narratives. Journal of the American Medical Informatics Association 17(1), 19–24 (2010)

32. Zhu, C., Tang, J., Li, H., Ng, H.T., Zhao, T.: A unified tagging approach to text normalization. In: The 45th Annual Meeting of the Association for Computational Linguistics, pp. 688–695 (2007)

33. Zsibrita, J., Vincze, V., Farkas, R.: magyarlanc: A Toolkit for Morphological and Dependency Parsing of Hungarian. In: Proceedings of Recent Advances in Natural Language Provessing 2013, Hissar, Bulgaria, pp. 763–771. Association for Computational Linguistics (2013)

# Detection and Expansion of Abbreviations in Hungarian Clinical Notes

Borbála Siklósi[2] and Attila Novák[1,2]

[1] MTA-PPKE Language Technology Research Group
[2] Pázmány Péter Catholic University, Faculty of Information Technology and Bionics,
50/a Práter Street, 1083 Budapest, Hungary
{surname.firstname}@itk.ppke.hu

**Abstract.** Processing clinical records is an important topic in natural language processing (NLP). However, for general NLP methods to work, a proper, normalized input is required, otherwise the system is overwhelmed by the unusually high amount of noise generally characteristic of this kind of text. One of the normalizing tasks is detecting and expanding abbreviations. In this paper, an unsupervised method to expand sequences of abbreviations in Hungarian medical records is presented. The implementation and evaluation of two methods are described. The first method relies on external resources: lists of medical concepts, and a manually created dictionary. The second method also utilizes these lexicons, but the quality is improved by using abbreviation interpretations automatically derived from the corpus itself.

**Keywords:** clinical text processing, abbreviation resolution.

## 1 Introduction

Processing medical texts is an emerging topic in natural language processing. There are existing solutions mainly for English to extract knowledge from medical documents, which thus becomes available for researchers and medical experts. However, locally relevant characteristics of applied medical protocols or information relevant to locally prevailing epidemic data can be extracted only from documents written in the language of the local community.

In Hungarian hospitals, clinical records are created as unstructured texts without using any proofing tools, resulting in texts full of spelling errors and nonstandard use of word forms in a language that is usually a mixture of Hungarian and Latin [11,10]. These texts are also characterized by a high ratio of abbreviated forms. The use of some of these abbreviations follows some standard rules, but most of them are used in an arbitrary manner. That is why simply matching these abbreviations to a lexicon is not satisfactory. Moreover, in most cases full statements are written in a special notational language [1] that is often used in clinical settings, consisting of only, or mostly abbreviated forms. Even for non-expert humans it is a hard task to find the phrase boundaries in a long sequence of shortened forms. A token-by-token lexicon matching would yield a

F. Castro, A. Gelbukh, and M. González (Eds.): MICAI 2013, Part I, LNAI 8265, pp. 318–328, 2013.

huge number of possible resolutions, but instead of disambiguating the meaning of these statements, only the noise would be increased. Thus processing such documents is not an easy task and resolving abbreviations is a prerequisite of further linguistic processing.

Another drawback of relying on external lexicons in order to find possible interpretations for abbreviations is the lack of such resources in Hungarian. There are the official descriptions for the ICD-10 coding system, but the matching pattern for abbreviations still must be defined in order to find resolution candidates. Thus it is not as reliable as some resources in English, such as the LABBR table of the UMLS (Unified Medical Language System), which already contains the most common medical abbreviated forms and their possible resolutions [2]. Even if there existed such a resource from which these candidates could be retrieved, the ranking of these candidates for finding the correct meaning in the actual context of the abbreviation would require a language model created from disambiguated texts. To the best of our knowledge, there is no such corpus available in Hungarian, and the manual creation of a gold standard with a size appropriate for training a supervised machine learning system would require a massive amount of expert knowledge, which is very expensive and is out of the scope of our work.

The goal of the research described in this paper is to resolve abbreviations of multiple tokens automatically by using the available lexical resources for medical phrases in Hungarian, while also relying on the clinical corpus itself. It is shown that although manually created lexical resources and ones derived from resources like medical dictionaries or ICD-10 terms are necessary but are not satisfactory to resolve abbreviations reliably. However, an unsupervised method that finds matching patterns within the corpus itself can significantly improve the quality of the resolution of abbreviations and also ensures the applicability of the method to other sub-domains.

## 2   Related Work

There are several studies, most of them applied to English texts, that address the specific task of medical language processing. One of the most challenging preprocessing steps is the detection and resolution of abbreviations found in the free-text parts of these documents. As opposed to biomedical literature, where the first mention of an abbreviated form is usually preceded by its expanded form or definition, in clinical records this is not the case. That is why simple abbreviation-definition patterns are not applicable to clinical notes as described by Hua et al. in [13]. The same study compares some machine learning approaches, all achieving considerable results, but even beside the use of already existing external resources, the authors admit the need of a manually created inventory. A recent study [12] compared the performance of some biomedical text processing systems trained on biomedical literature on the task of resolving abbreviations in clinical texts. All the systems (MetaMap, MedLEE and cTAKES) achieved suboptimal results calling for more advanced abbreviation recognition modules.

Most approaches to resolving clinical abbreviations are carried out in English relying on some very common medical lexical resources. Even though Hua in [13] showed that the sense inventories generated from the UMLS covered only about 35% of the abbreviations they had extracted from their corpus, these already contain definitions and possible interpretation candidates. Thus the problem can be reduced to abbreviation disambiguation, as it is carried out in [12,14,6]. These methods focus primarily on supervised machine learning approaches, where a part of the training corpus is labeled manually. Pakhomov in [5] described a semi-supervised method to build training data for Maximum Entropy modeling of abbreviations automatically. In most of these studies, both training and evaluation of the systems are performed on a few manually chosen abbreviations and their disambiguation.

In this work, a general evaluation is shown, without optimizing the system for just a few types of abbreviations. It also differs from other approaches in the use of external resources. The described method does not rely either on manually created sense inventories, or on manually labeled training data, the creation of which is very labor-intensive.

## 3   Characteristics of Clinical Abbreviations

The use of a kind of notational text is very common in clinical documents. This dense form of documentation contains a high ratio of standard or arbitrary abbreviations and symbols, some of which may be specific to a special domain or even to a doctor or administrator. These short forms might refer to clinically relevant concepts or to some common phrases that are very frequent in the specific domain. For the clinicians, the meaning of these common phrases is as trivial as the standard shortened forms of clinical concepts due to their expertise and familiarity with the context. Some examples for abbreviations falling into these categories are shown in Table 1.

The first problem of handling abbreviations found within running text is detecting them. Since these texts usually do not follow standard orthographic and punctuation rules, especially in the case of highly abbreviated notational text, the detection of abbreviations cannot be based on patterns formulated according to standard rules of forming abbreviations. The ending periods are usually missing, abbreviations are written with varying case (capitalization) and in varying length. For example the following forms represent the same expression, *vörös visszfény* 'red reflection': *vvf, vvfény, vörösvfény.*

From our anonymized clinical records corpus, which consists of 600,792 tokens, 3154 different abbreviations were extracted. A continuous series of shortened forms without any unabbreviated word breaking the sequence is also considered as a single abbreviation, in addition to considering its constituents each by themselves. Thus in the sentence

*Dg : Tu. pp. inf et orbitae l. dex. , Cataracta incip. o. utr. , Hypertonia,*

**Table 1.** Some examples for the use of simple abbreviations. Some of them are commonly known standard forms, usually of Latin origin, some others are, though related to the clinical domain, might have several meanings depending on the specific subdomain. The rest are abbreviated common words usually of Hungarian origin, and might also refer to both clinical phrases or common words.

| Domain | Abbreviation | Resolution | in Hungarian | in English |
|---|---|---|---|---|
| standard | o. d. | oculus dexter | jobb szem | right eye |
| | med. gr. | mediocris gradus | közepes fokú | medium grade |
| domain-specific | o. (ophthalmology) | oculus | szem | eye |
| | o. (general anatomy) | os | csont | bone |
| common domain | sü | saját szemüveg | saját szemüveg | own pair of glasses |
| specific phrase | fén | fényérzés nélkül | fényérzés nélkül | no sense of light |
| | n | normál | normál | normal |
| common words | köv | következő | következő | next |
| | lsd | lásd | lásd | see |

the abbreviation spans are:

$$Dg,$$
$$Tu.\ pp.\ inf,$$
$$l.\ dex.,$$
$$incip.\ o.\ utr..$$

In this example, the last section is misleading, since the token *incip.* is related to its preceding neighbour (*Cataracta*), which is not included in this list as part of an abbreviation. This mixed use of a phrase is very common in the documents, with a diverse variation of choosing certain words to be used in their full or shortened form. The individual constituents of such sequences of abbreviations are by themselves highly ambiguous, and even if there were an inventory of Hungarian medical abbreviations, which does not exist, their resolution could not be solved. Moreover, the mixed use of Hungarian and Latin phrases results in abbreviated forms of words in both languages, thus the detection of the language of the abbreviation is another problem.

Even though the standalone abbreviated tokens are highly ambiguous, they more frequently occur as members of such multiword abbreviated phrases, in which they are usually easier to interpret unambiguously. For example *o.* could stand for any word either in Hungarian or in Latin, starting with the letter *o*, even if limited to the medical domain. However, in our corpus of ophthalmology reports, *o.* is barely used by itself, but together with a laterality indicator, i.e. in forms such as *o. s.*, *o. d.*, or *o. u.* meaning *oculus sinister* 'left eye', *oculus dexter* 'right eye', or *oculi utriusque* 'both eyes', respectively. In such contexts, the meaning of the abbreviated *o.* is unambiguous. It should be noted, that these are not the only representations for these abbreviated phrases, for example *o. s.* is also present in the form of *o. sin.*, *os*, *OS*, etc. Statistics for some variations of these phrases are shown in Table 2.

The primary objective of the research described here is finding such spans in a sequence of abbreviations that can be unambiguously resolved together.

**Table 2.** Corpus frequencies of some variations for abbreviating the three phrases *oculus sinister, oculus dexter* and *oculi utrisque*, which are the three most frequent abbreviated phrases

| oculus sinister | freq | oculus dexter | freq | oculi utriusque | freq |
|---|---|---|---|---|---|
| o. s. | 1056 | o. d. | 1543 | o. u. | 897 |
| o.s. | 15 | o.d. | 3 | o.u. | 37 |
| o. s | 51 | o. d | 188 | o. u | 180 |
| os | 160 | od | 235 | ou | 257 |
| O. s. | 118 | O. d. | 353 | O. u. | 39 |
| o. sin. | 348 | o. dex. | 156 | o. utr. | 398 |
| o. sin | 246 | o. dex | 19 | o. utr | 129 |
| O. sin | 336 | O. dex | 106 | O. utr | 50 |
| O. sin. | 48 | O. dex. | 16 | O. utr. | 77 |

Since sometimes whole statements or even sentences are written using this kind of heavily abbreviated notation, the task of finding the optimal partitioning of the tokens to meaningful spans is of crucial importance. In the above example, the fragment *incip. o. utr.* should be divided into the spans of *incip.* and *o. utr.*, even if the abbreviation *incip.* is not relevant by itself, but still its meaning is not related to the rest of the abbreviation sequence.

## 4    Materials and Methods

In this research, anonymized clinical documents from the ophthalmology department of a Hungarian clinic are used. The first task was to collect abbreviations found in these documents. Then two methods were applied to find meaningful spans within longer statements and to resolve their meanings. The latter two problems in both methods are performed in one step, optimizing for the best coverage and interpretation at the same time.

### 4.1    Detection of Abbreviations

A general characteristic of the free-text parts of the documents is the non-standard use of language, lacking compliance with any orthographic standard. This applies to the abbreviated forms as well. One cannot rely on the standard markers of an abbreviation (such as the presence of a word-final period or words in all capitals, etc.). The description of a sophisticated algorithm for the detection task is out of the scope of this paper. We applied some heuristic rules, with features such as the presence or absence of a word-final period, the length of the token, the ratio of vowels and consonants within the token, the ratio of upper- and lowercase letters, and the judgment of a Hungarian morphological analyzer [4,7]. Using this method, a result of relatively higher recall and lower precision can be achieved, which is appropriate for further processing in this task for two reasons. The focus is not on retrieving individual tokens, but rather on finding sequences of abbreviations that will later be divided into semantically relevant spans. Thus if a single word, without any neighboring abbreviation is labeled as an abbreviation, it is not considered an abbreviation. On the other hand, if a word is part of a sequence and should not be resolved, then it will be untouched by the algorithm – since no relevant resolution can be applied to it – as if it had not been extracted. For example in the phrase *Exstirp. tu. et reconstr. pp. inf. l. d.*, the Latin word *et* is not an abbreviation, and will neither be attached to its preceding, nor to its following span during the resolution process.

## 4.2   Resolution of Abbreviations

**Lexical Lookup from External Resources.** In the first approach, once having a sequence of abbreviations, a maximum coverage resolution suggestion process is carried out. For each possible partitioning of the tokens into non-overlapping spans, a regular expression pattern is generated, which is then matched against lexicons. The patterns are created by general abbreviation rules, such as each letter in the abbreviated form represents the starting letter of each word in the expanded phrase. Or, in the case of multiword abbreviations, each member represents the beginning of each word (not just the first letter) in the interpretation. Some pattern generation rules are presented in Table 3.

**Table 3.** Some of the simplest patterns generated from two short abbreviated phrases. The complexity and variability of these patterns is proportional to the length of the original abbreviation sequence.

| abbr | regexp | matching expansion | regexp | matching expansion |
|------|--------|--------------------|--------|--------------------|
| o. s. | o[^ ]* s[^ ]* | oculus sinister | | |
| os | os[^ ]* | osteoporosis | o[^ ]* s[^ ]* | oculus sinister |

The lexicons where these patterns are looked up were created from the ophthalmology sections of the descriptions of the official coding system for diseases, anatomical structures and medical procedures, along with a medical dictionary. These resources were used to create a final list of phrases containing 3329 entries. The regular expressions are matched against possible resolution candidates from these lists. In addition to these official descriptions, a small domain-specific lexicon was also created manually with the help of a medical expert. This list contains frequent non-official abbreviations specific to the corpus. The resolution candidates generated for each span are ranked according to the source lexicon they originate from.

Finally, the different partitionings must be ranked according to three features, optimizing for the longest coverage and best resolution of the abbreviation sequence. The features used for ranking are 1) the number of all tokens in the sequence covered by a resolved form, 2) the size of the longest span covered, 3) the size of the shortest span covered. If the sequence *Exstirp. tu. et reconstr. pp.*

*inf. l. d.*, is partitioned as *Exstirp. tu. — et — reconstr. pp. inf. — l. d.*, with having a resolution candidate for each partition except for the word *et*, then the value of the features are 7, 3 and 2, respectively.

**Unsupervised, Corpus-Induced Resolution.** The main drawback of the previous method is that only official descriptions can be resolved. However, in clinical documents there are freestyle statements written in abbreviated forms that cannot be matched to any phrase in the lexicons. However, due to the limited domain of the corpus, one may assume that such statements, or at least some fragments, are contained within the corpus itself in their expanded form. Thus the second approach also utilizes the aforementioned corpus fragment matching strategy along with all partitioning possibilities. In the first round, however, the generated patterns are not matched against the lexicons, but are sought for in the corpus itself. In this case, single token fragments are not taken into account, which would rather increase the noise in the candidate list. During the generation of this list, the results are pruned using some threshold values based on the length of the covered span and the corpus frequency of the matched result.

Once this corpus-specific resolution is done, the lexicon lookup procedure is carried out, now on the partially resolved sequences, in order to finish the still improper resolutions or to find the missing ones. For example, the simple phrase *o. s.* is never present in the corpus as the fully resolved form of *oculus sinister*, but might be overwritten by the form *o. sin.* due to the much higher frequency of that variant of the abbreviation as part of the actual phrase. In either case, the lexicon lookup will find the full resolution. Replacing *o. s.* by *o. sin.* might also have an effect on covering the rest of the sequence that would in some cases not be matched if frequent subexpressions were not normalized first.

Using the corpus for normalizing the sequences is fully unsupervised, thus it can easily be applied to any other sub-domains that have a raw training corpus. As shown later in the evaluation section, this method of preprocessing before lexical lookup makes the system more robust by having a less significant drop in performance when using only a reduced version of our handmade, corpus-specific lexicon. This will be an important aspect in the extension of the described method to other domains in the future.

## 5   Evaluation

From our clinical corpus, 23 already tokenized documents (containing 4516 tokens) were separated for testing purposes. This test corpus contained 323 different, automatically detected abbreviations or abbreviation sequences. These were then manually filtered, and finally 44 unique abbreviation sequences (containing 140 tokens) were chosen, all of which occurred more than once in the test corpus and had a length of at least 2 tokens. Table 4 shows some example sequences with their fragmentation and resolution according to the two methods described above.

Evaluation was performed on the levels of both full multiword abbreviations and that of individual tokens. In the first case, a resolution of a sequence was

**Table 4.** Examples for expanding some abbreviation sequences with each method compared to the manually created gold standard

| | **Cat. incip. o. utr.** |
|---|---|
| 1st method | cat. incip. oculi utriusque |
| 2nd method | cataracta incipiens oculi utriusque |
| gold standard | cataracta incipiens oculi utriusque |
| | **Myopia c. ast. o. utr.** |
| 1st method | myopia kritikus fúziós frekvencia ast. oculi utriusque |
| 2nd method | myopia cum astigmia oculi utriusque |
| gold standard | myopia cum astigmia oculi utriusque |
| | **myop. maj. gr. o. u.** |
| 1st method | myop. maj. gr. oculi utriusque |
| 2nd method | myopia maj grad. oculi utriusque |
| gold standard | myopia major gradus oculi utriusque |
| | **med. gr. cum** |
| 1st method | med. gr. cum |
| 2nd method | med. gr. cum |
| gold standard | medium gradus cum |

considered correct if and only if the whole sequence was resolved correctly. In the second case, the number of correct individual tokens were considered, which naturally resulted in higher numbers. The performance was measured using the common metrics of precision, recall and f-measure with the following definitions. Precision is the number of correct interpretations over the number of somehow resolved elements (sequences or tokens), recall is the number of correct interpretations over the number of all elements (sequences or tokens), which corresponds to the definition of accuracy in this case. F-measure is derived as two times the product of precision and recall over the sum of these. Our methods were compared to a baseline system, in which no lexicons were used: this system resolved abbreviations using the corpus only. Table 5 shows the evaluation numbers.

It is clear from the results that relying only on the corpus itself, without any lexical resources results in very poor performance because the most frequent abbreviations are never resolved in the corpus. External lexicons are required to achieve an acceptable performance, but the method of using only external lexical resources performs significantly worse than applying the corpus search as a preprocessing step, even at the level of tokens. In addition to evaluating both methods both on individual tokens and full abbreviation sequences, the measurements were also carried out using a reduced version of our handmade lexicon. The original lexicon contained 97 different abbreviations with their resolution, while the reduced one contained only 70, i.e. the size was reduced by 28%. The other external resources were the same in both cases.

Although performance was adversely affected for both methods, the drop in performance is significantly lower in the second case, where much of the coverage

**Table 5.** Evaluation results for each method on both abbreviation and token levels with full (97 entries) and reduced (70 entries) lexicons

|  | precision | | recall | | f-measure | |
|---|---|---|---|---|---|---|
|  | abbr. | token | abbr. | token | abbr. | token |
| 1st method (full lexicon) | 46.34% | 78.57% | 43.18% | 55.79% | 44.70% | 65.25% |
| 1st method (reduced lexicon) | 39.02% | 68.04% | 36.36% | 47.82% | 37.64% | 56.17% |
| 2nd method (full lexicon) | 73.17% | 86.08% | 68.18% | 71.73% | 70.58% | 78.26% |
| 2nd method (reduced lexicon) | 68.29% | 85.08% | 63.63% | 70.28% | **65.88%** | **76.98%** |
| baseline (without lexicon) | 6.66% | 41.79% | 4.54% | 20.28% | 5.4% | 27.31% |

lost by deleting part of the manually created lexicon is regained dynamically by the system itself. Figure 1 shows the learning curve of the second method when gradually increasing the size of the training corpus. Point 0 on axis $x$ (i.e. corpus size 0) corresponds to the first method. At this point, the effect of reducing our lexicon is quite significant, however, this difference is made up by learning from the corpus.

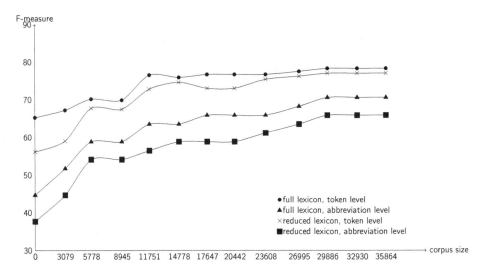

**Fig. 1.** The learning curve of each combination as a function of the size (in sentences) of the training corpus

This result provides the basis of extending the method to other domains as well, without using expensive human resources to build domain-specific lexicons manually.

# 6    Conclusion

The automatic interpretation of abbreviations in Hungarian clinical documents, though requires external lexical resources, can be efficiently improved using an unsupervised corpus-based method using abbreviation sequences and corpus frequencies of expanded forms instead of the laborious process of extending a strictly domain-specific manually created lexicon. It is shown that the ambiguity problem of short abbreviations can be handled by taking sequences of abbreviations corresponding to phrases or longer statements instead of creating a huge search space by generating resolution candidates for all individual constituents. Quantitative evaluation of the proposed system shows that although there is still some space for improvement regarding its accuracy, the system seems to adapt well to very domain-specific use of abbreviations.

**Acknowledgments.** This research was partially supported by the project grants TÁMOP–4.2.1./B–11/2-KMR-2011-0002 and TÁMOP–4.2.2./B–10/1-2010-0014.

# References

1. Barrows, J.R., Busuioc, M., Friedman, C.: Limited parsing of notational text visit notes: ad-hoc vs. NLP approaches. In: Proceedings of the AMIA Annual Symposium, pp. 51–55 (2000)
2. Liu, H., Lussier, Y.A., Friedman, C.: A study of abbreviations in the UMLS. In: Proceedings of the AMIA Annual Symposium, pp. 393–397 (2001)
3. Meystre, S., Savova, G., Kipper-Schuler, K., Hurdle, J.: Extracting information from textual documents in the electronic health record: a review of recent research. Yearb. Med. Inform. 35, 128–144 (2008)
4. Novák, A.: What is good Humor like? In: I. Magyar Számítógépes Nyelvészeti Konferencia, pp. 138–144. SZTE, Szeged (2003)
5. Pakhomov, S.: Semi-supervised maximum entropy based approach to acronym and abbreviation normalization in medical texts. In: Isabelle, P. (ed.) Proceedings of the 40th Annual Meeting on Association for Computational Linguistics (ACL), pp. 160–167. ACL Press, Philadelphia, USA, Rochester (2002)
6. Pakhomov, S., Pedersen, T., Chute, C.: Abbreviation and acronym disambiguation in clinical discourse. In: Friedman, C., Ash, J., Tarczy-Hornoch, P. (eds.) Proceedings of the AMIA Annual Symposium, Bethesda, MD, pp. 589–593. AMIA Press, Washington DC (2005)
7. Prószéky, G., Kis, B.: A unification-based approach to morpho-syntactic parsing of agglutinative and other (highly) inflectional languages. In: Proceedings of the 37th annual meeting of the Association for Computational Linguistics on Computational Linguistics, ACL 1999, pp. 261–268. Association for Computational Linguistics, Stroudsburg (1999)
8. Sager, N., Lyman, M., Bucknall, C., Nhan, N., Tick, L.J.: Natural language processing and the representation of clinical data. Journal of the American Medical Informatics Association 1(2) (March/April 1994)
9. Savova, G., Masanz, J., Ogren, P., Zheng, J., Sohn, S., Kipper-Schuler, K., Chute, C.: Mayo clinical Text Analysis and Knowledge Extraction System (cTAKES): architecture, component evaluation and applications. Journal of the American Medical Informatics Association 17(5), 507–513 (2010)

10. Siklósi, B., Novák, A., Prószéky, G.: Context-aware correction of spelling errors in Hungarian medical documents. In: Dediu, A.-H., Martín-Vide, C., Mitkov, R., Truthe, B. (eds.) SLSP 2013. LNCS, vol. 7978, pp. 248–259. Springer, Heidelberg (2013)
11. Siklósi, B., Orosz, G., Novák, A., Prószéky, G.: Automatic structuring and correction suggestion system for Hungarian clinical records. In: De Pauw, G., De Schryver, G.M., Forcada, M., Tyers, F., Waiganjo Wagacha, P. (eds.) 8th SaLT-MiL Workshop on Creation and Use of Basic Lexical Resources for Less-Resourced Languages, pp. 29–34 (2012)
12. Wu, Y., Denny, J.C., Rosenbloom, S.T., Miller, R.A., Giuse, D.A., Xu, H.: A comparative study of current clinical natural language processing systems on handling abbreviations in discharge summaries. In: Proceedings of the AMIA Annual Symposium 2012, pp. 997–1003 (2012)
13. Xu, H., Stetson, P., Friedman, C.: A study of abbreviations in clinical notes. In: Teich, J., Suermondt, J., Hripcsak, G. (eds.) Proceedings of the AMIA Annual Symposium, Bethesda, MD, pp. 821–825. AMIA Press, Washington DC (2007)
14. Xu, H., Stetson, P., Friedman, C.: Methods for building sense inventories of abbreviations in clinical notes. Journal of American Medical Informatics Association 16(1), 103–108 (2009)

# Composite Event Indicator Processing in Event Extraction for Non-configurational Language

Valery Solovyev[1] and Vladimir Ivanov[1,2]

[1] Kazan Federal University
420008 Kazan, Kremlevskaya st., 18
http://www.kpfu.ru
[2] National University of Science and Technology "MISIS"
119049 Moscow, Leninskiy pr., 4
http://www.misis.ru

**Abstract.** Using event indicators is a well-known approach for event extraction. However, in most cases, event indicators are represented as single isolated words. In this paper, we deal with composite event indicators consisting of two and more words. Composite indicators are crucial to track modality when extracting events (e.g., possible events, desirable events, etc.). We proposed algorithms for the extraction of composite indicators as well as algorithms for the extraction of event arguments from sentences with composite indicators. The research is focused on Russian as an example of non-configurational language.

**Keywords:** event extraction, non-configurational languages, composite event indicators.

## 1 Introduction

Fast retrieval of precise information about current business events is especially important for financial markets, which is particularly sensitive to news [12]. Ordinary information sources in Web—news feeds—usually provide only a rough categorization without the capability to select specific event types that traders and investors are interested in. A lot of research works are devoted to event extraction for English. Recent surveys and a classification of existing approaches can be found in [8] [7]. An approach using handcrafted text patterns and rules [7] [2] is mainstream in commercial information extraction systems. Text patterns and rules developed for English use important syntactic features based on the order of words in a sentence. In Russian, a non-configurational language with the free order of words, syntactic relations are marked with inflections. In Russian, in contrast to English, we have much less natural language processing (NLP) tools, including those for information extraction. One of the famous NLP tool kits for Russian, the AOT (http://aot.ru), includes part of speech (POS) tagger but it is not well documented and has no technical support. In [5], authors describe only a named entity recognition (NER) module for Russian. The two most prominent information extraction systems for Russian are the OntosMiner [3] and

F. Castro, A. Gelbukh, and M. González (Eds.): MICAI 2013, Part I, LNAI 8265, pp. 329–341, 2013.

RCO [4]. Both systems are commercial and unavailable for research. They are not described, studied, or tested systematically. In collaboration with HP Labs Russia, we have developed an event extraction system for the Russian language. The system is intended for real-time text processing and uses a knowledge-based approach with dictionaries and patterns. The input texts are retrieved from business news feeds. The system extracts five types of events, including the assignment of top managers in new positions in companies. Event participant type "organization" includes companies as well as noncommercial institutions like government agencies. We have exploited the Apache's Unstructured Information Management Architecture (UIMA) (`http://uima.apache.org/`) as a basic framework that provides a set of common NLP components such as tokenization and sentence splitting. In majority of information extraction (IE) systems ([14] [8]), events to be extracted are are represented in a sentence with a single word (an indicator word). Usually, it is a noun or a verb in noninfinite form. This corresponds to the common task of event extraction related to identification "who did what to whom", "when", "with what methods", "where" and "why" in texts. However, there might be categories of events (foreseen, desirable, etc.) that also may be of interest in event extraction. The following are examples:

(1)    a.   Владелец "Монако" предложил Моуринью возглавить команду.
            Owner of "Monaco" offered     Mourinho   to lead     the team.


       b.   Моуринью может возглавить команду.
            Mourinho   may    lead         the team.

In sentence above the infinitive represents an event and the verb "may" (syntactic head of the infinitive) represents modality. The study of modality in IE has been done in [14], where authors provide a comprehensive classification of modality types and their expressions in texts. The main result they obtained is an information extraction system that concerns two major types of modality expression: auxiliary verbs and subordinate clauses. Their approach is based on expert knowledge (e.g., patterns with auxiliary verbs are expressed using 140 rules). Usually, modality concern together with polarity which expresses event negation. In [14], only a simple case of negation is considered: "no" and "not". However, negation may be expressed in many other ways.

(2)    a.   X согласился принять  предложение Y.
            X has agreed  to accept an offer from  Y.

       b.   X отказался  принять  предложение Y.
            X has refused to accept an offer from  Y.

For the correct interpretation of such sentences, it is necessary to extract words semantically connected to the indicator word. In [6] authors describe an approach for the extraction of a modality of uncertainty for French. It is also based on patterns. In [1], an impact of different tasks to the whole IE system is evaluated. Authors mention the task of modality processing, but it is not sufficiently described. In our work, in contrast to [14], we discuss the case when the modality is expressed in a frame of a single sentence with common verbs, as in 1a or 1.b. We will call a chain the following sequence of words:

$$A_1 \rightarrow A_2 \rightarrow \cdots \rightarrow A_n, \qquad (*)$$

where $\rightarrow$ means the dependency relation between $A_i$ and $A_{i+1}$ (specifically, $A_{i+1}$ depends on $A_i$). Dependency hereafter is treated as in the dependency grammar theory [9] [16]. We are interested in chains consisting of verbs, nouns, pronouns, and adverbs. The chain should end with the indicator word and may be quite long, as in the following:

(3)  Путин согласился принять предложение возглавить список.
     Putin   agreed        to accept an offer      to head      the list.

Typically, event extraction deals with sentences that contain words indicating events of a particular type (indicator words) and detecting text spans covering the event participants. We suppose that an event is represented in a single sentence. To the best of our knowledge, none of the mentioned systems extract composite (not a single word) indicators and measure their impact on event extraction. The following are examples:

(4)  a.  X принял   предложение Y-ка  возглавить компанию.
         X accepted an offer from Y.gen to head      the company.

     b.  X сделал предложение Y-ку  возглавить компанию.
         X made   an offer to     Y.dat to head      the company.

Here to detect the leader of the company, extracting only one indicator is useless. One should also analyze the whole dependency chain and all the words that are dependent on the words from this chain. Both sentences have the same structure of dependencies and hence require additional morphological information to be considered. This situation is quite common for most non-configurational languages.

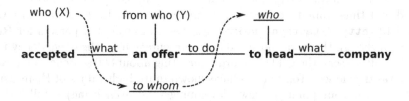

**Fig. 1.** Dependency relations and subject tracking in example 4a

In the figures above, lines without arrows denote syntax dependencies. Obligatory actants, which are not expressed on a shallow level [10], are underlined. These semantic actants are required for the correct interpretation of the situation.

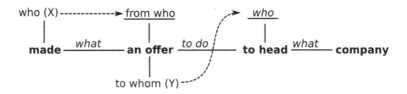

**Fig. 2.** Dependency relations and subject tracking in example 4b

Lines with arrows denote the transfer of a syntactic actant (expressed explicitly), which will fill the position of the semantic actant. Thus, the subject of the situation in both cases (4a and 4b) is taken from the actant of the noun «предложение» (an offer). But in 4b the actant is expressed on the shallow level and in (4a) it is taken from the actant «who» of the verb «make.» We will study the case where the indicator word is an infinitive verb. Basic observations show that up to 25% of sentences in Russian contain infinite forms of a verb. Indicators expressed as nouns are processed in a similar way, but this will require certain changes which we cannot describe here systematically because it is beyond the scope of the paper. Further, we will use the verb «возглавить» (to head, to lead) in examples throughout the paper. Of course, the whole approach is applicable to other verbs. The rest of the paper is organized as follows: an algorithm of chain reconstruction is represented in Section 2; an algorithm of event participant detection is described in Section 3; in Section 4 we propose a solutions for an ad hoc dictionary construction for event extraction based on composite indicators. Section 5 provides results and conclusions.

## 2 Reconstruction of a Composite Indicator Chain

In order to extract composite indicators, one needs to build a dependency chain that ends with an indicator word. We could use a common syntax parser to solve this task. However, on one hand, most parsers for Russian are either closed projects (with notable exceptions though, for example, [15]) or poorly documented and thus cannot be included in an IE pipeline. In 2012, the initiative RuEval-12 (http://testsynt.soiza.com) has run evaluated parsers for Russian. Even though there was no standard representation for the dependency tree shared by all parsers, the gold standard (consisting about 800 sentences) for evaluation was developed. Top parsers have shown quite high values of $F_1$-measure (94-96%). From our point of view, developing (and even using) a full-fledged parser for extraction of composite indicator chains appears to be an overkill. So we developed our own algorithm, which is much simpler and shows results competing with RuEval-12. The main idea is based on using the Google Books Ngram Viewer data set (GBD, Google Books data set) enriched with morphological information. The original data set contains statistics on occurences of n-grams (n=1 ... 5) as well as frequencies of binary dependencies between words (http://books.google.com/ngrams/). We use these binary dependencies to decide whether two words in a particular sentence are connected to each other with a syntactic link. As GBD stores all statistics on a year-by-year basis, we have preprocessed the original data set. For each 2-gram (binary dependency), we collect all its occurences on the whole data set and summate all frequency values since 1920. The resulting data set consists of pairs (n-gram, count). This data set is exploited in the algorithm of dependency chain reconstruction described below. In this section, we will describe an algorithm of composite indicator reconstruction. Let $h(w)$ be the head word and $w$ be the dependent word in a pair $h(w) \to w$. Input text is preprocessed using tokenization, sentence splitting, and POS tagging. Preprocessing includes an additional step of splitting sentences into smaller segments–text spans that do not contain any punctuation marks (,;:).

## 2.1 Dependency Chain Reconstruction Algorithm

In this subsection, we describe an algorithm for the reconstruction of a dependency chain constituting a composite indicator. We denote indicator word as $w_0$. Algorithm input involves the indicator word $w_0$ and $Seg$, a segment of the sentence with $w_0$. Algorithm output involves a chain $C = (w_{n-1}, w_{n-2}, ..., w_1, w_0)$, where each $w_{i-1}$ depends on $w_i$, where $i = 1..n$. The algorithm contains the following steps: GENERATE, RANK, FILTER, CHAIN. Further, we describe each step separately.

*GENERATE.* Generate set $P$ of word pairs in a segment $Seg$. When generating set $P$, we use simple rules discarding a certain pair $(w_i, w_{i+1})$ from the set $P$. The rules are as follows:

1. Forbid a certain part of speech for either $h(w)$ or $w$: $POS_{head}$. For example, the rule discarding conjunctions looks like the following: $CONJ_{head}$.

2. Forbid a certain part of speech to appear in a link: $(POS_{head}, POS_{dep})$. For example, the rule discarding pairs where a verb depends on a preposition looks like the following: $(PREP_{head}, VERB_{dep})$.

3. Forbid a word order (e.g., reverse order) for a certain dependency link: $(POS_{head}, POS_{dep})_{order}$. For example, a noun may not depend on a preposition that appears after the noun $(PREP_{head}, NOUN_{dep})_{reverse}$. We use about 100 rules in total. Each rule either describes what is nongrammatical in Russian or what pair is not relevant in a composite indicator chain.

*RANK.* The weight of each pair $(h(w), w)$ of $P$ is calculated using GBD. Weight is calculated according to the following formula:

$$weight(h(w), w) = \frac{F(h(w), w)}{S(h(w), w)D^2(h(w), w)},$$

where $F(h(w), w)$ is the frequency of pair $(h(w), w)$ in the GBD dependency data set, $D(h(w), w)$ is the distance (in words) between $h(w)$ and $w$ inside the segment, and $S(h(w), w)$ is calculated as follows:

$$S(h(w), w) = s_1(h(w)) + s_2(w),$$

where $s_1(x)$ is a number of pairs $(h(w), w)$ in the GBD dependency data set with the first element equaling to $x$ and with an arbitrary second element snd $s_2(x)$ is defined similarly, that is a number of pairs $(h(w), w)$ in the GBD dependency data set with the second element equaling to $x$ and with an arbitrary first element.

*FILTER.* Delete conflict pairs from $P$. In this step algorithm deletes from $P$ all the pairs that lead to one or more of the following conflicts:

1. Two words $h_1$ and $h_2$ are both the heads for one word $w$.
2. Two or more words form a cycle of dependencies.
3. The word $h$ is the head of two or more words (but only if it is forbidden in language's grammar; in Russian, for instance, a proposition may only be the head of a single word).

In all identified conflicts, the algorithm deletes a pair that weighs less.

*CHAIN.* Build a dependency chain $C$ using the filtered set $P$. The procedure for chain reconstruction is straightforward.

1. Insert $w_0$ in $C$, $i \leftarrow 0$.
2. If $P$ does not contain pair $(w_{i+1}, w_i)$, then construction of the chain $C$ is finished, or else
3. Insert $w_{i+1}$ in $C$ and delete pair $(w_{i+1}, w_i)$ from $P$, $i \leftarrow i + 1$, go to 2.

## 2.2   Evaluation of Chain Reconstruction

For the evaluation of the algorithm, we have selected 191 sentences from RuEval-12's gold standard. All these sentences contain at least one infinitive. The length of test chains vary from two to seven words. Most chains consist of two words. Using selected 191 sentences, we build a test set consisting of 238 pairs. The results of the parsers that participated in the initiative as well as the gold standard are also available on the website of RuEval-12 (`http://testsynt.soiza.com`). We use standard measures of precision and recall to evaluate the quality of the algorithm (Table 1).

# 3   Method for Extraction of Event Participants

We start with a simple case where all the words in a chain are verbs. We also require the verb valency to be either equal either two or three. This restriction comes from the fact that fourvalent verbs are rare, and their valencies starting from the fourth valency filled with dates and places, which are usually easy to

**Table 1.** Quality of composite indicator extraction

| Method Name | Precision | Recall | $F_1$ |
|---|---|---|---|
| Russian Malt | 0.79 | 1.0 | 0.88 |
| ETAP-3 | 0.78 | 1.0 | 0.87 |
| SyntAutom | 0.56 | 1.0 | 0.72 |
| SemSin | 0.83 | 0.95 | 0.89 |
| GBD based algoritm | 0.82 | 1.0 | 0.90 |

extract with special rules. Following [16], «subject» is said to be the first actant of the verb. If the verb is transformed into an infinitive, then its valencies change as follows: According to [16], all valencies stay unchanged except for the first valency (subject of the infinitive). The subject of the infinitive is not expressed on a syntactic level. The verb in an infinite form has an upcoming empty valency instead. This valency attaches to the dependency link from a head word the infinitive depends on. However, in order to get the correct interpretation of the sentence, one should find the subject of the infinitive (agent) on a semantic level. Considering the following example with verb «возглавлять» (to lead) in active voice we can observe that syntactic and semantic subjects are the same. The phrase «Моуринью возглавил команду» (Mourinho heads the team) describes the situation, where Mourinho is the leader of the team. But if we have an infinitive «возглавить» (as in examples 1a, 1b and 4a, 4b), then the noun group that might have become a subject is not connected to an indicator word. So one should develop special rules in this case. In a chain $A_1 \ldots A_n$, each of the verbs control the next one, and thus, only one or two valencies are filled with noun phrases. In a simple case of two words, this situation is well-known as the control of infinitive [17]. The control of infinitive has been described in a number of linguistic theories (HPSG [11], generative grammar [17], ECM [13], etc.) but it is still far from its solution. According to [17], obligatory control corresponds to the situations where the subject of an infinitive is unambiguously described by the controlling verb and its arguments. Arbitrary (nonobligatory) control corresponds mainly to depersonalized situations where the subject is not specified as in the following:

(5)  Запрещено курить  в  ресторанах.
     Forbidden   to smoke in restaurants.

We have randomly selected and manually checked about 500 sentences with the word «возглавить» in different grammatical forms. Nonobligatory control of infinitive was encountered only in one sentence. Various semantic and syntactic factors should be taken into account in order to decide which one of the verb's arguments will be the subject of the infinitive. The results in this field are derived for German [17], and we are not aware of similar works for Russian. However, we observed an interesting fact that in most cases the subject of an infinitive is defined using syntactic features only. Finally, the rules for the control of infinitive are the following:

(6)    a.  If the head verb has two valencies and is not an infinitive, then its
           subjective actant will be the subject for the dependent infinitive.

       b.  If the head verb has three valencies and is not an infinitive, then its
           second subjective actant (object) will be the subject for the dependent
           infinitive.

In 1b, the subject (which is the only subjective actant of the verb «may») acts
as the subject of the infinitive «to lead». The same is true for unpersonalized
sentences as in the following sentence:

(7)    Ему пришлось возглавить компанию.
       He   has        to lead     the company.

The verb «пришлось» (have to) in the sentence above does not have a subject, and the word «Ему» (he pronoun,dative) fills both the subject valencies of
«пришлось» and «возглавить». In 1a, in contrast, the noun phrase «Моуринью» (which acts as an object of the verb «предложил») is also the subject
of the infinitive «возглавить». This empirical rule does not depend on morphological features of object. For example, in the constructions «предложил Y-ку»
and «попросил Y-ка», grammatical cases of Y are different, but only Y (not X)
may be treated as the head of the company.

(8)    a.  X предложил Y-ку      возглавить компанию.
           X offered      Y.dative to lead     the company.

       b.  X попросил Y-ка       возглавить компанию.
           X asked       Y.genitive to lead    the company.

Here, only Y, and not X, may be treated as the possible new head of the company. This rule can be generalized for chains of arbitrary length in the following
manner:

(9)    a.  If all verbs $A_1 \ldots A_n$ in a dependency chain are two-valent, then the
           noun phrase that fills the subjective valency of A1 will also be the
           subject of $A_n$.

       b.  If there are three-valent verbs in a dependency chain, the subject
           of $A_n$ will be filled with the same noun phrase that fills the second
           subjective valency of the verb nearest (in the chain) to $A_n$.

Rules 9a and 9b may be simplified in the following rule:

(10)   A subjective actant of the verb nearest to $A_n$ will fill the position of the
       subject for $A_n$.

We illustrate this rule with the following sentence: «In 17th of July, Capello may agree to lead the Russian football team». All verbs in the chain «may → agree → to lead» are two-valent. So the name «Capello» is the subject of «lead». The next sentence contains a three-valent verb:

(11)    Президент Обама может предложить возглавить DARPA председателю сенатского комитета по иностранным делам Джону Керри.

President Obama may offer to lead DARPA to the chairman of the Senate Foreign Relations Committee, John Kerry.

The verb «offer» is three-valent, and its second valency is filled with «John Kerry», which will be the subject of «lead» as well (even though the phrase «John Kerry» is far from both the verbs «lead» and «offer»). Syntactic and semantic roles of the phrase are defined by case (dative), which is a normal way of expression for the second subjective valency in non-configurational languages.

Further, we discuss the case when the dependency chain contains nouns. Nouns used in such chains express the meaning of some action: "decision", "offer", etc. These nouns normally have two or three valences (e.g., «who» decided «what»). When the corresponding verb is transformed into a noun, the first valency is expressed by genitive case «X decided» ⇒ «decision of X». This valency we will call the first valency of the noun. All other valencies stay unchanged. The rule generalized for nouns looks as follows: (9) Given the word $A_i, (i = 1 \ldots n-1)$ nearest to $A_n$ with a subjective actant $S$, this actant will be the subject of the verb $A_n$. If the word $A_i$ has two subject actants, then the position of the subject for $A_n$ will be filled with the second actant.

In the phrase «X made an offer to Y to lead the company Z», the word ("offer") is the nearest to the indicator verb «lead» (in the dependency chain), has the second valency filled with Y, and Y acts as the head of the company. This rule works even if the position of the Y in the sentence will change. The observations given above led to the following algorithm for searching the noun phrase that will be the subject of the indicator verb (in infinitive form).

*Step 1.* Build the longest chain of verbs and nouns that will end with the indicator word.

*Step 2.* Recover the subjective actants for each word in the chain starting from the indicator word.

*Step 3.* Select the nearest word $A_i$ with the subjective actants. If the word $A_i$ has two actants, then the second actant will be the subject of the indicator $(A_n)$. On the other hand, if the word $A_i$ has only one subjective actant, then this actant will be the subject of the indicator.

Step 1 is described in Section 2, and Step 2 needs a model of the syntactic control for each word in the dependency chain. We treat the control model in a standard way, as in dependency grammar theory. For English, a number of resources such as FrameNet are developed. But for Russian, there is no FrameNet or similar resources that has been developed so far. That is why we propose an approximate solution. This solution is focused on the words that most frequently appear in chains and on building control•models for these words only. Given the models of control, we can find arguments compatible to morphological features (e.g., case) of a noun phrase head with the same features described in the model.

## 4     Frequency-Driven Approach to Dictionary Construction

As we have shown in Section 3, in order to properly define a subject of the indicator, one needs to build a dictionary to describe models for a limited set of indicator words that appear in dependency chains, each of which ends with an indicator word. Typically, processing modules of IE systems (e.g., NER) have recall at the level of 90%. We require the dictionary of models to provide recall at the same (or better) level. The idea of an approach for constructions of such a dictionary was tested on a single indicator word («возглавить»). To select certain control verbs, we used text collection of news feeds (cf. Section 2), Russian National Corpus (RNC) data and Google Books NGram Viewer data set (GBD). First, we selected a subset of sentences where the verb «возглавить» was used in the sense of leading a company (not in the sense of being at the top of a list or rating). Then we deleted duplicate sentences and ended up with 196 sentences. Most of the sentences (80%) contain the indicator verb in finite form. The remaining 20%, where the indicator was in infinite form, falls into three groups in 13%, the infinitive depends on a finite verb; in 6%, the infinitive depends on a noun; and in 1%, another construction is involved. We found the following control verbs:

It seens like the set of such verbs is restricted and limited in size. But this appears not to be true. In the RNC data set, we found 100 sentences (matched a syntactic pattern: verb → «возглавить») that contain 32 control verbs. Thus, we can use only frequent words for the dictionary of verbal control models. The comparison shows that only one word, «отказался», found in the news feeds collection is missing in the RNC data set. Manual analysis of both text collection and RNC data is time-consuming. This labor work could be facilitated using GBD. GBD statistics for dependency pairs have given the following results: The results of RNC and Google correspond to each other despite the differences between the two resources (i.e., same words are most frequent). In all cases, we observed obligatory control only. Note that 10 of the most frequent words from GBD cover lists retrieved from both the RNC data set and news feeds collection. Results for nouns that control the infinitive «возглавить» are presented in Table 3.

Again, six of most frequent words from GBD cover lists retrieved from both the RNC data set and news feeds collection (except for one word). Chains that consist of three and more words may contain almost any word that prevents to analyze such chains without a large dictionary of control models.

**Table 2.** Frequent verbs in composite indicators

| Verb | News | RNC | GBD [a] |
|------|------|-----|---------|
| может (may) | 11 | 17 | 0.000014 [b] |
| отказался (refuse) | 5 | - | 0.000003 |
| предложил (offer) | 5 | 24 | 0.00002 |
| согласился (agree) | 2 | 5 | 0.000006 |
| поручил (get) | 1 | 10 | 0.00001 |
| готов (ready) | 1 | - | 0.000002 |
| пригласил (invited) | 1 | - | - |
| должен был (have to) | - | 7 | 0.00001 |
| собирался (about to) | 5 | 6 | 0.000007 |
| решил (decide) | - | - | 0.000004 |
| хотел (want) | - | - | 0.000002 |

[a] Values are taken from books published in 2008.
[b] We aggregate all forms of the word.

**Table 3.** Frequent nouns in composite indicators

| Verb | News | RNC [a] | GBD |
|------|------|---------|-----|
| предложение (offer) | 6 | 15 | 0.000008 |
| приглашение (invitation) | 2 | 8 | 0.000002 |
| желание (desire) | 2 | 5 | 0.000001 |
| намерение (intension) | 1 | - | - |
| шансы (chance) | - | 8 | 0.000001 |
| согласие (agreement) | - | 6 | 0.000002 |
| право (right) | - | 5 | 0.000001 |

[a] In total, RNC data has 25 nouns; most of them are very rare.

Enumerating all pairs in such chains is also a laborious process. However, real texts contain less than 1% of chains with three verbs and about 7% of multiword chains with nouns. These basic observations led to an ad hoc methodology for event participant extraction. Given that the indicator word extracts the 10 most frequent verbs and the 10 most frequent nouns that control the indicator from GBD, experts can then build models for the selected words, which are then exploited in Step 2 of the algorithm described above. Given the chain C algorithm will consider only indicator word $A_2$ and the word $A_1$ that control the indicator. If $A_2$ has no arguments then the subject of $A_1$ will be the same as the subject in the sentence. This approach has shown 98% precision on 196 sentences with the word «возглавить». For other infinitives, we got about 90%.

# 5   Conclusion

The article is devoted to an extension for event extraction systems in the field of extraction of possible (incomplete or ceased) events. The approach presented is based on composite (multiword) event indicator extraction. We also proposed a method for tracking a subject of an infinitive indicator. This method is based on the control of infinitive theory and using Google Books Ngram data set. We evaluated the quality on a news feeds corpus. The final evaluation of the extraction system was postponed because of the low efficiency of other modules [1], such as NER. The study was carried out for Russian. However, this method is applicable to other non-configurational languages for which either a large corpus or a dictionary of control models is available.

**Acknowledgments.** This research was supported by Russian Foundation for Basic Research (grant 13-07-00773) and Ministry of Education and Science of the Russian Federation (project 8.3358.2011).

# References

1. Ahn, D.: The stages of event extraction. In: Proceedings of the Workshop on Annotating and Reasoning about Time and Events (2006)
2. Borsje, J., Hogenboom, F., Frasincar, F.: Semi-automatic financial events discovery based on lexico-semantic patterns. International Journal of Web Engineering and Technology 6(2), 115–140 (2010)
3. Efimenko, I.V., Khoroshevsky, V.F., Klintsov, V.P.: Ontosminer family: Multilingual ie systems. In: 9th Conference Speech and Computer (2004)
4. Ermakov, A.E., Pleshko, V.: Semantic interpretation in text analysis computer systems. Information Technologies 155(7) (2009) (in Russian)
5. Gareev, R., Tkachenko, M., Solovyev, V., Simanovsky, A., Ivanov, V.: Introducing baselines for russian named entity recognition. In: Gelbukh, A. (ed.) CICLing 2013, Part I. LNCS, vol. 7816, pp. 329–342. Springer, Heidelberg (2013)
6. Goujon, B.: Uncertainty detection for information extraction. In: The Proceedings of the International Conference RANLP, pp. 118–122 (2009)
7. Hogenboom, F., Frasincar, F., Kaymak, U., de Jong, F.: An overview of event extraction from text. In: Workshop on Detection, Representation, and Exploitation of Events in the Semantic Web (DeRiVE 2011) at Tenth International Semantic Web Conference (ISWC 2011), vol. 779, pp. 48–57 (2011)
8. Indurkhya, N., Damerau, F.J.: Handbook of natural language processing, vol. 2. CRC Press (2010)
9. Liu, H.: Dependency Grammar: from Theory to Practice. Science Press, Beijing (2009)
10. Mel'čnk, I.: Semantic description of lexical units in an explanatory combinatorial dictionary: Basic principles and heuristic criterial. International Journal of Lexicography 1(3), 165–188 (1988)
11. Metcalf, V.: Argument structure in hpsg as a lexical property: Evidence from english purpose infinitives. Locality of Grammatical Relationships (58) (2005)
12. Mitchell, M.L., Mulherin, J.H.: The impact of public information on the stock market. The Journal of Finance 49(3), 923–950 (1994)

13. Park, I.: A study on ecm infinitive structure. Studies in Generative Grammar 14(4), 497–517 (2004)
14. Saurı, R., Verhagen, M., Pustejovsky, J.: Annotating and recognizing event modality in text. In: The 19th International FLAIRS Conference, FLAIRS 2006 (2006)
15. Sharoff, S., Nivre, J.: The proper place of men and machines in language technology: Processing russian without any linguistic knowledge. In: Proceedings of the Annual International Conference "Dialogue", Computational Linguistics and Intellectual Technologies, vol. (10), pp. 657–670 (2011)
16. Tesnière, L., Fourquet, J.: Eléments de syntaxe structurale, vol. 1965. Klincksieck Paris (1959)
17. Wurmbrand, S.: Syntactic versus semantic control. In: Zwart, J.-W., Abraham, W. (eds.) Studies in Comparative Germanic Syntax: Proceedings of the 15th Workshop on Comparative Germanic Syntax, pp. 93–130 (2002)

# Exploration of a Rich Feature Set
# for Automatic Term Extraction

Merley S. Conrado, Thiago A. S. Pardo, and Solange O. Rezende

Instituto de Ciências Matemáticas e de Computação - ICMC,
Universidade de São Paulo - Campus de São Carlos - Caixa Postal 668
13560-970 São Carlos, SP, Brazil
{merleyc,taspardo,solange}@icmc.usp.br

**Abstract.** Despite the importance of the term extraction methods and
that several efforts have been devoted to improve them, they still have
4 main problems: (i) noise and silence generation; (ii) difficulty dealing
with high number of terms; (iii) human effort and time to evaluate the
terms; and (iv) still limited extraction results. In this paper, we deal with
these four major problems in automatic term extraction by exploring a
rich feature set in a machine learning approach. We minimized these
problems and achieved state of the art results for unigrams in Brazilian
Portuguese.

**Keywords:** Automatic term extraction, classification, machine learning.

## 1 Introduction

Terms (or terminological units) are lexical units of specialized meaning in a the-
matically restricted domain. A term may be: (i) simple (also called unigrams),
when it is lexically simple, i.e., formed by one singular element, such as *"biodi-
versity"*, or (ii) complex, when it is lexically complex, i.e., formed by more than
one element, such as *"aquatic ecosystem"* and *"natural resource management"*.
Automatic term extraction (ATE) methods aim to identify terms in specific domain corpora [1]. Such information is useful for building resources as dictionaries
and ontologies, and for improving results in applications of information retrieval,
extraction and summarization, for example.

Although ATE has been investigated for more than 20 years, there is still
room for improvement. There are four major ATE problems. The first problem
is that the ATE approaches may extract words that are not terms ("noise") or
do not extract all the terms ("silence"). As described in [2] and considering the
ecology domain, "an example of silence is when a term (e.g., *pollination*), with
low frequency, is not considered a candidate term (CT), and, therefore, it will not
appear in the extracted term list if we consider its frequency. Regarding noise, if
we consider that nouns may be terms and that adjectives may not, if an adjective
(e.g., *ecological*) is mistakenly tagged as a noun, it will be wrongly extracted as
a term." The second problem is the complexity of dealing with high number
of candidates (called the high dimensionality of candidate representation) that

F. Castro, A. Gelbukh, and M. González (Eds.): MICAI 2013, Part I, LNAI 8265, pp. 342–354, 2013.

requires time to process them. Since the ATE approaches generate large lists of candidate terms, the third problem is the huge human effort spent for validating the CTs, which is usually manually performed. The fourth problem is that the results are still not satisfactory and there is a natural ATE challenge due to the difficulty in obtaining a consensus among the experts about which words are terms of a specific domain [3].

Usually, the studies in the literature focus on extracting not only simple terms (unigrams), but also complex ones[1] [4–9]. In this paper, we focus on extracting unigrams. Despite the difficulty in comparing the ATE results due to variation (e.g., the size of the test corpora), we mention studies that have highlighted results for **unigrams**. When possible, we present the best precision (P) of the related work and its recall (R). Ventura and Silva [10] extracted terms using statistical measures that consider the predecessors and successors of CTs. They achieved, for English, P=81.5% and R=55.4% and, for Spanish, P=78.2% and R=60.8%. For Spanish, the Greek forms of a candidate and their prefix may help to extract terms (e.g., the Greek formant *laring* that belongs to the term *laringoespasm* in the medical domain) [3], achieving about P=55.4% and R=58.1%. For Spanish, Gelbukh et al. [11] compared the CTs of a domain with words of a general corpus using Likelihood ratio based distance. They achieved P=92.5%. For Brazilian Portuguese, the ExPorTer methods are the only previous work that uniquely extract unigrams [12]. Therefore, they are the state of the art for unigram extraction for Brazilian Portuguese (BP). The linguistic ExPorTer method considers terms that belong to some part of speech (POS) patterns and uses indicative phrases (such as *is defined as*) that may identify where terms are. It achieved P=2.74% and R=89.18%. The hybrid ExPorTer method uses the same linguistic knowledge with Frequency and Likelihood ratio. The latter obtained P=12.76% and R=23.25%.

In this paper[2], we present an approach that uses machine learning (ML), specifically the classification task, since it has been achieving high precision values [4, 5, 13]. Although the ML techniques may also generate noise and silence, they facilitate the use of a large number of candidate terms and their features, since they learn by themselves how to recognize a term and then they save time extracting them. Our approach differs from others because we explore a rich feature set using varied knowledge levels. With this, it is possible to decrease the silence and noise and, consequently, to improve the ATE results. Our features range from simple statistical (e.g., term frequency) and linguistic (e.g., POS) knowledge to more sophisticated hybrid knowledge, such as the analysis of the term context. As far as we know, the combination of this knowledge has not been applied before. Another difference is that we apply some statistical features (Term Variance [14], Term Variance Quality [15], Term Contribution [16], and n-gram length) that to date have not been used for ATE. We also propose new linguistic features for ATE. All these features are detailed in Section 2.

---

[1] It is not specified if Zhang et al. [4] extracted simple or complex terms.

[2] This paper is part of the ATE methodology proposed in [2].

Finally, for the first time, ML is applied to the ATE task for Brazilian Portuguese corpora, although our approach may be easily adapted to other languages. Focusing on extracting unigram terms, we run our experiments on 3 corpora of different domains. We compare our results with those produced by using frequency and TF-IDF information (that are commonly used for ATE) and by the only other work for ATE for unigrams in BP [12]. Comparing our results with [12], our main contribution is the improvement of precision (in the best case, we improve the results 11 times) and F-measure (in the best case, we improve 2 times).

Sections 2 and 3 describe our ATE approach and experimental setup. Section 4 presents the discussion of the results, conclusions, and future work.

## 2    Term Extraction Using Machine Learning

In order to model the ATE task as a machine learning solution, our approach considers each word in the input texts of a specific domain (except the stopwords) as a learning instance (candidate term). For each instance, we identify a set of features over which the classification is performed. The classification predicts which words are terms (unigrams) of a specific domain. We also test different attribute selection methods in order to verify which features are more relevant to classify a term.

We start by preprocessing the input texts, as shown in Figure 1. This step consists of POS tagging the corpora and normalizing[3] the words of the texts. The normalization helps to minimize the second ATE problem because it allows working with a lower CT representation dimensionality. When working with a lower dimensionality, there would be a smaller amount of CTs and, consequently, less candidates to be validated or refuted as terms (it would minimize the third ATE problem). In its turn, it might improve the quality of results (it handles the fourth ATE problem), and, definitely, it takes less time and fewer resources to carry out the experiments. By improving the results, consequently, we minimize silence and noise, which handles the first ATE problem. Still in the preprocessing, we remove stopwords. When removing these stopwords, we do not consider them as candidates, but we use the stopwords to identify the features.

We identify 19 features. 11 of these features are used for ATE in the literature, 3 features are normally applied to the attribute selection tasks (identified here by *), 5 new features were created (identified by **). These features are shown below, accompanied by the hypotheses that underlie their use. They are also divided into 3 levels of knowledge: statistical, linguistic, and hybrid. Our main hypothesis is that it is possible to improve the specific domain term identification by joining these features of different levels of knowledge.

---

[3] Normalization consists of standardizing the words by reducing their variations.

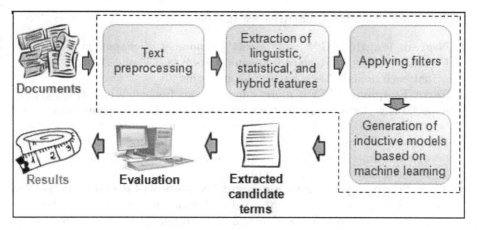

Fig. 1. The term extraction approach [2]

**The eight linguistic features we use are**

1. **Part-of-speech Pattern**: POS represents the linguistic category of the lexical items. A well-known **POS** pattern is *[Noun + Preposition + noun]*, which would extract the term *quality of education*. Usually, the unigram POS patterns are *noun* and *proper name*, but, according to [17], there are also adjective terms. So, we consider *noun, proper name,* and *adjectives*.

2. **Phrases**: are noun or prepositional phrases (**P**). We remove stopwords at the beginning and at the end of these phrases. Our hypothesis is that terms are normally noun phrases (or their kernels) and sometimes are prepositional phrases.

3. **Phrase kernel**: is the kernel of the noun or prepositional phrase (**PK**). For example, in the phrase *He is responsible for the quality of education*, the prepositional phrase (*for the quality of education*) would be identified, but only *quality of education* would be considered, because *for* and *the* are stopwords. We highlight that *of* is also a stopword, but in this case it is part of the POS pattern and must be preserved.

4. **Indicative Phrases (IP)** usually are near definitions or descriptions, because of that we expect they are close to terms. E.g., in *Ecology is defined as the study of body relationship*, we would consider *Ecology* and *study of body relationship* as CT.

5. **Words related to stem**: this one includes 3 features. When using a stemming technique to group similar meaning words in a stem, this stem has some words related to it. We consider the grammatical types of these words. For example, the words *educative, educators, education* and *educate* are originated from the stem *educ*. Therefore, the term *educ* may have as features **N_Noun\*\*** $= 2$ (*educators* and *education*), **N_Adj.\*\*** $= 1$ *educative*, **N_Verb\*\*** $= 1$ (*educate*), and **N_PO\*\*** $= 4$ (total number of words). Our hypothesis is that stemmed candidates that were originated from a higher number of nouns (instead of adjectives or verbs) are more probable to be terms.

**The seven statistical features we use are**

1. **N-gram length (SG\*\*):** represents the number of characters in a word. For example, the word *education* would have 9 as SG value. Our hypothesis is that each domain has a pattern for its terms.
2. **Term Frequency (TF):** represents the word frequency in a corpus. The hypothesis is that the candidates with low or very high frequencies may not be terms. In addition, TF is one of most used measures for ATE.
3. **Document Frequency (DF):** is the number of documents in which a word occurs. We expect that CT appears in at least some documents in order to be a representative term in the corpus.
4. **Term Frequency Inverse Document Frequency (TF-IDF):** [18] weights the word frequency according to its distribution along the corpus. Our hypothesis is that terms are well distributed throughout the corpus and have not very high frequencies. In addition, TF-IDF is a well-known ATE measure.
5. **Term Contribution (TCo\*):** [16] considers that the word importance is the contribution to the document similarity. We expect that terms help to distinguish one document from others.
6. **Term Variance (TV\*):** [14] assumes that important words do not have low frequency in documents and also maintain a non-uniform distribution throughout the corpus (higher variance). The hypothesis here is that terms may have higher variance.
7. **Term Variance Quality (TVQ\*):** [15] quantifies the quality of the word variance, following the same hypothesis above.

**The four hybrid features we use are:**

1. **General Corpus ($GC$):** whether a word occurs in a General Corpus. We expect that candidates that appear in a GC probably will not be a term in a specific domain.
2. **$GC$ Frequency ($GC\_Freq.$):** the frequency of a word in a GC. We expect that candidates with high frequencies in a GC will not be a term in a specific domain.
3. **C-value:** [19] analyzes the potential of a CT to be a term. For this analysis, C-value uses POS, the candidate frequency in the corpus and its frequency inside other bigger candidates terms. We believe that these analyses will help to extract terms.
4. **NC-Value** [19, 20] assumes that the context in which the candidate occurs is relevant to determine if it is a term.

See formal definitions of features in Figure 2. In this figure, $t$ corresponds to a CT; $N$ is the document number of the corpus; $f(t)$ is $t$ frequency in the corpus; $f_{ij}$ is the frequency of the $j^{th}$ CT in the $i^{th}$ document, as well as $f_{jx}$ is the frequency of the $j^{th}$ CT in the $x^{th}$ document; and $\bar{f}_j$ is the average of frequencies of the $j^{th}$ word in the corpus. On the other hand, for the C-value measure, $t$ corresponds to a noun phrase; $|t|$ is the $t$ length measured in grams;

$T_t$ is the CT set composed by CT that have the gram number bigger than $t$ and also that contain $t$; $P(T_t)$ is the number of such CT (types) including the $t$ type; and $\sum f(b)$ is the total number of $t$ as CT substring $b$ so that $|t| < |b|$. For the NC-value measure, $c_t$ is the contextual word set of the $t$ CT; $b$ is a contextual word of the $t$ candidate; and $f_t(b)$ is the frequency of $b$ as contextual word of the $t$ candidate.

| | | | |
|---|---|---|---|
| $TF_j = \sum\limits_{i=1}^{N} f_{ij}$ | $DF_j = \sum\limits_{i=1}^{N} (1\|f_{ij} \neq 0)$ | $TF - IDF_j = \sum\limits_{i=1}^{N} f_{ij} \times \log \dfrac{N}{DF_j}$ | $TC_j = \sum\limits_{x=1}^{N}\sum\limits_{y=1}^{N} f_{jx} \times IDF_j \times f_{jy} \times IDF_j$ |
| $TVQ_j = \sum\limits_{i=1}^{N} f_{ij}^2 - \dfrac{1}{N}\left[\sum\limits_{i=1}^{N} f_{ij}\right]^2$ | | $C\_value = \begin{cases} 1 + \log_2 \|t\| \times f(t) & t \text{ is not nested,} \\ 1 + \log_2 \|t\| \times \left(f(t) - \dfrac{1}{P(T_t)}\sum\limits_{b \in T} f(b)\right) & \text{, otherwise} \end{cases}$ | |
| $TV_j = \sum\limits_{i=1}^{N} [f_{ij} - \bar{f}_j]^2$ | | $NC\_value = 0.8 \times C\_value(t) + 0.2 \sum\limits_{b \in C_t} f_t(b) \times \dfrac{t(b)}{N}$ | |

**Fig. 2.** Objective measures used

Phrase (P), phrase kernel (PK), part-of-speech pattern (POS), indicative phrases (IP), and general corpus (GC) are discrete features (0 or 1) . For example, if the POS pattern of an unigram is noun, proper name, or adjective, the POS feature will be 1; otherwise, it will be 0. All other features are continuous (a real value obtained by computing the feature).

The candidates that have more chance of being a domain term are selected according to some criteria (see Section 3). Moreover, this selection minimizes the high dimensionality problem of CT representation. Finally, inductive models are generated based on machine learning aiming to identify terms, using the previous features. To evaluate the results, we used gold standard lists in order to calculate the precision, recall, and F-measure.

## 3   Experimental Setup

For the experiments, we used 3 corpora of different domains in the Portuguese language. The DE corpus [21] has 347 texts about distance education. For the preparation of the gold standard, noun phrases were considered as candidate terms if they: (i) had, at least, a pre-specified absolute frequency of one in the DE corpus; (ii) were not manually deleted by a linguist (the linguist deleted some proper names and noun phrases without terminological meaning (e.g., *19th century*); and, (iii) were unigrams and did not occur in a general corpus. Considering these candidates, a specialist decided for 118 terms to compose the unigram gold standard[4] [22]. The second one is the ECO[5] corpus [12]. It contains 390 texts of

---

[4] Di Felippo [22] stated that the DE unigram gold standard has 59 terms, but in this paper we used 118 unigrams that the authors provided us prior to their work.
[5] ECO corpus - http://www.nilc.icmc.usp.br/nilc/projects/bloc-eco.htm

ecology domain. The gold standard is composed of 322 unigrams that correspond to the intersection of terms extracted from 2 books, 2 glossaries, and 1 online dictionary (for the same domain), and the ECO corpus. The third corpus is the Nanoscience and Nanotechnology (N&N) corpus [23] that contains 1,057 texts. For the preparation of the gold standard, after removing stopwords, candidate terms were identified using statistical methods and some of these candidates were excluded manually by a linguist. Therefore, a specialist decided which of these candidates were terms of the gold standard, which resulted in a list of 1,794 unigrams [23, 24].

We POS tagged these corpora using the PALAVRAS[6] parser [25] and normalized their words. We chose the stemming[7] technique for the normalization because it helps to decrease representation dimensionality of CTs, as previously mentioned.

Afterwards, we identified and calculated 19 features, detailed in Section 2, in which 11 features are used for ATE in the literature, 3 features are normally applied to the attribute selection tasks (identified by *), 1 is usually used for Named Entity Recognition (identified by **), and 4 were created by us (identified by $^\Delta$).

Regarding the calculated features, we removed stopwords[8] at the beginning and at the end of the phrases. As an example of the IP feature, consider *are composed of* as an IP in *All organisms are composed of one or more cells*: in this case, we would consider *organisms* and *cells* as CTs. We used 40 IPs[8]. For *GC* and *GC_Freq.*, we used the NILC Corpus[9] as a general corpus, which contains 40 million words.

These features were calculated for each unigram in the corpus, except stopwords. These unigrams are considered candidate terms and they are called here **all CTs**. We also selected candidates by preserving only those that are noun phrases or prepositional phrases and also follow some of these POS: nouns, proper nouns, verbs, and adjectives [17]. The selected candidates are called here **selected CTs**. The total numbers of obtained candidates (stems) were 10,524, 14,385, and 46,203, for the ECO, DE, and N&N corpora, respectively. When we performed candidate selection, we decreased 63.10%, 63.18%, 66.94% in relation to the number of all the obtained candidates. Unfortunately, when applying this selection, 32, 23, and 159 true terms of the ECO, DE, and N&N corpora, respectively, were removed. On the other hand, the advantage of this selection was to be able to minimize the dimensionality of CT representation (the second ATE problem) and, therefore, the experiments took less time to be executed

---

[6] As all NLP tools for general domains, PALAVRAS is not excellent for specific domains. However, as it would be expensive (in terms of time and manual work) to customize it for each specific domain that we presented in this paper, we used it in its original version.

[7] We used PTStemmer, which is a stemming toolkit for the Portuguese language - http://code.google.com/p/ptstemmer/

[8] Available at http://sites.labic.icmc.usp.br/merleyc/micai2013/

[9] NILC Corpus - http://www.nilc.icmc.usp.br/nilc/tools/corpora.htm

and decreased the number of CTs that needed to be validate as terms (which correspond to the second and third ATE problems, respectively).

In order to identify which features must be used for ATE, we applied 2 attribute selection methods. Their evaluation is based on consistency (CBF) and correlation (CFS). The combination of these methods with search methods, available in WEKA [26], was: CFS with the RankSearch Filter (*CFS_R*) and BestFirst (*CFS_BF*), CBF with the Ranking Filter (*CBF_R*) and the Greedy Stepwise (*CBF_G*). These methods return feature sets that are considered the most representative ones for term classification. We also considered all the features (referred by *All*). For the DE corpus, the *CBF_G* attribute selection method did not select any feature.

In order to evaluate the ATE results[10] using **all CTs** and **selected CTs**, and evaluate the features used to extract terms, we chose largely known inductors in the machine learning area. They represent different learning paradigms: JRip (Rule Induction), Naïve Bayes (Probabilistic), J48 (Decision Tree) with confidence factor of 25% and 75%, and SMO (Statistical Learning). All of these algorithms are available in WEKA and described in [27]. We run the experiments on a 10 fold cross-validation strategy and calculated precision, recall, and F-measure scores of term classification in relation to the gold standard of unigrams for each corpus. The total number of experiments was 10 because we extracted terms using **all CTs** and **selected CTs** when considering all features and when considering only the features selected by each one of the combinations of attribute selection methods, previously mentioned.

In Tables 1 and 2, we present our best results (identified by *) for each corpus, comparing them with the baselines. We consider TF-IDF, Frequency, the linguistic ExPorTer method, and the hybrid ExPorTer method [12] as our baselines. The ExPorTer methods were briefly explained in the Section 1.

**Table 1.** The ATE results for the DE and ECO corpora

| The DE corpus | | | | The ECO corpus | | | |
|---|---|---|---|---|---|---|---|
| Method | Precision | Recall | F-Measure | Method | Precision | Recall | F-Measure |
| JRIP with CBF_R | **66.67** | 8.62 | 15.27 | JRIP with CBF_R | **62.50** | 6.67 | 12.05 |
| Naïve Bayes with CBF_R and All | 13.20 | 22.41 | 16.61 | Naïve Bayes with CBF_G and All | 25.54 | 19.67 | 22.22 |
| J48 with F.C. of 0.75 with CBF_R | 27.59 | 13.79 | **18.39** | Naïve Bayes with CFS_R and CFS_BF | 32.35 | 18.33 | **23.40** |
| Linguistic ExPorTer | 0.33 | **89.70** | 0.66 | Linguistic ExPorTer | 2.74 | **89.18** | 5.32 |
| Hybrid ExPorTer | 0.07 | 17.64 | 0.15 | Hybrid ExPorTer | 12.76 | 23.25 | 16.48 |
| Frequency | 5.9 | 50.86 | 10.57 | Frequency | 12.9 | 43.28 | 19.87 |
| TF-IDF | 6.1 | 52.58 | 10.93 | TF-IDF | 13.4 | 44.96 | 20.64 |
| All the corpus | 0.52 | 62.9 | 1.04 | All the corpus | 1.48 | 99.07 | 2.92 |

In Tables 1 and 2, for the DE corpus, the CBF_R attribute selection method chose the features: Freq, DF, TF-IDF, TV, TVQ, TCo, IP, GC, POS, GC_Freq., NC-value, C-value, N_Adj, N_Noun, N_Verb, and N_PO. For the ECO corpus, the CFS_R method selected TF-IDF, TV, TVQ, POS, and N_Noun; and the

---

[10] All the results are available at: http://sites.labic.icmc.usp.br/merleyc/micai2013/

CFS_BF method selected TF-IDF, TVQ, TCo, and POS. Although each attribute selection method chose different features, we observed that all of them selected a feature set that contains features of the three different levels of knowledge (linguistic, statistical, and hybrid). We highlight that, for calculating the recall score, we discounted the number of true terms of each corpus that were removed during candidate selection (previously explained). For example, for the DE corpus, 23 true terms were removed during candidate selection. After the term extraction, 26 candidate terms were correctly classified as terms, but it should be extracted 67 terms. Thus, the calculating of the recall score was $Recall = \frac{26}{26+67+23} = 22.41\%$ (see $3^{rd}$ line of Table 1).

With this, we confirmed our main hypothesis, which assumes that it is possible to improve the ATE results when joining features of different levels of knowledge. For example, for the N&N corpus, the best precision score (61.03%) was achieved when using all the features with the JRIP inductor. In Table 3, we show how the features of different levels of knowledge help

**Table 2.** The ATE results for the N&N corpus

| Method | Precision | Recall | F-Measure |
|---|---|---|---|
| JRIP with All | **61.03** | 25.42 | 35.90 |
| J48 with F.C. of 0.25 with All | 55.64 | 42.67 | **48.30** |
| Linguistic ExPorTer | 3.75 | **89.40** | 7.20 |
| Hybrid ExPorTer | 1.68 | 35.35 | 3.22 |
| Frequency | 31.6 | 20.83 | 25.1 |
| TF-IDF | 35.4 | 23.33 | 28.12 |
| All the corpus | 1.83 | 66.99 | 3.57 |

classifying terms. We also verified examples of noise, which shows that, although we improved the results, there is still room for improvement.

In a brief analysis, we observed that the P and N_Noun features, as we expected, help to identify terms, since the domain experts prefer terms that are nouns.

It is also interesting to analyze some instances. The word *fiber* has higher frequency in the corpus (the Freq feature) than *nanotecnology* and occurs 955 times in the general corpus (the GC_Freq. feature). The two last features could indicate that *fiber* would not be a term. However, other features might help to conclude that it is a term, since it occurs in 128 of 1057 texts (12.11% of the texts) and it is well distributed throughout the corpus and has not very high frequencies, if considering that non-terms might still have higher frequency, such as *innovation*. Although *nanotecnology* is lesser frequent than *fiber*, the first one maintains a non-uniform distribution throughout the corpus (it has high TV value) and does not occur in the general corpus (the GC feature), which help to classify it as a term.

If we compare *fiber* to *evolution*, the latter has a relatively similar DF value and also has high Freq, TF-IDF, and occurs in a general corpus. On the other hand, *evolution* probably is not defined or described in the texts, because it does not occur near some indicative phrase (the IP feature) neither it is a phrase kernel (the PK feature), which state that it is not a term. Finally, *innovation* was correctly classified as non-term because it has higher frequency than the other examples (the Freq feature), does not maintain a non-uniform distribution throughout the corpus (the TV feature), and does not occur near some indicative phrase (the IP feature), even thought it has some feature values that terms usually have (DF, TF-IDF, NC-value, P, PK, and POS). But, although it is a phrase kernel (the PK feature), when considering its stem (*innov*), there are more adjectives and verbs (respectively, the N_Adj and N_Verb features) than nouns (the N_Noun feature) that originated its stem. This might indicate that their feature values that depend on its frequency might not refer to the noun.

**Table 3.** Result examples for the N&N corpus

| Candidates | nanotecnology | fiber | evolution | innovation |
|---|---|---|---|---|
| SG | 7 | 4 | 6 | 4 |
| Freq | 67 | 868 | 589 | 1268 |
| DF | 39 | 128 | 120 | 264 |
| TF-IDF | 96.01 | 795.84 | 556.54 | 763.93 |
| TV | 12365.31 | 5507.98 | 31.9 | 9.97 |
| TVQ | 11132.97 | 4095.55 | 12 | 1 |
| TCo | 66810.58 | 63433.89 | 183.81 | 76.26 |
| GC | 0 | 1 | 1 | 1 |
| GC_Freq. | 0 | 955 | 40 | 561 |
| IP | 1 | 1 | 0 | 0 |
| C-value | 67 | 868 | 589 | 1268 |
| NC-value | 2.49 | 0.81 | 1.74 | 1.64 |
| P | 1 | 1 | 1 | 1 |
| PK | 1 | 1 | 0 | 1 |
| POS | 1 | 1 | 1 | 1 |
| N_Noun | 1 | 4 | 2 | 2 |
| N_Adj | 0 | 4 | 0 | 7 |
| N_Verb | 0 | 0 | 0 | 5 |
| N_PO | 4 | 9 | 2 | 16 |
| Is it a term? | Yes | Yes | No | No |

Still analysing Tables 1 and 2, the best precision value obtained for the DE corpus using the term classification, 66.67%, was achieved by the *CBF_R* attribute selection method using the JRIP inductor. Our best recall score, 22.41%, was obtained using Naïve Bayes with the *CBF_R* method or with all features (referred in the Table 1 by *All*). The best F-measure value was 18.39% when using the J48 inductor with confidence factor of 75% with *CBF_R*.

For the ECO corpus, the best precision score was 62.50% obtained using the JRIP inductor with the *CBF_R* method. The best recall score was 19.67% using Naïve Bayes with the *CBF_G* method or with all features (*All*). Our best F-measure score was 23.40% obtained with Naïve Bayes with the *CFS_R* method or with the *CFS_BF* method.

For the N&N corpus (Table 2), the best precision score was 61.03% using the JRIP inductor. Our best recall was 52.53% and the best F-measure score was 42.67%, both using J48 inductor with confidence factor of 25%. The last three results used all features (*All*).

## 4    Conclusions and Future Work

In this paper we explored a rich feature set in a machine learning solution to the ATE task. We showed that features of different knowledge leves are useful and that they may generate state of the art results, improving some previous results in the area and dealing with some well-known problems in this task.

It is important to notice that some features were used for the first time in the ATE task. It is also interesting to identify features that are better for ATE. All the tested attribute selection methods indicated the TF-IDF as an essential feature for ATE. 90.9% of the methods selected N_Noun and TVQ, and 81.81% selected TV, IP, N_adj, and POS as relevant features. However, only one of these methods chose GC_Freq., and none of these methods chose the SG feature. Regarding the levels of knowledge - statistical, linguistic, and hybrid - in which each feature was classified, at least 45.45% of the methods chose 6 statistical, 5 linguistic, and 3 hybrid features. We also observed that the best F-measures were obtained when using at least linguistic and statistical features together.

For future work, we intend to use instance selection techniques as well as to explore new features that may represent other knowledge levels, e.g., features from Wikipedia and ontologies that might codify semantic restrictions on what may be considered terms.

**Acknowledgment.** Grants 2009/16142-3, 2011/19850-9, 2012/03071-3, and 2012/09375-4, from Sao Paulo Research Foundation (FAPESP).

## References

1. Cabré, M.T., Estopà, R., Vivaldi, J.: Automatic term detection: a review of current systems. In: Bourigault, D., Jacquemin, C., L'Homme, M.-C. (eds.) Recent Advances in Computational Terminology, pp. 53–88. John Benjamins, Amsterdam (2001)
2. Conrado, M.S., Pardo, T.A.S., Rezende, S.O.: A machine learning approach to automatic term extraction using a rich feature set. In: Proceedings of the 2013 NAACL HLT Student Research Workshop, Atlanta, USA, pp. 16–23 (2013)
3. Vivaldi, J., Rodríguez, H.: Evaluation of terms and term extraction systems: A practical approach. Terminology 13(2), 225–248 (2007)
4. Zhang, X., Song, Y., Fang, A.: Term recognition using conditional random fields. In: Proc. of IEEE NLP-KE, pp. 333–336 (2010)
5. Zhang, Z., Iria, J., Brewster, C., Ciravegna, F.: A comparative evaluation of term recognition algorithms. In: Calzolari, N., Choukri, K., Maegaard, B., Mariani, J., Odjik, J., Piperidis, S., Tapias, D. (eds.) Proc. of the 6th on LREC, pp. 2108–2113. ELRA, Marrakech (2008)

6. Foo, J., Merkel, M.: Using machine learning to perform automatic term recognition. In: Bel, N., Daille, B., Vasiljevs, A. (eds.) Proc. of the 7th LREC - Wksp on Methods for automatic acquisition of Language Resources and their Evaluation Methods, pp. 49–54 (2010)
7. Nazar, R.: A statistical approach to term extraction. Int. Journal of English Studies 11(2) (2011)
8. Vivaldi, J., Cabrera-Diego, L.A., Sierra, G., Pozzi, M.: Using wikipedia to validate the terminology found in a corpus of basic textbooks. In: Calzolari, N., Choukri, K., Maegaard, B., Mariani, J., Odjik, J., Piperidis, S., Tapias, D. (eds.) Proc. of the 8th Int. CNF on LREC. ELRA, Istanbul (2012)
9. Lopes, L.: Extração automática de conceitos a partir de textos em língua portugesa. Ph.D. dissertation, PUCRS. RS, Brazil (2012)
10. Ventura, J., Silva, J.F.: Ranking and extraction of relevant single words in text. In: Rossi, C. (ed.) Brain, Vision and AI, pp. 265–284. InTech, Education and Publishing (2008)
11. Gelbukh, A., Sidorov, G., Lavin-Villa, E., Chanona-Hernandez, L.: Automatic term extraction using log-likelihood based comparison with general reference corpus. In: Hopfe, C.J., Rezgui, Y., Métais, E., Preece, A., Li, H. (eds.) NLDB 2010. LNCS, vol. 6177, pp. 248–255. Springer, Heidelberg (2010)
12. Zavaglia, C., Oliveira, L.H.M., Nunes, M.G.V., Aluísio, S.M.: Estrutura ontológica e unidades lexicais: uma aplicação computacional no domínio da ecologia. In: Proc. of the 5th TIL Wksp, pp. 1575–1584. SBC, RJ (2007)
13. Loukachevitch, N.: Automatic term recognition needs multiple evidence. In: Calzolari, N., Choukri, K., Declerck, T., Dogan, M., Maegaard, B., Mariani, J. (eds.) Proc. of the 8th on LREC, pp. 2401–2407. ELRA, Turkey (2012)
14. Liu, L., Kang, J., Yu, J., Wang, Z.: A comparative study on unsupervised feature selection methods for text clustering. In: Proc. of IEEE NLP-KE, pp. 597–601 (2005)
15. Dhillon, I., Kogan, J., Nicholas, C.: Feature selection and document clustering. In: Berry, M.W. (ed.) Survey of Text Mining, pp. 73–100. Springer (2003)
16. Liu, T., Liu, S., Chen, Z.: An evaluation on feature selection for text clustering. In: Proceedings of the 10th Int. CNF on Machine Learning, pp. 488–495. Morgan Kaufmann, San Francisco (2003)
17. Almeida, G.M.B., Vale, O.A.: Do texto ao termo: interação entre terminologia, morfologia e linguística de corpus na extração semi-automática de termos. In: Isquerdo, A.N., Finatto, M.J.B. (eds.) As Ciências do Léxico: Lexicologia, Lexicografia e Terminologia, 1st edn., vol. IV, pp. 483–499. UFMS, MS (2008)
18. Salton, G., Buckley, C.: Term weighting approaches in automatic text retrieval, Ithaca, NY, USA, Tech. Rep. (1987)
http://ecommons.library.cornell.edu/bitstream/1813/6721/1/87-881.pdf (October 10, 2008)
19. Frantzi, K.T., Ananiadou, S., Tsujii, J.: The $C - value/NC - value$ method of automatic recognition for multi-word terms. In: Nikolaou, C., Stephanidis, C. (eds.) ECDL 1998. LNCS, vol. 1513, pp. 585–604. Springer, Heidelberg (1998)
20. Barrón-Cedeño, A., Sierra, G., Drouin, P., Ananiadou, S.: An improved automatic term recognition method for spanish. In: Gelbukh, A. (ed.) CICLing 2009. LNCS, vol. 5449, pp. 125–136. Springer, Heidelberg (2009)
21. Souza, J.W.C., Di Felippo, A.: Um exercício em lingüística de corpus no âmbito do projeto TermiNet. University of Sao Paulo (ICMC-USP), SP, Brazil, Tech. Rep. NILC-TR-10-08 (2010)

22. Gianoti, A.C., Di Felippo, A.: Extração de conhecimento terminológico no projeto TermiNet. University of Sao Paulo (ICMC-USP), SP, Brazil, Tech. Rep. NILC-TR-11-01 (2011), http://www.ufscar.br/~letras/pdf/NILC-TR-11-01_GianotiDiFelippo.pdf (April 4, 2013)
23. Coleti, J.S., Mattos, D.F., Genoves Junior, L.C., Candido Junior, A., Di Felippo, A., Almeida, G.M.B., Aluísio, S.M., Oliveira Junior, O.N.: Compilação de Corpus em Língua Portuguesa na área de Nanociência/Nanotecnologia: Problemas e soluções, 192nd ed., L. e. C. H. F. U. Humanitas/Faculdade de Filosofia, Ed. SP, Brazil: Tagnin and Vale, vol. 1 (2008)
24. Coleti, J.S., Mattos, D.F., Almeida, G.M.B.: Primeiro dicionário de nanociência e nanotecnologia em língua portuguesa. In: Pecenin, M.F., Miotello, V., Oliveira, T.A. (eds.) II Encontro Acadêmico de Letras (EALE), Caderno de Resumos do II EALE, pp. 1–10 (2009)
25. Bick, E.: The Parsing System "PALAVRAS". Automatic Grammatical Analysis of Portuguese in a Constraint Grammar Framework, Aarhus Universitetsforlag (2000)
26. Hall, M., Frank, E., Holmes, G., Pfahringer, B., Reutemann, P., Witten, I.H.: The WEKA data mining software: An update. In: SIGKDD-ACM, vol. 11, pp. 10–18 (2009)
27. Witten, I.H., Frank, E.: Data Mining: Practical Machine Learning Tools and Techniques, 2nd edn. Morgan Kaufmann Series in Data Management Systems. Morgan Kaufmann Publishers Inc., San Francisco (2005)

# A Pseudo-Relevance Feedback Based Method to Find Comprehensive Web Documents

Rajendra Prasath  and  Sudeshna Sarkar

Department of Computer Science and Engineering
Indian Institute of Technology, Kharagpur - 721 302, India
{drrprasath,shudeshna}@gmail.com

**Abstract.** In web search, given a query, a search engine is required to retrieve a set of relevant documents. We wish to rank documents based on the content and look beyond mere relevance. Often there is a requirement that users want comprehensive documents containing variety of aspects of information relevant to the query topic. Given a query, a document is considered to be *comprehensive* only if the document covers more number of aspects of the given query. The comprehensiveness of a web document may be estimated by analyzing various parts of its content, and checking diversity, coverage of the content and the relevance as well. In this work, we have proposed an information retrieval system that ranks documents based on the comprehensiveness of the content. We use pseudo relevance feedback to score the comprehensiveness of web documents as well as their relevance. Experiments show that the proposed method effectively identifies documents having comprehensive content.

## 1   Introduction

A search engine is required to retrieve relevant information given the query. While using a search engine, people require different aspects of information at different times. Often there is a requirement that user wants comprehensive documents containing various aspects of information relevant to the query topic.

Consider the query "New Delhi". The WIKIPEDIA page on "New Delhi" is an example of a comprehensive document. This page covers information on different subtopics such as *overview, geography, climate, transport, demographics, culture, cityscape, historic sites, museums, sports, economy, sister cities, service sectors* and so on. Since this WIKIPEDIA page covers many subtopics, it is a comprehensive document. These subtopics may be different for other relevant documents retrieved for the same query. Consider another web page of lonelyplanet.com retrieved for the same query. This document contains information associated with a single aspect - history of New Delhi. Even though this page has relevant information, its content is not comprehensive. So users have to visit many web pages to identify the content on various aspects of the query, instead of visiting a single web page having various aspects of information.

In the health domain, consider the query, "lung cancer". To this query, the document[1] belonging to the medlineplus site contains information on only one

---

[1] http://www.nlm.nih.gov/medlineplus/lungcancer.html

F. Castro, A. Gelbukh, and M. González (Eds.): MICAI 2013, Part I, LNAI 8265, pp. 355–366, 2013.
© Springer-Verlag Berlin Heidelberg 2013

aspect associated with causes and symptoms of lung cancer. This document is relevant but does not have diverse information on lung cancer. Hence it is not comprehensive. For the same query, consider another web document[2] belonging to the medicalnewstoday domain. This document covers information on different subtopics such as *overview, types of lung cancer, causes, cancer cell evolutions, symptoms, diagnosis, treatment* - including surgery and radiation, *prevention*, and recent news. Hence this document is more comprehensive than the first one.

In this work, we propose a method to compute a score of each document based on the number and variety of aspects covered by it pertaining to the query. This scoring method finds documents that are comprehensive to the query.

This paper is organized as follows: Section 2 presents the past work. Section 3 describes the proposed method to find comprehensive documents. Experimental results are given in Section 4. Finally, Section 5 concludes the paper.

## 2    Related Work

Lipshutz and Taylor[1] proposed a formalism for comprehensive document representation based on a five dimensional space: *physical organization* - refers to the document appearance and layout of contents, *logical organization* - refers the reading order of information with their continuity across pages, *functional organization* - conveys the intent of the document, *topical organization* - points to the referential links across components like from a body of text to a photograph, and *document class* - refers to the general characterization of a document.

Many researchers have proposed documents retrieval methods based on clustering of documents. Lee *et al.*[2] proposed a two-step model for document re-ranking using document clusters. In this method, an initial set of documents is retrieved based on the vector space model [3] and then retrieved documents are analyzed based on the context of all terms in a document and query terms via *clustering*. Makrehchi [4] proposed an approach that applies the query-based text clustering to learn the taxonomy and then to generate relevant queries. Recently Krikon [5] proposed a language-model-based approach to re-ranking search results by integrating whole-document information with that induced from inter-passage, inter-document, and query-based similarities.

Relevance Feedback (RF) based approaches are quite popular in Information Retrieval. Xu and Yin[6] proposed an approach based on implicit relevance feedback to capture the subjectivity and dynamics of topicality and novelty in relevant judgments. They studied the possibility of enhancing topicality-based relevance judgment of users with subjective novelty judgment in an interactive IR system. Clarke *et al.*[7] presented a pseudo relevance based framework that models user information needs as a set of *nuggets*, each represents a fact or similar piece of information or topicality. A particular document is relevant if it contains at least one nugget pertaining to the query. This framework rewards novelty and diversity of information based on the cumulative gain.

---

[2] http://www.medicalnewstoday.com/info/lung-cancer/

Nuray and Can[8] proposed relevance feedback based data fusion methods for ranking in which the retrieval results of multiple systems are merged using the Rank Position, Borda Count, and Condorcet methods to determine the pseudo relevance. Top-ranked documents are considered as the "(pseudo) relevant documents" and used to evaluate and rank the retrieval systems. Wu et al.[9] proposed a relevance feedback algorithm that uses document-contexts by splitting the retrieved documents into sub-lists of document-contexts for different query term patterns including single query term occurrence, a pair of query terms that occur either in a phrase or in proximity. Scores of top ranking document-contexts for the same document are summed together to form the document score. The document with the highest score is used for feedback. Document-contexts are finally re-ranked in each sub-list to find relevant documents with high diversity.

Many researchers have contributed to diversifying results in web search[10,11,12]. Most of these papers discussed diversification of content across multiple documents and no single work focused on the diversity of content within a document. Welch et al.[13] proposed a search diversification algorithm for informational queries by explicitly modeling the requirements that needs multiple pages, each may focus on a few subtopics. They attempted to find a set of documents together having diverse information on various subtopics. This diversification algorithm defines a measure of satisfaction with respect to the query. Recently Santos et al.[14] assessed the diversification performance of : *Bing* and *Google* in the context of the diversity task of the TREC[3] 2009 and 2010 Web tracks. The results show that these web search engines are very effective at diversifying search results for ambiguous queries.

## 3 Comprehensive Content Search

In this work, we develop a method, namely *SAC* (*Segment And Cluster*), that finds individual documents covering information on various aspects. Instead of finding diverse information across search results, we wish to find each individual document that contains diverse information on various topics.

### 3.1 Overview

The objective of the proposed approach is to find documents that are comprehensive. Given a collection, many documents may have content that covers different aspects. Usually comprehensive documents are long in size and may have different sections. These sections refer to diverse aspects and are relevant to the query. So the content of a document has to be analyzed to know whether it contains different sections. It may be also require to identify how far a section is relevant to the query and how important it is to the query. For this, we make an assumption that if a particular subtopic is relevant, it will be represented

---

[3] Text REtrieval Conference (TREC) - http://trec.nist.gov/

in many of the top relevant documents. If we can find a subtopic which is represented many times in the top $n$ documents, then such a subtopic is referred as an important subtopic. The measure of document importance is considered by the number of subtopics covered by it and the number of documents having that subtopic. Based on this, we propose a framework using Pseudo Relevance Feedback (PRF) to estimate the comprehensive score of the documents.

## 3.2   Pseudo Relevance Feedback

Documents retrieved by an IR system pertaining to a query may either be relevant or irrelevant. Relevance Feedback (RF) systems require users to mark the initial set of retrieved documents as relevant or irrelevant. IR system uses such feedback from users to further improve the performance of documents retrieval. To get improved retrieval performance without an extended interaction of users, Pseudo Relevance Feedback (PRF) [15] based methods have been proposed. The idea of PRF is to provide a mechanism for automatic local analysis that helps to find a better representative set of documents for the given query[15]. The PRF does documents retrieval to find an initial set of documents for a given query. The evidence captured from the content analysis of the initial set of retrieved documents is considered as PRF to the IR system that ranks top $k$ documents based on PRF as the final set of relevant results.

## 3.3   Diverse Aspects of a Document

Suppose we consider a large number of top relevant documents retrieved for a given query. We assume that these documents cover all important aspects of the query. We also assume that if there exists a subtopic which is represented in many of these documents, then it is probably relevant to the query. Subtopics which are irrelevant to the query will not occur in many documents. We also recognize that some documents are diverse because of many different sections and some documents have a few sections. We assume that we can segment the document into sections, and each section contains a coherent subtopic. If a subtopic is important, similar sections will occur in many documents in the total collection. While segmenting the content of documents and analyzing all segments across the collection, we can find out the important subtopics. Manually doing this task for subtopic identification is laborious and not scalable in practice. So we need a mechanism that automatically identifies the diverse information that come from different important subtopics.

## 3.4   SAC: The Proposed Method

In this section, we describe the proposed SAC method. Given a collection of documents pertaining to a query, we wish to assign a score to each document which measures the comprehensiveness of the document content.

At first, documents retrieved for a query are divided into text segments which are then clustered. We hope that segments belonging to one cluster will have similar content and will pertain to one subtopic. A relevant document may describe one or more such subtopics. Since we assume that segments of many relevant documents are available, larger sized clusters may be assumed to correspond to important subtopics whereas smaller clusters may either contain information that are either irrelevant or of not much importance to the query because they have a fewer segments across the collection. For each document, we will identify the distribution of its segments so as to identify the subtopics (clusters) covered by it. The documents, whose segments belong to many important clusters, will contain comprehensive information. Based on this hypothesis, this proposed SAC method uses cluster based subtopic information as PRF to identify comprehensive documents.

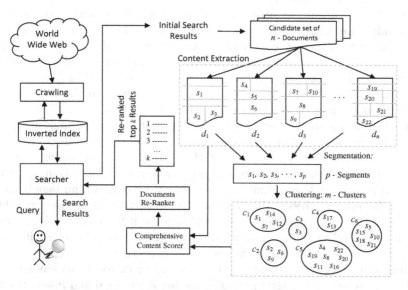

**Fig. 1.** The architecture of the proposed IR system

## 3.5   System Architecture

The proposed IR system, given in Figure. 1, contains the following components:

- **Search Engine:** Given a query, a search engine is required to retrieve a large number of relevant documents; we assume that the majority of documents retrieved are relevant.
- **Content Extraction:** This module takes the web page and removes noise, and filters the relevant content.
- **Comprehensive Content Scorer:**
  - **Segmentation:** Divides the filtered content into segments.
  - **Clustering:** Text segments are clustered to get important subtopics.
  - **Scoring:** This module assigns a score to each document based on its content covering important subtopics

– **Re-ranking:** This module re-ranks documents based on their comprehensive content score.

The components of the proposed system are described below.

### 3.5.1  Search Engines

Instead of building a separate search engine, one of the popular search engines may be used to retrieve an initial pool of relevant documents given a query. In this work, we have, for each query, retrieved top $n$ documents from Google to form a pool of relevant documents pertaining to the query.

### 3.5.2  Content Extraction

A typical web document contains information, along with various parts having advertisements, banners, forms, RSS news feeders, images, links or horizontal/vertical menus, copyright / site ownership information, etc. Many of these parts may have no information with respect to the actual content of the document. Such blocks are assumed to be noisy blocks. To identify and remove noisy blocks, we use *link-to-text* ratio [16] which is defined as the ratio between the length of the text tagged with and without hyperlinks.

Web documents are created in different layouts ( using html markups ) with customized cascaded style sheets(css). Some of these web documents are either semi- or ill-structured due to the fact that the tags in the underlying html markups are not balanced. So we perform content extraction from each web document as follows: Using HtmlCleaner[4] Library, we obtain html tags-balanced DOM ( Document Object Model ) like tree structure from the given html markups of the relevant web document and traverse it to identify noisy contents at each node level by applying *link-to-text* ratio heuristic. After removing noisy blocks, the rest is considered as the cleaned web content.

While extracting the content, more focus was given to blocks having table, div, lists, page break, paragraph break, heading levels 1 - 6 and finally the rest of document content. The content extraction module extracted 409 / 476 noisy blocks and achieved the overall accuracy of 85.92% in filtering noisy contents.

### 3.5.3  Document Segmentation

The document segmentation module is to divide the document into parts such that each part corresponds to one coherent segment. We assume that the blocks identified using the hierarchical structure of a document are independent semantic units which mostly correspond to a single subtopic. Segmentation of a document can be done at any heading levels especially in a web document.

The noise filtered web document may contain various informative sections, paragraphs, page breaks, headings, sections, subsections, tables. So the filtered content is divided into smaller segments at the following tag levels: div, table, header, paragraph, page breaks, line breaks and tags that support emphasize, italics, font size, font face. If subheadings covered by these tags are either larger in size

---

[4] HtmlCleaner 2.2 - http://htmlcleaner.sourceforge.net/

or contain more than two levels then the recursive segmentation is applied at selected inner tags until the lowest heading level, that contains a fewer child nodes and enough text content, is reached. Then the text content from each document segment is extracted. The number of text segments extracted per document may vary across the collection of relevant documents. This can be improved by dynamically calculating the ideal segmentation level using suitable techniques that could identify coherent segments starting at any given heading.

### 3.5.4   Clustering Text Segments

This module takes document segments and groups them into clusters, each contains similar document segments. All document segments present in a cluster are pertaining to a single subtopic. We also maintain the information of document segments and their associated clusters after segments are clustered.

Subtopics covered by a document can be identified by grouping the document segments into clusters. Many clustering algorithms are popularly known in the literature[17]. Dhillon et al.[18] proposed a fast graph clustering algorithm that first takes the input in the form of a graph whose nodes are terms and edge weights are co-occurrence statistics and then performs clustering in 3 steps: *coarsening, initial clustering* and *refining*. This algorithm is applied on the input term - co-occurrence graph to obtain a fixed set of clusters of terms. Using clustered terms, text segments are re-represented in the space of clusters that finds different aspects of text segments in each document.

In this work, we apply the graph clustering algorithm to group similar text segments. Suppose that there are $m$ clusters, then let $C = \{c_1, c_2, \cdots, c_m\}$ be the set of clusters. Since we assumed that larger clusters will correspond to important subtopics, we estimate the importance of each cluster, as $S_1(c_j)$, based on the number of segments it contains, as follows: Let $|c_j|$ be the number of segments in cluster $c_j$. Then the total number of segments in all clusters is the sum of all segments present in all clusters. So $S_1(c_j)$ can be defined as:

$$S_1(c_j) = \frac{|c_j|}{\sum_1^m |c_j|} \tag{1}$$

Large $S_1(c_j)$ indicates that it is probably an important subtopic, provided the segments are contributed by majority of documents. Least value of $S_1(c_j)$ indicates that the corresponding cluster $c_j$ may be less important or an outlier.

Alternatively we analyze the importance of a document via its segments spanning over several clusters. This phenomenon signifies diverse aspects of a document in terms of the number of subtopics covered by it. Since a comprehensive document will have many important sections, each belongs to a subtopic, in turn, to a different cluster. So the document having text segments in different clusters may tend to have diverse information. Now we derive the score of a cluster having segments from different documents, $S_2(c_j)$, as follows: Let $|d(c_j)|$ be the number of documents containing the subtopic - cluster $j$. Then for each document in the collection, consider the total number of such clusters across all documents. So $S_2(c_j)$ can be defined as:

$$S_2(c_j) = \frac{|d(c_j)|}{\sum_1^m |d(c_j)|} \qquad (2)$$

---

**Algorithm 1.** Finding documents having comprehensive content

---

**Input:** Query $q$

**Description:**

1: **Initial Set**: Input the query $q$ to search engine and retrieve the initial set of top $n$ documents: $D = \{d_1, d_2, \cdots, d_n\}$
2: **for** each retrieved document $d_i$, $1 \leq i \leq n$ **do**
3:     **Content Filtering**: Identify and remove noisy blocks and get filtered content;
4:     **Segmentation**: Use segmentation algorithm to divide the filtered content into text segments; Let these segments corresponding to $d_i$ be $s_i^1, s_i^2, \cdots, s_i^p$, $p \geq 0$
5: **end for**
6: **Clustering**: Apply a clustering algorithm on extracted text segments and group them into clusters. Suppose that there are $m$ clusters, then $C = \{c_1, c_2, \cdots, c_m\}$.
7: **for** each cluster $c_j$, $1 \leq j \leq m$ **do**
8:     Compute $score(c_j)$, of cluster $c_j$ using Equation. 3
9: **end for**
10: **for** each document $d_i$, $1 \leq i \leq n$ **do**
11:     **Document Scoring**: Compute comprehensive content score, $\text{CCS}(d_i)$, for document $d_i$ using Equation. 4
12: **end for**
13: **Re-Rank**: Sort the documents in decreasing order of their CCS scores.
14: **return** top $k$ documents ($k \leq n$) as comprehensive documents

**Output:** The re-ordered list of top $k \leq n$ comprehensive documents

---

Either or combinations of these two equations may be used to score the importance of the document clusters. Combining equation. 1 and equation. 2, we get $score(c_j)$ - as the relative importance between the number of segments in cluster $c_j$ and documents covering distinct clusters as follows:

$$score(c_j) = \sqrt{S_1(c_j) \times S_2(c_j)} \qquad (3)$$

### 3.5.5 Comprehensive Content Scoring

This component computes the comprehensive content score (CCS) of each document in the initial retrieved set pertaining to the query. Two stages are involved in this computation. At first, $score(j)$ - the score of each cluster $j$, $1 \leq j \leq m$ is computed as follows: First we find the cluster importance by counting the number of text segments belonging to cluster $j$. This measure on cluster $j$ is indirectly taken as its relative importance across the initial set of documents. Additionally more number of documents having text segments belonging to cluster $j$ signify the relative importance of the aspect associated with cluster $j$ pertaining to the query. Using these two measures, we compute $score(c_j)$ for $j$th cluster using Equation. 3.

Suppose that there are $l$ clusters containing segments of $d_j$. Now the comprehensive content score $\text{CCS}(d_i)$, for document $d_i$ is computed as follows:

$$\text{CCS}(d_i) = \sum_{r=1}^{l} score(c_r) \tag{4}$$

Based on the computed CCS, documents are re-arranged to place comprehensive documents on the top of the ranked list. The steps in the proposed approach are given in Algorithm. 1.

## 4   Experimental Results

We have selected a set of 15 queries listed below with their IDs: [1] - kaziranga national park, [2] - mahatma gandhi, [3] - delhi metro rail, [4] - sachin tendulkar, [5] - leptospirosis, [6] - jawaharlal nehru fellowship, [7] - pallavas stone sculptures, [8] - viswanathan anand, [9] - eiffel tower, [10] - cauvery water dispute, [11] - philosophy of plato, [12] - cure for lung cancer, [13] - bilateral network, [14] - shimla toy train, [15] - kolkata eden gardens. Using this set of queries, we have used Google to get the initial pool of relevant documents and an average of top 54 documents have been considered in Google results for each query.

A document having lengthy content would probably contain more information irrespective of its diverse aspects. Based on this, the baseline system with length based approach has been built using the initial pool of results retrieved by Google for each query. In this method, each document content has been scored based on the number of words in the content as the selected feature. We have stripped out stopwords from the document content and only the number of content words are considered for scoring comprehensiveness of each document. Then we applied the scoring of documents with the proposed SAC method to find the comprehensive content among the pool of retrieved documents. Finally we have provided three lists, each having top 10 documents retrieved by Google, length based and the proposed SAC methods, to evaluators.

### 4.1   Evaluation Methodology

The focus is on evaluating the quality or goodness of the document content in terms of the coverage of informative subtopics pertaining to the query. We have used 2 evaluators to judge the quality of the content of top 10 documents retrieved by Google, content length based system and the proposed SAC method. The guidelines for comprehensive content evaluation are given in Table 1.

Evaluators are instructed to perform the systematic evaluation on the comprehensiveness of the document content as follows:

- Evaluators picked up each of top 100 documents, evaluated by reading its content and observed the number of subtopics covered by each document pertaining to the query. Then depending on the maximum coverage of subtopics and their importance pertaining to the query, the quality of the content is scored in the 4 points scale as outlined in Table. 1.

Table 1. Guidelines for Comprehensive Content evaluation

| Score | Type | Description |
|---|---|---|
| 3 | Comprehensive | Doc. content covers many aspects of the query |
| 2 | Less Comprehensive | Doc. content covers one or two aspect(s) of the query |
| 1 | Relevant but not Comprehensive | Doc. content covers no specific aspects of the query, but contains only links, short snippets, reviews |
| 0 | Irrelevant | Document contains noisy or irrelevant information |

– The evaluators were given the ranked search results returned by (i) Google
  (ii) Baseline - content length based approach (iii) the proposed SAC method.
  Based on the given guidelines, evaluators carried out the scoring of the
  content of search results to find documents covering various aspects.
– Find the average of CCS scores over top $k$ ( = 10, 20, 30, 50, 100) results.

Table 2. Comparison of Comprehensive Content Scores of top 10 search results from: Baseline, Google, the proposed SAC methods

| | | CC Scores (Average) | | |
|---|---|---|---|---|
| QID | Query | Google | Length Based Approach | Proposed SAC |
| 1 | kaziranga national park | 1.00 | 1.50 | 2.40 |
| 2 | mahatma gandhi | 0.90 | 1.40 | 1.30 |
| 3 | delhi metro rail | 0.60 | 0.40 | 1.10 |
| 4 | sachin tendulkar | 0.70 | 0.90 | 1.80 |
| 5 | leptospirosis | 0.90 | 1.10 | 1.50 |
| 6 | jawaharlal nehru fellowship | 1.00 | 1.20 | 1.30 |
| 7 | pallavas stone sculptures | 0.90 | 1.30 | 2.00 |
| 8 | viswanathan anand | 1.10 | 1.20 | 1.70 |
| 9 | eiffel tower | 0.90 | 1.60 | 1.50 |
| 10 | cauvery water dispute | 1.00 | 1.10 | 1.40 |
| 11 | philosophy of plato | 1.80 | 1.90 | 1.90 |
| 12 | cure for lung cancer | 1.60 | 2.20 | 2.00 |
| 13 | bilateral network | 0.40 | 0.30 | 1.10 |
| 14 | shimla toy train | 0.70 | 0.70 | 1.30 |
| 15 | kolkata eden gardens | 0.80 | 0.70 | 1.60 |
| | **Overall Average** | **0.95** | **1.17** | **1.59** |

## 4.2 Effects of Comprehensive Content Scoring

Table. 2 presents the querywise results of comprehensive content evaluation
of top 10 search results. We have given a few querywise observations from
comprehensive content evaluation. For the query, "pallavas stone sculptures"
(ID: 7), the proposed approach effectively identified various aspects like: types of
sculptures, materials used, stone work, places of interests, architecture, temples,
and so on. For the query, "sachin tendulkar", pages having photos and debated
articles on "whether Sachin will score 100 100s?", have been retrieved. The content

of these pages focused on awards and practice session photos having text captions that contribute to multiple clusters. Similar effects observed in pages retrieved for queries like "eiffel tower", "delhi metro rail". The proposed method is unable to find enough content to judge the comprehensiveness of these documents. For the health related query, "leptospirosis" (ID: 5), the proposed method identified comprehensive documents present in lower rank and brings it to top 10 documents. Documents retrieved for the query ID. 8 contain Viswanath Anand's recent games and achievements. Many documents described the news related to his nationality but most of them discussed his career highlights.

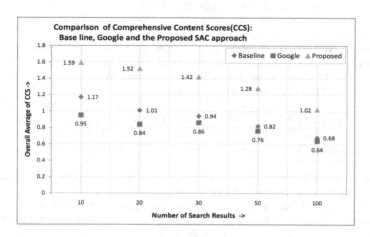

**Fig. 2.** Comparison of CCS of top $k$ results from: Baseline, Google, Proposed SAC

For query ID. 10 (cauvery water dispute), most of the documents present snippets of recent talks held by both the states involved in this dispute. For the query ID. 13 (bilateral network), most of the top 10 documents are from forums dealing with Interview Questions & Answers like content. But the proposed system identified the segments that effectively describe the aspects of bilateral network among the forum answers. We have performed similar analysis on the comprehensive content of top 20, 30, 50 and 100 documents and presented the overall average of the comprehensive content scores of three methods: baseline, Google and the proposed SAC approach in Figure 2.

## 5   Conclusion

In this work, we have proposed an approach to find comprehensive documents in terms of distinct subtopics covered by it. We performed the content analysis of documents using segments based clustering to estimate various aspects covered by them. Subtopics associated information are used as pseudo relevance feedback to find comprehensive documents covering diverse aspects pertaining to the query. Experimental results on web documents retrieved for the selected set of queries show that the proposed method effectively identifies comprehensive documents. In future, we plan apply the proposed method on FIRE or CLEF corpora to improve the ordering of comprehensive documents.

# References

1. Lipshutz, M., Taylor, S.: Comprehensive document representation. Mathematical and Computer Modelling 25(4), 85–93 (1997)
2. Lee, K.S., Park, Y.C., Choi, K.S.: Re-ranking model based on document clusters. Inf. Process. Manage. 37(1), 1–14 (2001)
3. Salton, G., Wong, A., Yang, A.C.S.: A vector space model for automatic indexing. Communications of the ACM 18, 229–237 (1975)
4. Makrehchi, M.: Query-relevant document representation for text clustering. In: ICDIM, pp. 132–138 (2010)
5. Krikon, E., Kurland, O., Bendersky, M.: Utilizing inter-passage and inter-document similarities for reranking search results. ACM Trans. Inf. Syst. 29(1), 1–3 (2010)
6. Xu, Y., Yin, H.: Novelty and topicality in interactive information retrieval. J. Am. Soc. Inf. Sci. Technol. 59(2), 201–215 (2008)
7. Clarke, C.L., Kolla, M., Cormack, G.V., Vechtomova, O., Ashkan, A., Büttcher, S., MacKinnon, I.: Novelty and diversity in information retrieval evaluation. In: Proceedings of the 31st Annual International ACM SIGIR Conference on Research and Development in Information Retrieval, SIGIR 2008, pp. 659–666. ACM, New York (2008)
8. Nuray, R., Can, F.: Automatic ranking of information retrieval systems using data fusion. Inf. Process. Manage. 42(3), 595–614 (2006)
9. wU, H., Luk, R., Wong, K., Nie, J.: A split-list approach for relevance feedback in information retrieval. Information Processing & Management (2012) (to appear)
10. Chapelle, O., Ji, S., Liao, C., Velipasaoglu, E., Lai, L., Wu, S.L.: Intent-based diversification of web search results: metrics and algorithms. Inf. Retr. 14(6), 572–592 (2011)
11. Rafiei, D., Bharat, K., Shukla, A.: Diversifying web search results. In: Proceedings of the 19th International Conference on World Wide Web, WWW 2010, pp. 781–790. ACM, New York (2010)
12. Agrawal, R., Gollapudi, S., Halverson, A., Ieong, S.: Diversifying search results. In: Proceedings of the Second ACM International Conference on Web Search and Data Mining, WSDM 2009, pp. 5–14. ACM, New York (2009)
13. Welch, M.J., Cho, J., Olston, C.: Search result diversity for informational queries. In: Proceedings of the 20th International Conference on World Wide Web, WWW 2011, pp. 237–246. ACM, New York (2011)
14. Santos, R.L., Macdonald, C., Ounis, I.: How diverse are web search results? In: Proc. of the 34th Int. ACM SIGIR Conference, SIGIR 2011, pp. 1187–1188. ACM, New York (2011)
15. Manning, C.D., Raghavan, P., Schtze, H.: Introduction to Information Retrieval. Cambridge University Press, New York (2008)
16. Gupta, S., Kaiser, G.E., Grimm, P., Chiang, M.F., Starren, J.: Automating content extraction of html documents. World Wide Web 8(2), 179–224 (2005)
17. Jain, A.K., Murty, M.N., Flynn, P.J.: Data clustering: a review. ACM Comput. Surv. 31(3), 264–323 (1999)
18. Dhillon, I.S., Guan, Y., Kulis, B.: Weighted graph cuts without eigenvectors a multilevel approach. IEEE Trans. Pattern Anal. Mach. Intell. 29(11), 1944–1957 (2007)

# Enhancing Sentence Ordering by Hierarchical Topic Modeling for Multi-document Summarization

Guangbing Yang[1], Kinshuk[2], Dunwei Wen[2], and Erkki Sutinen[1]

[1] School of Computing, University of Eastern Finland,
P.O. Box 111 80101 Joensuu, Finland
{yguang,erkki.sutinen}@cs.joensuu.fi
[2] School of Computing and Information Systems, Athabasca University, 1 University
Drive, Athabasca, Alberta T9S 3A3, Canada
{dunweiw,kinshuk}@athabascau.ca

**Abstract.** The sentence ordering is a difficult but very important task in multi-document summarization. With the aim of producing a coherent and legible summary for multiple documents, this study proposes a novel approach that is built upon a hierarchical topic model for automatic evaluation of sentence ordering. By learning topic correlations from the topic hierarchies, this model is able to automatically evaluate sentences to find a plausible order to arrange them for generating a more readable summary. The experimental results demonstrate that our proposed approach can improve the summarization performance and present a significant enhancement on the sentence ordering for multi-document summarization. In addition, the experimental results show that our model can automatically analyze the topic relationships to infer a strategy for sentence ordering. Human evaluations justify that the generated summaries, which implement this strategy, demonstrate a good linguistic performance in terms of coherence, readability, and redundancy.

**Keywords:** sentence ordering, hierarchical topic model, text summarization, machine learning.

## 1 Introduction

The concerns of how to alleviate the oft-decried information overload problem have recently given rise to interest in research of multi-document summarization, especially in extractive multi-document summarization. The extractive multi-document summarization can be simply described as a group of processes that automatically extract and synthesize source texts to summaries by identifying the importance and coherence of sentences from a set of documents. One of the main tasks is to determine the important sentences from the multiple documents, and another one is to make the summary sentences ordered properly. Many solutions have been provided to tackle with the first task, normally by using either statistics-based methods or Bayesian based language models to produce summaries. However, little attention has been given to the task of sentence

F. Castro, A. Gelbukh, and M. González (Eds.): MICAI 2013, Part I, LNAI 8265, pp. 367–379, 2013.
© Springer-Verlag Berlin Heidelberg 2013

ordering for generating more readable summaries [3],[6],[7],[11]. Based on the experimental results of previous research [3],[6],[11], the sentence ordering is a very important but difficult task in multi-document summarization.

The problem of the sentence ordering in multi-document summarization is more critical than in single document settings. In single document summarization, the summary sentences are naturally ordered by human authors and can be determined from the original document. In multi-document context, however, the summary sentences normally come from different documents written by different authors with various writing styles, and normally without natural coherence between these sentences. Furthermore, according to the research results from [2], multi-document based summaries written by humans do not follow the trend of cutting and pasting in the extractive based single-document summarization [9]. This makes it extremely hard to trace a sentence order from a human summary to optimize the coherence of the summary generated automatically.

Some approaches have recently been proposed to address the problem of sentence ordering. These approaches include the preference learning [6], spanning tree algorithms for regeneration of sentence in a dependency tree [19], probabilistic ordering [11], statistical coherence optimization [10], the rhetorical structure based approach [22], and so on. Although some improvements in sentence ordering have been achieved, these methods do not always yield coherent summaries. Most of them rely on the investigation of sentence features by using either naïve ordering algorithms or the surface and entity level features of documents (e.g., the majority ordering and chronological ordering, etc.). In addition, a lack of training data restricts the research and data usage to conclude a strategy for sentence ordering [3]. Existing corpus-based methods, such as supervised learning, are not easily apt to address a fully statistical approach due to the difficulty of constructing a corpus of training sets that cover many acceptable orderings for each single text. Thus, a new approach is recommended for identifying the sentence ordering properly by automatically analyzing the contents of articles to create more coherent summaries in multi-document summarization.

In this paper, a novel approach is proposed to the problem of sentence ordering in multi-document summarization. Our idea came from the previous research [3,6] that indicated the importance of the topical relatedness in the evaluation of sentence ordering. Considering the significant achievement of the Bayesian based topic modeling in the research of natural language processing and machine learning, our model is built upon the hierarchical Latent Dirichlet Allocation model (hLDA) [4] with a hierarchical prior defined by nested Chinese Restaurant Process (nCRP), which provides tree topologies for topics, and integrates the concepts of topic over time (TOT) model [20]. By investigating hierarchical topics and their correlations, this model is able to identify sentence ordering in a summary.

The rest of the paper is organized as follows: Section 2 discusses our new model in details. Section 3 discusses the experiments and results. Section 4 presents concluding remarks with discussion.

## 2     Sentence Ordering by Hierarchical Topic Model

### 2.1     Core Concept

Coherent sentences connect topics consistently and focus on the important content for a reader. Normally, an important idea is described in a topic sentence and supported by following details in a paragraph. Thus, a hierarchical relationship between topics and subtopics may reveal the connections of sentences in documents. The higher level of topics in this hierarchy may represent more general ideas presented in content, and lower level of topics may describe more specific content. Sentences share these relevant topics normally tended to appear together [3]. Based on this hypothesis, it is possible to group sentences under the same topic hierarchy and catch the sentence ordering from the hierarchical relationships between topics. In other words, the topic correlations discovered in topic hierarchies may associate with sentence ordering. Thus, the problem of how to discover sentence ordering can be transferred to the problem of how to learn the topic hierarchy from documents.

To deal with the problem of learning the topic hierarchy from documents, a hierarchical Latent Dirichlet Allocation (hLDA) model [4] is employed to organize topics into a hierarchy. The nested Chinese restaurant process (nCRP) is used to sample the prior on tree topologies for topic allocation. In this hierarchical structure, each node is associated with a topic, which is sampled over words. Along a path from the root node to a leaf node, the model can generate a sentence by repeatedly sampling topics, and then sampling the words from the selected topics. The nCRP provides a tree topology. A general topic is closer to the root than a specific one. Following this tree topology, a sentence that consists of more general topics normally has a shorter path and its average sum of the levels for corresponding topics is small. If a sentence includes more specific topics, it will have a longer path in this tree. In addition, each level assignment of the topic that associates with an individual word in a sentence can also be used to determine the entire level of the sentence. The details of the algorithm for sentence ordering will be discussed in Section 2.5.

In addition, the concept of topics over time model [20] is adapted in our model to arrange the sentence order by analyzing the chronological order of publication timestamps. However, the chronological ordering of sentences is mainly useful for news and scientific articles, but shows a significant limitation for other kinds of documents. Based on this situation, using publication timestamps to decide the chronological order among sentences is an auxiliary for sentence ordering in our model.

### 2.2     Hierarchical Sentence Coherence Topic Model

The nested Chinese restaurant process (nCRP) is the prior of the topics in our case and can be expressed as follows:

$$p(z_i|s_{-i}) = \frac{n_i}{\gamma + n - 1}, p(z_{i+1}|s_{-i}) = \frac{\gamma}{\gamma + n - 1} \tag{1}$$

where $z_i$ represents a topic in certain level of the tree, $s_i$ is the new sentence and $s_{-i}$ represents the previous sentences, $\gamma$ is the parameter that controls the tendency of the sentences (e.g., customers) in a path (e.g., a restaurant) of the tree to share topics (e.g., tables). For details about the nCRP, one can refer [4].

In this model, three distributions are mixed together to represent the distribution of the topic hierarchy. These three distributions are: path allocation, level allocation, and timestamp allocation, which represent the probabilities of topic hierarchy, the probabilities of topics, and the probabilities of topic over time, respectively. By observing sentences in which their initial orders are indicated by the path distribution, the posterior of the level distribution represents the topic allocation and the posterior of the path distribution represents the allocation of the topic correlation.

The collapsed Gibbs sampling algorithm [13] is employed in this model to sample the path $c_s$ and the level allocations to topic $z_{s,n}$ in those paths where $z_{s,n}$ is allocated. A sentence is generated by first randomly choosing an L-level path through the topic hierarchy and then sampling the words from the L-dimensional topics that are associated with nCRP prior along that path. One can refer the original work [4] for more details about this generative process. The graphical representation for our model, namely Hierarchical Sentence Coherence Topic Model (HSCTM) is presented in Figure 1. In this graphic model, $s_m = \{s_1, s_2, \ldots, s_L\}$ are latent variables that represent the nodes in L-level trees and associate with the nCRP prior. Each level is sampled from the LDA [5] hidden variables $\mathbf{z}$. Thus, the posterior conditional distribution for $s_m$, which is associated with the L topics sampled from words $\mathbf{w}$ in the sentence $\mathbf{s}$, allocates the topics along the path of the sentence generation.

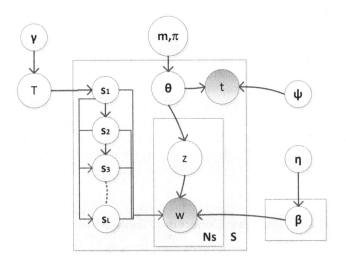

**Fig. 1.** The graphical model representation of HSCTM

The joint distribution $P(w, s, z, t | \gamma, m, \pi, \eta, \psi)$ can be expressed as follows:

$$P\left(w, s, z, t | \gamma, m, \pi, \eta, \psi\right) = P\left(w, s, z | \gamma, m, \pi, \eta\right) P\left(t, w, z | m, \pi, \eta, \psi\right)$$

$$\propto \underbrace{P\left(z | w, s, m, \pi, \eta\right)}_{level-allocation} \times \underbrace{P\left(s | w, z, \gamma, \eta\right)}_{path-allocation} \times \underbrace{P\left(z | t, w, m, \pi, \eta, \psi\right)}_{timestamp-allocation} \quad (2)$$

where w, s, z, and t are vectors of distributions of words, paths, topics (or levels of paths) and timestamps.

In the right side of the Equation (2), three distributions represent the level allocation, path allocation, and timestamp allocation, respectively, as the results of the collapsed Gibbs sampling. For details about the process of sampling for each allocation, one can refer the original work from [4],[20]. Here, we discuss the probabilistic inference, hyperparameter estimation, and the method to compute the sentence ordering.

## 2.3   Probabilistic Inference

The posterior inference is the inverse step of the generative process described above for estimating the hidden structure of a corpus (e.g., a set of sentences) [4]. As described above, the entire probabilistic inference can be processed as three separated Gibbs samplings, and then combined these three steps into an overall process to infer the mode of the posterior distribution. The sampling processes of the level allocation and the path allocation are identical to the original hierarchical topic model [4]. Here we only discuss the sampling of the timestamps because the topic prior, which is the distribution of GEM [16], is different from the original topic over time model [20].

**Sampling Timestamps.** With a Beta prior $\psi$, the timestamp allocation for each sentence given all other timestamps and observed words can be described as: $p\left(z_{s,n} = k | t, w, z_{s,-n}, m, \pi, \eta, \gamma\right)$, which can be expressed as a joint distribution:

$$p\left(t_{s,n} | z_{s,n}, w_{s,-n}, \eta\right) p\left(z_{s,n} | z_{s,-n}, \psi\right) \propto \left(N\left(z_{s,-n} = k\right) + (1-m)\pi - 1\right)$$

$$\times \frac{N\left(z_{s,-n} = k\right) + \eta_{w_{s,-n}} - 1}{\sum_{v=1}^{V} N\left(z_{s,-n} = k\right) + \eta_{w_{s,-n}} - 1} \times \frac{(1 - t_{s,n})^{\psi_{1,z_{s,n}}^{-1}} t_{s,n}^{\psi_{2,z_{s,n}}^{-1}}}{B\left(\psi_{1,z_{s,n}}, \psi_{2,z_{s,n}}\right)} \quad (3)$$

where $N\left(z_{s,-n} = k\right)$ is the number of topics for all words in sentence s excluding the word n, V represents the vocabulary, m and $\pi$ are hyperparameters of topic prior, which is the distribution of GEM [16]. $B\left(\psi_{1,z_{s,n}}, \psi_{2,z_{s,n}}\right)$ is the Beta factor and the hyperparameter $\psi$ is estimated by calculating the moments during each Gibbs sampling. For details about the estimation of $\psi$, one can refer[20].

## 2.4   Hyperparameter Inference

The hyperparameters $\gamma$, $\eta$, m, $\pi$, and $\psi$ can be estimated by using a Gibbs EM algorithm [1] during the inference process. The values of hyperparameters are usually prior distributions that contain parameters called hyper-hyperparameters

[4]. Normally, the hyper-hyperparameters are given fixed values in practical application, and the hyperparameters can be approximated by computing the mode of the joint distribution in Eq. (2) when the Markov chain is in a stationary state. The highest logarithm of the probability of the posterior mode or the logarithm of the maximum likelihood in this stationary state can be used to determine the values of hyperparameters. Other methods for hyperparameter estimation are fixed-point iteration and Newton-Raphson iteration [14],[15],[18].

For practical convenience, the Gibbs EM algorithm is employed in our model for hyperparameter estimation because the process of EM can be accomplished during the posterior inference performed by the collapsed Gibbs sampler. Algorithm 1 in Figure 2 shows the steps of Gibbs EM for estimating the hyperparameter $\eta$. The other hyperparameters can be obtained in the same way.

---

**Algorithm 1. The Gibbs EM algorithm for hyperparameter $\eta$**

1. Initialize z, s, and $\eta$

2. **E Step**: Sample $\{z^{(w)}\}_{w=1}^{\omega} \sim P\left(z|w, s, t, \gamma, m, \pi, \eta, \psi\right)$, where $\Omega$ denotes the Gibbs sampling space.

3. **M Step**:

$$\hat{\eta} := \underset{\eta}{argmax} \frac{1}{\Omega} \sum_{\Omega} log\left(p\left(w_{s,n}|z, s, w_{-(s,n)}, \eta\right)\right)$$

$$= \underset{\eta}{argmax} \frac{1}{\Omega} \sum_{\Omega} log\left(N\left(z_{s,n}, s_{s,z_{s,n}}, w_{s,n}\right) + \eta\right), \text{ where } \Omega \text{ is the}$$

sample size, compute $\hat{\eta}$ with number of samples when $z_{-(s,n)} = z_{s,n}$, $s_{z_{s,n}} = s_{s,z_{s,n}}$, and $w_{-(s,n)} = w_{s,n}$.

4. Repeat **E Step** until converged.

---

**Fig. 2.** Algorithm of Gibbs EM for estimating the hyperparameter $\eta$

## 2.5   Sentence Ordering

To evaluate the sentence ordering, a sentence order score is defined as the sum of the level assignment for each word divided by the probabilistic value of its topic in the sentence, and then averaged out over the number of words, plus the path allocation of this sentence for a summary. The equation for this calculation is given as follows:

$$SO = \frac{1}{N_s} \sum_{n}^{N_s} \frac{p\left(z_{s,n}\right)}{L_{z_{s,n}}} + p\left(s_s\right) \tag{4}$$

where $p\left(z_{s,n}\right)$ is the posterior distribution value of topic $z_{s,n}$ defined in Equation (2), which includes both level allocation and timestamp allocation for the topic $z_{s,n}$ that associates with the word n in the sentence s, $L_{z_{s,n}}$ represents the level assignment for the topic $z_{s,n}$ and its value ranges from 1 to the depth of the tree. Thus, the low value of the level assignment suggests that the topic is general. $N_s$ is the total number of words for a sentence, and $p\left(s_s\right)$ is the path allocation for this sentence. Based on this formula, a higher sentence ordering score indicates that the sentence consists of more general topics and has a short path to the root, and as a result, this sentence may position at the front of the generated summary.

# 3   Experiments and Results

It is a difficult task to automatically justify the sentence ordering of a summary generated by a summarization system. A semi-automatic evaluation approach is widely employed to measure the performance of the algorithms used in sentence ordering [6],[11]. Our experiment adapts the same evaluation measures used in [6]: the Kendall's rank correlation coefficient ($\tau$) and Spearman's rank correlation coefficient ($\rho$).

## 3.1   Evaluation Metrics and Experimental Data

These two methods are statistic measures that evaluate the association between two sentence orderings, which are ranked by a summarization system and human summarizers respectively. One can refer Bollegalas work [6] for detailed discussions on how to use them to evaluate the sentence ordering in multi-document summarization.

In our experiment, three hundred summaries were selected to build a testing data set. This data set included two hundred human summaries provided by Document Understanding Conference (DUC) 2006 corpus (in which there were total fifty clusters, and each cluster had four summaries written by human experts) plus one hundred system summaries generated by two summarization systems, in which one was the benchmark system on DUC 2006 and another one was the system that was built upon a topical n-grams model [21]. There were total 4,106 sentences and 82,051 words in the testing data set. The vocabulary size was 10,099.

Our hierarchical sentence coherence topic model (HSCTM) was trained by using DUC 2006 corpus, which contained 50 clusters and each cluster included 25 articles, and the initial values for the hyperparameters used in the experiments were: $\eta$=1.0,0.5,0.25,0.125, $\gamma$=0.5, m=0.35 (the GEM mean), $\pi$=100 (the GEM variance), $\psi$=0.01. The depth for the tree structure was 4, and the burning time was 10,000 for the Gibbs sampling. After the training, the hyperparameters with the best performance for our model were: $\eta$=0.00148, $\gamma$=0.94, m=2.57 (the GEM mean), $\pi$=100 (the GEM variance), $\psi$=0.51. These updated hyperparameters were used in our testing. During the testing, those three hundred summaries were sampled by our HSCTM model and sentences were reordered based on the score calculated using Equation (4). After this process, two sentence ordering quantities processed by our model, namely the original ordering quantities of those summaries and the ordering quantities of the summaries, were used in the Kendall's $\tau$ and Spearman's $\rho$ analysis.

## 3.2   Experimental Results

The experimental results are shown in Table 1. The mean value and the value of standard deviation are computed based on these three hundred results of Kendall's $\tau$ and Spearman's $\rho$ analysis. Comparing with the experimental results that were analyzed by the method of probabilistic ordering (PO) discussed in

Bollegala [6], our average Kendall's $\tau$ and Spearman's $\rho$ are 0.095 and 0.169, and increase 1.37 and 1.7 times over the values obtained in Bollegala's experiment (average $\tau = 0.040$ and $\rho = 0.062$), respectively [6].

**Table 1.** Correlation between original sentence ordering and new sentence ordering generated by HSCTM model

| Metric | Mean | Std.Dev |
|---|---|---|
| Results including topic over time model | | |
| Kendall's $\tau$ | 0.095 | 0.221 |
| Spearman's $\rho$ | 0.169 | 0.279 |
| Results excluding topic over time model | | |
| Kendall's $\tau$ | 0.094 | 0.248 |
| Spearman's $\rho$ | 0.167 | 0.282 |

Although the corpus used in our experiment is different from the dataset used in the experiment discussed in [6], the comparison is still meaningful because our dataset contains 300 summaries from DUC rather than 60 summaries manually created by two human subjects [6]. Our experimental results seem more plausible that can be easily compared with results of experiments conducted by other researchers in future.

In order to justify the effectiveness of the timestamps to the sentence ordering, the similar testing was done by our model without counting the topics over time model [20]. The experimental results are listed in Table 1 (lower panel) and show that the topics over time model has no obvious contributions to the overall performance. As discussed previously, the chronological order performs poorly when summarized information was collected from various sources and not event based, such as in our case.

### 3.3 ROUGE Evaluation and Results

This experiment used ROUGE [12], the official evaluation toolkit for text summarization in DUC, to evaluate the performance of our HSCTM model. The evaluation metrics: ROUGE-1, ROUGE-2, and ROUGE-SU4 were investigated during the experiment, and the recall, precision, and F measures of these metrics were reported in this experiment.

Table 2 shows the system comparison results of ROUGE-1, ROUGE-2, and ROUGE-SU4 on DUC 2006 data. In order to evaluate the performance of the summarization approach addressed in this study, the results of one of the benchmark summarizers in DUC2006 are also listed in Table 2. System ID (S-ID) 24 represents this system, namely IIITH-Sum [8]. S-ID T1 represents the summary generated by the Topical n-grams model based summarizer, which performed better than system IIITH-Sum both in ROUGE-1 and ROUGE-2 evaluations. For detailed system comparisons, one can refer [23]. S-ID A to J represents human summaries in DUC 2006. Our HSCTM model reordered the sentences and did not alter any other features of the generated summary, such as words, phrases, a sentence length, and word sequences in a sentence, and so on. Thus, the ROUGE-1 measures for reordered summaries should be the same as the results of ROUGE-1 evaluation for original summaries.  Table 2 only shows

**Table 2.** Experimental results on the data of DUC 2006

| S-ID | R-1 | | R-2 | | R-SU4 | |
|---|---|---|---|---|---|---|
| | Original | Reorder | Original | Reorder | Original | Reorder |
| 24 | 0.41017 | 0.41017 | 0.09513 | 0.09713 | 0.15478 | 0.15583 |
| T1 | 0.40541 | 0.40541 | 0.09386 | 0.09716 | 0.14905 | 0.15410 |
| A | 0.45864 | 0.45864 | 0.10358 | 0.10493 | 0.16812 | 0.16948 |
| B | 0.46845 | 0.46845 | 0.11681 | 0.11903 | 0.17500 | 0.17612 |
| C | 0.47110 | 0.47110 | 0.13210 | 0.13340 | 0.18279 | 0.18429 |
| D | 0.47008 | 0.47008 | 0.12368 | 0.12874 | 0.17803 | 0.17968 |
| E | 0.44870 | 0.44870 | 0.10472 | 0.10847 | 0.16393 | 0.16598 |
| F | 0.42866 | 0.42866 | 0.10666 | 0.10719 | 0.15777 | 0.15777 |
| G | 0.45598 | 0.45598 | 0.11247 | 0.11472 | 0.16946 | 0.17107 |
| H | 0.45995 | 0.45995 | 0.11015 | 0.11142 | 0.17007 | 0.17094 |
| I | 0.45347 | 0.45347 | 0.10654 | 0.10633 | 0.16810 | 0.16844 |
| J | 0.45623 | 0.45623 | 0.10671 | 0.11087 | 0.16750 | 0.16891 |

the F-measures of ROUGE evaluation on metrics ROUGE-1, ROUGE-2, and ROUGE-SU4 (corresponds to the column R-1, R-2, R-SU4 in the table respectively), but does not give recall and precision results due to the space limitations. The values of F-measures for the original summaries are listed under the column Original in the table, and the values of F-measures for the summaries with reordered sentences are shown in the column Reorder. As we analyzed previously, the values of ROUGE-1 evaluation did not change for all summaries. The values of ROUGE-2 and ROUGE-SU4 for all summaries increased slightly in a range of 1.05% to 4.1%. The amount of increases is not statistically significant in this experiment. However, the trend of this increase indicates that the effectiveness of the sentence ordering presented by our model is positive for multi-document summarization.

## 3.4   Human Evaluation and Results

In this experiment, a subjective evaluation was also conducted for further comparison to evaluate the performance of our HSCTM model. Three university students in Computer Science participated in this experiment. Sixty summaries were randomly selected from our testing dataset, half of them were human summaries and half were system summaries. Both their sentences were reordered by our model. During the experiment, those three human judges were asked to read these summaries and reorder sentences necessarily to make the summaries more readable and coherent based on their understanding. The original summaries and articles were also given to them for reference. The Kendall's $\tau$ and Spearman's $\rho$ were calculated for each pair of quantities of sentence ordering and the averages and standard deviations are listed in Table 3. The results are slightly higher than the values listed in Table 2, but verify that our model has performed consistently.

**Table 3.** Kendall's $\tau$ and Spearman's $\rho$ between human evaluation and ROUGE evaluation

|  |  | Correlation on Human Summaries |
|---|---|---|
|  | **Kendall's $\tau$** | **Spearman's $\rho$** |
| Mean | 0.149 | 0.252 |
| Std.Dev | 0.261 | 0.306 |
|  |  | Correlation on System Summaries |
|  | **Kendall's $\tau$** | **Spearman's $\rho$** |
| Mean | 0.137 | 0.244 |
| Std.Dev | 0.267 | 0.341 |

Note that the average values of Kendall's $\tau$ and Spearman's $\rho$ are quite small and not statistically significant. Thus, a further analysis was performed using Lapata's judgment elicitation study [11] to allocate $\tau$ values into various bins based on their value range. A histogram showed the range of $\tau$ values in Figure 3. Based on this histogram, one can see the most $\tau$ coefficients are ranged from: -0. 5 < $\tau$ < -0.25, -0.25 < $\tau$ < 0.0, 0.0 < $\tau$ < 0.25, and 0.25 < $\tau$ < 0.5. To simplify the comparison, those $\tau$ value bins were combined into four groups: $\tau$ < 0.0, 0.0 < $\tau$ < 0.25, 0.25 < $\tau$ < 0.5, and $\tau$ > 0.5. Then, a variance analysis (ANOVA) was given to compare the correlations between human and system summaries. The ANOVA results for these binned $\tau$ values showed in Table 4.

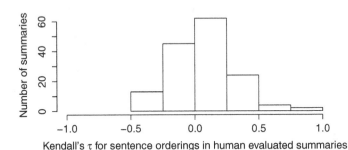

Kendall's $\tau$ for sentence orderings in human evaluated summaries

**Fig. 3.** The histogram of binned Kendall's $\tau$ values

There was only one factor, $\tau$, in this ANOVA analysis with four levels corresponding to the four bins of $\tau$ values. The ANOVA showed that when $\tau$ value was less than zero and between 0.25 to 0.5, the $\tau$ values from these two bins for the system evaluations of sentence orderings were significantly different from the values from the human evaluations. When $\tau$ value was between zero to 0.25 and above a half of the maximum $\tau$ value (which is one), there were no significant differences in sentence orderings between human and system evaluations.

Table 4. ANOVA results for binned Kendall's $\tau$

| Kendall's $\tau$ Range | F | p | Significant |
|---|---|---|---|
| $0.0 < \tau$ | 11.378 | <0.001 | ** |
| $0.0 < \tau < 0.25$ | 0.118 | 0.732 | |
| $0.25 < \tau < 0.5$ | 18.756 | <0.0001 | *** |
| $0.5 < \tau$ | 0.352 | 0.561 | |

## 4 Discussion and Conclusion

In this paper a Bayesian based topic hierarchy model was proposed for solving the problem of sentence ordering in multi-document summarization. The constraints of the sentence ordering in multi-document summarization are learned from the topic hierarchies of the corpus. The experimental results showed that the topics and topic hierarchies were important constraints for the ordering task. Both results from human evaluation and ROUGE testing indicated that our Hierarchical Sentence Coherence Topic model (HSCTM) could successfully evaluate the sentence ordering and order sentences to generate a summary with high coherence and sufficient cohesion.

In addition, the variance analysis showed significant differences in sentence orderings between the human and system evaluations, although this significance occurred only in certain range of Kendall's $\tau$ coefficients. By reviewing these sentences, we found that humans performed better ordering judgment when $\tau$ value was less than zero. In this case, the correlations between the hierarchical topics were not obvious. A similar situation occurred in the case when $\tau$ value ranged from 0.25 to 0.5. In this case, many topics discovered in the sentences were layered in the same level so that there was no distinction between the topics. In this particular example, humans were able to find out semantic associations among sentences and ordered them properly, but the system was lack of abilities to determine such semantic difference or similarity. For the other two bins of $\tau$ values, the system evaluation had no significant difference from the human evaluation because the hierarchical relationships between topics were clearly allocated. The similar evaluation result demonstrated that our model was able to determine the sentence ordering from the topic hierarchies. Nevertheless, this analysis result indicated that our proposed approach was suitable for the problem of the sentence ordering in multi-document summarization.

Our model can obtain ordering information automatically. Thus, it is particularly suitable for tasks in multi-document summarization and provides alternative strategies to sentence ordering especially for documents that are not event based and have unavailable publishing date or relevant timestamps. The evaluation results of Kendall's $\tau$ and Spearman's $\rho$ indicated that our model performed much better than other probabilistic ordering methods even through the values of $\tau$ and $\rho$ themselves were not always significant from the statistical perspective. In addition, the ROUGE evaluation demonstrated that our model was able to improve the summarization performance and the method of sentence ordering made our summarizer comparable to the benchmark systems in DUC.

However, a number of issues in practice need to be addressed in future work. First, our Hierarchical Sentence Coherence Topic model (HSCTM) only considered the topic correlation from the perspective of topic hierarchy without examining the topic relatedness in the same hierarchical level. Some models, such as the dependency tree in the spanning tree algorithms for regeneration of sentence [19] and a hierarchical Pitman-Yor dependency model [17] in generative dependency modeling, addressed approaches to deal with this dependency problem. Second, from the perspective of the computing performance, the tree structure of the model is not suitable for a larger dataset. For example, in our case, the total number of sentences is 4,106, which is not big, but the number of possible permutations for these sentences in a 4-level tree is very big. If the trees depth increases doubly to eight, the number of the possible permutations for a sentence and the number of tree nodes will become too huge to be processed efficiently. In this situation, the training and testing become extremely hard tasks because they require a huge amount of computer memory spaces and processor time. However, if the model is trained based on a small dataset, the topic hierarchies found from the corpus will not reflect the real associations of topics. Therefore, a better algorithm needs to be studied in order to improve the computing performance significantly. Third, the topics discovered in a topic model typically represent the general concepts abstracted from a group of documents. Sometimes, this generalization may disperse the process for importance discovery. For a practical application, such as the text summarization, a strategy (e.g., query-focused) is essential to supervise the topic model by specifying a topic theme to increase the accuracy. The dependency modeling and query-focused strategy could be potential improvements to take place with respect to the model in future work.

**Acknowledgments.** This research was supported by the NSERC, iCORE, Xerox, and the research related funding by Mr. A. Markin. This work was also supported by a Research Incentive Grant (RIG) of Athabasca University.

# References

1. Andrieu, C., De Freitas, N., Doucet, A., Jordan, M.I.: An introduction to mcmc for machine learning. Machine Learning 50, 5–43 (2003)
2. Banko, M., Vanderwende, L.: Using n-grams to understand the nature of summaries. In: Proceedings of HLT-NAACL 2004: Short Papers. HLT-NAACL-Short 2004, pp. 1–4. Association for Computational Linguistics, Stroudsburg (2004)
3. Barzilay, R., Elhadad, N., McKeown, K.R.: Inferring strategies for sentence ordering in multidocument news summarization. J. Artif. Int. Res. 17(1), 35–55 (2002)
4. Blei, D.M., Griffiths, T.L., Jordan, M.I.: The nested chinese restaurant process and bayesian nonparametric inference of topic hierarchies. J. ACM 57(2), 7:1–7:30 (2010)
5. Blei, D.M., Ng, A.Y., Jordan, M.I.: Latent dirichlet allocation. The Journal of Machine Learning Research 3, 993–1022 (2003)
6. Bollegala, D., Okazaki, N., Ishizuka, M.: A preference learning approach to sentence ordering for multi-document summarization. Information Sciences 217, 78–95 (2012)

7. Celikyilmaz, A., Hakkani-Tür, D.: Discovery of topically coherent sentences for extractive summarization. In: ACL, pp. 491–499 (2011)
8. Jagarlamudi, J., Pingali, P., Varma, V.: Query independent sentence scoring approach to duc 2006. In: Proceeding of Document Understanding Conference (DUC 2006) (2006)
9. Jing, H.: Using hidden markov modeling to decompose human-written summaries. Computational linguistics 28(4), 527–543 (2002)
10. Kim, H.D., Park, D.H., Vydiswaran, V.V., Zhai, C.: Opinion summarization using entity features and probabilistic sentence coherence optimization: Uiuc at tac 2008 opinion summarization pilot. Urbana 51, 61801 (2008)
11. Lapata, M.: Automatic evaluation of information ordering: Kendall's tau. Computational Linguistics 32(4), 471–484 (2006)
12. Lin, C.Y.: Rouge: A package for automatic evaluation of summaries. In: Text Summarization Branches Out: Proceedings of the ACL 2004 Workshop, pp. 74–81 (2004)
13. Liu, J.S.: The collapsed gibbs sampler in bayesian computations with applications to a gene regulation problem. Journal of the American Statistical Association 89(427), 958–966 (1994)
14. MacKay, D.J., Peto, L.C.B.: A hierarchical dirichlet language model. Natural Language Engineering 1(3), 289–308 (1995)
15. Minka, T.: Estimating a dirichlet distribution (2000)
16. Pitman, J.: Combinatorial stochastic processes, vol. 1875. Springer (2006)
17. Pitman, J., Yor, M.: The two-parameter poisson-dirichlet distribution derived from a stable subordinator. The Annals of Probability 25(2), 855–900 (1997)
18. Wallach, H.M.: Topic modeling: beyond bag-of-words. In: Proceedings of the 23rd International Conference on Machine Learning, pp. 977–984. ACM (2006)
19. Wan, S., Dras, M., Dale, R., Paris, C.: Spanning tree approaches for statistical sentence generation. In: Krahmer, E., Theune, M. (eds.) Empirical Methods. LNCS, vol. 5790, pp. 13–44. Springer, Heidelberg (2010)
20. Wang, X., McCallum, A.: Topics over time: a non-markov continuous-time model of topical trends. In: Proceedings of the 12th ACM SIGKDD International Conference on Knowledge Discovery and Data Mining, pp. 424–433. ACM (2006)
21. Wang, X., McCallum, A., Wei, X.: Topical n-grams: Phrase and topic discovery, with an application to information retrieval. In: Seventh IEEE International Conference on Data Mining, ICDM 2007, pp. 697–702. IEEE (2007)
22. Wolf, F., Gibson, E.: Paragraph-, word-, and coherence-based approaches to sentence ranking: A comparison of algorithm and human performance. In: Proceedings of the 42nd Annual Meeting on Association for Computational Linguistics, p. 383. Association for Computational Linguistics (2004)
23. Yang, G., Chen, N.S., Kinshuk, S.E., Anderson, T., Wen, D.: The effectiveness of automatic text summarization in mobile learning contexts. Computers & Education 68, 233–243 (2013)

# An Enhanced Arabic OCR Degraded
# Text Retrieval Model

Mostafa Ezzat, Tarek ElGhazaly, and Mervat Gheith

Computer Sciences Department, Institute of Statistical Studies & Research,
Cairo University, Egypt
{Mostafa.Ezzat,Tarek.Elghazaly}@cu.edu.eg,
MGheith@issr.cu.edu.eg

**Abstract.** This paper provides a new model enhancing the Arabic OCR degraded text retrieval effectiveness. The proposed model based on simulating the
Arabic OCR recognition mistakes on a word based approach. Then the model
expands the user search query using the expected OCR errors. The resulting expanded search query gives higher precision and recall in searching Arabic
OCR-Degraded text rather than the original query. The proposed new model
showed a significant increase in the degraded text retrieval effectiveness over
the previous models. The retrieval effectiveness of the new model is %97, while
the best effectiveness published for word based approach was %84 and the best
effectiveness for character based approach was %56. In addition, the new model
overcomes several limitations of the current two existing models.

**Keywords:** Arabic OCR Degraded Text Retrieval, Orthographic Query Expansion, Synthesize OCR-Degraded Text.

## 1 Introduction

The amount of printed material increased tremendously in the fifteenth century. Many
documents continue to be available only in print, although the number of documents
available as character-coded text is now increasing as a result of electronic publishing,
especially for Arabic. There were unusual technological hurdles until recently, including limited computer infrastructure and lack of Arabic support in Web browsers and
popular operating systems. Further, different proprietary formats for Arabic text encoding were done in many. All these factors mean that users often access only the
printed documents or images (scanned images of the printed documents). In fact,
finding character-coded Arabic text instead of Arabic document images on the Web is
still uncommon. This makes searching documents by user query very complicated.

Without automated process, the user would be only able to manually find the desired documents or consult a person who is familiar with the searched documents.
Since such search can easily be done by searching character coded documents, and we
can automate the process by generating the character-coded representations of the
documents. In principal, we can generate the character-coded representation of the
documents by rekeying the documents' text or creating metadata about the documents

F. Castro, A. Gelbukh, and M. González (Eds.): MICAI 2013, Part I, LNAI 8265, pp. 380–393, 2013.

such as titles, summaries, or keywords. But these approaches would be labor intensive and impractical for large numbers of documents. Another automated way to produce a character-coded representation is to scan the documents and then use Optical Character Recognition (OCR), which is an automated process that converts document images into character-coded text. However, the results often contain errors. Further, Arabic properties like orthography, which is how words are written and complex morphology, which is how words are constructed, adversely affect the accuracy of OCR. On the other hand, the OCR process is inexpensive and thus well suited for large document collections.

## 1.1    Orthographic Properties of Arabic

Arabic is a right-to-left connected language that uses 28 letters, and its shapes change depending on their positions in words. Fifteen letters contain dots to differentiate them from other letters. And depending on the discretion of the document producer, these letters may or may not have diacritics (short vowels). Ligatures, which are special forms for some character sequences, and kashidas, which are symbols that extend the length of words, are often employed in printed text. Having a connected script that uses ligatures and kashidas complicates isolation of individual letters in OCR, and dots and diacritics make OCR sensitive to document noise and speckle. Figure 1 shows some examples of letters with different dots, diacritic, and letters in different positions, kashida, and ligature [3]. Most Arabic OCR systems segment characters [4, 5, 6, 7], while a few opted to recognize words without segmenting characters [8, 9], and another system developed by BBN avoids character segmentation by dividing lines into slender vertical frames (and frames into cells) and uses an HMM recognizer to recognize character sequences [10].

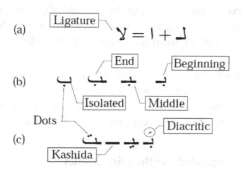

**Fig. 1.** (a) A ligature, (b) Shapes of the letter "ba" and (c) a diacritic and kashida[23]

This paper presents OCR-Degradation synthesizing model that is trained on different shapes of the words generated from the OCR recognition process and the model is independent of the technique used in the OCR process itself. Then using the training information, we reformat the user search query by inserting all the possible shapes of each query word to generate the search query that will return all the documents related to the original search query.

In the following section we will introduce the previous work done in this direction and also we will compare two different models that use a similar approach to enhance the degraded text information retrieval.

## 2     Comprehensive Study for the Previous Work

Building a model that simulates the OCR-Degraded text covers an important part of information retrieval when the retrieved text is returned from the OCR process. The OCR process in this case is affected by many factors like the Paper quality which is affected by the time, human errors done during the scanning process, the accuracy of the OCR system used and the font which the document was initially printed with.

All these factors and others affects the information retrieval process done on the text resulted from the OCR process.so modeling the OCR-Degraded text is a major part in any research that deals with information retrieval. In this section we will present two models were developed by ElGhazaly and Darwish as parts of their research in the information retrieval in the same language or in different languages. To the best of our knowledge, they are the only models built specially or Arabic OCR-Degraded Text retrieval.

### 2.1     ElGhazaly OCR-Degraded Synthesizing Model

The model is a Word Based model that is trained and tested on complete words. ElGhazaly generated documents of single word per line, and then print, scan and OCR these documents using Sakhr OCR, then he manually align the OCR recognition results with the clean text document. During this manual alignment he checked if there is a deformation of the OCR-Degraded word, then he stored the deformed OCR-Degraded Word and its original word as a training pair in the OCR Errors Database [2, 22].

Then ElGhazaly used this OCR Error model to expand the query used in the information retrieval. This Orthographic Query Expansion approach attempts to find different misrecognized versions of a query word in the collection being searched. But ElGhazaly didn't proof the retrieval effectiveness of his model.

### 2.2     Darwish OCR-Degraded Synthesizing Model

Darwish model is based on the character level not the word level as ElGhazaly. The main idea of the model was based on the fact that the context affects the character shape in a word, because Arabic letters are connected and change shape depending on their position in the word and some special shapes are formed when special characters are sequenced in the same word, so his assumption was that the position of a letter being recognized and the letters surrounding it ("context") would be important in developing a good model.

The model was simply based on aligning the OCR recognition results from the print(300X300), 200x200, and 200x100 versions of the Zad collection (the training and testing data set as we will mention later in this section ) with the associated clean text version of the same collection. The alignment was done using SCLITE which is an application from the National Institute of Standards and Technology (NIST), which employs a dynamic programming string alignment algorithm that attempts to minimize the edit distance between two strings. Basically, the algorithm uses identical matches to anchor alignment, and then uses word position with respect to those anchors to estimate an optimal alignment on the remainder of the words. Two factors affected his alignment process. The printed and clean text versions in the Zad collection were obtained from different sources that exhibited minor differences (mostly substitution or deletion of particles such as in, from, or, and then), and secondly some areas in the scanned images of the printed page exhibited image distortions that resulted in relatively long runs of OCR errors.

Based on the alignment done using the SCLITE and the other algorithm Darwish implemented, he built a "garbler" tool which reads in the clean word $C1..Ci..Cn$ and synthesize OCR degradation to produce a garbled word $D'1..D'j..D'm$. This "garbler" chooses and perform a random edit operation (insertion, substitution or deletion) based on the probability distribution for the possible edit operations. The garbler was the tool that simply takes any word and generates the different error shaped that would be produced if this word was printed and OCR-ed.

## 2.3     The Model Training

The training data is one of the most important factors that affects the success or failure of any experiment, if we designed the correct model but used bad data to train the model, the result will be the failure of the model, and in the other hand if we choose good training data for the model, this will raise the success rate of the model. In this section we will compare between the training data used by both ElGhazaly and Darwish with training their models.

**ElGhazaly Training Data.** ElGhazaly took 200 documents from the corpus documents he constructed, and then he formatted them to keep only one word per line. Then he used the "Adobe Acrobat printer driver to convert the plain text documents into PDF format. Then based on his tests on the different OCR systems- he decided to use Sakhr Arabic OCR as the recognition system for the rest of the experiment. He then applied the OCR process on the 200 documents, with average 30 pages; the total number of pages was about 30,000 pages with single word per line.

The result was having the original text for the documents and the result text from the OCR (the OCR-Degraded Text).Then he aligned manually the degraded documents returned from the OCR with the original clean text documents to have both Original & Degraded Text with the same line number.

**Darwish Training Data.** Darwish used Arabic book "Zad Al-Me'ad" which is available as a printed book and also available as electronic version for free. The book consists of 2,730 separate documents that address a variety of topics such as mannerisms, history, jurisprudence and medicine. Darwish scanned the printed version of Zad Al-Me'ad at 300x300 dpi (dots per inch) resolution, and then he manually zoned the images into multipage file to correspond exactly to the 2,730 documents in the character-coded clean copy of the collection.

Then Darwish used Sakhr's Automatic Reader version 4.0 OCR engine to convert the images into plain text. Darwish measured the accuracy for the OCR-degraded text and it was computed with reference to the clean text using software from the University of Nevada at Las Vegas [11], obtaining 18.7%, for the images with 300 X 300 resolutions.

## 2.4    The Test Data

This section illustrates the test data collection that has been developed by both researchers in order to illustrating the success of their models.

**ElGhazaly Test Data.** ElGhazaly generated two data test sets selected from the training and testing pool, the first data set included 50 long documents consists of 26,579 words. The second test group contains 100 long documents consists of 51,765 words, and as ElGhazaly mentioned in his dissertation that there is no intersection between the training data sets and the test data sets collection.

**Darwish Test Data.** Darwish main goal for the OCR degradation model testing was to verify that the modeled OCR degradation and real OCR degradation have similar effects on information retrieval operation. Darwish decided to validate the effect of synthesized OCR degradation on retrieval effectiveness for the TREC collection [12] at the print (300X300) and 200x200 resolutions. TREC collection is the LDC LDC2001T55 collection, which was used in the Text REtrieval Conference (TREC) 2002 cross-language track. And for brevity Darwish called it TREC collection. The TREC collection contains 383,872 articles from the Agency France Press (AFP) Arabic newswire. Darwish indexed the synthetically degraded TREC collections using words, lightly stemmed words, character n-grams- where n ranged between 3 and 5-, and combinations of n-grams and lightly stemmed words [23].

**The Accuracy of the Models.** It was important for us to see the accuracy of both models, because this will show us the direction of our research. Because each model has a different direction, one of them is based on word based approach and the other one is based on character based approach.

After training the model on 53,787 words, ElGhazaly model produced accuracy of 84.74% on test set contains 51,658 words [21]. Elghazaly introduced his own accuracy measure, which is the number of accurate replacements (with respect to the training set size) divided by the total number of OCR-Degraded words. In other words, if the mistaken OCR-degraded word is available in the training set with the correct original word, then this will be considered as accurate replacement. Otherwise, it will be considered as not accurate one. But ElGhazaly didn't actually indexed and search his test data set calculate the precision, recall   and mean average precision of his model [21].

On the other hand Darwish model produced accuracy for 3- gram or 4 gram character indexing was 87% [1, 24], but here we must illustrate the difference in both accuracy measurements, because Darwish was measuring according to the character level which means, For example, consider a page of 20 lines, each line has on average 10 words, and each word has on average 5 characters. This means the page has 1000 characters in 200 words. If we consider the OCR output of this page to have only 20 character errors each in a separate word, this means character accuracy of 98% where it means word accuracy of 90%. Darwish Also illustrated that the best mean average precision of his model which was "0.56" [1, 25].

# 3     The Proposed OCR-Degraded Arabic Text Retrieval Model

Our Proposed OCR-Degraded Arabic Text Retrieval model is based on two steps, the first step is synthesize the OCR-Degraded text, and then expands the user search query using the expected OCR error generated from the Arabic OCR error simulation. The first step in the model, which is, modeling the OCR degradation is an important point when handling electronic library information retrieval, unfortunately, despite the claims of commercial vendors; OCR error rates are far from perfect, particularly for challenging languages like Arabic [13]. The result is that the low accuracy of the Arabic OCR text affects directly the accuracy of the online retrieval process regarding these documents.

There are many challenges for the OCR to give accurate outputs. Also, there are many models for correcting the OCR outputs. Many models for simulating the OCR errors have been analyzed. They are mainly depending on 1-gram and sometimes n-gram character replacement algorithm. However, in Arabic, as character shape defers up to its position in the words (begin, middle, end, Isolated). So, it is too difficult to include all these variables (7-gram character for example) plus the character position in one model. However, even if the 7-gram is reached, the 8-grams will not be covered and so on. The next section (3.1) describes the OCR-Degradation synthesizing model, which is a word based model trained and tested on complete words. This model supports the maximum n-grams in the training set with respect to the words' positions. Then in section 3.2 we will show how we used this model to enhance Arabic OCR Degraded Text retrieval.

## 3.1     The OCR-Degradation Synthesizing Model

As we mentioned, the proposed OCR-Degradation synthesizing model is a word based model that is trained and tested on complete words. This model supports the maximum n-grams in the training set with respect to the characters' positions. The model main idea is to align the OCR degraded words and the clean text words, the alignment operation is done based on the edit distance which is the insertions, deletions, and substitutions operations required to correct the degraded text. Calculating the edit distance between two Arabic words requires caution, because Arabic words may be formatted with prefix letters which sometimes forms half the word length, which means, if we calculated the edit distance between two words contains the same prefixes but the remaining of the two words is completely different, our model will consider them as the same word but some degradation happened while the OCR. To solve this problem our model ignores the Arabic prefixes letters while computing the edit distance between any words.

The model is built to accept any recognition accuracy that may result from the OCR system; this is done using the edit distance. which means specifying the deformation level the user of the model wants to cover in his training data set .The model checks each word in each document of the OCR-Degraded documents' set against the corresponding original word, if the edit distance between the two words less than or equal a selected value, the model stores the deformed shape linked with the original word as a training pair in the OCR errors database. Otherwise the model ignores these words and fetches the next words from the OCR-Degraded and cleans text files. Figure 2 illustrates the OCR-degradation synthesizing model.

And to test our proposed model we built a software application we called The "Aligner", which performs all the actions illustrated in the model and constructs the training database. The "Aligner" takes both Original and OCR-ed text files and tokenize them into words, then based on the edit distance between them, the tool updates our training database that stores the original word shape and the corresponding shapes of the words appeared in the OCR version. Figure 3 displays the aligner application interface.

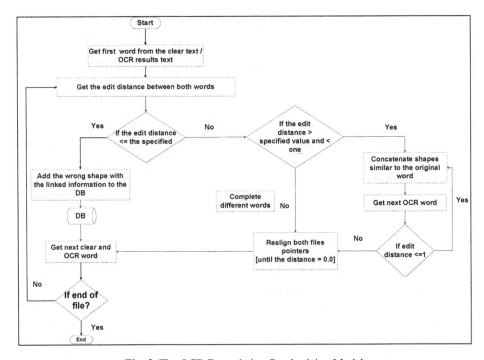

**Fig. 2.** The OCR Degradation Synthesizing Model

The model starts by fetching the first word from the clean the OCR-Degrade text files, and then the model calculates the edit distance between both words. Here we have three cases we shall handle, the first case, the edit distance value is less than or equal the accepted value, the second case, the value is larger than the accepted value but less than or equal one, and the third and final case, the value is larger than one. The first case means that the edit distance is within the accepted value specified by the model user in the application interface; so the model adds both words to the training database.

The second case means that either the degraded word is part of the original word, but the OCR application split it while the recognition process, which happens sometimes for long words, or the recognition process was bad for this word and the system recognized only few characters of the word. This point formed a limitation in the word based models we checked, they didn't consider if the word was recognized as two and sometimes three parts [2,22].

We decided to cover this limitation in our model. This means, if the OCR system recognized one word into two or three words, our system will consider these parts as one word and store them in the training database as one shape corresponding to the original shape. Finally, the third case , if the edit distance between both words is larger than one, which means that both words and completely different, this means that the model has lost the correct position of anchors corresponding to each file, in this case our model realign the anchors until both files anchors are pointing on the same word.

The "Aligner" updates the training database with degraded shapes with its corresponding original shapes; the database structure was designed to keep only one entry of the original word and any number, but unique, of the deformed shapes of this word. The database also stored the context of the deformed shapes, like the preceding word and the succeeding word. This information will be used in our future work which is checking how the OCR-Degraded word context affects the retrieval effectiveness.

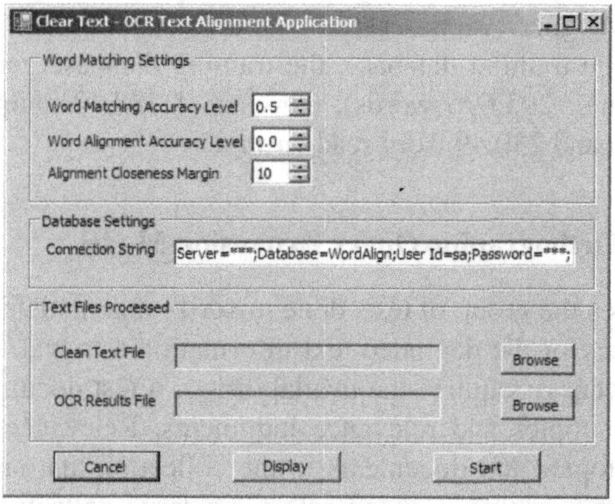

**Fig. 3.** The "Aligner" Application interface

## 3.2     Orthographic Query Expansion

After synthesizing the OCR-Degraded text, here comes the second step of the ortho-graphic query expansion model, which is expanding the user search using the expected OCR error simulation model. To expand the user query we built a query generation tool, this tool takes the original user query and generates the deformed OCR- Degraded query. The following figure (Figure 4) illustrates the Query Genera-tion user interface.

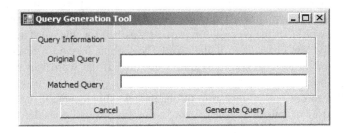

**Fig. 4.** Query Generation Tool

## 3.3     Training the OCR Degradation Synthesizing Model

The model was trained on the electronic version of the Arabic three volume book "Abgad El Eloum" or "Alphabet of science" and for short naming we will call it "ABGAD". For the experiment we printed the first two volumes of the book, which contained 205,761 words, then we scanned and OCR-ed the first two volumes using the best Arabic OCR  application, Sakhr Automatic reader version 10.Sakhr OCR produces 99.8% accuracy for high-quality documents 96% accuracy for low-quality documents [14]. In this stage we have the original electronic version of the book, and the corresponding OCR-ed version of the same electronic text.

Then using the "Aligner" we processed both the clean text and the OCR generated text and generates the training database, the training database generated constructed from 1500 documents (205,696 words), consists of 388,40 unique words, 182,647 words read correctly and 230,49 word read wrong.

## 3.4     Testing the Orthographic Query Expansion Model

This section describes the group of tests done to verify that modeled OCR degradation increases the accuracy of the degraded text information retrieval. Generally; evaluat-ing retrieval effectiveness requires the availability of a test document collection with an associated set of topics and relevance judgments. Relevance judgments are the mappings between topics and documents in the collection that are relevant to them. The cost of producing relevance judgments for a large collection is very high and dominates the cost of developing test collections [15].

There are three ways to produce relevance judgment, the first one is "pooling" , which is assessing manually the relevance of the union of the top n documents from multiple retrieval systems for every topic [16]. The second way is manual user-guided search, where a relevance judge manually searches and assesses documents for a topic until the judge is convinced that all relevant documents are found [17]. The third way is exhaustively searching the documents for relevant documents [18].

These three ways often miss some relevant documents, and assessment of relevance is necessarily subjective, but studies shown that relevance judgments can be reliably used to correctly differentiate between retrieval systems provided that a sufficient number of queries are used [4, 19, 16]. Voorhees estimated the number of sufficient queries to be about 25 [16]. But here in our test we extended the search query to be 35 queries to collect more data about the retrieval accuracy.

**Orthographic Query Expansion Model Test Set Statistics.** We based our test on two test sets have been selected from the Training and test pool. The first one includes 20 documents (66,985 words), which is the third volume of "ABGAD". And to memorize the training set was the first two volumes only of the book. And the second data test set contains 2,730 long documents containing 621,763 words. There is no intersection between the Training and Test sets.

The second test data is "ZAD" data collection ,which is a 14th century religious book called Zad Al-Me'ad, which is free of copyright restrictions and for which an accurately character-coded electronic version exists [20]. We here must illustrate that this is the same test set used by Darwish in his model [1].

### 3.5    Testing the Orthographic Query Expansion Model Accuracy

This section describes the development of a test collection that can be used to evaluate alternative techniques for searching scanned Arabic text and a set of experiments that were designed to identify the effect of the proposed model on retrieval effectiveness. IR evaluation measures are concerned with precision and recall given:

|              | Relevant | Not Relevant |
|--------------|----------|--------------|
| **Retrieved** | A | B |
| **Not Retrieved** | C | D |

$$\text{Percision} = \frac{A}{(A+B)} \qquad \text{Recall} = \frac{A}{(A+C)}$$

Precision measures the fraction of retrieved documents that are relevant. Recall measures the fraction of all relevant documents that are actually retrieved. IR-effectiveness measures use precision and recall in different ways. For example, precision at n measures the precision after a fixed number of documents have been retrieved. Another is precision at specific recall levels, which is the precision after a fraction of relevant documents are retrieved.

For our experiment we indexed our clean and OCR-Degraded documents on the best Arabic search engine, IDRISI 6.0[14]. One of IDRISI features is creating separate search collection for different group of documents depending on the user requirements. So we created a separate collection for the clean text documents and another collection for the OCR-Degraded documents. The author of the paper, a native speaker of Arabic, developed 35 topics and exhaustively searched the collection for relevant documents.

Then using the "Query Generation" tool that takes the user clean text query and based on the training database generates the relevant OCR-Degraded text query, we passed both the original search query and the OCR degraded query to IDRISI to search the clean text collection and the OCR-Degraded text collection separately. Using this way we can compare the results of both collections and get the precision and recall to check our model accuracy.

After completing the experiment on the thirty five queries we analyzed the results and found that. For test data set 1, the number of relevant documents per topic ranged from one (for one topic) to eighteen, averaging 14. For test data set 2 the number of relevant documents per topic ranged from two (for one topic) to 224, averaging 121. The average query length used for the test data set 1 is 4 .1 words and for test data set 2 is 5.2 words. The following figure displays the search precision and recall returned from the search engine relevant to the number of retrieved document for test data set 1.

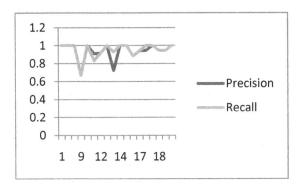

**Fig. 5.** Test Data Set 1 Precision and Recall relevant to no. of documents retrieved

And the following figure (figure 6) displays the search precision and recall returned from the search engine relevant to the number of retrieved document for test data set 2.

The figure shows that the recall and precision values returned from searching OCR-Degraded text relative to the number of returned document in the test data set 2. Unfortunately  Darwish didn't mention the precision and recall measurements for his model. He was most concerned with the mean average precision value of his information revival system, the mean average precision is the most commonly used evaluation metric which eases comparison between systems [16]. The best mean average precision resulted by Darwish was "0.56" [1] for 3-Gram and 4-gram steamed words,

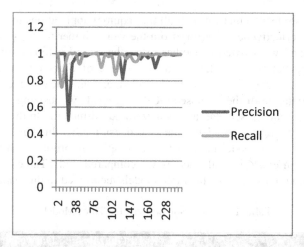

**Fig. 6.** Test Data 2 Precision and Recall relevant to no. of documents retrieved

in the other hand the mean average precision resulted by the proposed model for test data set 1 is "0.96" and for test data set 2 is "0.97".which means a significant improvement in the information retrieval effectiveness.

# 4    Conclusion

In the second section we provided a comprehensive study of the previous models designed to simulate OCR-Degraded text, to the best of our knowledge Darwish and Elghazaly models are the only models designed especially for Arabic recognition, then we provided our model which we consider advanced the state of the art for Arabic OCR-Degraded text retrieval in specific and IR in general. Perhaps the most challenging contribution was the development of new OCR degraded synthesizing model that improves information retrieval effectiveness. The proposed new model has shown high effectiveness than the previously developed n-gram or either word level models.

The model was trained on 1500 documents containing 205,696 words, consists of 38,840 unique words, 182,647 words read correctly and 230,49 word read wrong. And the model was tested on two different data sets, on the first data set, which consisted only of 20 documents containing 66,985 words.

And the second test data set were 2,730 separate documents containing 621,763 words. There were no intersection between the training data sets and test data sets. When the model was applied on the first data set ,The mean average precision produced was  "0.96" , and when the model applied on the second data set the mean average precision produced was "0.97".In the other hand Darwish shown that the best mean average precision produced by his model for 3–gram indexed data set was "0.56" [1]. We here must illustrate that ElGhazaly didn't measure his model performance against indexed data set [2] and he depended only on calculating the number of OCR-Degraded words in the training set as an accuracy measurement.

We must illustrate also that we built all the required applications to proof the model accuracy and effectiveness, starting from the word aligner to the query expansion. On the other hand we showed that other researchers used external applications like SCLITE an application from the National Institute of Standards and Technology (NIST) or manual alignment to align the degraded text with the clean text.

The main limitation of the proposed OCR-Degraded synthesizing model is its dependency on the training set size, as it's a word based model. On the other hand the character based model proposed by Darwish doesn't have this limitation. Also we must illustrate that our model handles the word splitting problem while recognition and this limitation exists in both models we compared with. Table 1 illustrates the main comparison points between the three models mentioned in this paper.

**Table 1.** Comparison between the Three Models

| Comparison Point | ELGhazaly Model | Darwish Model | Proposed Model |
|---|---|---|---|
| The model considered word context error that may affect the recognition operation. | ✓ | ✗ | ✓ |
| The model is word based and covers any word with any length once it was trained on it | ✓ | ✗ | ✓ |
| The accuracy measurement used based on the word level not on character level | ✓ | ✗ | ✓ |
| The model solved the word concatenation problem | ✗ | ✓ | ✓ |
| The model tried to simulate different degradation levels | ✗ | ✓ | ✓ |
| The model idea can potentially be useful in widespread applications | ✓ | ✓ | ✓ |
| The model retrieval effectiveness is tested on indexed data set | ✗ | ✓ | ✓ |
| The model considered enhancing the scanned images before OCR | ✗ | ✗ | ✓ |
| The model accuracy is not affected by the training set size | ✗ | ✓ | ✗ |

# References

[1] Darwish, K.: Probabilistic Methods for Searching OCR-Degraded Arabic Text, A PhD Dissertation, University of Maryland, College Park (2003)

[2] Elghazaly, T.: Cross Language Information Retrieval (CLIR) for digital libraries with Arabic OCR-Degraded Text, A PhD Dissertation, Cairo University, Faculty of Computers and Information (2009)

[3] Chen, A., Gey, F.: Building an Arabic Stemmer for Information Retrieval. In: TREC, Gaithersburg, MD (2002)

[4] Burgin, B.: Variations in Relevance Judgments and the Evaluation of Retrieval Performance. Information Processing and Management 28(5), 619–627 (1992)

[5] Callan, P., Lu, Z., Croft, B.: Searching distributed collections with inference networks. In: SIGIR (1995)

[6] Blando, L.R., Kanai, J., Nartker, T.A.: Prediction of OCR accuracy using simple image features. In: Proceedings of the Third International Conference on Document Analysis and Recognition, August 14-16, vol. 1, pp. 319–322 (1995)

[7] Chen, S., Subramaniam, S., Haralick, R.R., Phillips, I.: Performance Evaluation of Two OCR Systems. In: Annual Symp. on Document Analysis and Information Retrieval (1994)

[8] Darwish, K., Oard, D.: CLIR Experiments at Maryland for TREC 2002: Evidence Combination for Arabic-English Retrieval. In: TREC, Gaithersburg, MD (2002)

[9] Cole, A., Graff, D., Walker, K.: Arabic Newswire Part 1 Corpus (1-58563-190-6), Linguistic Data Consortium (LDC)

[10] Darwish, K.: Building a Shallow Morphological Analyzer in One Day. In: ACL Workshop on Computational Approaches to Semitic Languages (2002)

[11] Rice, S., Jenkins, F., Nartker, T.: The fifth annual test of OCR accuracy. Information Science Research Institute, University of Nevada, Las Vegas (1996)

[12] Harman, D.K.: Overview of the first Text REtrieval Conference (TREC-1). In: Proceedings of the First Text Retrieval Conference (TREC-1). pp. 1–20. NIST Special Publication 500-207 (March 1993)

[13] Kanungo, T., Marton, G.A., Bulbul, O.: OmniPage vs. Sakhr: Paired model evaluation of two Arabic OCR products. In: Proc. of SPIE Conf. on Document Recognition and Retrieval (1999)

[14] http://WWW.SAKHR.COM (last visited on June 2013)

[15] Soboroff, I., Nicholas, C., Cahan, P.: Ranking retrieval systems without relevance judgments. In: SIGIR (2001)

[16] Voorhees, E.: Variations in Relevance Judgments and the Measurement of Retrieval Effectiveness. In: SIGIR, Melbourne, Australia (1998)

[17] Wayne, C.: Detection & Tracking: A Case Study in Corpus Creation & Evaluation Methodologies. In: Language Resources and Evaluation Conference, Granada, Spain (1998)

[18] Tseng, Y., Oard, D.: Document Image Retrieval Techniques for Chinese. In: Symposium on Document Image Understanding Technology, Columbia, MD (2001)

[19] Salton, G., Lesk, M.: Relevance Assessments and Retrieval System Evaluation. Information Storage and Retrieval 4, 343–359 (1969)

[20] Publishers, Al-Areeb Electronic

[21] Elghazaly, T., Fahmy, A.: Query Translation and Expansion for Searching Normal and OCR-Degraded Arabic Text. In: Gelbukh, A. (ed.) CICLing 2009. LNCS, vol. 5449, pp. 481–497. Springer, Heidelberg (2009)

[22] Elghazaly, T.A., Fahmy, A.A.: English/Arabic Cross Language Information Retrieval (CLIR) for Arabic OCR-Degraded Text. Communications of the IBIMA 9(25), 208–218 (2009); ISSN 19437765

[23] Darwish, K., Oard, D.: CLIR Experiments at Maryland for TREC 2002: Evidence Combination for Arabic-English Retrieval. In: TREC, Gaithersburg, MD (2002)

[24] Darwish, K., Oard, D.: Term Selection for Searching Printed Arabic. In: SIGIR (2002)

[25] Darwish, K., Oard, D.: Probabilistic Structured Query Methods. In: To appear in SIGIR (2003)

# ELEXR: Automatic Evaluation of Machine Translation Using Lexical Relationships

Alireza Mahmoudi[1], Heshaam Faili[1],
Mohammad Hossein Dehghan[1], and Jalal Maleki[2]

[1] University of Tehran, Tehran, Iran
School of Electrical and Computer Engineering
College of Engineering
{ali.mahmoudi,hfaili,mh.dehghan}@ut.ac.ir
[2] Linköping University, Linköping, Sweden
Dept of Computer and Information Science
jalal.maleki@liu.se

**Abstract.** This paper proposes ELEXR[1], a novel metric to evaluate machine translation (MT). In our proposed method, we extract lexical co-occurrence relationships of a given reference translation (Ref) and its corresponding hypothesis sentence using hyperspace analogue to language space matrix. Then, for each term appearing in these two sentences, we convert the co-occurrence information into a conditional probability distribution. Finally, by comparing the conditional probability distributions of the words held in common by Ref and the candidate sentence (Cand) using Kullback-Leibler divergence, we can score the hypothesis. ELEXR can evaluate MT by using only one Ref assigned to each Cand without incorporating any semantic annotated resources like WordNet. Our experiments on eight language pairs of WMT 2011 submissions[2] show that ELEXR outperforms baselines, TER and BLEU, on average at system-level correlation with human judgments. It achieves average Spearman's rho correlation of about 0.78, Kendall's tau correlation of about 0.66 and Pearson's correlation of about 0.84, corresponding to improvements of about 0.04, 0.07 and 0.06 respectively over BLEU, the best baseline.

**Keywords:** Automatic Evaluation, Machine Translation, Evaluation Metrics, BLEU, TER, Lexical Relationships, Machine Translation Evaluation.

## 1 Introduction

Evaluating a translation is not a trivial task. Since machine translation (MT) systems have been developed rapidly in recent years, quality evaluation of these systems has been considered as an important issue. One way to evaluate such a system accurately is to hire human expert evaluators to measure the quality of a system in a systematic approach. But this method is quite expensive and

---

[1] ELEXR: Evaluation using Lexical Relationships.
[2] They are available at http://www.statmt.org/wmt11.

F. Castro, A. Gelbukh, and M. González (Eds.): MICAI 2013, Part I, LNAI 8265, pp. 394–405, 2013.
© Springer-Verlag Berlin Heidelberg 2013

time consuming, because it takes days or weeks to finish. This problem could be serious when it is necessary to frequently evaluate a developing system.

Common automatic evaluation metrics evaluate MT based on measures like precision, recall and edit distance. In this paper we propose a new metric for MT evaluation using lexical co-occurrence information (LCI) of a reference translation (Ref) and its corresponding candidate sentence (Cand). The main idea of our proposed method is to extract LCI of a Ref and its Cand using hyperspace analogue to language (HAL) space matrix [1] incorporating a sliding window. Then LCI is converted into a conditional probability distribution. Finally, by comparing the conditional probability distribution of the words held in common by Ref and Cand using Kullback-Leibler (KL) divergence [2], we can score the hypothesis.

This paper is organized as follows. The next section briefly describes some existing MT evaluation metrics. In Section 3, we introduce HAL space matrix and then, we explain how to extract LCI of sentence words using this matrix. Section 4 explains our method to evaluate MT. Our experiments and evaluations are presented in Section 5. Finally, we describe conclusion in Section 6.

## 2   Related Work

In this section, we focus on some well-known metrics that have received a lot of research interests in several studies in particular Workshop on Statistical Machine Translation (WMT), which compares different evaluation metrics [3–5].

BLEU [6] is a widely used metric that counts and compares $n$-gram overlaps between Cand and one or more Refs. This metric is similar to precision measure, such that, precision is computed for all higher order of $n$. Two aspects of translation are obtained by means of this modified n-gram precision scoring function: *adequacy* and *fluency*. m-BLEU [7], an enhanced version of BLEU, is another metric that uses flexible word matching, which is based on stemming and WordNet rather than exact word matching. Clearly, using an external language resource such as WordNet is considered as a weakness for this metric in some languages that do not have such a resource.

AMBER [8] is another automatic evaluation metric, which is a modified version of BLEU. In fact, it incorporates recall and some other features like extra penalties and some text processing variants to match the human judgment. Like BLEU, AMBER is language independent and its calculation can be done quickly. An enhanced version of AMBER [9] has two modifications. The important one is the use of new ordering penalty, which helps to evaluate free-word-order languages.

PORT [10] is another metric that is proposed especially for tuning MT systems. It uses precision, recall, strict brevity penalty, strict redundancy penalty and ordering metric without incorporating any external language resources, and like AMBER, it is quick to compute.

METEOR [7, 11, 12] computes a lexical similarity score for a given Cand and Ref using word-to-word alignments. This metric uses three matchers to build alignments incrementally in a series of stages. At each stage, these matchers are used to identify pair words not aligned in previous stages, to match between Ref and Cand. At the end of each stage, the largest subset of these matches is selected as an alignment such that each word in the candidate sentence aligns to at most one word in Ref. Then matched words are marked to avoid reconsideration in the later stages. Finally a union of all stages alignments is considered as a result of these stages. In situations when there are multiple reference sentences, the candidate is scored against each reference sentence independently and the maximum score is selected as a score of the candidate. Although METEOR tries to overcome some of weaknesses of BLEU, like m-BLEU it is not feasible to use this metric for languages such as Persian, which lacks a suitable language resource like Princeton WordNet. Thus, this issue remains as a weakness of METEOR and other metrics such as TESLA [13], ROSE [14], MPF [15] and TINE [16] that need language resource or suitable language processing tools to evaluate MT.

TER [17] is a metric using the minimum number of edits performed on Cand to be converted into Ref exactly. There are several metrics such as mTER [7], TER-Plus [18], WER, mWER [19], CDER [20], PER and mPER [21] that use edit distance to evaluate MT in some different ways. SPEDE [22] is another metric for sentence level MT evaluation that is based on probabilistic finite state machine (PFSM) model. By learning weighted edit distance in a PFSM, and by computing probabilistic edit distance as predictions of translation quality, each translation is evaluated. It has been proposed to overcome some short comings which standard edit distance models have in capturing long-distance word swapping or cross alignments.

There are some other metrics which consider different measures such as syntactic structure of Cand and one or more corresponding Refs to evaluate MT systems [23], or those which consider the fact that each word contributes a different amount of information to the meaning of a sentence [24] and use several measures to find out the information loads of terms, called term informativeness measures. Almost all of these metrics use human produced reference sentences to score a candidate sentence, however there is a metric based on IBM1 lexicon probabilities which does not need any reference translations [25].

## 3    Extracting Word Relationship Using HAL Space Matrix

If the co-occurrence relationships among sentence terms are produced, the similarity of a given sentence can be measured by comparing these relationships. As mentioned above, the main idea of this article is to produce lexical co-occurrence information of a given MT output and corresponding one or more reference sentences, using a sliding window. The window moves over Ref and Cand and produces word co-occurrence statistical information. This information is in the numerical form, which refers to the number of co-occurrence of a term and any other term in the sentence.

Now, using their word co-occurrence statistical information, any two arbitrary terms could be compared. More precisely, each term has a set of co-occurrence words in a sentence and this set with its related words, could be interpreted as a probability distribution. Therefore by comparing the probability distribution of any common word between Cand and Ref, the similarity of the given sentences could be measured to score each candidate sentence. In the next subsections we will see how HAL space matrix is generated and word relationships are computed using this matrix.

## 3.1 HAL Space Matrix

HAL is a model of semantic space for deriving word co-occurrence relationships (word co-occurrence statistical information). HAL space has been developed to extract LCI of the words appearing in a text. The calculation of HAL space is based on a $n \times n$ matrix where $n$ is the number of distinct words in the text. A sliding tunable-fixed-length window is used to fill this matrix. As this window moves across the text, an accumulated co-occurrence matrix is produced for all distinct words appearing in the text from a certain vocabulary.

The main approach to produce HAL space matrix of a text is direction sensitive. It means that the co-occurrence information produced for a specific word in its row is related to the words occurring before it in some windows. The co-occurrence information produced in its column is also related to the words occurring after it. However, it does not need to account word order to extract word relationship in our method. Instead, we consider different word orders with different scores according to their distance, which explain in Section 4.1. An example to show HAL space matrix produced for the sentence "*I read the best book of the world*" using a 4-sized sliding window is presented in Table 1. Note that, we consider distinct words in this matrix.

**Table 1.** HAL space matrix for the sentence "*I read the best book of the world*" using a 4-sized window

|        | I | read | the | best | book | of | world |
|--------|---|------|-----|------|------|----|-------|
| I      |   |      |     |      |      |    |       |
| read   | 4 |      |     |      |      |    |       |
| the    | 3 | 4    | 1   | 2    | 3    | 4  |       |
| best   | 2 | 3    | 4   |      |      |    |       |
| book   | 1 | 2    | 3   | 4    |      |    |       |
| of     |   | 1    | 2   | 3    | 4    |    |       |
| world  |   |      | 4   | 1    | 2    | 3  |       |

This is how HAL matrix is generated: suppose we want to compute value of the cell in the row of "*read*" and the column of "*I*" in Table 1. Before the HAL's window begins to move, it contains "*I*" (now the length of the window is considered 0). At the first step, the window moves for the first time and the word "*read*" enters the window. Now, the window contains two words, "*I*" and "*read*" (the length of the window is 1). This process is continued as long as the window contains the next four (due to the size of the window which is 4) words after "*I*". In this step the word "*I*" goes out and the word "*of*" enters. So, "*read*" appears four times (or in four steps) after "*I*" and the value of the cell related to row of "*read*" and column of "*I*" is 4. Table 2 presents the first five steps to compute the value of this cell in more detail.

**Table 2.** The first four steps to compute the value of the cell in the row of "*read*" and the column of "*I*" in Table 1 using a 4-sized window

| step | content of the window | value |
|------|----------------------|-------|
| initial | I | 0 |
| 1 | I, read | 1 |
| 2 | I, read, the | 2 |
| 3 | I, read, the , best | 3 |
| 4 | I, read, the, best, book | 4 |
| 5 | read, the, best, book, of | 4 |

During this process the values of all the cells are computed and finally the HAL matrix is generated for a given sentence. Note that the cells with value of 0 are left blank in this matrix.

### 3.2 Word Relationship

Using HAL space matrix the conditional probability of a word $t_j$ can be computed by normalizing HAL vector by the sum of all dimension weights:

$$P(t_i|t_j) = \frac{HAL(t_i|t_j)}{\sum_k HAL(t_k|t_j)} \qquad (1)$$

Where $HAL(t_i|t_j)$ is the sum of the weights of $t_i$ in the row related to $t_j$ and the weight of $t_i$ in the column related to $t_j$. For example the conditional probability of $P(best|book)$ obtained from our simple example is computed easily using Equation (1) as follows: $P(best|book) = \frac{4}{1+2+3+4+3+4+2} \approx 0.21$. This probability demonstrates the degree of relationship between "*best*" and "*book*".

## 4    ELEXR

We believe that, if the lexical relationships obtained from Cand are similar to those obtained from Ref for the words held in common, they are probably similar in words appearing in the sentence and word order. The main steps done by ELEXR to score a Cand against its corresponding Ref are explained in the next three subsections.

## 4.1   Modified HAL Space Computations

In order to compute word relationships more accurately, we modify HAL space computation. In fact, because the strength of the association between two words is inversely proportional to their distance, we increment the value of a cell related to two co-occurred words of $t_i$ and $t_j$ using $Inc_{t_i,t_j}$, which is defined as follows:

$$Inc_{t_i,t_j} = \frac{1}{distance(t_i, t_j)} \tag{2}$$

Where $distance(t_i, t_j)$ refers to the number of words placed between $t_i$ and $t_j$ plus one. Thus, in Table 2 in the second step when "*the*" appears for the first time in the window, the value of $HAL(the|I)$ is incremented by 0.5 instead of 1, due to their distance ($Inc_{I,the} = \frac{1}{distance(I,the)} = \frac{1}{2} = 0.5$). Equation (2) is somehow inspired by reciprocal rank in which the relevant result is scored based on its position in the results.

## 4.2   Generating and Comparing Conditional Probability Distributions

Using Equation (1), ELEXR generates all conditional probabilities related to Ref and Cand. These probabilities make a probability distribution for each word appearing in Ref and Cand. Now, we use KL-divergence to compare conditional probability distribution of the words held in common by Ref and Cand using the following equation, which computes total KL-divergence score:

$$D_{KL}(P\|Q) = \sum_{t_j \in C} \sum_{t_i \in Ref} P(t_i|t_j) \log \frac{P(t_i|t_j)}{Q(t_i|t_j)} \tag{3}$$

Where $C$ refers to the set of terms held in common by Ref and Cand. For each term $t_j$, we consider only those words that co-occurr with it in $P$, where $P$ and $Q$ are the conditional probability distributions of $t_j$ in Ref and Cand respectively. Thus, it is not required to smooth $P$ values. But it is possible that no words are held in common between Ref and Cand. In such a case, the words that are not in common with Ref, are added to Cand and additive smoothing (add-$\delta$) is used to estimate $Q(t_i|t_j)$. We have used Equation (4) to smooth $Q(t_i|t_j)$.

$$Q'(t_i|t_j) = \frac{Q(t_i|t_j) + \delta}{1 + n \times \delta} \tag{4}$$

Where $n$ refers to the total number of the words that appear in Cand plus the number of uncommon words added to Cand. The smoothing parameter $\delta$, is tuned using a data set containing more than 1000 sentences.

## 4.3   Sentence and System Scoring

In this step, first we compute *Norm*, the arithmetic average number of unmatched words in Ref and Cand normalized by their length (LEN) which is defined as follows:

$$Norm = \frac{\left(\frac{unm_{Ref}}{Ref_{LEN}} + \frac{unm_{Cand}}{Cand_{LEN}}\right)}{2} \tag{5}$$

Where $Ref_{LEN}$ and $Cand_{LEN}$ refer to the number of the words appearing in Ref and Cand. $unm_{Ref}$ and $unm_{Cand}$ also refer to the number of unmatched words in Ref and Cand respectively. When all of the quantities are computed, we divide $D_{KL}(P\|Q)$ by the total number of common words in Ref and Cand to compute $D_{Avg}$, the arithmetic average of total KL-divergence obtained using Equation (3). Actually, $Norm$ is a coefficient to increase or decrease the impact of $D_{Avg}$. Then, we use the following formula to score each Cand against its corresponding Ref:

$$score(Cand|Ref) = D_{Avg} \times Norm \tag{6}$$

The *score*, which is considered as a sentence-level score, theoretically is a value ranging from 0 to positive infinity, for the same sentences and completely different sentences respectively. However, in practice and in our experiments there are no scores more than 1000. Finally, for a given set of Cands (MT outputs) and their corresponding Refs, ELEXR scores each Cand and the final score (system-level score) over all sentences is computed by means of the following equation as the system score (The lower the score, the better MT system is):

$$ELEXR = \frac{\sum_{All(Cand,Ref)} score(Cand|Ref)}{N} \tag{7}$$

Where $N$ refers to the total number of translations and $(Cand|Ref)$ is a pair of one Cand and its corresponding Ref.

## 5    Experiments

We used data from the last two years (2011 and 2012) of WMT shared task, where there are five source languages in the submissions, French (FR), Spanish (ES), German (DE), English (EN) and Czech (CZ). Some statistics about the submissions of WMT 2011 and 2012 are presented in Table 3.

We used submissions of WMT 2012 to tune the window size of HAL space matrix for each of the eight language pairs based on Spearman's rho correlation coefficient with human judgments. Fig. 1 demonstrates detailed results for six language pairs including CZ-EN, DE-EN, EN-CZ, EN-FR, ES-EN and FR-EN. For each language pairs, we have investigated the effect of different window sizes on the Spearman's rho correlation coefficient and selected the window size corresponding to the best result. Two other language pairs have different scales and could not be shown well in this Figure. According to Fig. 1, the most improvement appears for the window sizes of less than 6 and after that there are not a significant changes in the Spearman's rho correlation coefficient. This phenomenon is related to the average length of sentences. In other words, windows with size greater than 6 almost contain all terms of the sentence and increasing the size of the window does not improve performance.

**Table 3.** Some statistics about eight language pairs and the number of systems participating in WMT 2011 and 2012 [4, 5]

| Language Pair | # System-2011 | # System-2012 |
|:---:|:---:|:---:|
| CZ-EN | 8 | 6 |
| EN-CZ | 10 | 13 |
| DE-EN | 20 | 16 |
| EN-DE | 22 | 15 |
| ES-EN | 15 | 12 |
| EN-ES | 15 | 11 |
| FR-EN | 18 | 15 |
| EN-FR | 17 | 15 |
| overall | 125 | 103 |

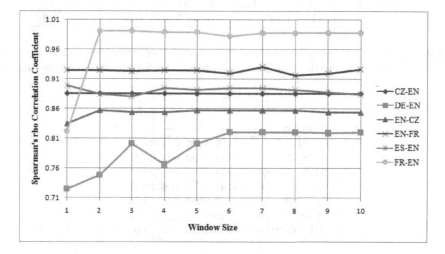

**Fig. 1.** Effect of the window size on Spearman's rho correlation coefficient

Submissions of WMT 2011 are used to evaluate the performance of ELEXR. For each language pair, we measured the correlation with human judgments based on three correlation coefficients: Spearman's rho, Kendall's tau and Pearson's r. We use BLEU and TER as our main baselines because they do not use any external resources either. These metrics also are used as two main baselines in WMT metric tasks. Table 4 shows the results of our system-level experiments for each correlation coefficient on each language pair. The last column shows the results averaged across all language pairs for each metrics. According to these results, ELEXR achieves average Spearman's rho correlation of about 0.78, Kendall's tau correlation of about 0.66 and Pearson's r correlation of about 0.84, corresponding to improvements of about 0.04, 0.07 and 0.06 respectively over BLEU, the best baseline. It means that ELEXR outperforms baselines on average at system-level correlation with human judgments.

**Table 4.** Absolute values of system-level Spearman's rho, Kendall's tau and Pearson's r correlation coefficients of the automatic evaluation metrics with the human judgments for all language pairs

|  | Metric | EN-CZ | EN-DE | EN-ES | EN-FR | CZ-EN | DE-EN | ES-EN | FR-EN | Average |
|---|---|---|---|---|---|---|---|---|---|---|
| | ELEXR | 0.58 | 0.43 | **0.91** | **0.89** | **0.98** | **0.67** | **0.96** | 0.84 | **0.78** |
| Spearman's rho | BLEU | **0.65** | **0.44** | 0.87 | 0.86 | 0.88 | 0.48 | 0.9 | **0.85** | 0.74 |
| | TER | 0.50 | 0.12 | 0.81 | 0.84 | 0.83 | 0.33 | 0.89 | 0.77 | 0.64 |
| | ELEXR | 0.47 | 0.32 | **0.75** | **0.75** | **0.93** | **0.52** | **0.85** | 0.65 | **0.66** |
| Kendall's tao | BLEU | **0.51** | **0.34** | 0.71 | 0.66 | 0.71 | 0.37 | 0.71 | **0.67** | 0.59 |
| | TER | 0.33 | 0.12 | 0.64 | 0.71 | 0.71 | 0.27 | 0.73 | 0.56 | 0.35 |
| | ELEXR | **0.70** | **0.63** | **0.91** | 0.94 | **0.97** | **0.71** | **0.99** | **0.90** | **0.84** |
| Pearson's r | BLEU | 0.63 | 0.62 | 0.86 | 0.93 | 0.89 | 0.46 | 0.95 | 0.89 | 0.78 |
| | TER | 0.45 | 0.21 | 0.84 | **0.95** | 0.79 | 0.23 | 0.78 | 0.75 | 0.62 |

**Table 5.** Absolute values of system-level Spearman's rho correlation coefficients of the automatic evaluation metrics with the human judgments for translation out of English

| Metric | EN-CZ | EN-DE | EN-ES | EN-FR | Average |
|---|---|---|---|---|---|
| TESLA-M | - | **0.90** | **0.95** | **0.96** | **0.94** |
| TESLA-B | - | 0.81 | 0.90 | 0.91 | 0.87 |
| MPF | **0.72** | 0.61 | 0.87 | 0.89 | 0.78 |
| ROSE | 0.65 | 0.41 | 0.90 | 0.86 | 0.71 |
| ELEXR | 0.58 | 0.43 | 0.91 | 0.89 | 0.70 |
| AMBER | 0.56 | 0.53 | 0.87 | 0.84 | 0.70 |
| METEOR | 0.65 | 0.3 | 0.74 | 0.85 | 0.63 |

Although the proposed metric should be compared with other metrics which do not require more resources, to compare our metric with some other metrics reported in the results of WMT 2011, we have also used other metrics including the best ones as additional baselines, considering translation both to and from English separately. We only used Spearman's correlation coefficients which are reported officially in the results of WMT 2011. Note that, some of these metrics use external language resources, so, this comparison is not really fair. Table 5, shows the result of this experiment for translation out of English including metrics such as TESLA-M, TESLA-B, MPF, ROSE, AMBER and METEOR. Table 6, also shows the result of the same experiment for translation into English including metrics such as MTERATER-PLUS [26], TINE-SRL-MATCH [16], TESLA-F, TESLA-B [13], ROSE and AMBER.

To show that the variance of the ELEXR scores and the difference in ELEXR metric is reliable, we have set up another experiment. In this experiment system submissions of WMT 2011 are used as our test sets. First, one system was selected

**Table 6.** Absolute values of system-level Spearman's rho correlation coefficients of the automatic evaluation metrics with the human judgments for translation into English

| Metric | CZ-EN | DE-EN | ES-EN | FR-EN | Average |
|---|---|---|---|---|---|
| MTERATER-PLUS | 0.95 | **0.90** | 0.91 | 0.93 | **0.92** |
| TESLA-B | **0.98** | 0.88 | 0.91 | 0.91 | **0.92** |
| TESLA-F | 0.95 | 0.79 | **0.96** | 0.90 | 0.90 |
| TINE-SRL-MATCH | 0.95 | 0.69 | 0.95 | 0.87 | 0.87 |
| ELEXR | **0.98** | 0.67 | **0.96** | 0.84 | 0.86 |
| AMBER | 0.88 | 0.59 | 0.86 | **0.95** | 0.82 |
| ROSE | 0.88 | 0.48 | 0.90 | 0.85 | 0.78 |

**Table 7.** The standard deviation and paired t-statistics for 80 blocks

| System name | online-A (EN-ES) | jhu (EN-FR) | systran (FR-EN) | jhu (DE-EN) | upm (ES-EN) | cst (CZ-EN) | udein (EN-DE) | cu-zeman (EN-CZ) |
|---|---|---|---|---|---|---|---|---|
| ELEXR | 148.376 | 163.145 | 180.626 | 211.297 | 231.056 | 273.043 | 286.440 | 337.693 |
| Stdev | 63.363 | 68.348 | 64.916 | 49.739 | 71.127 | 66.005 | 58.737 | 66.868 |
| t | - | 2.753 | 4.800 | 5.379 | 3.067 | 5.328 | 1.724 | 5.482 |

from each language pair randomly. These eight systems were sorted based on their ELEXR scores to present an order of the systems from the worst to the best. Then, we divided sentences of each system into blocks of 25 sentences each. Finally, ELEXR scored each block separately and the variance and paired t-statistics are computed. Each system is compared by the t-statistic with its left system in the ELEXR order. The results of this experiment are presented in Table 7. As shown in Table 7, all t-statistics are above of 1.7 and since a paired t-statistic of 1.7 or above is 95% significant, thus, the differences between the systems scores are statistically very significant and accordingly reliable. The same experiments are performed separately for all language pairs and all systems and similar results are obtained, however due to space limitations they have been omitted.

# 6 Conclusion

In this paper we proposed ELEXR, a novel metric for automatic evaluation of machine translation. ELEXR is a language independent metric that uses only one reference translation without incorporating any external resources like WordNet.

We showed that ELEXR outperforms AMBER, BLEU, METEOR, ROSE and TER in term of system-level correlation with human judgments on average. Also, we showed that ELEXR scores and the differences between the system-level scores are statistically very significant and accordingly reliable.

# References

1. Lund, K., Burgess, C.: Producing high-dimensional semantic spaces from lexical co-occurrence. Behavior Research Methods 28, 203–208 (1996)
2. Kullback, S., Leibler, R.A.: On information and sufficiency. The Annals of Mathematical Statistics 22, 79–86 (1951)
3. Callison-Burch, C., Koehn, P., Monz, C., Peterson, K., Przybocki, M., Zaidan, O.F.: Findings of the 2010 joint workshop on statistical machine translation and metrics for machine translation. In: Proceedings of the Joint Fifth Workshop on Statistical Machine Translation and Metrics MATR, pp. 17–53. Association for Computational Linguistics (2010)
4. Callison-Burch, C., Koehn, P., Monz, C., Zaidan, O.F.: Findings of the 2011 workshop on statistical machine translation. In: Proceedings of the Sixth Workshop on Statistical Machine Translation, pp. 22–64. Association for Computational Linguistics (2011)
5. Callison-Burch, C., Koehn, P., Monz, C., Post, M., Soricut, R., Specia, L.: Findings of the 2012 workshop on statistical machine translation. In: Proceedings of the Seventh Workshop on Statistical Machine Translation. Association for Computational Linguistics (2012)
6. Papineni, K., Roukos, S., Ward, T., Zhu, W.J.: Bleu: a method for automatic evaluation of machine translation. In: Proceedings of the 40th Annual Meeting on Association for Computational Linguistics, pp. 311–318. Association for Computational Linguistics (2002)
7. Agarwal, A., Lavie, A.: Meteor, m-bleu and m-ter: Evaluation metrics for high-correlation with human rankings of machine translation output. In: Proceedings of the Third Workshop on Statistical Machine Translation, pp. 115–118. Association for Computational Linguistics (2008)
8. Chen, B., Kuhn, R.: Amber: A modified bleu, enhanced ranking metric. In: Proceedings of the 6th Workshop on Statistical Machine Translation, pp. 71–77 (2011)
9. Chen, B., Kuhn, R., Foster, G.: Improving amber, an mt evaluation metric. In: NAACL 2012 Workshop on Statistical Machine Translation (WMT 2012), pp. 59–63 (2012)
10. Chen, B., Kuhn, R., Larkin, S.: Port: a precision-order-recall mt evaluation metric for tuning. In: Proceedings of the 50th Annual Meeting of the Association for Computational Linguistics (ACL 2012) (2012)
11. Banerjee, S., Lavie, A.: Meteor: An automatic metric for mt evaluation with improved correlation with human judgments. In: Proceedings of the ACL Workshop on Intrinsic and Extrinsic Evaluation Measures for Machine Translation and/or Summarization, pp. 65–72 (2005)
12. Lavie, A., Denkowski, M.J.: The meteor metric for automatic evaluation of machine translation. Machine Translation 23, 105–115 (2009)
13. Dahlmeier, D., Liu, C., Ng, H.T.: Tesla at wmt 2011: Translation evaluation and tunable metric. In: Proceedings of the Sixth Workshop on Statistical Machine Translation, pp. 78–84. Association for Computational Linguistics (2011)

14. Song, X., Cohn, T.: Regression and ranking based optimisation for sentence level machine translation evaluation. In: Proceedings of the Sixth Workshop on Statistical Machine Translation, pp. 123–129. Association for Computational Linguistics (2011)

15. Popović, M.: Morphemes and pos tags for n-gram based evaluation metrics. In: Proceedings of the Sixth Workshop on Statistical Machine Translation, pp. 104–107. Association for Computational Linguistics (2011)

16. Rios, M., Aziz, W., Specia, L.: Tine: A metric to assess mt adequacy. In: Proceedings of the Sixth Workshop on Statistical Machine Translation, pp. 116–122. Association for Computational Linguistics (2011)

17. Snover, M., Dorr, B., Schwartz, R., Micciulla, L., Makhoul, J.: A study of translation edit rate with targeted human annotation. In: Proceedings of Association for Machine Translation in the Americas, pp. 223–231 (2006)

18. Snover, M., Madnani, N., Dorr, B., Schwartz, R.: Fluency, adequacy, or hter? exploring different human judgments with a tunable mt metric. In: Proceedings of the Fourth Workshop on Statistical Machine Translation, vol. 30, pp. 259–268. Association for Computational Linguistics (2009)

19. Nieen, S., Och, F.J., Leusch, G., Ney, H.: An evaluation tool for machine translation: Fast evaluation for mt research. In: Proceedings of the 2nd International Conference on Language Resources and Evaluation, pp. 39–45 (2000)

20. Leusch, G., Ueffing, N., Ney, H.: Cder: Efficient mt evaluation using block movements. In: Proceedings of the Thirteenth Conference of the European Chapter of the Association for Computational Linguistics, pp. 241–248 (2006)

21. Tillmann, C., Vogel, S., Ney, H., Zubiaga, A., Sawaf, H.: Accelerated dp based search for statistical translation. In: European Conf. on Speech Communication and Technology, pp. 2667–2670 (1997)

22. Wang, M., Manning, C.D.: Spede: Probabilistic edit distance metrics for mt evaluation. In: Proceedings of WMT (2012)

23. Kahn, J.G., Snover, M., Ostendorf, M.: Expected dependency pair match: predicting translation quality with expected syntactic structure. Machine Translation 23, 169–179 (2009)

24. Wong, B., Kit, C.: Atec: automatic evaluation of machine translation via word choice and word order. Machine Translation 23, 141–155 (2009)

25. Popović, M., Vilar, D., Avramidis, E., Burchardt, A.: Evaluation without references: Ibm1 scores as evaluation metrics. In: Proceedings of the Sixth Workshop on Statistical Machine Translation, pp. 99–103. Association for Computational Linguistics (2011)

26. Parton, K., Tetreault, J., Madnani, N., Chodorow, M.: E-rating machine translation. In: Proceedings of the Sixth Workshop on Statistical Machine Translation, pp. 108–115. Association for Computational Linguistics (2011)

# Modeling Persian Verb Morphology to Improve English-Persian Machine Translation

Alireza Mahmoudi, Heshaam Faili, and Mohsen Arabsorkhi

School of Electrical and Computer Engineering,
College of Engineering,
University of Tehran, Tehran, Iran
{ali.mahmoudi,hfaili}@ut.ac.ir, marabsorkhi@ece.ut.ac.ir

**Abstract.** Morphological analysis is an essential process in translating from a morphologically poor language such as English into a morphologically rich language such as Persian. In this paper, first we analyze the output of a rule-based machine translation (RBMT) and categorize its errors. After that, we use a statistical approach to rich morphology prediction using a parallel corpus to improve the quality of RBMT. The results of error analysis show that Persian morphology comes with many challenges especially in the verb conjugation. In our approach, we define a set of linguistic features using both English and Persian linguistic information obtained from an English-Persian parallel corpus, and make our model. In our experiments, we generate inflected verb form with the most common feature values as a baseline. The results of our experiments show an improvement of almost 2.6% absolute BLEU score on a test set containing 16 K sentences.

**Keywords:** Morphology, Machine Translation, Persian Verb Morphology, SMT, Rule-based MT, Parallel Corpus, Decision Tree.

## 1 Introduction

Translation from or into a morphologically rich language, where a word stem appears in many completely different surface forms, deals with many challenges. "The sensitivity to data sparseness" is known as one of the main limitations of statistical machine translation (SMT). Generally, SMT uses word-based or phrased-based approach [1], and though a target side word form has been seen in the train data, translation model is not able to translate corresponding source side word to a correct one in a different situation. This problem becomes severe in translation of verbs, where by changing some of the sentence components such as the subject of a verb, the verb form accordingly changes. This problem can be partially overcome in a rule-based machine translation (RBMT) using a large number of rules and states. But the number of these rules and their corresponding complexity are related directly to the morphologically richness of the language [2]. So, morphological analysis is an important process in translating from or into such languages, because it reduces the sparseness of the model.

In this paper, we select a rule-based English-Persian machine translation as a baseline for our approach. First, we analyze the output of this RBMT to

F. Castro, A. Gelbukh, and M. González (Eds.): MICAI 2013, Part I, LNAI 8265, pp. 406–418, 2013.

categorize errors. Based on the results of our error analysis, verb conjugation has been found as the most important and problematic phenomenon in the context of MT. Also, the verbs are known as a highly inflecting class of words and an important part of morphological processing in Persian. So, in this paper we focus on the verb to improve English-Persian RBMT. In other words, we use a novel approach to statistically rich morphology prediction for Persian verbs and compare this technique with rule-based ones. We predict morphological features of the verb using statistical model incorporating decision tree classifier (DTC) [3], which is an approach to multistage decision making. In order to train DTC, we use an English-Persian parallel corpus, which contains linguistic information such as syntactic parse tree and dependency relations on English side, as well as linguistic information to generate an appropriate inflected Persian verb on Persian side. Morphological features which we predict and use to generate the inflected form of a verb are voice (VOC), mood (MOD), number (NUM), tense (TEN), negation (NEG) and person (PER).

The reminder of the paper is organized as follows: in Section 2 we describe related works; Section 3 briefly reviews some challenges in the translation of English to Persian and Persian verb conjugation; Section 4 presents rule-based morphology generation, the baseline, and our proposed approach to statistically generate rich morphology; in Section 5 our experiments and the results are presented; and finally, in Section 6 we cover conclusions and future work.

## 2    Related Work

Modeling rich morphology in machine translations has received a lot of research interest in several studies. In this section we review the main efforts which are morphologically trying to improve MT. The main approach used in SMT model is based on factored models, an extension of phrased-based SMT model [4]. Morphology generation in this approach focuses on words instead of phrases (which is known as a limitation for this approach). In other words, each word is annotated using morphology tags on morphologically rich side and the model is trained to generate morphology. A similar approach is used in [5] to translate from English into Greek and Czech languages. They especially focus on noun cases and verb persons. Mapping from syntax to morphology in factored model is used in [6] to improve English-Turkish SMT. Hierarchical phrase-based translation, an extension of factored translation model, proposed in [7] to generate complex morphology using a discriminative model for Czech as the target language.

Segmentation is another approach that improves MT by reducing the data sparseness of translation model and increasing the similarity between two sides [8–10]. This method analyzes morphologically rich side and unpacks inflected word forms into simpler components. In [8] it is shown that modifying Czech as the input language using 'pseudowords' improves the Czech-English machine translation system. Similar approaches are used in [10] for English to Turkish SMT, in [9] for translating from English into Finnish and in [11] to improve Persian-English SMT.

Maximum entropy model is another approach used in [12] for English-Arabic and English-Russian MT. They proposed a post-processing probabilistic framework for morphology generation utilizing a rich set of morphological knowledge sources. There are some similar approaches used in [13] for Arabic and Russian as the target languages and in [14] for English-Finnish SMT. In these approaches, the model of morphology prediction is an independent process of the SMT system.

Recently, a novel approach to generate rich morphology is proposed in [15]. They use SMT to generate inflected Arabic tokens from a given sequence of lemmas and any subset of morphological features. They also have used their proposed method to model rich morphology in SMT [15, 16]. Since we use lemma with the most common feature values as our baseline, the results of their experiments is somewhat comparable to ours. However, they use only lemma with no prediction as their baseline. So, our baseline is more stringent than the baseline used in [15].

Our work is conceptually similar to that of [17], in which they incorporate a morphological classifier for Spanish verbs and define a collection of context dependent linguistic features (CDLFs), and predict each morphology feature such as PER or NUM. However, we use a different set of CDLFs and incorporate DTC to predict the morphology features of the Persian verbs.

## 3    Persian Challenges

Persian language is known as a highly inflected and morphologically rich language. So, translating from a morphologically poor language such as English into such a language is not a trivial task. In this language, in translation process, for example, there are some words that are produced by combining more than one word in the source. Hence, for such a translation becomes more complex. This complexity makes many problems and errors that affect directly the quality of MT output. To investigate the errors and the importance of each, we have selected 1000 sentences from the output of an English-Persian RBMT. These sentences have been analyzed and corresponding errors have been classified as suggested in [18]. In the next subsection, we will discuss our MT error analysis and the results in more details to show the most prominent source of errors.

### 3.1    Error Analysis

In order to investigate the errors appearing in an English-Persian RBMT, we have selected 1000 sentences randomly from our RBMT output. In [18] the MT errors are classified into five types: Missing Words, Word Order, Incorrect Words, Unknown Words and Punctuations. According to these error types, each sentence has been checked separately and all errors within it have been detected (finally, 5223 errors have been detected). Table 1 shows error types and sub-types and the results of this experiment. As indicated in Table 1, the most problematic error type is the use of incorrect form which is known as the widest category of

**Table 1.** Error statistics of our RBMT which is selected as the baseline

| Error types | Error sub-types | | Count | E to P % |
|---|---|---|---|---|
| Missing words | | | 548 | 10.50 |
| | | content words | 203 | 3.89 |
| | | filler words | 345 | 6.61 |
| Word order | | | 563 | 10.78 |
| | | Word local range | 150 | 2.88 |
| | | Word long range | 285 | 5.46 |
| | | Phrase local range | 31 | 0.59 |
| | | Phrase long range | 97 | 1.86 |
| Incorrect words | | | **3877** | **74.23** |
| | sense | | 833 | 15.95 |
| | | word lexical choice | 472 | 9.04 |
| | | disambiguation | 361 | 6.91 |
| | incorrect form | | 1110 | 21.25 |
| | extra words | | 285 | 5.46 |
| | Style | | 1065 | 20.39 |
| | idioms | | 584 | 11.18 |
| Unknown words | | | 133 | 2.55 |
| | unknown stems | | 121 | 2.32 |
| | unseen forms | | 12 | 0.23 |
| Punctuations | | | 102 | 1.95 |

error. This error refers to that one, when MT cannot find a correct or at least an appropriate translation for a given word. In fact, this type of error is related to a bad use of cases such as person, tense, gender, number etc. in output. In Persian, these cases mostly appear in building of a verbs and nouns (including pronoun), however the latter case is in minority. This issue reveals that verbs have an important role in translation quality, if a MT can provide correct form of a given verb in the output by using correct person, tense, number, voice, mood and negation. Based on this, we have decided to focus on the verb as an important linguistic structure in Persian. By selecting the verb as the goal of this research, another important challenge appears, Persian verb morphology. This problem is investigated in the next subsection.

## 3.2 Persian Verb Morphology

The verb in Persian has a complex inflectional system [19]. This complexity appears in the following aspects: Different verb forms, Different verb stems, Affixes marking inflections and Auxiliaries used in certain tenses.

*Simple* form and *compound* form are two forms used in Persian verbal system. Simple form is broken into two categories according to the stem used in its formation. Two stems used to construct a verb are the followings: the present stem and the past stem. Each of which is used in creating of specific tenses.

**Table 2.** Inflections and morphological features of ن + می + فروش + یم /n+my+frvŝ+ym (we are not selling) and است + شده + ه + فروخت /frvxt+h+ŝdh+ast (it has been sold)

| feature | nmyfrvŝym | frvxth ŝdh ast |
|---|---|---|
| verb form | simple | compound |
| stem | frvŝ(present) | frvxt(past) |
| prefix | n, my | - |
| suffix | ym | h |
| auxiliary | - | ŝdh, ast |
| VOC | active | passive |
| ASP | subjunctive | indicative |
| NUM | plural | singular |
| TEN | simple present | present perfect |
| NEG | negative | positive |
| PER | first | third |

**Table 3.** Morphological features of the verb and their corresponding values

| Feature | Values |
|---|---|
| VOC | active, passive |
| ASP | imperative, subjunctive, indicative |
| NUM | singular, plural |
| TEN | simplepast, pastperfect, future, simplepresent, presentperfect, progressivepast, progressivepresentperfect |
| NEG | negative, positive |
| PER | p1,p2,p3 |

We cannot derive the two stems from each other due to different surface forms they usually have. Therefore, they treated as distinct characteristics of verb [19].

Compound form refers to those that require an auxiliary to form a correct verb. Several affixes are combined with stems to mark MOD, NUM, NEG and PER inflections. Auxiliaries are used to make a compound form in certain tenses to indicate VOC and TEN inflections, similar to "HAVE" and "BE" in English. Two examples are given in Table 2 for نمیفروشیم /nmyfrvŝym[1] /nemiforushim (we are not selling) and فروخته شده است /frvxth ŝdh ast/ forukhte shode ast (it has been sold), which both of them have the same infinitive form.

## 4   Approach

In this section we will discuss two techniques to generate inflected verb form. The first one is based on a rule-based approach in which a lot of linguistic

---

[1] The short vowels such as *o, a, e* are not generally transcribed in Persian.

rules are written to detect six morphological features of the verb using linguistic information obtained from the source side. In the second approach which is the propose of this paper, we introduce a statistical approach to rich morphology generation. As stated above, morphological features of the verb are VOC, MOD, NUM, TEN, NEG and PER respectively, which we predict and use to generate the inflected form of the verb. Table 3 reports all feature values. At the end of this section these two techniques are compared and the results are presented.

## 4.1 Rule-Based Morphology Generation

In this approach for a given English sentence (source side) Stanford Parser [20] is used to produce syntactic parse tree of a sentence, dependency relationships and part of speech tag (POS) of each word within the sentence. A verb is detected using its POS and the value of a specific feature is detected using corresponding dependencies. For example if a verb has a dependency relationship with "will" the feature value of TEN is "future"[2].

As another example, if a verb has a dependency relationship called "subj with a word such as "I the feature value of the PER is "p1 and the feature value of the NUM is "singular. However there are a lot of situations in which no rules can be found to detect a feature value for a specific morphological feature. For example, in an imperative sentence there is no way to detect any feature value for NUM (singular? or plural?). These cases could be handled using the context of the text which the given sentence is known as a part of it. But in a translation task, a sentence is treated solely without considering surrounding sentence or corresponding context. In these cases, we have defined a default value for each feature. These values are the following:

- VOC: active
- ASP: indicative
- NUM: singular
- TEN: simplepast
- NEG: positive
- PER: p3

After detecting six morphological features of a given verb, we can generate a verb form using a finite state automaton (FSA) [19]. This FSA has more than 500 states (however there are final states that are not reachable) and uses the values of VOC, ASP, TEN, NEG, NUM and PER respectively to generate an inflected verb form using coresponding lemma. We consider this technique (generating an inflected verb form using a rule-based approach) as one of the baseline for our statistical method.

## 4.2 Statistical Morphology Generation

Our proposed approach is broken into two main steps: DTC training and Morphology prediction. These steps will be described more precisely bellow.

---

[2] Due to space constraints and a large number of the rules, our sets of rules are omitted.

**Table 4.** Some statistics about English-Persian parallel corpus [21]

|  | English | Persian |
|---|---|---|
| # Sentences | 399,000 | 399,000 |
| # Tokens | 6,528,241 | 6,074,550 |
| # Unique tokens | 65,123 | 101,114 |
| # Stems | 40,261 | 91,329 |

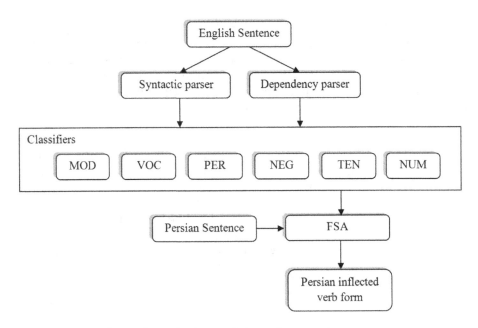

**Fig. 1.** General schema of the verb generation process

**DTC Training.** To make train and test sets, we used an English-Persian parallel corpus [21] containing 399 K sentences (367 K to train, 16 K to validate and 16 K to test). More details about this corpus, which is used by [21] to build an SMT, are presented in Table 4. Giza++ [22] was used to word alignment. Among all alignments assigned to each verb, we have only selected such an alignment with a high probability to translate both from English to Persian and Persian to English. With this heuristic we ignore a lot of alignments to produce a high quality data set. We have selected 100 sentences randomly and evaluated the alignments manually, so that 27% recall and 93% precision were obtained.

Then, we define a set of syntactic features on English side as DTC learning features. These features consist of several language-specific features such as POS of the verb, dependency relationships of the verb and POS of subject of the verb. English side is parsed using Stanford Parser [20]. Then, we can produce training data set by analyzing Persian verb aligned to each English verb using [23], in which two unsupervised learning methods have been proposed to

**Table 5.** CCR (%) of six DTCs and corresponding improvements

| Features | Baseline | Rule-Based | Prediction | Improvement |
|----------|----------|------------|------------|-------------|
| ASP | 78.26 | 80.99 | **91.44** | 10.45 |
| NUM | 69.07 | 79.19 | **86.86** | 7.67 |
| VOC | 86.23 | 86.39 | **88.38** | 1.99 |
| TEN | 46.53 | 67.8 | **79.83** | **12.03** |
| PER | 51.62 | 94.78 | **97.93** | 3.15 |
| NEG | 83.21 | 97.81 | **97.94** | 0.13 |

identify compound verbs with their corresponding morphological features. The first one which is extending the concept of pointwise mutual information uses a bootstrapping method and the second one uses K-means clustering algorithm to detect compound verbs. However, as we have the verb, we only use their proposed method to determine VOC, MOD, NUM, TEN, NEG and PER for a given verb as the class labels.

**Morphology Prediction.** In [13] fully inflected word form is predicted and in [14] morphemes are predicted. Unlike these approaches, we predict morphological features like that of presented in [15, 16]. Using our training data set, we build six language specific DTCs to predict each of the morphological features. Each DTC uses a subset of our feature set and predicts corresponding morphology feature independently. Then, we use a FSA to generate an inflected verb form using these six morphological features. This FSA is an extension of the FSA used by the rule-based method. Fig. 1, shows the general schema of the verb generation process.

Table 5 shows the Correct Classification Ratio (CCR) of each DTC learned on our train data containing 178782 entries and evaluated on a test set containing more than 20 K verbs. The most common feature value is used as a baseline for rule-based and statistical approaches, for each classifier. The most improvement is achieved in the prediction of PER in comparison with this baseline. Others have high CCR but they also have high baselines. In comparison with rule-based morphology generation our statistical approach performs better and the CCRs in Table 5 show improvement in all cases, which the best one is related to TEN.

# 5 Experiments

In this section, we present our experiments and the results on a test set containing 16K sentences selected from an English-Persian parallel corpus. As the first goals of our experiments, we are interested in knowing the effectiveness of our approach to rich morphology prediction and the contribution each feature has. To do so, like [12] and [15], where use aligned sentence pair of reference translations instead of the output of an MT system as input (reference experiments), we also perform reference experiments because they are golden in terms of word order, lemma choice and morphological features. Table 6 shows the detailed n-gram BLEU [24]

**Table 6.** Morphology generation results in our reference experiments using gold Persian lemma plus different set of gold morphological features. When we add a feature to the previous feature set we use "++" notation. RB refers to the results of verb generation using the rule-based approach.

| Generation Input | BLEU-1 | BLEU-2 | BLEU-3 | BLEU-4 | BLEU | TER |
|---|---|---|---|---|---|---|
| Baseline | 96.8 | 93.4 | 91.7 | 89.9 | 91.46 | 0.0473 |
| RB Baseline | 98.2 | 96.5 | 95.4 | 94.5 | 95.82 | 0.0252 |
| LEM+ASP | 96.3 | 93.0 | 91.2 | 89.4 | 91.67 | 0.0505 |
| LEM+NUM | 96.9 | 93.7 | 91.8 | 90.1 | 91.76 | 0.0407 |
| LEM+VOC | 97.1 | 94.1 | 92.3 | 90.6 | 92.25 | 0.0416 |
| LEM+TEN | 96.8 | 94.2 | 92.5 | 91.0 | 93.61 | 0.0324 |
| LEM+PER | 96.9 | 93.6 | 91.8 | 90.0 | 91.73 | 0.0447 |
| LEM+NEG | 96.9 | 93.7 | 91.8 | 90.1 | 91.76 | 0.0446 |
| LEM+ASP+NUM | 96.8 | 93.9 | 92.3 | 90.7 | 92.63 | 0.0462 |
| ++VOC | 97.1 | 94.5 | 93.0 | 91.6 | 93.31 | 0.0422 |
| ++TEN | 99.0 | 98.0 | 97.3 | 96.6 | 97.71 | 0.0099 |
| ++PER | 99.1 | 98.3 | 97.7 | 97.0 | 98.03 | 0.0086 |
| ++NEG | **99.3** | **98.5** | **98.0** | **97.4** | **98.28** | **0.0074** |

precision (for n=1,2,3,4), BLEU and TER [25] scores for morphology generation using gold lemma with the most common feature values (Baseline) and other gold morphological features and their combinations as our reference experiments.

In this experiment, we replace each sentence verb, with predicted verb generated by FSA using lemma plus the most common feature values as the baseline. In comparison with the baseline used in [15], this one is more stringent. As another baseline we use the rule-based approach, which determines morphological features of the verb grammatically and generates inflected verb form. We use each gold feature separately to investigate the contribution each feature has. Finally, we combine the gold features incrementally. Adding more features improve BLEU and TER scores. Since, there are some cases in which with the same morphological features it is possible to generate different but correct verb forms, the maximum BLEU score of 100 is hard to be reached even if we are given the gold features. So, the best results (98.28 of BLEU and 0.0074 of TER) could be considered as an upper bound for proposed approach. As indicated in Table 6, or statistical model produces a better output. It means that generation process using improved FSA performs well. Note that, these results are obtained from our reference experiments in which a reference is duplicated and on of them modified by our approach and evaluated with another one using automatic evaluation metric. In fact, there is no a real translation task here and a reference is evaluated by its modified version.

We have performed the same reference experiments on the same data using predicted features instead of gold features. Table 7 reports the results of detailed n-gram BLEU precision, BLUE and TER scores. According to the results, our approach outperforms the baseline in all configurations. The best configuration uses all predicted features and shows an improvement of about 2.6% absolute

**Table 7.** Morphology generation results in our reference experiments using gold Persian lemma plus different set of predicted morphological features. When we add a feature to the previous feature set we use "++" notation. RB refers to the results of verb generation using the rule-based approach.

| Generation Input | BLEU-1 | BLEU-2 | BLEU-3 | BLEU-4 | BLEU | TER |
|---|---|---|---|---|---|---|
| Baseline | 96.8 | 93.4 | 91.7 | 89.9 | 91.46 | 0.0473 |
| RB Baseline | 96.8 | 93.7 | 91.7 | 89.8 | 91.99 | 0.0474 |
| LEM+ASP | 96.3 | 93.0 | 91.1 | 89.2 | 91.54 | 0.0498 |
| LEM+NUM | 96.9 | 93.7 | 91.9 | 90.1 | 91.81 | 0.0443 |
| LEM+VOC | 96.8 | 93.6 | 91.8 | 90.0 | 91.86 | 0.0448 |
| LEM+TEN | 96.2 | 93.3 | 91.5 | 89.8 | 92.67 | 0.0422 |
| LEM+PER | 96.8 | 93.5 | 91.7 | 89.9 | 91.65 | 0.0451 |
| LEM+NEG | 96.9 | 93.6 | 91.8 | 90.0 | 91.71 | 0.0448 |
| LEM+ASP+NUM | 96.4 | 93.2 | 91.3 | 89.5 | 91.72 | 0.0489 |
| ++VOC | 96.4 | 93.2 | 91.3 | 89.5 | 91.91 | 0.0487 |
| ++TEN | 97.0 | 94.5 | 92.9 | 91.4 | 93.90 | 0.0350 |
| ++PER | 97.0 | 94.6 | 93.0 | 91.5 | 94.00 | 0.0345 |
| ++NEG | **97.2** | **95.0** | **93.5** | **92.0** | **94.04** | **0.0343** |

BLEU score and 0.0130% absolute TER against our first baseline. Also, in comparison with our second baseline, rule-based approach, we achieve improvements of about 2.05% absolute BLEU score and 0.0131% absolute TER.

These results indicate that our proposed approach to predict morphological features of the verb using DTC and generate inflected verb form using FSA outperforms the baselines. In order to study the performance of our statistical model in a real translation process, we have used our model as a morphological analyzer component in our RBMT that we used it as a baseline.

In this experiment the output of RBMT is evaluated using detailed n-gram BLEU precision and BLUE in two different cases: verbs have been generated using the rule-based approach and verbs have been generated using our statistical model. In both cases lemma is selected using an English-Persian dictionary. It means that unlike our reference experiments, lemma is not golden here. So, according to BLEU, our evaluation metric, in comparison with reference experiments, salient improvement will not be achieved. The output of RBMT is evaluated using two test sets which are used in [21] as test sets to evaluate their SMT. The first one contains about 2500 sentences extracted from the book "English Grammar In Use" (EGIU). This test set also has two reference sets. The latter test set contains about 400 sentences extracted from a parallel corpus (PCTS) (the corpus which we have selected to make our train data). This test set also has four reference sets. In addition, a test set containing about 800 sentences extracted from a news corpus. This test set has four reference sets. The results of this experiment are presented in Table 8. According to Table 8, our proposed approach outperforms RBMT, the baseline that generates inflected verb form using a rule-based approach, and improves the output of this RBMT

**Table 8.** Detailed n-gram BLEU precision and BLUE scores for three test sets on the RBMT

|      | Method | BLEU-1 | BLEU-2 | BLEU-3 | BLEU-4 | BLEU |
|------|--------|--------|--------|--------|--------|------|
| EGIU | Statistical | **68.2** | **35.5** | **19.7** | **11.3** | **26.63** |
|      | RBMT | 67.7 | 35.0 | 19.6 | **11.3** | 26.57 |
| NEWS | Statistical | **67.3** | **27.8** | **12.2** | **5.4** | **18.09** |
|      | RBMT | 66.9 | 27.5 | 12.0 | 5.3 | 17.93 |
| PCTS | Statistical | **61.2** | **26.5** | **11.2** | **4.8** | **17.20** |
|      | RBMT | 60.8 | 26.3 | 11.1 | 4.7 | 17.01 |

in all cases. As regards PCTS has been selected from the parallel corpus that we used to make train data, the most improvement is achieved in this case due to the same context and domain.

## 6    Conclusions

In this paper we present a supervised approach to statistically rich morphology generation that improves MT output. We focus on the verb inflections as a highly inflecting class of words in Persian. Using different combination of morphological features to generate inflected verb form, we evaluate our approach on a test set containing 16 K sentences and obtain better BLEU and TER scores compared with our baselines, morphology generation with lemma plus the most common feature values and rule-based morphology generation.

Our proposed model can be used as a component to generate rich morphology for any kind of languages and MTs. Also, our proposed approach predicts each morphological feature independently. In the future, we plan to investigate how the features affect each other to present an order in which a predicted morphological feature is used as a learning feature for the next one.

**Acknowledgment.** This work has been partially funded by Iran Telecom Research Center (ITRC) under contract number 9513/500.

## References

1. Koehn, P., Och, F.J., Marcu, D.: Statistical phrase-based translation. In: Proceedings of the 2003 Conference of the North American Chapter of the Association for Computational Linguistics on Human Language Technology, vol. 1, pp. 48–54. Association for Computational Linguistics (2003)
2. Somers, H.: Review article: Example-based machine translation. Machine Translation 14, 113–157 (1999)
3. Quinlan, J.R.: Induction of decision trees. Machine Learning 1, 81–106 (1986)
4. Koehn, P., Hoang, H.: Factored translation models. In: Proceedings of the 2007 Joint Conference on Empirical Methods in Natural Language Processing and Computational Natural Language Learning (EMNLP-CoNLL), vol. 868, p. 876 (2007)

5. Avramidis, E., Koehn, P.: Enriching morphologically poor languages for statistical machine translation. In: Proceedings of the 46th Annual Meeting of the Association for Computational Linguistics (ACL): Human Language Technologies, pp. 763–770 (2008)

6. Yeniterzi, R., Oflazer, K.: Syntax-to-morphology mapping in factored phrase-based statistical machine translation from english to turkish. In: Proceedings of the 48th Annual Meeting of the Association for Computational Linguistics(ACL): Human Language Technologies, pp. 454–464 (2010)

7. Subotin, M.: An exponential translation model for target language morphology. In: Proceedings of the 49th Annual Meeting of the Association for Computational Linguistics(ACL): Human Language Technologies (2011)

8. Goldwater, S., McClosky, D.: Improving statistical mt through morphological analysis. In: Proceedings of the Conference on Human Language Technology and Empirical Methods in Natural Language Processing, pp. 676–683. Association for Computational Linguistics (2005)

9. Luong, M.T., Nakov, P., Kan, M.Y.: A hybrid morpheme-word representation for machine translation of morphologically rich languages. In: Proceedings of the 2010 Conference on Empirical Methods in Natural Language Processing, pp. 148–157. Association for Computational Linguistics (2010)

10. Oflazer, K.: Statistical machine translation into a morphologically complex language. In: Gelbukh, A. (ed.) CICLing 2008. LNCS, vol. 4919, pp. 376–387. Springer, Heidelberg (2008)

11. Namdar, S., Faili, H.: Using inflected word form to improve persian to english statistical machine translation. In: Proceedings of the 18th National CSI (Computer Society of Iran) Computer Conference (2013)

12. Minkov, E., Toutanova, K., Suzuki, H.: Generating complex morphology for machine translation. In: Proceedings of the 45th Annual Meeting of the Association for Computational Linguistics (ACL): Human Language Technologies, vol. 45, p. 128 (2007)

13. Toutanova, K., Suzuki, H., Ruopp, A.: Applying morphology generation models to machine translation. In: Proceedings of the 46th Annual Meeting of the Association for Computational Linguistics(ACL): Human Language Technologies, vol. 8 (2008)

14. Clifton, A., Sarkar, A.: Combining morpheme-based machine translation with postprocessing morpheme prediction. In: Proceedings of the 49th Annual Meeting of the Association for Computational Linguistics (ACL): Human Language Technologies, vol. 1, pp. 32–42 (2011)

15. El Kholy, A., Habash, N.: Rich morphology generation using statistical machine translation. In: Proceedings of the 7th International Natural Language Generation Conference (INLG), p. 90 (2012)

16. El Kholy, A., Habash, N.: Translate, predict or generate: Modeling rich morphology in statistical machine translation. In: Proceedings of European Association for Machine Translation (EAMT), vol. 12 (2012)

17. de Gispert, A., Marino, J.: On the impact of morphology in english to spanish statistical mt. Speech Communication 50, 1034–1046 (2008)

18. Vilar, D., Xu, J.: dHaro, L.F., Ney, H.: Error analysis of statistical machine translation output. In: Proceedings of the International Conference on Language Resources and Evaluation (LREC), pp. 697–702 (2006)

19. Megerdoomian, K.: Finite-state morphological analysis of persian. In: Proceedings of the Workshop on Computational Approaches to Arabic Script-based Languages, pp. 35–41. Association for Computational Linguistics (2004)

20. Klein, D., Manning, C.D.: Accurate unlexicalized parsing. In: Proceedings of the 41st Annual Meeting of the Association for Computational Linguistics(ACL): Human Language Technologies, pp. 423–430 (2003)

21. Mansouri, A., Faili, H.: State-of-the-art english to persian statistical machine translation system. In: 2012 16th CSI International Symposium on Artificial Intelligence and Signal Processing (AISP), pp. 174–179. IEEE (2012)

22. Och, F.J., Ney, H.: A systematic comparison of various statistical alignment models. Computational Linguistics 29, 19–51 (2003)

23. Rasooli, M., Faili, H., Minaei-Bidgoli, B.: Unsupervised identification of persian compound verbs. In: Batyrshin, I., Sidorov, G. (eds.) MICAI 2011, Part I. LNCS, vol. 7094, pp. 394–406. Springer, Heidelberg (2011)

24. Papineni, K., Roukos, S., Ward, T., Zhu, W.J.: Bleu: a method for automatic evaluation of machine translation. In: Proceedings of the 40th Annual Meeting of the Association for Computational Linguistics (ACL): Human Language Technologies, pp. 311–318 (2002)

25. Snover, M., Dorr, B., Schwartz, R., Micciulla, L., Makhoul, J.: A study of translation edit rate with targeted human annotation. In: Proceedings of Association for Machine Translation in the Americas, pp. 223–231 (2006)

# An XML Based TBX Framework to Represent Multilingual SNOMED CT for Translation

Olatz Perez-de-Viñaspre and Maite Oronoz

IXA NLP Group,
University of the Basque Country UPV/EHU,
Donostia
operezdevina001@ikasle.ehu.es,
maite.oronoz@ehu.es
http://ixa.si.ehu.es

**Abstract.** In this paper we show a schema to represent the SNOMED CT (Systematized Nomenclature of Medicine-Clinical Terms) ontology's multilingual terminology. In this case, our objective is the representation of the source SNOMED CT descriptions in English and Spanish, and their translations into the Basque Language. The annotation formalism we defined represents not only the terms but also the metadata needed in order to translate the SNOMED CT descriptions and the information generated from those translations. It has been used to store 276,427 Concepts and 882,003 Descriptions in English, Spanish and Basque. We adapted the TML (Terminological Markup Language) module of the TBX (TermBase eXchange) standard for that purpose. This standard is based on XML.

**Keywords:** SNOMED CT, XML, Multilingual Medical Terminology, Knowledge Representation.

## 1 Introduction

Correct and suitable representation of data is a necessary task when working in natural language processing in general, and in the gathering of lexical information in particular. In this paper we describe an adaptation of the TermBase eXchange International Standard to represent a clinical terminology called SNOMED CT [3]. According to the multilingual nature of SNOMED CT, each concept has terms in different languages. Thus, we represent multilingual terminological content of the medical domain maintaining the references to its ontological structure. In addition, metadata for describing the information concerning to the translations into Basque is represented too, in the proposed framework.

The "Systematized Nomenclature of Medicine-Clinical Terms" (SNOMED CT) is a comprehensive clinical ontology that provides clinical content for clinical documentation and reporting. It can be used to code, retrieve, and analyze clinical data. The terminology comprises Concepts, Descriptions and Relationships

F. Castro, A. Gelbukh, and M. González (Eds.): MICAI 2013, Part I, LNAI 8265, pp. 419–429, 2013.

with the objective of precisely representing clinical information across the scope of health care [6]. SNOMED CT is widely recognized as the leading global clinical terminology for use in Electronic Health Records. It is maintained and developed by an International body: the "International Health Terminology Standards Development Organization" or IHTSDO [5]. Although the SNOMED CT source language is English it has already been translated to other languages like Spanish. There are released guidelines for the translation of it [4].

Being aware of the importance of SNOMED CT for managing and extracting medical information, one of our objectives is the semi-automatic translation of a part of SNOMED CT to our language, Basque. Basque is a minority language spoken in the Basque Country. It is an isolate language, but today holds co-official language status in the Basque Country. It is a highly inflected language with free order of sentence constituents. We know that the general objective of the translation of SNOMED CT is ambitious but at the same time necessary in the process of normalization of the language.

As mentioned before, Basque is a minority language. Thus, the resources to translate SNOMED CT into it are not enough for a manual translation of the Concepts, as recommended in [4]. We propose a semi-automatic translation of its terminology, by means of NLP techniques, so the manual work done by experts will be focused on the validation and correction of the terms generated.

Thus, in this paper we show a formalism to represent the English and Spanish versions of SNOMED CT, as well as the corresponding Basque terms obtained semi-automatically. Furthermore, as our aim is to obtain a multilingual terminology, we use the TermBase eXchange standard, that among others, has been defined for that purpose.

The International Release of SNOMED CT is represented in tab-delimited text. In order to translate its terminological content semi-automatically, additional structured information is needed for the translated Basque terms, such as the translation method or the source term.

SNOMED CT is included in the Metathesaurus of UMLS (*Unified Medical Language System*) [2], and the Methathesaurus, including SNOMED CT, is stored in Rich Release Format (RFF) files or relations of a relational database. Anyway, in order to translate SNOMED CT, we are more interested in its terminology, and less than in the relations between them. Thus, we need a rich representation of SNOMED CT, that allows us to maintain the original structure, but to add structured information for translation purposes.

XML allows to represent data in a semi-structured way. In addition it adds semantics to the data by means of the element tags. In this way, it is possible to adequate the structure of each element to the data related to it. In the near history many standards have been defined in order to represent terminology. It is worth to point out the importance of XML among those standards, being the base of many of them such as XML representation of Lexicons and Terminologies (XLT) [12], Lexical Markup Framework (LMF) (ISO-24613:2008) [7], Dictionary Markup Language (DML) [10] or TermBase eXchange (TBX) (ISO-30042:2008) [8] [11].

The remainder of the paper is as follows. After this introduction, section 2 describes the main specifications of SNOMED CT and section 3 briefly describes TBX. Section 4 exposes the data model adopted to represent the terminology content of SNOMED CT. Finally, conclusion and future work are exposed in section 5.

## 2   SNOMED CT Structure

The essential components of SNOMED CT are the Concepts, the Descriptions and the Relationships. A Concept is a clinical idea to which a unique SNOMED CT identifier has been assigned. Each Concept is associated to a set of Descriptions, that have representations such as synonyms and translations to different languages. The Concept is logically defined by its Relationships to other Concepts. All the Concepts in SNOMED CT are organized into 19 Top Level Hierarchies with different semantic tags. The semantic tag indicates the semantic category and hierarchy where the Concept belongs. For example, the hierarchy named "Body structure" groups the semantic tags "body structure", "morphologic abnormality", "cell" and "cell structure".

There are three types of Descriptions: *Fully Specified Name* (FSN), *Preferred Term* (PT) and *Synonyms*. The *Fully Specified Name* makes Concepts readable for humans and they usually finish with a "semantic tag" in parenthesis. In the Technical Implementation Guide [6] it is fixed that "a particular language Reference Set will only contain a single FSN" and it will not be used in a clinical record. *Preferred Terms* are common words or phrases used by clinicians to name that Concept. *Synonyms* are terms that are acceptable alternatives to the

**Table 1.** An example of the Descriptions of the concept "Obstruction of pelviureteric junction"

| Concept: 95575002 - Obstruction of pelviureteric junction | |
|---|---|
| Descriptions in English | |
| *Description* | Type |
| Obstruction of pelviureteric junction (disorder) | FSN |
| Obstruction of pelviureteric junction | Preferred Term |
| PUJ - Pelviureteric obstruction | Synonym |
| PUO - Pelviureteric obstruction | Synonym |
| Pelviureteric obstruction | Synonym |
| UPJ - Ureteropelvic obstruction | Synonym |
| Ureteropelvic obstruction | Synonym |
| Descriptions in Spanish | |
| obstrucción de la unión pelviureteral (trastorno) | FSN |
| obstrucción de la unión pelviureteral | Preferred Term |
| obstrucción ureteropelviana | Synonym |
| obstrucción ureteropélvica | Synonym |

Preferred Term as a way of expressing a Concept. As specified in the Technical Implementation Guide, "Synonyms and Preferred Terms (unlike FSNs) are not necessarily unique. More than one concept might share the same Preferred term or Synonym".

Table 1 shows an example in which the Concept with the identifier "95575002" has in its upper side the Descriptions of the English version, being the *Fully Specified Name* "Obstruction of pelviureteric junction (disorder)" with the semantic tag *disorder* and the *Preferred Term* "Obstruction of pelviureteric junction". It has five *Synonyms* in English. In the same table 1 we can see that the number of *Synonyms* for the Spanish version is quantitatively different as it has only two of them. In the case of the synonyms it is easy to understand as each language has its own synonym sets.

The terminological information from SNOMED CT, as shown in Table 1, is stored in a TBX framework described in section 3.

# 3   TermBase eXchange Standard

TermBase eXchange (TBX) is an International Standard based on XML that defines a framework with the purpose of representing structured terminological data. It is designed to support different processes, such as analysis or descriptive representation. The main objective of TBX is the interchange of terminological data.

In order to support different types of terminological data used in termbases, TBX includes two modules expressed in XML: a core structure and a formalism to identify the terminological data and their constraints (XCS, eXtensible Constraint Specification). This terminological data is expressed by means of data-categories, that are represented as the value of the "type" attribute in XML. The term TBX implies the result of the interaction of both modules.

The XCS mechanism allows the definition of data-categories to adjust to the requirements of different users. By means of defining the data-categories and the constraints among categories, each user-group can define its own TML (Terminological Markup Language) (ISO-11642:2003). This characteristic of TBX is very useful as it is not usual to find terminology collections that share the exact same data-categories. Anyway, TBX provides a default set of data-categories in order to maximize the interoperability among currently existing terminological data. This set of data-categories is defined and constrained by the default XCS. Thus, TBX provides a blind representation mechanism, so users are able to interpret data without consulting providers.

For getting the Basque translation of SNOMED CT there are available among others some specialized glossaries of the bio-medical domain for Basque. Those have been compiled at the University of the Basque Country and have the aim of reflecting the terminology used by experts in a real context. All these glossaries are gathered in a system called TZOS [1]. TZOS is an On-Line System for Terminology Service that has been designed as a tool for the creation and spreading of Basque terminology in the University environment. TZOS represents those glossaries following the TBX framework, and that is one of the reasons for adapting the TML used in TZOS to represent SNOMED CT terminology content.

## 4   Our Approach

In this section we describe the data model adopted from TZOS to represent the terminology content of the English and Spanish versions of SNOMED CT as well as to include the additional information needed for translation purposes. That is, having as basis the model used in TZOS, we define and use the new data model exposed in the following lines.

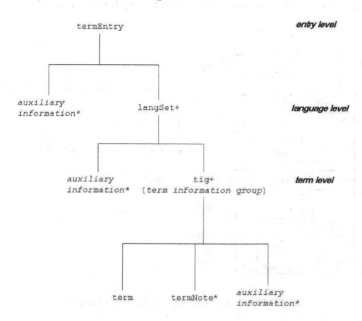

**Fig. 1.** Structure and levels of a terminological entry in TZOS

A terminological entry in TZOS has the structure shown in Figure 1. There are three levels having associated its own information:

- *Entry level:* it corresponds to the concept, representing the concept-related information.
- *Language level:* information about the concept is expressed in different languages, that is, a `langSet` for each language (in the figure 1, the symbol + indicates that it can occur once or more times).
- *Term level:* it represents the term itself (`term`) and the associated information by means of a `tig` element. There is a `tig` element for each synonym-term of the concept. By means of the auxiliary information, descriptive features of the term, administrative information or other kind of information can be represented at any level (the symbol * indicates that it can occur 0 or more times).

In the following lines we describe how we reused this structure of TBX in order to represent SNOMED CT Concepts, Descriptions and the corresponding Basque terms.

### 4.1   Representation of SNOMED CT

For each SNOMED CT Concept we define a `termEntry`. This `termEntry` is complemented by the hierarchy, the semantic tag and the English *Fully Specified Name*. Information regarding the transaction is also represented, such as the person in charge of the generation or edition of the term or the date and time that it was done. This information is helpful in order to manage the database itself.

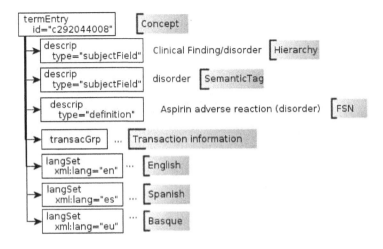

**Fig. 2.** Structure of a SNOMED CT Concept

In the Figure 2 we show an example that corresponds to the SNOMED CT Concept with the FSN "Aspirin adverse reaction (disorder)". This information is represented by the data-category *definition* that is the value of the "type" attribute in the `descrip` element. Its Concept identifier is "292044008" (`termEntry` element's id attribute) and the hierarchy to it belongs "Clinical Finding/disorder", being "disorder" the semantic tag (both of them through the *subjectField* data-category). Regarding the languages, on the one hand, in the English and Spanish language sets (`langSet`) we store the PTs and Synonyms from SNOMED CT; on the other hand, Basque terms are represented with additional descriptive metadata as shown in section 4.2.

We have located the English FSN of the Concept in the entry level instead of in the term level because FSNs are not found in clinical reports and, in consequence, we have decided not to translate them. Furthermore, FSNs are used to identify Concepts so locating them at the entry level is more adequate to SNOMED CT's philosophy.

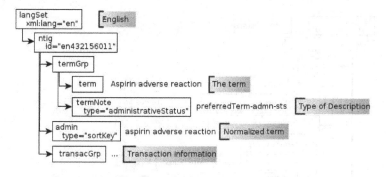

**Fig. 3.** Structure of an English SNOMED CT term

To represent a SNOMED CT Description, we store the term itself and also other descriptive metadata. Following the example shown in Figure 3 (that continues the example shown in Figure 2), the term is "Aspirin adverse reaction", its Description type a *Preferred Term* ("preferredTerm-admn-sts" in TBX as the value of the *administrativeStatus* data-category), the normalized term is "aspirin adverse reaction" (through the *sortKey* data-category) and transaction information is also stored.

The design presented in this section allows the representation of the terminology content of SNOMED CT. The structure of SNOMED CT that is obtained by means of Relationships is not represented in TBX but it is accessible using the Concept and Descriptions identifiers in the International Release of SNOMED CT.

## 4.2   Representation of Basque Terms

As mentioned before, our aim is to get Basque terms from the SNOMED CT terminology, so we could obtain a semi-automatic translation to Basque. To represent those terms, we need additional metadata such as the concept source term or the resource from where it has been obtained.

The process to obtain those Basque terms is based on four main resources: i) specialized dictionaries, ii) finite state transducers and word-level morphosemantic rules [13], iii) shadow syntax-level rules and iv) adapted machine translation. The way the term is generated is represented in the *entrySource* data-category. The origin of the SNOMED CT term is represented with the *conceptOrigin* data-category.

Depending on the resource used, word-level or syntax-level information is also represented. That is, by means of the `termCompList` element, we can split the term into syllables, morphemes, words or chunks. This is useful for the correction of the Basque terms. Let us see the example shown in Figure 4 that complites the previous

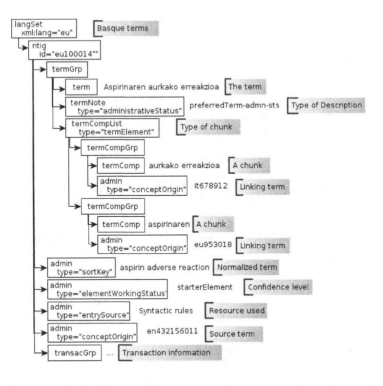

**Fig. 4.** Structure of a Basque term

example (Figures 2 and 3). The Basque word *"aspirinaren"* ("of the aspirin") is linked to the Basque term identified by "eu953018", *"aspirina"*. So, if an expert corrects the Basque term *"aspirina"*, by *"azido azetilsaliziliko"* ("acetylsalicylic acid"), for instance, this is also applied to *"aspirinaren aurkako erreakzioa"* ("aspirin adverse reaction"), obtaining *"azido azetilsalizilikoaren aurkako erreakzioa"* ("acetylsalicylic acid adverse reaction"). This update of changes on the Basque terms is possible thanks to the linking between terms.

In this case, we also need to store the confidence level we give to the obtained term. That is, through the *elementWorkingStatus* data-category we differentiate the Basque term obtained from a specialized dictionary or from word-level or syntax-level rules, giving them a different value. For example, terms extracted from dictionaries have a higher value than the ones generated using finite state transducers because experts have checked them to create the dictionary.

Figure 5 shows the XML representation of the example shown above by the Figures 2, 3 and 4.

```
<termEntry id="c292044008">
 <descrip type="subjectField">010</descrip>
 <descrip type="subjectField">011</descrip>
 <descrip type="definition">Aspirin adverse reaction (disorder)</descrip>
 <transacGrp>...</transacGrp>
 <langSet xml:lang="en">
  <ntig id="en432156011">
   <termGrp>
    <term>Aspirin adverse reaction</term>
    <termNote type="administrativeStatus">preferredTerm-admn-sts</termNote>
   </termGrp>
   <admin type="sortKey">aspirin adverse reaction</admin>
   <transacGrp>...</transacGrp>
  </ntig>
 </langSet>
 <langSet xml:lang="es">...</langSet>
 <langSet xml:lang="eu">
  <ntig id="eu100014">
   <termGrp>
    <term>Aspirinaren aurkako erreakzioa</term>
    <termNote type="administrativeStatus">preferredTerm-admn-sts</termNote>
    <termCompList type="termElement">
     <termCompGrp>
      <termComp>aurkako erreakzioa</termComp>
      <admin type="conceptOrigin">it678</admin>
     </termCompGrp>
     <termCompGrp>
      <termComp>aspirinaren</termComp>
      <admin type="conceptOrigin">eu953018</admin>
     </termCompGrp>
    </termCompList>
   </termGrp>
   <admin type="sortKey">aspirinaren aurkako erreakzioa</admin>
   <admin type="elementWorkingStatus">starterElement</admin>
   <admin type="entrySource">102</admin>
   <admin type="conceptOrigin">en432156011</admin>
   <transacGrp>...</transacGrp>
  </ntig>
 </langSet>
</termEntry>
```

**Fig. 5.** An example of the XML structure

## 5    Conclusions and Future Work

We defined a formalism to represent SNOMED CT terms through the TBX International Standard. Thus, each SNOMED CT Concept is stored with its English and Spanish terms and also with the Basque terms obtained by a semi-automatic translation process. The role of metadata is essential in order to maintain the relationship to the SNOMED CT ontological graph (we use the Concept and Description identifiers) and also to manage the translation and correction processes (origin of translation, word-level splitting...).

Even the formalism exposed is based on the English and Spanish versions for translating SNOMED CT into Basque, it can be used for any other languages as all the defined adaptations are language independent.

Due to the wide terminology of SNOMED CT the XML generated is so large that we had split it by the hierarchy the concepts belongs to. Thus, we obtain one XML document for each High level SNOMED CT hierarchy. In the case of "Clinical Finding/disorder" the XML document is still too large, so we divided it by the semantic tag ("finding" and "disorder") of the concept's FSN. We have been able to represent 296,427 SNOMED CT Concepts, 476,356 English Descriptions, 379,977 Spanish Descriptions and in the first steps of the translation to Basque, 25,670 terms in Basque.

The first steps towards the semi-automatic translation have been successfully performed obtaining promising results. Regarding the formalism here described, we have probed the appropriateness of it in order to represent SNOMED CT terminology content, as well as to store the Basque terms obtained from the specialized dictionaries.

The XML documents generated following this formalism, are well-formed. Besides, they were validated using both the standard TBX Relax NG schema [9] and the one defined for TZOS. Those two schemes mainly differ in the definition of a new "dateTime" data-category, which allows a better manage of the data generated on-line.

Although the big data already gathered and represented by this formalism asures its robustness, a step forward will be made in a near future by representing the shadow syntax of complex terms.

# References

1. Arregi, X., Arruarte, A., Artola, X., Lersundi, M., Zabala, I.: TZOS: An On-Line System for Terminology Service. In: Centro de Lingüística Aplicada, pp. 400–404. Actualizaciones en Comunicacin Social (2013)
2. Bodenreider, O.: The Unified Medical Language System (UMLS): integrating biomedical terminology. Nucleic Acids Research 32, 267–270 (2004)
3. College of American Pathologists: The Systematized Nomenclature of Human and Veterinary Medicine: SNOMED International (1993)
4. Høy, A.: Guidelines for Translation of SNOMED CT. Tech. Rep. version 2.0, International Health Terminology Standards Development Organization IHTSDO (2010)
5. IHTSDO: International Health Terminology Standards Development Organisation (IHTSDO) (2013), http://www.ihtsdo.org/
6. International Health Terminology Standards Development Organisation IHTSDO: SNOMED CT Technical Implementation Guide. July 2012 International Release. Tech. rep., International Health Terminology Standards Development Organisation IHTSDO (2012)
7. ISO: Language Resource management – Lexical Markup Framework (LMF). Tech. rep., International Organization for Standarization, Geneva, Switzerland (June 2008)

8. LISA: Systems to manage terminology, knowledge, and content - TermBase eXchange (TBX). Tech. rep. Localization Industry Standards Association (2008)

9. (LISA), L.I.S.A.: TermBase eXchange (TBX),
   http://www.ttt.org/oscarstandards/tbx/ (2008)

10. Mangeot, M.: An XML Markup Language Framework for Lexical Databases Environments: the Dictionary Markup Language. In: LREC Workshop on International Standards of Terminology and Language Resources Management, Las Palmas, Spain, pp. 37–44 (May 2002)

11. Melby, A.K.: Terminology in the age of multilingual corpora. The Journal of Specialised Translation 18, 7–29 (2012)

12. SALT project: SALT project – XML representations of Lexicons and Terminologies (XLT) – Default XLT Format (DXLT). Tech. rep., SALT project (2000), reference name of working document: DXLT specification draft 1b

13. de Viaspre, O.P., Oronoz, M., Aguirrezabal, M., Lersundi, M.: A Finite-State Approach to Translate SNOMED CT Terms into Basque Using Medical Prexes and Sufxes. In: The 11th International Conference on Finite-State Methods and Natural Language Processing (FSMNLP 2013) (2013)

# The Twin Hypotheses

## Brain Code and the Fundamental Code Unit: Towards Understanding the Computational Primitive Elements of Cortical Computing

Newton Howard

Massachusetts Institute of Technology
nhmit@mit.edu

**Abstract.** The Brain Code (BC) relies on several essential concepts that are found across a range of physiological and behavioral functions. The Fundamental Code Unit (FCU) assumes an abstract code unit to allow for a higher order of abstractions that informs information exchanges at the cellular and genetic levels, together the two hypotheses provide a foundation for a system level understanding and potentially cyphering of the Brain Code [1–3]. This paper discusses an organizing principle for an abstract framework tested in a limited scope experimental approach as a means to show an empirical example of cognitive measurement as well as a framework for a Cortical Computation methodology. Four important concepts of the BC and FCU are discussed. First, the principle of activation based on Guyton thresholds. This is seen in the well-known and widely documented action potential threshold in neurons, where once a certain threshold is reached, the neuron will fire, reflecting the transmission of information. The concept of thresholds is also valid in Weber minimum detectable difference in our sensing, which applies to our hearing, seeing and touching. Not only the intensity, but also the temporal pattern is affected by this [4]. This brings insight to the second important component, which is duration. The combination of both threshold crossing and duration may define the selection mechanisms, depending on both external and intrinsic factors. However, ranges exist within which tuning can take place. Within reason it can be stated that no functional implication will occur beyond this range. Transfer of information and processing itself relies on energy and can be described in waveforms, which is the third concept. The human sensing system acts as transducer between the different forms of energy, the fourth principle. The aim of the brain code approach is to incorporate these four principles in an explanatory, descriptive and predictive model. The model will take into account fundamental physiological knowledge and aims to reject assumptions that are not yet fully established. In order to fill in the gaps with regards to the missing information, modules consisting of the previous described four principles are explored. This abstraction should provide a reasonable placeholder, as it is based on governing principles in nature. The model is testable and allows for updating as more data becomes available. It aims to replace methods that rely on structural levels to abstraction of functions, or approaches that are evidence-based, but across many noisy-elements and assumptions that outcomes might not reflect behavior at the organism level.

F. Castro, A. Gelbukh, and M. González (Eds.): MICAI 2013, Part I, LNAI 8265, pp. 430–463, 2013.
© Springer-Verlag Berlin Heidelberg 2013

**Keywords:** The Brain Code (BC), Fundamental Code Unit, (FCU), brain language, Cortical Computing, primitives, the abstract code unit, brain algorithms.

# 1    Introduction

Structures that are inherently simple are most often sufficiently sophisticated to represent complex systems, including networks of neurons, neurotransmitter proteins, or chemical receptors on the neurons themselves. There is a seemingly contradictory characteristic of complex systems, whereby they appear strikingly simple at the unit level, but can achieve unparalleled complexity at higher orders. This is the basis of the Fundamental Code Unit (FCU) argument; an assumed abstract code unit to allow for higher order of abstractions, and provide a foundation for the Brain Code [1, 2, 5] organizing principle model. This paper presents a low-level analysis of the phenomena that compose cognition, and the means by which we can better understand it. Here we begin with a discussion of the potential applicability of Brownian motion formulas to the uncertainty inherent in protein-driven neurotransmissions, for protein exchange occurs at a lower level than neural activation and is often a causal agent in neural activity. For instance, Rubinsztein [6] demonstrates that the ubiquitin–proteasome and autophagy–lysosome pathways are the primary means of protein transmission into the organelles of neurons. The former are multiprotein complexes whose function is to degrade nuclear and cytosolic proteins. Rubinsztein also details the process of endoplasmic-reticulum-associated degradation (ERAD), in which misfolded protein is retrotranslocated back into the cytosol, where the proteasome pathway degrades them.

In a hypothetical model offered, each of these events can be appropriately captured by the introduction of Brownian motion methods, which currently have wider applications to models in imaging technology. The "Brain Code" is a higher-level analysis. The data processing methods that can be used to assemble it can come from neurological, chemical and psychological components. That is, a computational method whereby cognitive events such as neural spikes, network activation, and memory recall can be understood in terms of the simultaneous physical phenomena that cause them. The Brain Code is thus described as cumulative cognitive output, of which natural language is just one product. Ultimately, a "brain language" is decoded from a combination of inputs (natural language, behavioral outputs and electrical activities of the brain) yielding a comprehensive cognitive picture. Thus, the process described is essentially one of deriving enhanced insight from a series of fragmented, often incomplete streams of data. I offer reviews of several different analytical methods, along with examples of phenomena applications for each. Brain codes, such as cognitive state signatures or behavioral indicators such as movements and other behavioral expressions, continue to provide valuable insight into the patient's cognitive state even after higher motor and cognitive functions are significantly impaired. Thus, brain codes remain a common output to both functioning and impaired neural systems, unlike natural language expressions if used alone [7].

# 2    Background

In order to study brain function, some researchers have attempted to reverse-engineer neuronal networks and even the brain itself. This approach is based on the assumption that neurons in-vivo act just like simple transistors in-silico. Unfortunately, both network and whole-brain modeling have led to very little insight into actual brain function. This is largely because transistor-based computing reacts to static events whilst neurons can react to processes. In contrast to transistors, neurons can establish and change their connections and vary their signaling properties according to a variety of rules, allowing them to adapt to circumstances, self-assemble, auto-calibrate and store information by changing their properties according to experience.

The central question of the Mind Machine Project at MIT in 2007 was: how does our brain and the nervous system take patterns of light at the eye, sound at the ear, or touch on the skin and determine properties of the surrounding environment? How does our brain react to emotions manifested through expressions, symbols and languages? How are patterns of various energy scales combined then transduced by multitudes of sensory systems that lead to the perception of a coherent multi-dimensional world and recognition of objects of reality and fictional existence. How are the ordered and the disordered mind both capable of those amazing faculties? How do they support adaptive behaviors of desisted and functional responses, articulated by majuscules? To understand the brain requires an investigation of the problem at several levels simultaneously: from elector-physiology observable to molecular mechanisms of information storage and signaling, to the multi-scale neural network formation and trends. From a code and process to an automata of sensory information, from the functional processes of perception, recognition, and behavioral control that must be implemented by the brain to the language expressed by higher intelligence and adaptation.

## 2.1    Fundamental Code Unit Defined

To understand the FCU approach, we need to establish a mutual understanding of the nature of sensory information processing in the brain. Brain information processing of incoming sensory information (such as speech sounds) can be viewed as the following step by step process:  Sensory transduction—e.g., converting speech sounds into electrical information transmitted to the brain via the auditory nerves. Conversion of that information into intelligible language that our mind (whatever that may be) can comprehend as records of events, concepts, stories, and so on.  For the visual system, that language is a series of images, discerned as objects that may move, emit light, etc. These patterns provide an understanding of our physical surroundings.  Analogously for the auditory system the conversion process to language can be considered as discerning a series of sounds as speech, expressed in patterns that consistently correlate with specific objects, feelings and thoughts. Those meaningful representations can be communicated to and from others, based on a common understanding of what those speech sounds signify—language. Storage of those meaningful patterns as meaningful thoughts, as a series of both images and auditory language representations of somewithin the brain. Retrieval of those meaningful thought patterns, either at will or involuntarily.  The latter case refers to spontaneous thoughts, our constant internal dialog which can at times be distracting and prevent us from concentrating on what we find meaningful and important. To offer an example, Autism Spectrum Disorders (ASD) are strongly tied to genetic identity. However, like many others such as ADHD, schizophrenia and certain other disorders, it's underlying cause is not tied to a single gene as is the case in Huntington's Disease which belongs to another class of NDD with complexity in cause in symptomology.

On the cellular & molecular level, the etiology of the disorder appears equally diverse and complex. Adding to the challenges of developing new therapies for ASD--or improving current ones—is the fact that the key underlying cellular & molecular mechanisms—such as those responsible for transducing speech sounds into mutually understood and remembered language within the brain—have not yet been clearly defined. Using the advances in AI techniques that are increasingly grounded in the reality of brain physiology, such as new neural network algorithms NLP or others briefly discussed here will greatly benefit and aid the discovery of new methods and processes to reach meaningful solutions. We will have distinct categories based on their underlying etiology, more intimately correlated to each of the multiplicity of mechanisms that can give rise to the speech and behavioral abnormalities characteristic of many of those brain disorders.

It should also serve as a guide to the development of new therapeutic strategies on an accelerated time frame, based on the ability of the brain to rewire itself in response to experience--neuroplasticity.  Such neuroplasticity-based therapies do not require detailed mechanistic knowledge of brain function abnormalities. In certain forms of ASD, there appears to be hyperactivity of spontaneous internal thoughts, images, and ideas, and this may contribute to the observed symptomatology.  *In all forms of ASD,* language deficits and image recognition deficits (e.g. the inability to make sense of subtleties of human facial expression) are hallmarks of that symptomatology.

In the 19th century, Darwin's insightful outside-in observations of life's diversity in time and space gave rise to the notion of inheritable characteristics that could change over time—genes, a fundamental coding unit dictating those characteristics that could change (mutate) over time, giving rise to systematic changes promoting environmental adaptability, and eventually giving rise to new life forms—i.e., evolution.  Also in the 19th century the outside-in research of Gregor Mendel and others homed in further on the nature of the gene, specifically its role in the expression of discernible characteristics by parental inheritance.

By the 1930's, long before DNA was discovered, those fundamental units were shown by light microscopy to reside on chromosomes, and we had a basic view of the cellular phenomenology of genetic inheritance and genetic abnormalities. In genetics, long before our current detailed cellular and molecular-level view of genetics was obtained—before DNA was discovered to be the unit of genetic information coding, storage and expression—a great deal was known about the nature of the gene as a discrete, fundamental coding element, dictating a wide variety of inherited characteristics, both physical and mental. Long before we had an inside, molecular level view of the fundamental coding unit, DNA, we had a detailed outside-in view of the gene, a view that proved quite useful in many ways.

How might this historical analogy to the field of genetics relate to brain information processing? This question is key to the FCU-based strategy for understanding brain information processing and its abnormalities, by analogy with the historical success of understanding the properties of genetic information encoding in the brain, the FCU-based strategy is based on this premise:   In the face of limited but advancing understanding of brain information processing on a molecular & cellular level, our novel FCU approach addresses the problem from an entirely different direction.

To help appreciate this dualistic approach, by analogy we can compare the FCU brain information strategy to the field of genetics, as viewed from the outside in (observations of the evolving characteristics of organisms) vs. the inside out (the structure of DNA and the dynamics of its translation into the protein elements comprising the organism's structure and metabolism, etc).   FCU-based strategy for understanding brain information processing may reveal fundamental properties of brain information processing, long before the molecular and neurophysiological complexities of the brain's information processing pathways and processes are fully revealed. The practical advantages of viewing human consciousness as an abstract concept, as well as a biological entity embedded in the brain— Isaac Newton's discernment of universal laws governing motion. In his 17$^{th}$ century world, the motions of heavenly bodies seemed unmanageably complicated. Astronomers such as Kepler developed elaborate schemes to describe such motions, but such schemes offered little in the way of fundamental understanding of said complexity. Newton came along, and used his mathematical talents together with other gifts to propose that these motions could be more meaningfully described if one were to postulate the existence of an all pervasive, universal force—gravity—that exerted its actions on heavenly bodies by universal laws that could be represented mathematically. As we know, this insight greatly simplified the apparent complexity of planetary motion, and to this very day has proved of great value in predicting the orbital trajectory of satellites, etc. All this was done in the face of a lack of knowledge (strikingly incomplete to this very day) of the physical nature and origin of this gravitational force. Gravitational field theory was developed solely by—yet again, as in the discovery of the gene—the outside-in approach of observing its effect on bodily motion.

How does Isaac Newton's approach bear relation to FCU-based approach to deciphering the complexity of information processing in the brain? Again in this case, neuroscience has told us a great deal about the brain's molecular and cellular pathways and processes associated with information processing, but the inside view is still too incomplete to provide a unified view of the coding and handling of information in the brain. By viewing the brain's ability to import information and process it into thought patterns and concepts meaningful to human conscious awareness as an abstract concept—approaches akin to force field theory of physics, cutting edge tools of mathematics and computer science can be productively brought to bear on human neural information coding research in health and disease.

We can usefully model human consciousness as a mathematical abstraction, whose underlying properties can be revealed through an analysis of its manifestations in the form of language and behavior.

A prerequisite for the connectivity analysis proposed above is the ability to define networks, in terms of foci where activity relevant to a task is to be found and the connections between these areas as they are defined anatomically and functionally. There are many ways of defining how nodes are related, e.g., through phase relationship or amplitude modulations, directed or undirected and with or without time delays. Each of the different sensible ways of defining a metric for the inter-dependence between nodes poses a distinct question and many such questions must be addressed at any one time. We have used tomographic analysis of MEG data to identify the nodes of the network since we have already demonstrated that we can identify activity from the MEG data with high accuracy [8].

Recent work has focused on eye movement in awake state and sleep processing in the visual system [9, 10], because eye movement and the visual system are the only systems we understand reasonably well to attempt a serious modeling with the graph theory as outlined in Ioannides [11] and [12]. Studies in the visual system have covered a wide range of stimuli including simple stimuli like checker board patterns [8, 13, 14] occluded figures [15, 16] illusory contours [17] and a series of studies on face and face affect recognition, both on control [18, 19] and schizophrenic subjects [20].

It was clear from these studies that it would be necessary to also deal with controlling the state of the subject. For these reasons a series of studies was undertaken on sleep [10, 21] and attention [22, 23]. Finally two cases were studied where the visual system was studied in extreme conditions, where damage probed its operations under conditions that were beyond what the system was optimized for evolution for maximum efficiency. In the first case the hemianopic subject GY was studied with stimuli presented to the intact and damaged hemisphere, and thus allowing the identification of spatiotemporal profiles of visual processing with and without primary visual cortex [24].

Research by Ioannides and his team was based on the observation that simple and complex tasks alike (regardless of whether they involve motion, concept processing or both) necessarily involve the activation of and communication between multiple brain areas. While some neural networks are permanent in structure and function, most of the ones involved in these tasks contain components, whether individual cells or sub-networks, which are members of multiple larger networks.

Complex and dynamic information and data networks such as the human brain share many characteristics in common, such as recurring patterns, as well as sudden changes, or shocks, that can redefine the structure of the network, or simply alter it. Ioannides et al. used a modified functional coupling measure method in order to take "snapshots" of neural connectivity from signal.

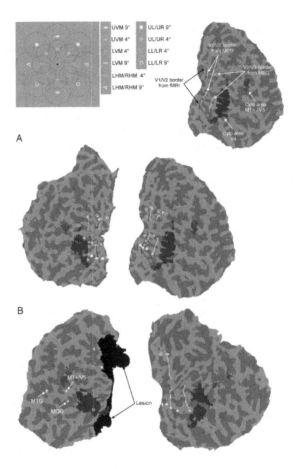

**Fig. 1.** (Fig. 2. in Ioannides et al. (2012)) Shows distribution of the ROIs on the flattened occipital cortex. The left hemisphere flattened patches are shown on the left and the right hemisphere patches on the right. Colored shapes mark centers of ROIs obtained in response to stimuli presented in different parts of the visual field, as depicted on the upper right part of the figure. Cyan and yellow shapesmark ROIs corresponding to stimuli presented at eccentricities of 4° and 9° respectively. Triangles, rhombi and circles indicate ROIs for stimuli presented on the horizontal meridian, vertical meridian and in the quadrants respectively. Filled and empty shapes indicate ROIs for stimuli presented in the upper and lower visual fields respectively. The markings for estimated visual area borders are indicated on the example flattened patch on the upper right part of the figure. White lines indicate borders between early visual areas estimated based on source analysis of MEG data alone. Black lines indicate the borders between areas V1 and V2 estimated in independent fMRI experiments. Putative V4 and V5 areas obtained from the above 50% cytoarchitectonic probabilistic maps are also indicated on the flattened patches. (A) shows distribution of ROIs in a typical control subject. (B) shows distribution of ROIs in GY. Crosses mark the locations of the three high-level ROIs in the ipsilesional hemisphere. The black patches show the lesioned portion of the left occipital cortex.

These snapshots usually consisted of time windows in the 100ms range, which were then progressively moved forward to track the change in computed values (local efficiency between attended and ignored conditions) over time. Time-window width was calculated to be 2 cycles of the lower frequency. The work of Ioannides et al. is particularly relevant to cortical computing and the brain abstract code because it helps bridge the analytical gap between computational networks and structures outside the human brain, such as man-made data representations, and the neural processes that occur within the brain.

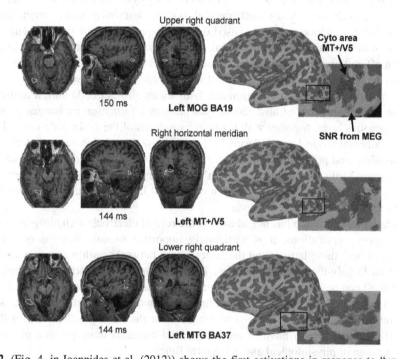

**Fig. 2.** (Fig. 4. in Ioannides et al. (2012)) shows the first activations in response to "unseen" stimuli in the blind hemifield of GY. The first activations (SNR>0.2) elicited by stimuli presented in the UR quadrant (upper row, MOG BA19), on the RHM (middle row, MT+/V5) and in the LR quadrant (lower row, MTG BA37) are shown on the MRI and lateral aspect of the inflated cortical surfaces of the left hemisphere. Note that the first responses to all three "unseen" stimuli were in the ipsilesional hemisphere. Axial (left), sagittal (middle) and coronal (right) MRI slices best covering the relevant activations are shown. The yellow contours on each MRI view encompass the regions with SNR>0.2. Activation latencies are given below the sagittal views. The black rectangles on the inflated cortical surfaces indicate the zoomed areas shown in their lower right part. Putative V5 area obtained from the 50% cytoarchitectonic probabilistic maps is also shown in the inflated maps and they are captured also on the first and second zoomed views.All the mentioned studies can be considered as preparatory for the implementation of the approach outlined in Ioannides (2007) "Dynamic Functional Connectivity." It represents a solid volume of work demonstrating that the elements to build a proper graph theoretical approach are in place.   It also testifies an unparalleled wealth of MEG data already collected that can provide the foundation for the more extensive work on subcortical functional interaction and connectivity.

By modeling both types of systems using similar methods (i.e. graph theory) to describe similar phenomena, they demonstrate that the network-based methodology used by the brain code to describe brain activity is sufficiently complex and efficient to accommodate neural activation, even in highly volatile states.

Where the primary objective of Ioannides et al. was to provide a network-centric model of brain processes, [25] show a biochemical basis for understanding those same changes in neural networks over time. While both of these authors lend implicit support for the cortical theorem, Marx & Gilon show a physical basis for theoretical underpinnings, such as a unary mathematical system describing neural connectivity. Marx & Gilon's method, which is based on a three-part model of memory engrams, focuses on individual neurons and neural neurons, extracellular matrices, and chemicals that affect the activity of these matrices as a means to prove the brain code algorithm to reach a Fundamental Code Unit (FCU) as proposed by Howard [1].

Where a proposed cognitive minimum assumes an abstract code unit, a minimum to allow for higher order of abstractions that informs information exchanges at cellular and genetics level, together with his twin hypothesis of the brain code method and the Fundamental Code Unit, Howard [27] provided a foundation for a system level understanding and potentially cyphering of the Brain Code. Termed "Neural extracellular matrices" (nECM's) Marx and Gilon's (2013) method for describing chemically encoded information transfer is based on a hydrated lattice structure manipulated by neurons using electro-elastic processes.

While current research has not addressed the role of electroelastichydrogels in specific memory applications, it is particularly important to note that the networked structure of both these lattices and the larger neural networks with which they interact operate on largely the same set of rules. Thus, the same based cortical mathematical system used can be applied to hydrated lattices. Furthermore, the multilevel analytical function is born out of the independent arrival of two disparate research efforts focused on different brain phenomena which arrive at the same conclusion. If a Brain Code (BC) exists it will have to rely on several essential concepts that are found across a range of physiological and behavioral functions.

Modeling with the graph theory as outlined by Ioannides in [11] and [12] offers a data driven proven and tested methodology towards empirical evidence that supports the existence of cortical microcircuits that implement these models of computing primitives, as disused in aspects of the models where microcircuits in the brain have been examined and modeled. Our current method if further supported could yield significant advances towards identifying what is the minimum set of new information about cortical microcircuits that would significantly advance the state of the art connectivity, synaptic weights, glial distribution, neuromodulator state, gene expression, neural activity patterns, etc.

## 2.2    The Energy Paradox

Economy and efficiency are guiding principles in physiology [28]. We thus argue that understanding the design rules that shaped neuronal function and network organization will help us in the understanding and modeling of brain function. This notion was already recognized about 100 years ago by Cajal, who stated "all of the formations of the neuron and its various components are simply morphological adaptations governed by the laws of conservation for time, space and material" [29]. The structural and physiochemical relationships that connect resources used in brain performance are determined by three major constraints: geometrical limitations on packaging and wiring, energy consumption considerations, and energy-efficient neural codes. One obvious difference between current in-silico technology and the brain is their three-dimensional organization. Most microprocessor chips use a small number of layers of planar wiring. In contrast, neurons wire in a complete 3D fashion. Various studies have examined optimal geometric patterns of connectivity and find that neurons, arranged in cortical columns, strike the optimum balance between two opposing tendencies: transmission speed and component density [30, 31].

Understanding the design rules underlying the micro-level columnar organization will thus be crucial for a better understanding of the brain as a whole. Energy usage poses another conspicuous difference between neural networks in-silico and in-vivo. The Blue Gene/IP supercomputer, used to model a cat's cerebral cortex, requires orders of magnitude more energy than an actual cat brain and still runs about 100 times slower [32]. The main issue is that transistor based networks convert most of the energy used into heat. Brains make considerably more efficient use of the energy they consume (about 20% of the resting metabolism) [33–35], about 50% is used to drive signals across synapses with the remainder supporting the maintenance of resting membrane potentials and the vegetative function of neurons and glia.

It should be noted that cortical gray matter consumes a higher proportion of energy (75%) than white matter [36] highlighted by the fact that global connectivity in the cortex is very sparse: the probability of any two neurons having a direct connection is around 1:100 for neurons in vertical columns 1 mm in diameter but only 1:1,000,000 for distant neurons. These findings point to another major design rule: use the majority of resources for modular, local signaling and computing (gray matter) and spend the rest on long-range communication (myelinated axons: white matter) linking the distributed computational units. Finally, energy constraints also govern the optimal coding schemes. It is well established that redundancy reduction is a major design principle in the cortex [37]. By maximizing the ratio between information coded and energy expended for signal transmission and resting state maintenance, sparse coding regimes improve energy efficiency [38–40].

Sparse coding regimes, in which a small proportion of neurons signal at any one time, have the additional benefit of a large representational capacity [41]. An improved appreciation of the geometrical and energy constraints that are fundamental to the functioning of the brain should provide a valuable guide for the study of neuronal network architecture and coding. We have already learned that neurons do not statically integrate information as transistors do and also that the electric fields generated by neuronal activity, in turn can affect neuronal activity itself [42]. We should thus ask whether it is appropriate to assume a binary code for neural networks or whether a more holistic view is required. Current attempts to computationally mimic brain function attempt to do so by fitting form to expected function; our unitary system proposal offers an alternative to persisting in a computer hardware-inspired understanding of the human brain by asserting the necessity of comprehending the physical expression cognition on each medium at which it operates at level that reveals the cognitive min and the cortical primitives .

A forthcoming article "How much information should we drop to become intelligent?" [43] explores a simulation model that is based on the idea of payment as a means that could be defined as processing cost. It could reflect that cognitive processing for categorizing comes at an energy cost. This works well under the following thought experiment: All objects are placed in one category → no processing needed for categorizing → "low entropy." All objects are placed in own category → processing needed for categorizing → "high entropy." A fundamental question remains: why would dispersal of energy (entropy) be the price to pay for categorizing? It is, of course an abstract question, but otherwise it might be any cost function. In addition, dispersion would be the natural tendency of a system. This work would also imply that it is "harder" (costs more energy) to classify an object as a member of a group rather than a group itself (higher abstraction), and would simultaneously explain why good ideas yield more questions than answers.

Consider how energy usage poses a conspicuous difference between neural networks in-silico and in-vivo. This leads me to assert that an energy paradox exists in the brain, whereby energy usage poses another conspicuous difference between neural networks in-silico and in-vivo. But more specifically a paradox in which energy use is not equal to cognitive throughput (ct), between neural networks in-silico and in-vivo, where ct is always > eMax, and CMax sits at the parallel operation of large data. Energy constraints are governed by optimal coding principles and it is well established that redundancy reduction is a major design principle in the cortex. By maximizing the ratio between information coded, and energy expended for signal transmission and resting state maintenance, sparse coding regimes can improve energy efficiency. Sparse coding regimes, in which a small proportion of neurons signal at any one time, have the additional benefit of a large representational capacity [43–45].

## 3    The Brain Code

Morse code is an appropriate metaphor to express Brain Code paradigm, for it describes a simple code to express meaning and concepts however complex they may be. Yet it is basic in its structure. If we assume a Morse code is transmitted via many multiple modalities, and subsystems of the cortical universe, it will survive the molecular pathway journey and reach a higher function, such as language. Also, there is uniformity, as the structure must remain the same throughout any transmission. The unitary basis for conceptualizing the brain's combined throughputs uses the etymology of the Brain Code and the Fundamental Code Unit to offer a theoretical framework that supports advances of cortical computing. Essentially, the FCU hypothesis is an attempt to offer a system of code-methodology, which governs fundamental neuron communication across all brain activities, that which formed the fundamental unit of thought through evolution. Therefore, it is hypothesized that behavior, intelligence, cognition and conscience are all products of and expressed using the same schema of coding in both stimulus processing and decoding.

A comprehensive model that can explain how high level functioning is affected by biological coding is currently underdeveloped. Encoding behavioral information from cognitive states is computationally possible using the "Brain Code" model. The Brain Code is designed to enhance our study and understanding of human cognition. Anderson [46] proposes neural reuse as a fundamental organizational principle of neural networks in the brain.

In particular, he suggests that structures and resources within the brain are often allocated according to current needs, rather than created on an ad-hoc basis. Functions sharing cognitive resources include "evolution and development of the brain, including (for instance) the evolutionary-developmental pathway supporting primate tool use and human language; the degree of modularity in brain organization; the degree of localization of cognitive function; and the cortical parcellation problem and the prospects (and proper methods to employ) for function to structure mapping." Anderson thus provides further support for the notion that the key to deciphering cognition lies in the ability to properly understand brain networks in their specific temporal contexts. To provide a superior understanding of cognition, one must demonstrate not only that these processes are related, but show how they relate to one another.

To that end, the Brain Code (BC) framework we propose is a unified analysis of patterns in neural oscillation, linguistics, behavior enabled by simultaneous data stream acquisition and analysis. By causally linking sensory stimuli, cognitive activity, and cognitive outputs such as language and behavior, the BC framework maintains the networked structure of the brain, but is populated with units specifically relevant to cognition. Because we don't yet possess the ability to manipulate and interact directly with these networks, the Brain Code framework interpolates multiple data streams and modalities, including electroencephalography (EEG), speech recording and analysis, and movement analysis, to provide an accurate portrayal of the inner workings of the brain. This data fusion is superior to single-stream analyses for two primary reasons.

The first is the incomplete and largely uncertain picture painted by many such methods. Linguistic analysis, for instance, can only reveal so much about the cognitive state of the individual, because language is a voluntary act that is controlled and regulated by conscious thought. Thus, cognitive state will not always be evident in speech. By expanding cognitive state and cognitive analysis to realms that are less under conscious control, such as recurring movements behavioral and neural oscillation patterns, it is possible to develop a more complete picture of the mind, as well as deviations between conscious and unconscious mind processes to discern state of order or disorder. The brain code will initially apply machine learning. Despite the limitations it will provide a means to determine the most relevant features and provide a prediction of future behavior. Future work will evaluate additional methods to include the testing of additional BC specific wavelets.

## 3.1    Brain Code Defined

While Brain Code is an abstract phenomenon in that it is a human cognitive construct, it is composed of physical and chemical phenomena whose interactivity is still not well understood. By designing data units, data acquisition hardware, and novel cognitive data structures, we intend to demonstrate in this section that, given high quality properly formatted data, we can shed light on this interactivity. In addition to the methods outlined in this paper for analyzing individual data streams, a key component of brain code derivation is tracing the relationship each of these data streams has with the others. Shibata et al. [47] present an FMRI neurofeedback method for inducing visual perceptual learning that bears relevance to my position in that their findings contain two important implications first, visual perceptual learning (VPL) in the early visual cortex of adult primates is sufficiently malleable so that fMRI feedback can influence the acquisition of new information and skills when applied to the correct region of the brain [47].

Second, these methods can induce not only the acquisition of new skills and on formation but can aid in the recovery of neurological connections that have been damaged by accident or disease. For instance, a trauma victim suffering from language skill loss can potentially recover those skills through fMRI neurofeedback induction. BC method seeks the same state clarity in cognition, but further proposes that cognition on process level must be based on some finite number of neurological connections – those same connections influenced by the activity of fMRI neurofeedback. This process does not target a single neuron, but a locality of connected neurons, and based on its positive effects on the conscious process of Visual Perceptual Learning.

Shibata's fMRI could be an induction research that could provide powerful evidence for the composition of thought because it can be used to determine the minimum amount of neuronal connectivity for the formation of thoughts. In today's state of the art technology, our primary means of monitoring activity within the brain is to measure the electromagnetic phenomena produced by the brain's activities. Electroencephalography, for instance, allows identification of the brain areas and networks activated by the patient's responses to specific stimuli. In most research settings, these stimuli include hyperventilation, visual stimuli such as flashing lights, directed mental activity, and sleep pattern manipulation. While EEG and similar real-time brain monitoring methods may appear to be the most promising avenue of clinical brain and cognitive research, technology has not yet matured to the point of providing sufficient spatial resolution to identify specific neural webs that are being activated by certain stimuli. For that reason, EEG is often used in broad category diagnosis such as the identification of comas, encephalopathies, and, in some cases, brain death.

These disparate methods beg an important question: how do we extract brain code from these data streams? Because none of these methods can provide a complete brain code by themselves, it is important to develop a method that allows each to compensate for the others' shortcomings. For instance, EEG monitoring alone cannot reveal the precise conceptual neural webs being activated during exposure to a stimuli.

However, as quantities of data rise, pattern analysis based on a combination of electroencephalographic monitoring, linguistic assessment and behavioral tracking can identify those concepts from a cognitive perspective, as well as the neurological phenomena related to them. For example, a patient suffering from cynophobia (abnormal fear of dogs) will reveal aberrant EEG readings when shown a picture of a dog. However, EEG alone will do little more than to identify a disorder that is already obvious to a clinician. If we combine behavior and linguistics into this assessment, we can create an "informed self-report" based on a brain code, in which cognitive state analysis is conducted alongside the patient's own speech output.

Self-reporting may reveal a traumatic incident with a dog early in the patient's life, and linguistic analysis of that self-report, along with behavioral data can identify further the source of the cynophobia, whether it was the result of a single experience, long-term conditioning, or concept conflation. A brain code analysis of a patient such as this would include thorough EEG testing using a broad spectrum of dog-related sensory stimuli, in addition to linguistic analysis of the patient's self-report and an IMU-based assessment of body language.

In the cynophobia example, we expect that a patient shown pictures of dogs as stimuli (or perhaps shown a live dog in a controlled environment) would have EEG signatures pointing to an activation of the amygdala (recalling a remembered fear reaction such as anticipatory anxiety), as well as activation of the hypothalamus. Behavioral analysis based on movement patterns captured with inertial measurement units (IMU's) would distinguish the patient's behavior as part of a learned pattern or spontaneous, and mind-state analysis of the context and content of the patient's linguistic output would yield further insight about the nature of the patient's fear.

# 4    Brain Code Multimodal Fusion Model Case Study

Understanding cortical computing is crucial for addressing several scientific and medical challenges such as the expected increase in the prevalence of neurodegenerative diseases. The growing understanding of brain-like computations suggests that at the strategic level this challenge should be addressed from a fresh perspective. A Brain Code Platform (BCP) has been proposed as an integrative environment for measuring brain activity. The BCP will focus on cheap and noninvasive measurement of brain-activity at (1) several complementary levels of analysis, in (2) naturalistic settings (3) by fusing brain related activities such as speech and movement and by (4) using novel mathematical tools for understanding these activities, fusing different measurements of the brain and brain-related activities, and using this information fusion for early warning signals for the outburst of neurodegenerative diseases. This platform is based on analysis of brain primitives through spontaneous patterns of activation. A growing understanding in the field of brain-like computations is the critical importance that a-priory information plays in the generation of computational primitives. We would like to review the growing evidence that such a-priory information is readily available for examination in the human brain- through the newly discovered phenomena of spontaneously emerging neuronal activity patterns. These patterns offer a unique window into in-built, a-priory information that plays a critical role in cortical networks on the one hand, and in allowing powerful and optimal computational processes that are inherent in human cognition. Such a-priory information has been amply recognized as playing a critical role in numerous cognitive functions- from perception to motor control [48-69].

An important set of computational failures concerns cases where cognitive biases are distorted to such an extreme level that they lead to cortical mal-function. We argue that the resting state patterns should recapitulate the typical functional abnormalities encountered by patients suffering from brain pathologies. Although a large body of data is rapidly accumulating with regards to abnormalities of spontaneous patterns (SPs) associated with various brain pathologies- surprisingly few studies have attempted to directly compare task-related abnormalities with their corresponding SPs [70-72].

The BCP will allow us to measure the spontaneous patterns of subjects at different levels of analysis in a non-invasive way. The information gained through this measurement will be integrated with the measurement of speech and movement that have been found to be efficient indicators of pathologies in neurodegerative disease [7, 73-89]. Novel mathematical tools and methodologies, such as the affine invariance [90] and dynamic graph methods will be used to identify patterns in the data, pattern that through Machine Learning algorithms aim to predict the outburst of the neurode-gerative disease.

Here we review a cognitive load experiment, evaluating the effect of everyday living behavior on cognitive processing [91, 92]. A spatial auditory Stroop task was used. The input signal consisted of a spatial signal (sound in left or right ear) with a sound ("Left" or "right"). After cognitive processing was assessed using the Stroop task a simple behavioral response was required depending on if the sound and spatial orientation matched or differed, by shaking the head. It has been shown that the planum temporale region is responsible for perceiving the location of sounds [93]. The neurons in this region represent, in a non-intentional or pre-attentive fashion, the location of sound sources in the environment. Space representation in this region may provide the neural substrate needed for an orientation response to critical auditory events and for linking auditory information with information acquired through other modalities. This indicates a neural basis that can be linked with the defined brain encoding for this example. A connection between different modalities has been shown between e.g. speech and vision [94]. This link can be structural, but the brain code provides a more abstract approach. The concept relies on the well-known phenomenon of resonance [95]. The resonance transfer of energy between molecules, or between sites within a large molecule, plays a central role in many areas of modern chemistry and physics [96]. There is evidence that stochastic resonance within the human brain can enhance behavioral responses to weak sensory inputs [97].

Both speech and intended movement can be transformed to wavelets to provide a signal that can resonate [98, 99]. The fundamental frequency of speech is roughly 50–210 Hz [100] and for movement the relevant physiological range is .5–10 Hz [101]. Signals are normalized against those ranges generating a unitary pseudo frequency. The association between these modalities can be determined based on the coherence between wavelets from normalized signals. We performed a brain code analysis by extracting each of these data streams, performing interdependent time series analysis on each, A machine learning approach is currently used as placeholder for linking the different data streams. Once specific features start to emerge a unitary method will be introduced. This replacement of machine learning with unitary math provides a generalization across data streams, which allows for further direct linkage between modalities.

# 5     Examining the Brain Code Principles

A growing understanding in the field of brain-like computations is the critical importance that a-priory information plays in the generation of computational primitives. For example in [102]—a critical parameter in developing brain-inspired visual recognitions algorithm is the incorporation of a-priory information about informative vs. uninformative primitives of visual recognition. Such extensive information, which typically can be derived either through evolutionary processes or through daily experience, is available to the system a-priori—i.e. even before it interacts with the optical information. By embedding vast levels of such a-priory information in the computational primitives- the task of recognition systems becomes much more efficient and performance is greatly improved. The critical question that is still unclear is to what extent the human brain actually makes use of such information, whether it is acquired only during early development, and whether it extends throughout all cognitive processes.

Contrary to previous concepts- the incorporation of a-priory information is an extremely pervasive process, that occurs throughout all daily life, extends to all cognitive and neuronal aspects- and can explain both the outstanding computational capabilities of the human brain on the one hand, but also its devastation in various brain pathologies on the other. There is growing evidence that such a-priory information is readily available for examination in the human brain- through the newly discovered phenomena of spontaneously emerging neuronal activity patterns.

## 5.1     Spontaneously Emerging Spatiotemporal Neuronal Activity Patterns

While traditionally most cognitive neuroscience research has focused on mapping the details of task-induced activation patterns, more recently it is becoming evident that highly informative activity goes on also in the absence of such overt tasks.

Thus, it is now becoming quite clear that even during rest the brain is active- and not in a random manner, but in a highly complex rich and robust pattern of activity [103]. Furthermore, these activity patterns have now been documented not only in brain imaging but in single units and -LFP recordings as well [104-106], showing ultra-slow dynamics [107].

The functional role of these spontaneous (also termed "resting state") patterns (SP) remains elusive. However, regardless of their function we can ask- what can these patterns tell us about the underlying cortical function? I would like to propose here that these patterns offer a unique window into in-built, a-priory information that plays a critical role in cortical networks on the one hand, and in allowing powerful and optimal computational processes that are inherent in human cognition.

Since the pioneering work of Hebb (1949) it has been realized that such a-priory biases are embodied in the synaptic efficacies of synaptic connections in cortical networks. SPs uncover the underlying structure of synaptic connectivity in cortical networks and thus offer us a unique window into the a-priory information stored in the cortex. More generally- these a-priory tendencies are an essential component in determining individual traits and sensitivities in typical and individuals suffering from brain pathologies. Thus, the SPs may provide an important and unique window into deciphering such biases in individual brains.

Such a-priory information has been amply recognized as playing a critical role in numerous cognitive functions—from perception to motor control [48-69].

### 5.2    A Toy Model of A-Priory Biases

Why should SPs reflect the cortical a-priory network biases? To illustrate how the hypothetical link comes about we will consider a highly simplified "toy" model (Figure 3). We start by considering a simple feed-forward circuit, consisting of four V1-like "line detectors" that feed converging inputs into a target high order neuron. Following Hebbian learning we expect the training pattern to generate a corresponding modification of synaptic efficacies—essentially embedding a trace of the average co-activations in the network connections (red plus signs). Importantly, note that the restructuring of the connectivity strength of this simple circuit now endows it with a-priory sensitivity towards a triangle shape.

The crucial question to consider with regards to the SPs is what happens to this simple toy model when sensory inputs are blocked—i.e., in a state of "rest"? Making the simplest assumption of residual internal noise that uniformly drives cortical neurons- it is not difficult to see (bottom panel)—that under the impact of uniform random activations, the tendency of the red neurons will be to co-activate- due to their strong excitatory connectivity, while the red and blue neurons will be de-correlated given the weak synaptic biases in this case.

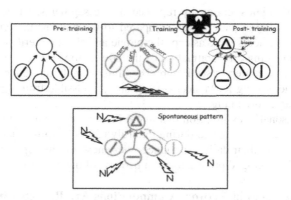

**Fig. 3.** Toy model

Thus, the spontaneous activity will uncover the pattern underlying connectional structure—essentially recapitulating the trained trace of a-priory network biases. Simply put- the inherent, spontaneously generated, noise in the system is sufficient to uncover the a-priory synaptic biases of cortical networks. Such biases could then be measured by mapping the correlation structures (also termed "Functional Connectivity", FC) in the spontaneous activity fluctuations—the spontaneous patterns—that emerge during rest.

### 5.3    Experimental Support for the Hypothesis

While this is of course a highly over-simplified model, it contains within it three main testable predictions that we will review below. First, we expect that the SPs will generally correspond to the average "training" of cortical networks during natural daily life. Second, we would expect the SPs to reflect individual differences in network and cognitive biases, including reflection of cortical abnormalities. Finally, given the dependence of a-priory biases on prior training- it should be possible to re-shape the structure of SPs through controlled focused task-activation under laboratory conditions. Below we consider the experimental evidence pertinent to each of these predictions.

**Spontaneous Patterns Reflect Daily Activation Patterns.** The first prediction is based on the assumption illustrated in Figure 3—that the structure of the SPs reflects the average "training" patterns that cortical networks exhibit in the course of daily life. Given the methodological limitations of our ability to follow cortical activations during natural conditions, this prediction cannot be precisely tested using current methodologies. However, first order approximations are abundant.

As previously argued by [108], a fruitful methodology for approximating naturalistic stimuli, at least within the domain of audio-visual cortical systems, could be the use of movies. Following this logic, and taking advantage of the fact that during sleep SPs appear to be as informative as during the wake resting state [107, 109], Ramot et al [110] have used ECOG recordings in patients to map the correlation structure generated in the patients' cortex by repeated movie segments. Critically, when this movie-driven correlation pattern was compared to the patterns that emerged spontaneously when the patients were asleep- the movie and sleep patterns were significantly correlated- indicating a recapitulation of the correlation structure of the movie driven and spontaneous patterns (see Figure 3).    Interestingly the range of patterns was significantly richer during REM sleep—suggesting a possible from the typical resting state statistics during dreaming.

Under the reasonable assumption that approximately the same networks were activated during movie watching and during the truly natural audio-visual stimulation the patients underwent in their daily experience- then these results support the notion that the SPs reflect the averaged prior activation patterns of the patients.

**Individual Differences in Network Computations Are Reflected in Spontaneous Patterns.** While the main body of brain imaging research has focused on mapping common principles of human cortical function- an important complementary aspect relates to individual differences- how unique cognitive biases and traits of individuals are reflected in their cortical organization. A number of studies reveal that these patterns should provide a potentially powerful method to map such cognitive traits across individuals and unique groups.

Important set of computational failures concerns cases where cognitive biases are distorted to such an extreme level that they lead to cortical mal-function. In this case the STR hypothesis predicts that the resting state patterns should recapitulate the typical functional abnormalities encountered by patients suffering from brain pathologies. Although a large body of data is rapidly accumulating with regards to abnormalities of SPs associated with various brain pathologies- surprisingly few studies have attempted to directly compare task-related abnormalities with their corresponding SPs [70-72].

In the visual domain, Gilaie-Dotan et al [70] have compared visual activation patterns in an individual suffering from a developmental form of object agnosia with his SPs. A striking abnormality in the visual activation pattern in this individual was manifested in a profound inactivation of mid-hierarchy visual areas during processing of a variety of visual stimuli. Such inactivation is expected to produce a strong decorrelation between these mid-areas and the rest of visual areas during naturalistic viewing. As expected from the STR hypothesis—examining the SPs revealed a similar disruption in FC of the SPs in this individual (see Figure 4).

In an important study Baldassarre et al. [111] a correlation between individual differences in resting state FC and individual differences in performance of a subsequent novel perceptual task. According to Zou et al intrinsic resting state activity (ALFF – amplitude of low-frequency fluctuations) can predict subsequent task-evoked brain responses and behavioral performance in a working memory task [112]. ALFF-behavior correlations were also described for object color knowledge tasks [113] and resting state FC has been shown to predict cognitive control and intelligence [114, 115], as well as reading competency [116, 117] and pain perception [118, 119]. A number of other studies have demonstrated similar predictive properties of spontaneous ongoing activity on individual performance [67, 69, 116, 120-129] and even personality traits [130].

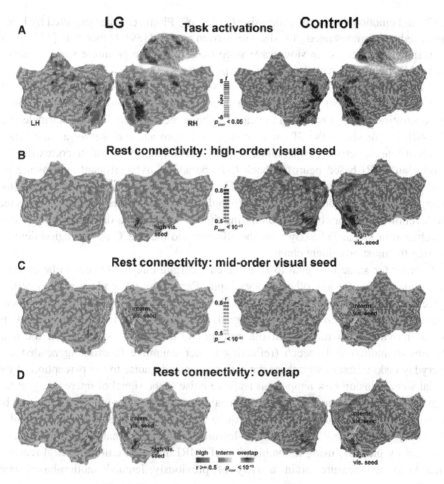

**Fig. 4.** Task activation and rest connectivity [70]

## 5.4    Examining Storage of A-Priory Information under Laboratory Conditions

Finally, the most direct mean studying the dynamic storage of a-priory information is to inject such information under laboratory conditions. A number of recent studies have indeed addressed this possibility under carefully controlled experiments. Thus, it was shown that prolonged exposure to distinct categories of visual information causes differential coupling of frontal networks with posterior category-selective visual regions during subsequent rest [131]. A connection between mechanisms of learning and resting state activity was also described for associative encoding [129], visual perceptual learning [132], motor learning [133-135], semantic matching [136], language comprehension

[137], and emotional and pain processing [118, 138]. Plastic changes triggered by learning have been demonstrated  for sleep regulation as well [139]. Huber et al. [139] found have shown an increase in slow-wave sleep localized to the premotor site that underwent TMS-induced potentiation during the previous wakefulness.

If indeed the SPs reflect past cortical activations—the a-priory information should, in principle, be present at a fairly long delay after the original activation. A direct demonstration that this is indeed the case has been recently provided by Harmelech et al [140]. In this study, the SPs were compared before and *a day after* a single short epoch of intense activation was induced in the dorsal anterior cingulate cortex (dACC ) using an fMRI-based neurofeedback (NF) paradigm. A significant and lasting restructuring of the SPs according to a Hebbian-like rule was observed. Thus, the change (increase and decrease) in FC strength of cortical voxels during rest reflected the level of their prior co-activation during the NF epoch. Data-driven examination of the change in global FC a day after the NF revealed the dACC as the region demonstrating the most prominent change.

In order for an audio signal to be detected a certain threshold needs to be crossed. The same applies for any other sensory input. Perception takes place when a certain perceptual dynamic threshold is crossed. However, capacity might already have been taken up for proper perception of the signal, due to additional tasks such as speaking and/or moving. This means that the perceptual "threshold" is reliant on the data streams of motion and speech (reflecting higher cognitive functioning needed e.g. everyday tasks). Essentially, these data streams can add noise to the perception of the initial signal. Fusion now happens as additive noise to the signal of interest (e.g. audio signal "left"). Subsequently, this will mean that a particular signal "left" can be drowned out if too many other things require attention/cognitive function. Werheid et al. [141] investigated implicit rule learning in a combination of Parkinson's and healthy patients, using a combination of fMRI and a variation of serial reaction time tasks to measure brain activity of previously learned motion-based task sequences.

The results of this study suggest that activations in the frontomedian and posterior cingulate cortex, instead of random blocks, are linked to a larger role for the frontomedian cortex in stimulus prediction, an area of cognitive deficit in Parkinson's patients. Patients with early-stage Parkinson's disease experienced difficulties in the pre-training phase of the experiment, but rule-learning remained intact during fMRI data acquisition when the rules had been instilled and stimulus prediction was taken out of the equation. fMRI results showed very little difference between the PD and control patients in terms of frontomedian and posterior cingulate activations, and that the effect on patients with early stage PD of the disease progression is primarily limited to lateral striatofrontal dopaminergic projections, because medial dopaminergic projections, which are used in the application of previously known "rules," or routines, are not significantly affected by the disease in this stage.

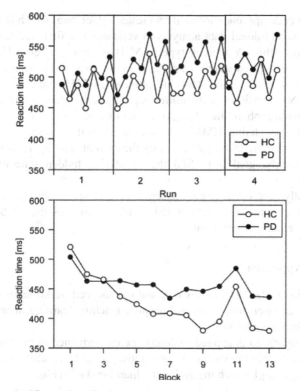

**Fig. 5.** There is a significant disparity between reaction times for healthy controls (white) and patients with Parkinson's disease (black)

Figure 5 depicts Z-maps that show the contrast between 'Sequence' and 'Random' condition for healthy controls and patients with Parkinson's disease. Note that in patients with PD, the activity level decreases in the transition from sequence to random activities, suggesting greater difficulty with stimuli for which the patients are unprepared. This phenomenon is notably absent in the healthy control component. Their findings are in agreement with the results of the cognitive load experiment previously discussed [91]. The fMRI study confirms that processing will show differential indicators during task load conditions.

## 6    Discussion

Python codes developed to date based on the Brain Code methodology contain two functions for time-frequency analysis and machine learning classifiers. It is necessary to show in a single equation or method that there is utility in using a brain code approach instead of current machine learning (ML) methods; here I have suggested the use of wavelets to show where the work will progress after ML. Wavelets are more specific to the application of BC. Work done to date on fusing multiple data streams within the brain code approach focused and tested affect data, which is easily extendable, but requires additional data analysis to validate. The first step was to focus on the predictive algorithm. A specific type of Markov chain, called a Hidden Markov Model (HMM) was applied where the states are unknown, and therefore are "hidden", however the emissions from the states are observed. HMMs are composed of hidden states, $S=\{1,...,N\}$, transition probabilities, $a_{ij}$ = transition probability from state i to state j, and emission probabilities, $b_j(o_m) = P(\text{emitting } o_m | S=j)$.

Similar to Markov chains, HMMs also are based on the property that at each time step t, the future state $S_{t+1}$ is only affected by the current state $S_t$. Therefore, given the visible emissions, the goal is to find the underlying hidden state of each of the emissions.

Mathematically, for each given sequence of emissions $O=\{o_1,o_2,...o_t\}$, the sequence of hidden states S is determined which maximizes the probability of the hidden states given the observations.

## 6.1    Tested Approach

Attempts to train an HMM from raw data did not succeed, scikit-learn was used (scikit-learn.org) as an open source general-purpose machine learning library for Python, and using the Gaussian HMM.

The Viterbi algorithm is applied to determine the sequence of hidden states S contained in S which makes the visible states O most probable, resulting in a set of Viterbi paths $Q=\{q_1,q_2,...,q_t\}$ which maximize the likelihood of $P(E|\lambda)$.

Formally,

$$P(O|\lambda) = \pi_{q1}b_{q1}(o_1)a_{q1q2}b(o_2)\,...\,a_{qt-1qt}b_{qt}(o_t)$$
$$= \pi_{q1}b_{q1}(o_1)\prod_{(k)=2}^{t} a_{q(k)-1q(k)}b_{q(k)}\big(o_{(k)}\big) = f(\pi,a)\prod_{(k)=1}^{t} b_{q(k)}\big(o_{(k)}\big)$$

*(Equation 3.1 from Xydeas et al., 2006)*

The method was tested on upper limb data [91]. The upper limb motion patterns were obtained by an IMU sensor attached to the wrist. The Euclidian norm of the acceleration signal was used as main feature, as accelerations can be applied to differentiate between different motions [142] The norm was determined by

$$\|a\| = \sqrt{a_x^2 + a_y^2 + a_z^2}$$

with $a$ as the 3D acceleration vector $[a_x\ a_y\ a_z]$. The norm was computed for each index point and the signal was subsequently segmented in 1-second windows. It has already been shown that smooth eye movements require cognitive attention during selective tracking tasks (Barnes 2008). The smoothness of other selective tasks, as seen in everyday living, might also have a similar cognitive component which could affect smoothness. The Hurst parameter ($H$) describes the sharpness of the acceleration signal, with a higher value indicating a smoother motion. Parameter estimation of fractional Brownian motion based on wavelets can be applied in order to approximate $H$.

The first assumption for the presented task would be that smoothness starts to vary more as cognitive loading is introduced. However, relying more on an automated movement process when an additional cognitive task is introduced might also have the opposite effect. Therefore, the exact change of the signal is likely to be subject dependent. The changes in the parameter are described by obtaining the standard deviation of several 1-second windows. The threshold value ($T_h$) was computed for each subject by taking the average of the standard deviation found for one loaded and one unloaded condition. Data from 10 subjects containing two loaded and two unloaded conditions, which were needed for determining a subject dependent threshold (training set), as well as an additional data set for testing the accuracy of the prediction. The described approach aimed to correctly predict cognitive loading based only upon the estimated variation of $H$ during the movement task. The results show that the model makes a better than chance prediction (Table 1). This particular method provided an accuracy of 65% (Table 1). The test results for the prediction of 10 subjects who performed an everyday living activity, with or without an additional stroop task.

**Table 1.** Performance outcomes for the different tasks

|  | Loaded condition | Unloaded condition |
|---|---|---|
| Loaded prediction | 9 | 1 |
| Unloaded prediction | 6 | 4 |
|  | Sensitivity 60% | Specificity 80% |

The outcomes show that we could predict with a sensitivity of 60% and specificity of 80% if the auditory stroop task was introduced just by looking at an accelerometer on the wrist during a normal everyday task.

The single loaded tasks consisted either of speaking or preparing the meal, while the dual task required both while performing the Stroop task. The results are given in Table 2. No statistically significant differences in reaction time were seen between the three conditions.

**Table 2.** Performance outcomes for the different tasks

|  | Speech (n = 66) | Motion (n = 66) | Speech + motion (n = 99) |
|---|---|---|---|
| Missing data   (%) | 5 | 6 | 1 |
| Correct responses   (%) | 88 | 94 | 77 |
| Reaction time(s) Mean ± standard deviation | 2.15 ± 0.75 | 1.80 ± 0.47 | 2.11 ± 1.53 |

# 7    Conclusion and Future Work

While the complexity of systems that are not inherently linear lends itself to difficulty in expressing the physical phenomena within itself.t o those structures, I propose the methodology of the Brain Code, a representation scheme designed initially to enhance our study of human brain disorders, mainly the early detection of neurodegenerative disease. The properties of codes and their fitness for a specific application, in this case the biological solution of the human brain, requires an accurate but also relevant and energy efficient description. Applying machine learning as placeholder in order to identify relevant features and subsequently introducing unitary math as a proper interface between in- and output provides the base for the brain code. The Brain Code offers a theoretical framework that bridges the gap between cognitive outputs—the mind—and the biological, chemical, and physical source of those processes—the brain. The "Brain Code" framework is a large task to accomplish; it is attractive for an open source scale approach. Thus BC is argued as a design principle that leads to a framework. As the initial task requires the construction of a wavelet function or set of wavelets for each modality possibly one mother wavelet for a combined modality should also be tested. Because wavelets can describe audio / speech / movement and brain activity in same domains, this also allows all modalities to be described in the "same" way. After testing a mother wavelet, links to resonance and energy input and output should be investigated.

Neural algorithms that form the basis of inference and recognition in the brain are a potential basis for creating new types of machine learning algorithms that potentially meet human-like performance characteristics better than today's leading systems, like the model for parallel processing in neural systems and computers [143]. The Brain Code suggests that within a given cortical region or cognitive/sensory domain, the brain employs hierarchical algorithms composed of repeated instances of a limited set of computing "primitives" or modular constructs.

These primitives are further theorized to be embodied in cortical microcircuits at various scales, as part of the evolutionary method of solving this biological solution through nature. Although there has been significant progress in understanding multiple aspects of cortical microcircuits and the larger networks in which they are embedded, a comprehensive description of their structure, function, and interconnectivity remains elusive. Consequently, a myriad of mathematical, computational, conceptual, and schematic models have been proposed to describe the nature of the cortical computing primitives and the hierarchical algorithms that employ mathematical, computational, or otherwise executable models of cortical computing supported by neuroanatomy.

Most models are purely conceptual, schematic, or descriptive, for example a framework that simultaneously acquires and analyzes multiple cognitive and behavioral data streams. Specifically, those presenting analytical models to combine neural models and cognitive models, as well as offer a means to infer "relationships that might exist between the biological and physical properties of the brain and higher-level cognitive processes [144].

Very little is known about the underlying processes that drive cognition. Thus, an effective model of cognition, which can be used to both interpret and interact with cognition in-vivo, must be able to link each natural process involved in cognition, from behavior to language to individual neural activations, in a coherent manner. Such a joint modeling framework would account for the necessity of a unified "timeline" through which meaningful experimental analysis can be performed. This information may be used to formulate a new program aimed at developing novel machine learning algorithms based on high fidelity representations of cortical microcircuits [44].

**Acknowledgement.** Section 2.1, and section 5 were largely contributions from Andreas Ioannides and Rafael Malach, respectively, for a proposal submitted to IARPA-RFI-13-05: Cortical Computing. This paper also includes contributions from John F. Stein, Yair Neuman and Jeroen Bergmann thank you all so much for your valuable input. This paper benefited from editing efforts of Rebecca Howard and Alexis Stern. I am also thankful to Alexander Gelbukh, who provided valuable feedback and assistance with the publication process. I would also like to thank all researchers and consultants at Biological Coprocessors Inc.  who participated in this. This work was made possible in part by funding from The Brain Sciences Foundation (Providence, RI) and DOD funding, as well as IARPA funding under the metaphor research program.

# References

1. Howard, N.: Brain Language: The Fundamental Code Unit. The Brain Sciences Journal 1(1), 4–45 (2012)
2. Howard, N.: The Fundamental Code Unit of the Brain: Deciphering the DNA of Cognition. Frontiers Systems Neuroscience (commissioned, in preparation, 2013)
3. Howard, N., Rao, D., Fahlstrom, R., Bergmann, J., Stein, J.: The Fundamental Code Unit-Applying Neural Oscillation Detection Across Clinical Conditions. Frontiers (commissioned, in Preparation, 2013)
4. Howard, N., Rao, D., Fahlstrom, R., Stein, J.: The Fundamental Code Unit: A Framework for Biomarker Analysis. In: Proc. The 2nd Neurological Biomarkers Conference at the 2013 Biomarker Summit, San Francisco, California, March 20-22 (2013)
5. Fitzgibbons, P.J., Wightman, F.L.: Gap detection in normal and hearing-impaired listeners. J. Acoust. Soc. Am. 72(3), 761–765 (1982)
6. Rubinsztein, D.C.: The roles of intracellular protein-degradation pathways in neurodegeneration. Nature 443(7113), 780–786 (2006)
7. Howard, N., Bergmann, J., Stein, J.: Combined Modality of the Brain Code Approach for Early Detection and the Long-term Monitoring of Neurodegenerative Processes. Frontiers Special Issue INCF Course Imaging the Brain at Different Scales (2013)
8. Moradi, F., Liu, L.C., Cheng, K., Waggoner, R.A., Tanaka, K., Ioannides, A.A.: Consistent and precise localization of brain activity in human primary visual cortex by MEG and fMRI. Neuroimage 18(3), 595–609 (2003)
9. Ioannides, A.A., Fenwick, P.B.C., Liu, L.: Widely distributed magnetoencephalography spikes related to the planning and execution of human saccades. The Journal of Neuroscience 25(35), 7950–7967 (2005)

10. Ioannides, A.A., Corsi-Cabrera, M., Fenwick, P.B.C., del Rio Portilla, Y., Laskaris, N.A., Khurshudyan, A., Theofilou, D., Shibata, T., Uchida, S., Nakabayashi, T.: MEG tomography of human cortex and brainstem activity in waking and REM sleep saccades. Cerebral Cortex 14(1), 56–72 (2004)

11. Ioannides, A.A.: Dynamic functional connectivity. Current Opinion in Neurobiology 17(2), 161–170 (2007)

12. Ioannides, A.A., Liu, L., Poghosyan, V., Saridis, G.A., Gjedde, A., Ptito, M., Kupers, R.: MEG reveals a fast pathway from somatosensory cortex to occipital areas via posterior parietal cortex in a blind subject. Front. Hum. Neurosci. 7, 429 (2013)

13. Tzelepi, A., Ioannides, A.A., Poghosyan, V.: Early (N70m) neuromagnetic signal topography and striate and extrastriate generators following pattern onset quadrant stimulation. NeuroImage 13(4), 702–718 (2001)

14. Poghosyan, V., Ioannides, A.A.: Precise mapping of early visual responses in space and time. Neuroimage 35(2), 759–770 (2007)

15. Plomp, G., Liu, L., van Leeuwen, C., Ioannides, A.A.: The "mosaic stage" in amodal completion as characterized by magnetoencephalography responses. J. Cogn. Neurosci. 18(8), 1394–1405 (2006)

16. Liu, L.C., Plomp, G., van Leeuwen, C., Ioannides, A.A.: Neural correlates of priming on occluded figure interpretation in human fusiform cortex. Neuroscience 141(3), 1585–1597 (2006)

17. Bakar, A.A., Liu, L., Conci, M., Elliott, M.A., Ioannides, A.A.: Visual field and task influence illusory figure responses. Human Brain Mapping 29(11), 1313–1326 (2008)

18. Liu, L., Ioannides, A.A., Streit, M.: Single trial analysis of neurophysiological correlates of the recognition of complex objects and facial expressions of emotion. Brain Topography 11(4), 291–303 (1999)

19. Ioannides, A.A., Liu, L.C., Kwapien, J., Drozdz, S., Streit, M.: Coupling of regional activations in a human brain during an object and face affect recognition task. Human Brain Mapping 11(2), 77–92 (2000)

20. Ioannides, A.A., Poghosyan, V., Dammers, J., Streit, M.: Real-time neural activity and connectivity in healthy individuals and schizophrenia patients. Neuroimage 23(2), 473–482 (2004)

21. Ioannides, A.A., Kostopoulos, G.K., Liu, L., Fenwick, P.B.C.: MEG identifies dorsal medial brain activations during sleep. Neuroimage 44(2), 455–468 (2009)

22. Poghosyan, V., Ioannides, A.A.: Attention modulates earliest responses in the primary auditory and visual cortices. Neuron 58(5), 802–813 (2008)

23. Ioannides, A.A., Poghosyan, V.: Spatiotemporal dynamics of early spatial and category-specific attentional modulations. NeuroImage 60(3), 1638–1651 (2012)

24. Ioannides, A.A., Poghosyan, V., Liu, L., Saridis, G., Tamietto, M., de Beeck, M.O., De Tiège, X., Weiskrantz, L., De Gelder, B.: Spatiotemporal profiles of visual processing with and without primary visual cortex. Neuroimage (2012)

25. Marx, G., Gilon, C.: The molecular basis of memory. Part 2: chemistry of the tripartite mechanism. ACS Chem. Neurosci. 4(6), 983–993 (2013)

26. Marx, G., Gilon, C.: The Molecular Basis of Memory. ACS Chemical Neuroscience 3(8), 633–642 (2012)

27. Howard, N.: The Twin Hypotheses: Brain Code and the Fundamental Code Unit. Springer Lecture Notes in Artificial Intelligence (in press, 2013)

28. Ramon Cajal, S.: Histology of the nervous system of man and vertebrates. Oxford Univ. Press, New York (1995)

29. Koulakov, A.A., Chklovskii, D.B.: Orientation preference patterns in mammalian visual cortex: a wire length minimization approach. Neuron 29(2), 519–527 (2001)

30. Mitchison, G.: Neuronal branching patterns and the economy of cortical wiring. Proceedings of the Royal Society of London. Series B: Biological Sciences 245(1313), 151–158 (1991)

31. Gara, A., Blumrich, M.A., Chen, D., Chiu, G.L.T., Coteus, P., Giampapa, M.E., Haring, R.A., Heidelberger, P., Hoenicke, D., Kopcsay, G.V., Liebsch, T.A., Ohmacht, M., Steinmacher-Burow, B.D., Takken, T., Vranas, P.: Overview of the Blue Gene/L system architecture. IBM Journal of Research and Development 49(2.3), 195–212 (2005)

32. Rolfe, D.F., Brown, G.C.: Cellular energy utilization and molecular origin of standard metabolic rate in mammals. Physiological Reviews 77(3), 731–758 (1997)

33. Kety, S.S.: The general metabolism of the brain in vivo. Metabolism of the Nervous System, 221–237 (1957)

34. Sokoloff, L.: The metabolism of the central nervous system in vivo. Handbook of Physiology-Neurophysiology 3, 1843–1864 (1960)

35. Aiello, L.C., Bates, N., Joffe, T.: In defense of the expensive tissue hypothesis. In: Evolutionary Anatomy of the Primate Cerebral Cortex, pp. 57–78. Cambridge University Press, Cambridge (2001)

36. Simoncelli, E.P., Olshausen, B.A.: Natural image statistics and neural representation. Annual Review of Neuroscience 24(1), 1193–1216 (2001)

37. Baddeley, A.: The central executive: A concept and some misconceptions. Journal of the International Neuropsychological Society 4(5), 523–526 (1998)

38. Balasubramanian, V., Kimber, D., Berry Ii, M.J.: Metabolically efficient information processing. Neural Computation 13(4), 799–815 (2001)

39. Field, D.J.: What is the goal of sensory coding? Neural Computation 6(4), 559–601 (1994)

40. Levy, W.B., Baxter, R.A.: Energy efficient neural codes. Neural Computation 8(3), 531–543 (1996)

41. Fröhlich, F., McCormick, D.A.: Endogenous electric fields guide neocortical network activity. Neuron 67(1), 129–143 (2010)

42. Nave, O., Neuman, Y., Perlovsky, L., Howard, N.: How much information should we drop to become intelligent? Applied Mathematics and Computation (under review, 2013)

43. Howard, N.: Methods for Cortical Computing. IARPA RFI 13-05 Cortical Computing Primitives and Connectomics (submitted, 2013)

44. Anderson, M.L.: Neural reuse: A fundamental organizational principle of the brain. Behavioral and Brain Sciences 33(4), 245 (2010)

45. Howard, N.: Mathematical Review for Cortical Computation Proposition for Brain Code Hypothesis. Frontiers Systems Neuroscience (commissioned, in preparation 2013)

46. Busch, N.A., Dubois, J., VanRullen, R.: The phase of ongoing EEG oscillations predicts visual perception. The Journal of Neuroscience 29(24), 7869–7876 (2009)

47. Laughlin, S.B., Sejnowski, T.J.: Communication in Neuronal Networks. Science 301(5641), 1870–1874 (2003)

48. Shibata, K., Watanabe, T., Sasaki, Y., Kawato, M.: Perceptual learning incepted by decoded fMRI neurofeedback without stimulus presentation. Science 334(6061), 1413–1415 (2011)

49. Sadaghiani, S., Hesselmann, G., Friston, K.J., Kleinschmidt, A.: The relation of ongoing brain activity, evoked neural responses, and cognition. Frontiers in Systems Neuroscience 4 (2010)

50. Wang, X.-J.: Decision making in recurrent neuronal circuits. Neuron 60(2), 215–234 (2008)
51. Barraclough, D.J., Conroy, M.L., Lee, D.: Prefrontal cortex and decision making in a mixed-strategy game. Nature Neuroscience 7(4), 404–410 (2004)
52. Arieli, A., Sterkin, A., Grinvald, A., Aertsen, A.: Dynamics of ongoing activity: explanation of the large variability in evoked cortical responses. Science 273(5283), 1868–1871 (1996)
53. Ploner, M., Lee, M.C., Wiech, K., Bingel, U., Tracey, I.: Prestimulus functional connectivity determines pain perception in humans. Proceedings of the National Academy of Sciences 107(1), 355–360 (2010)
54. Kayser, C., Montemurro, M.A., Logothetis, N.K., Panzeri, S.: Spike-phase coding boosts and stabilizes information carried by spatial and temporal spike patterns. Neuron 61(4), 597–608 (2009)
55. Arnal, L.H., Giraud, A.-L.: Cortical oscillations and sensory predictions. Trends in Cognitive Sciences 16(7), 390–398 (2012)
56. Stefanics, G., Hangya, B., Hernádi, I., Winkler, I., Lakatos, P., Ulbert, I.: Phase entrainment of human delta oscillations can mediate the effects of expectation on reaction speed. The Journal of Neuroscience 30(41), 13578–13585 (2010)
57. SanMiguel, I., Widmann, A., Bendixen, A., Trujillo-Barreto, N., Schröger, E.: Hearing Silences: Human Auditory Processing Relies on Preactivation of Sound-Specific Brain Activity Patterns. The Journal of Neuroscience 33(20), 8633–8639 (2013)
58. Kok, P., Jehee, J.F., de Lange, F.P.: Less is more: expectation sharpens representations in the primary visual cortex. Neuron 75(2), 265–270 (2012)
59. de Lange, F.P., Rahnev, D.A., Donner, T.H., Lau, H.: Prestimulus oscillatory activity over motor cortex reflects perceptual expectations. The Journal of Neuroscience 33(4), 1400–1410 (2013)
60. Chavan, C.F., Manuel, A.L., Mouthon, M., Spierer, L.: Spontaneous pre-stimulus fluctuations in the activity of right fronto-parietal areas influence inhibitory control performance. Frontiers in Human Neuroscience 7 (2013)
61. Köver, H., Bao, S.: Cortical plasticity as a mechanism for storing Bayesian priors in sensory perception. PloS One 5(5), e10497 (2010)
62. Fiser, J., Berkes, P., Orbán, G., Lengyel, M.: Statistically optimal perception and learning: from behavior to neural representations. Trends in Cognitive Sciences 14(3), 119–130 (2010)
63. Drewes, J., VanRullen, R.: This is the rhythm of your eyes: the phase of ongoing electroencephalogram oscillations modulates saccadic reaction time. The Journal of Neuroscience 31(12), 4698–4708 (2011)
64. Schurger, A., Sitt, J.D., Dehaene, S.: An accumulator model for spontaneous neural activity prior to self-initiated movement. Proceedings of the National Academy of Sciences 109(42), E2904–E2913 (2012)
65. Fried, I., Mukamel, R., Kreiman, G.: Internally generated preactivation of single neurons in human medial frontal cortex predicts volition. Neuron 69(3), 548–562 (2011)
66. Soon, C.S., Brass, M., Heinze, H.-J., Haynes, J.-D.: Unconscious determinants of free decisions in the human brain. Nature Neuroscience 11(5), 543–545 (2008)
67. Engel, A.K., Fries, P., Singer, W.: Dynamic predictions: oscillations and synchrony in top–down processing. Nature Reviews Neuroscience 2(10), 704–716 (2001)
68. Hesselmann, G., Kell, C.A., Eger, E., Kleinschmidt, A.: Spontaneous local variations in ongoing neural activity bias perceptual decisions. Proceedings of the National Academy of Sciences 105(31), 10984–10989 (2008)

69. Boly, M., Balteau, E., Schnakers, C., Degueldre, C., Moonen, G., Luxen, A., Phillips, C., Peigneux, P., Maquet, P., Laureys, S.: Baseline brain activity fluctuations predict somatosensory perception in humans. Proceedings of the National Academy of Sciences 104(29), 12187–12192 (2007)

70. Gilaie-Dotan, S., Hahamy-Dubossarsky, A., Nir, Y., Berkovich-Ohana, A., Bentin, S., Malach, R.: Resting state functional connectivity reflects abnormal task-activated patterns in a developmental object agnosic. Neuroimage 70, 189–198 (2013)

71. Watkins, K.E., Cowey, A., Alexander, I., Filippini, N., Kennedy, J.M., Smith, S.M., Ragge, N., Bridge, H.: Language networks in anophthalmia: maintained hierarchy of processing in 'visual'cortex'. Brain 135(5), 1566–1577 (2012)

72. Liu, J., Qin, W., Yuan, K., Li, J., Wang, W., Li, Q., Wang, Y., Sun, J., von Deneen, K.M., Liu, Y.: Interaction between dysfunctional connectivity at rest and heroin cues-induced brain responses in male abstinent heroin-dependent individuals. PloS One 6(10), e23098 (2011)

73. Fahn, S.: Description of Parkinson's disease as a clinical syndrome. Annals of the New York Academy of Sciences 991(1), 1–14 (2003)

74. Jankovic, J.: Parkinson's disease: clinical features and diagnosis. Journal of Neurology, Neurosurgery & Psychiatry 79(4), 368–376 (2008)

75. Aarsland, D., Brønnick, K., Ehrt, U., De Deyn, P.P., Tekin, S., Emre, M., Cummings, J.L.: Neuropsychiatric symptoms in patients with Parkinson's disease and dementia: frequency, profile and associated care giver stress. Journal of Neurology. Neurosurgery & Psychiatry 78(1), 36–42 (2007)

76. Aarsland, D., Andersen, K., Larsen, J.P., Perry, R., Wentzel-Larsen, T., Lolk, A., Kragh-Sorensen, P.: The rate of cognitive decline in Parkinson disease. Archives of Neurology 61(12), 1906 (2004)

77. Aarsland, D., Larsen, J.P., Lim, N.G., Janvin, C., Karlsen, K., Tandberg, E., Cummings, J.L.: Range of neuropsychiatric disturbances in patients with Parkinson's disease. Journal of Neurology, Neurosurgery & Psychiatry 67(4), 492–496 (1999)

78. Bottini Bonfanti, A.: More than movement: the importance of the evolution of mild cognitive impairment in Parkinson's disease. Journal of Neurology, Neurosurgery & Psychiatry (2013)

79. Chaudhuri, K., Healy, D.G., Schapira, A.H.V.: Non-motor symptoms of Parkinson's disease: diagnosis and management. The Lancet Neurology 5(3), 235–245 (2006)

80. de la Monte, S.M., Wells, S.E., Hedley-Whyte, E.T., Growdon, J.H.: Neuropathological distinction between Parkinson's dementia and Parkinson's plus Alzheimer's disease. Annals of Neurology 26(3), 309–320 (1989)

81. Hu, M., Cooper, J., Beamish, R., Jones, E., Butterworth, R., Catterall, L., Ben-Shlomo, Y.: How well do we recognise non-motor symptoms in a British Parkinson's disease population? J. Neurol. 258(8), 1513–1517 (2011)

82. Riedel, O., Klotsche, J., Spottke, A., Deuschl, G., Förstl, H., Henn, F., Heuser, I., Oertel, W., Reichmann, H., Riederer, P.: Cognitive impairment in 873 patients with idiopathic Parkinson's disease. Journal of Neurology 255(2), 255–264 (2008)

83. Starkstein, S., Preziosi, T., Berthier, M., Bolduc, P., Mayberg, H., Robinson, R.: Depression and cognitive impairment in Parkinson's disease. Brain: a Journal of Neurology 112, 1141–1153 (1989)

84. Wertman, E., Speedie, L., Shemesh, Z., Gilon, D., Raphael, M., Stessman, J.: Cognitive disturbances in parkinsonian patients with depression. Cognitive and Behavioral Neurology 6(1), 31–37 (1993)

85. Bavelier, D., Newport, E.L., Hall, M.L., Supalla, T., Boutla, M.: Persistent Difference in Short-Term Memory Span Between Sign and Speech Implications for Cross-Linguistic Comparisons. Psychological Science 17(12), 1090–1092 (2006)

86. Tsanas, A., Little, M.A., McSharry, P.E., Ramig, L.O.: Nonlinear speech analysis algorithms mapped to a standard metric achieve clinically useful quantification of average Parkinson's disease symptom severity. Journal of the Royal Society Interface 8(59), 842–855 (2011)

87. Tsanas, A., Little, M.A., McSharry, P.E., Spielman, J., Ramig, L.O.: Novel speech signal processing algorithms for high-accuracy classification of Parkinson's disease. IEEE Trans. Biomed. Eng. 59(5), 1264–1271 (2012)

88. Skodda, S., Grönheit, W., Schlegel, U.: Impairment of Vowel Articulation as a Possible Marker of Disease Progression in Parkinson's Disease. PloS One 7(2), e32132 (2012)

89. Howard, N., Stein, J., Aziz, T.: Early Detection of Parkinson's Disease from Speech and Movement Recordings. Oxford Parkinson's Disease Center Research Day (2013)

90. Pham, Q.-C., Bennequin, D.: Affine invariance of human hand movements: a direct test. arXiv preprint arXiv:1209.1467 (2012)

91. Bergmann, J., Fei, J., Green, D., Howard, N.: Effect of Everyday Living Behavior on Cognitive Processing. PloS One (in preparation, 2013)

92. Bergmann, J., Langdon, P., Mayagoita, R., Howard, N.: Exploring the use of sensors to measure behavioral interactions: An experimental evaluation of using hand trajectories. PloS One (under review, 2013)

93. Deouell, L.Y., Heller, A.S., Malach, R., D'Esposito, M., Knight, R.T.: Cerebral responses to change in spatial location of unattended sounds. Neuron 55(6), 985–996 (2007)

94. Blank, H., Anwander, A., von Kriegstein, K.: Direct structural connections between voice-and face-recognition areas. The Journal of Neuroscience 31(36), 12906–12915 (2011)

95. Spiegler, A., Knösche, T.R., Schwab, K., Haueisen, J., Atay, F.M.: Modeling brain resonance phenomena using a neural mass model. PLoS Computational Biology 7(12), e1002298 (2011)

96. Andrews, D.L., Demidov, A.A.: Resonance energy transfer. Wiley (1999)

97. Kitajo, K., Nozaki, D., Ward, L.M., Yamamoto, Y.: Behavioral stochastic resonance within the human brain. Physical Review Letters 90(21), 218103 (2181)

98. Howard, N., Pollock, R., Prinold, J., Sinha, J., Newham, D., Bergmann, J.: Effect of impairment on upper limb performance in an ageing sample population. In: Stephanidis, C., Antona, M. (eds.) UAHCI 2013, Part II. LNCS, vol. 8010, pp. 78–87. Springer, Heidelberg (2013)

99. Kronland-Martinet, R., Morlet, J., Grossmann, A.: Analysis of sound patterns through wavelet transforms. International Journal of Pattern Recognition and Artificial Intelligence 1(02), 273–302 (1987)

100. Traunmüller, H., Eriksson, A.: The frequency range of the voice fundamental in the speech of male and female adults, Manuscript, Department of Linguistics, University of Stockholm (1994), http://www.ling.su.se/staff/hartmut/aktupub.htm (accessed May 8, 2004)

101. Barnes, G.R., Benson, A.J., Prior, A.R.: Visual-vestibular interaction in the control of eye movement. Aviat. Space Environ. Med. 49(4), 557–564 (1978)

102. Lerner, Y., Epshtein, B., Ullman, S., Malach, R.: Class information predicts activation by object fragments in human object areas. J. Cogn. Neurosci. 20(7), 1189–1206 (2008)

103. Nir, Y., Hasson, U., Levy, I., Yeshurun, Y., Malach, R.: Widespread functional connectivity and fMRI fluctuations in human visual cortex in the absence of visual stimulation. Neuroimage 30(4), 1313–1324 (2006)
104. He, B.J., Snyder, A.Z., Zempel, J.M., Smyth, M.D., Raichle, M.E.: Electrophysiological correlates of the brain's intrinsic large-scale functional architecture. Proceedings of the National Academy of Sciences 105(41), 16039–16044 (2008)
105. Manning, J.R., Jacobs, J., Fried, I., Kahana, M.J.: Broadband shifts in local field potential power spectra are correlated with single-neuron spiking in humans. The Journal of Neuroscience 29(43), 13613–13620 (2009)
106. Nir, Y., Dinstein, I., Malach, R., Heeger, D.J.: BOLD and spiking activity. Nature Neuroscience 11(5), 523–524 (2008)
107. Nir, Y., Mukamel, R., Dinstein, I., Privman, E., Harel, M., Fisch, L., Gelbard-Sagiv, H., Kipervasser, S., Andelman, F., Neufeld, M.Y.: Interhemispheric correlations of slow spontaneous neuronal fluctuations revealed in human sensory cortex. Nature Neuroscience 11(9), 1100–1108 (2008)
108. Hasson, U., Nir, Y., Levy, I., Fuhrmann, G., Malach, R.: Intersubject synchronization of cortical activity during natural vision. Science 303(5664), 1634–1640 (2004)
109. Dinstein, I., Pierce, K., Eyler, L., Solso, S., Malach, R., Behrmann, M., Courchesne, E.: Disrupted neural synchronization in toddlers with autism. Neuron 70(6), 1218–1225 (2011)
110. Ramot, M., Fisch, L., Davidesco, I., Harel, M., Kipervasser, S., Andelman, F., Neufeld, M.Y., Kramer, U., Fried, I., Malach, R.: Emergence of Sensory Patterns during Sleep Highlights Differential Dynamics of REM and Non-REM Sleep Stages. The Journal of Neuroscience 33(37), 14715–14728 (2013)
111. Baldassarre, A., Lewis, C.M., Committeri, G., Snyder, A.Z., Romani, G.L., Corbetta, M.: Individual variability in functional connectivity predicts performance of a perceptual task. Proceedings of the National Academy of Sciences 109(9), 3516–3521 (2012)
112. Zou, Q., Ross, T.J., Gu, H., Geng, X., Zuo, X.N., Hong, L.E., Gao, J.H., Stein, E.A., Zang, Y.F., Yang, Y.: Intrinsic resting-state activity predicts working memory brain activation and behavioral performance. Human Brain Mapping (2012)
113. Wang, X., Han, Z., He, Y., Caramazza, A., Bi, Y.: Where color rests: Spontaneous brain activity of bilateral fusiform and lingual regions predicts object color knowledge performance. Neuroimage (2013)
114. Cole, M.W., Yarkoni, T., Repovš, G., Anticevic, A., Braver, T.S.: Global connectivity of prefrontal cortex predicts cognitive control and intelligence. The Journal of Neuroscience 32(26), 8988–8999 (2012)
115. van den Heuvel, M.P., Stam, C.J., Kahn, R.S., Pol, H.E.H.: Efficiency of functional brain networks and intellectual performance. The Journal of Neuroscience 29(23), 7619–7624 (2009)
116. Wang, X., Han, Z., He, Y., Liu, L., Bi, Y.: Resting-state functional connectivity patterns predict Chinese word reading competency. PloS One 7(9), e44848 (2012)
117. Koyama, M.S., Di Martino, A., Zuo, X.-N., Kelly, C., Mennes, M., Jutagir, D.R., Castellanos, F.X., Milham, M.P.: Resting-state functional connectivity indexes reading competence in children and adults. The Journal of Neuroscience 31(23), 8617–8624 (2011)
118. Riedl, V., Valet, M., Wöller, A., Sorg, C., Vogel, D., Sprenger, T., Boecker, H., Wohlschläger, A.M., Tölle, T.R.: Repeated pain induces adaptations of intrinsic brain activity to reflect past and predict future pain. Neuroimage (2011)

119. Wager, T.D., Atlas, L.Y., Leotti, L.A., Rilling, J.K.: Predicting individual differences in placebo analgesia: contributions of brain activity during anticipation and pain experience. The Journal of Neuroscience 31(2), 439–452 (2011)
120. Martin, A., Barnes, K.A., Stevens, W.D.: Spontaneous neural activity predicts individual differences in performance. Proceedings of the National Academy of Sciences 109(9), 3201–3202 (2012)
121. Freyer, F., Becker, R., Dinse, H.R., Ritter, P.: State-dependent perceptual learning. The Journal of Neuroscience 33(7), 2900–2907 (2013)
122. Barttfeld, P., Wicker, B., McAleer, P., Belin, P., Cojan, Y., Graziano, M., Leiguarda, R., Sigman, M.: Distinct patterns of functional brain connectivity correlate with objective performance and subjective beliefs. Proceedings of the National Academy of Sciences 110(28), 11577–11582 (2013)
123. Ventura-Campos, N., Sanjuán, A., González, J., Palomar-García, M.-Á., Rodríguez-Pujadas, A., Sebastián-Gallés, N., Deco, G., Ávila, C.: Spontaneous Brain Activity Predicts Learning Ability of Foreign Sounds. The Journal of Neuroscience 33(22), 9295–9305 (2013)
124. Zhu, Q., Zhang, J., Luo, Y.L., Dilks, D.D., Liu, J.: Resting-state neural activity across face-selective cortical regions is behaviorally relevant. The Journal of Neuroscience 31(28), 10323–10330 (2011)
125. Coste, C.P., Sadaghiani, S., Friston, K.J., Kleinschmidt, A.: Ongoing brain activity fluctuations directly account for intertrial and indirectly for intersubject variability in Stroop task performance. Cerebral Cortex 21(11), 2612–2619 (2011)
126. Mennes, M., Kelly, C., Zuo, X.-N., Di Martino, A., Biswal, B.B., Castellanos, F.X., Milham, M.P.: Inter-individual differences in resting-state functional connectivity predict task-induced BOLD activity. Neuroimage 50(4), 1690–1701 (2010)
127. Hampson, M., Driesen, N.R., Skudlarski, P., Gore, J.C., Constable, R.T.: Brain connectivity related to working memory performance. The Journal of Neuroscience 26(51), 13338–13343 (2006)
128. Seeley, W.W., Menon, V., Schatzberg, A.F., Keller, J., Glover, G.H., Kenna, H., Reiss, A.L., Greicius, M.D.: Dissociable intrinsic connectivity networks for salience processing and executive control. The Journal of Neuroscience 27(9), 2349–2356 (2007)
129. Tambini, A., Ketz, N., Davachi, L.: Enhanced brain correlations during rest are related to memory for recent experiences. Neuron 65(2), 280–290 (2010)
130. Adelstein, J.S., Shehzad, Z., Mennes, M., DeYoung, C.G., Zuo, X.-N., Kelly, C., Margulies, D.S., Bloomfield, A., Gray, J.R., Castellanos, F.X.: Personality is reflected in the brain's intrinsic functional architecture. PloS One 6(11), e27633 (2011)
131. Stevens, W.D., Buckner, R.L., Schacter, D.L.: Correlated low-frequency BOLD fluctuations in the resting human brain are modulated by recent experience in category-preferential visual regions. Cerebral Cortex 20, 1997–2006 (2010)
132. Lewis, C.M., Baldassarre, A., Committeri, G., Romani, G.L., Corbetta, M.: Learning sculpts the spontaneous activity of the resting human brain. Proceedings of the National Academy of Sciences 106(41), 17558–17563 (2009)
133. Albert, N.B., Robertson, E.M., Miall, R.C.: The resting human brain and motor learning. Current Biology 19(12), 1023–1027 (2009)
134. Taubert, M., Lohmann, G., Margulies, D.S., Villringer, A., Ragert, P.: Long-term effects of motor training on resting-state networks and underlying brain structure. Neuroimage 57(4), 1492–1498 (2011)
135. Yoo, K., Sohn, W.S., Jeong, Y.: Tool-use practice induces changes in intrinsic functional connectivity of parietal areas. Frontiers in Human Neuroscience, 7 (2013)

136. Wang, Z., Liu, J., Zhong, N., Qin, Y., Zhou, H., Li, K.: Changes in the brain intrinsic organization in both on-task state and post-task resting state. Neuroimage 62(1), 394–407 (2012)

137. Hasson, U., Nusbaum, H.C., Small, S.L.: Task-dependent organization of brain regions active during rest. Proceedings of the National Academy of Sciences 106(26), 10841–10846 (2009)

138. Eryilmaz, H., Van De Ville, D., Schwartz, S., Vuilleumier, P.: Impact of transient emotions on functional connectivity during subsequent resting state: A wavelet correlation approach. Neuroimage 54(3), 2481–2491 (2011)

139. Huber, R., Esser, S.K., Ferrarelli, F., Massimini, M., Peterson, M.J., Tononi, G.: TMS-induced cortical potentiation during wakefulness locally increases slow wave activity during sleep. PloS One 2(3), e276 (2007)

140. Harmelech, T., Preminger, S., Wertman, E., Malach, R.: The Day-After Effect: Long Term, Hebbian-Like Restructuring of Resting-State fMRI Patterns Induced by a Single Epoch of Cortical Activation. The Journal of Neuroscience 33(22), 9488–9497 (2013)

141. Werheid, K., Zysset, S., Müller, A., Reuter, M., von Cramon, D.Y.: Rule learning in a serial reaction time task: an fMRI study on patients with early Parkinson's disease. Cognitive Brain Research 16(2), 273–284 (2003)

142. Spulber, I., Georgiou, P., Eftekhar, A., Toumazou, C., Duffell, L., Bergmann, J., McGregor, A., Mehta, T., Hernandez, M., Burdett, A.: Frequency analysis of wireless accelerometer and EMG sensors data: Towards discrimination of normal and asymmetric walking pattern. In: Book Frequency Analysis of Wireless Accelerometer and EMG Sensors Data: Towards Discrimination of Normal and Asymmetric Walking Pattern, pp. 2645–2648. IEEE (2012)

143. Eckmiller, R., Hartmann, G., Hauska, G.: Parallel processing in neural systems and computers. Elsevier Science Inc. (1990) (1990)

144. Turner, B.M., Forstmann, B.U., Wagenmakers, E.-J., Brown, S.D.: A Bayesian framework for simultaneously modeling neural and behavioral data. NeuroImage 72, 193–206 (2013)

# Predicting Metabolic Syndrome with Neural Networks

Miguel Murguía-Romero[1,*], Rafael Jiménez-Flores[2],
A. René Méndez-Cruz[2], and Rafael Villalobos-Molina[1,3]

[1] Unidad de Biomedicina,
[2] Carrera de Médico Cirujano,
Universidad Nacional Autónoma de México,
Ave. de los Barrios 1, Los Reyes Iztacala, Tlalnepantla 54090, México
[3] Instituto de Ciencias Biomédicas, Universidad Autónoma de Ciudad Juárez,
Chihuahua, México
miguelmurguia@ciencias.unam.mx

**Abstract.** Metabolic syndrome (MetS) is a condition that predisposes individuals to acquire diabetes and cardiovascular disease. The prevalence of MetS among young Mexicans (17-24 years old) is high (14.6%), and is an important risk factor to develop more serious impairments. Thus, it is crucial to detect MetS in young as they could be alerted to modify their life habits to revert or delay further health complications. One barrier to identify the MetS in large young populations is the high costs and complex logistics involved. The aim of this study was to build a tool to predict MetS in young Mexicans using noninvasive data, such as anthropometrics (waist circumference, height, weight, or body mass index), family-inherited background (diseases of parents), or life and eating habits, but excluding laboratory data such as blood glucose, cholesterol or triglycerides that implies to withdraw blood samples incurring in costs and nuisance for people. We evaluated 826 Mexican undergraduate students collecting both, invasive and noninvasive data and determined whether each one bears or not MetS. Then we build neural networks (NN) using only noninvasive data, but with the output class known (with and without MetS). Noninvasive data were classified into six groups, and arranged into ten sets as input layer. We generated 10 NN's taking 70% of record as training set, and the 30% as validation records. We used the positive predictive value (PPV) as classifier efficiency of the NN's. The PPV of the NN's vary from 38.2% to 45.4%, the last from a NN including those anthropometrics variables (sex, waist circumference, height, weight, body mass index) as input variables, and the hours per week of physical exercise. Comparing percentage of true positive (students with MetS) detected with the NN vs. a random selection, i.e., 45.4% of PPV vs. 14.6% of MetS prevalence in the objective population, it is expected to improve the MetS identification by three fold.

**Keywords:** Neural network, obesity, metabolic syndrome, young Mexicans.

---

* Corresponding author.

F. Castro, A. Gelbukh, and M. González (Eds.): MICAI 2013, Part I, LNAI 8265, pp. 464–472, 2013.

# 1  Introduction

The metabolic syndrome (MetS) is an impairment that involves dyslipidemia (high triglycerides, low HDL cholesterol) high blood glucose, high blood pressure and central obesity [1,2]. MetS is considered a risk factor to acquire diabetes mellitus type II, and cardiovascular disease, the two main causes of death in Mexico [3]. It is known that the prevalence of MetS among Mexican young population (17-24 years old) is about 14.6% [4], this imply that more than 2.5 millions of young have MetS [5]. To formally identify whether a young bears or not MetS it is indispensable to measure blood levels of HDL cholesterol, triglycerides, and fasting glucose, that implies to take a blood sample, thus if a public health strategy is implemented to detect MetS, it will be required a complex logistics and a not low economic cost associated. So, a tool that would estimate if a young bears or not MetS will be beneficial to public health strategies that intend to address the problem of the high prevalence of diabetes and atherosclerosis.

There are some works describing NN to identify MetS, but including clinical parameters that implies to withdraw blood samples  [6,7], such as insulin and cholesterol, among others.

The aim of this study was to build a neural network as a tool to predict the presence of MetS in young population, which assumes themselves as being healthy, that do not require the clinical parameters obtained from a blood sample, and using only noninvasive data, such as anthropometric data and life and nutrition habits.

# 2  Positive Predictive Value

The objective of the analysis was to select a sample of individuals and hence candidates to perform laboratory analyses, involving the withdraw of blood samples. In that context, a good classifier is one that will maximize the percentage of young with MetS out of all identified by such classifier, i.e., that will maximize the positive predictive value (PPV) [8]. As for a clinical test there have been defined more than one efficiency measures, next we give definition of three of them in order to precise the criteria to measure the efficiency of the built neural network.

## 2.1  Definitions

- Sensitivity. The proportion of positive cases, i.e., who have the disease, identified by the test.
- Specificity. The proportion of negative cases, i.e., who do not have the disease, identified by the test.
- Positive predictive value. The proportion of positive cases identified by the test of all positives estimated by the test.

Graphically, those three concepts can be illustrated as in Figure 1.

**Table 1.** Reference values of clinical and anthropometric parameters to define the metabolic syndrome. Cut-off points of metabolic syndrome parameters are based on [1].

| Parameter | Categorical cut-off point |
|---|---|
| HDL Cholesterol | $<50$ mg/dL in women |
| | $<40$ mg/dL in men |
| Waist circumference | $\geq 80$ cm in women |
| | $\geq 90$ cm in men |
| Triglycerides | $\geq 150$ mg/dL |
| Blood pressure | $\geq 130$ mmHg systolic |
| | $\geq 85$ mmHg diastolic |
| Fasting glucose | $\geq 100$ mg/dL |

## 3   Method

### 3.1   Sample Data

We invited 1000 students of first grade to participate in the project, consisting in evaluate their physical health. All students accepted to participate in the study and signed an informed consent. The study was divided into two stages: first, the students filled a web questionnaire, MiSalud (www.misalud.abacoac.org), consisting of several sections, where they recorded its life and nutritional habits, hereditary background, and sports or physical activity. At the second stage, the students were cited with the physicians of the group to perform anthropometric measures (waist circumference, height, weight, and blood pressure) and blood samples were taken by personnel of CARPERMOR, S.A. de C.V., an international reference laboratory, to determine blood levels of glucose, HDL cholesterol, and triglycerides, among other molecules. The information collected in both stages was integrated into a database, and the presence or absence of MetS was assigned to the database record of each student applying international criteria (Table 1); this classification, presence/absence of MetS, was taken as the desired output of the neural network. After this process the records with missing answers in the questionnaire were eliminated from the database, so the final database included records of 826 students.

### 3.2   Input Variables

We considered a total of 14 variables, all noninvasive, as input (Table 2). To facilitate the combinatory to use as input layers, the variables were grouped into six classes: anthropometrics, physical activity, beverages, smoking, meals, and heredity history. A total of ten combinations of variables were used as input layer (Table 3). Beverages variables are reported in liters per week, calculated based on question such as: How many glasses of water you drink per day? Vegetables and carbohydrates variables were also summarized to number of meals per week that the student reported to include some food of that kind. Metabolic impairments included the number of impairments reported by the student herself/himself, and also the family-inherited background included the total of diseases related to MetS that the student reports to has her/his mother and father.

## 3.3   Neural Networks Building

We used the functions included in the nnet package of the R language [9] (Figure 2) to build the NN's that uses the back propagation algorithm with a single hidden layer. The architecture of all the networks included three layers: input layer, output layer, and one hidden layer. The input layer vary from 5 to 14 neurons (see Table 3), the hidden layer were fixed in 25 neurons, and output layer in two neurons, one each indicating one of two possible outputs: with MetS and without MetS. Considering an input set or variables, say WC + SEX + HEIGHT + WEIGHT + BMI (Table 2), different training sets were defined, so one NN were build based on each training set, obtaining ten NN's for each set of variables. The cases of training sets were selected randomly taking 70 cases of every 100 cases (Figure 2); the remaining 30% of cases were used as validation set. Also, ten different set of variables were defined as input (Table 3), and the averages of PPV for ten training sets were reported as a measure of efficiency of the NN as a classifier.

# 4   Results

## 4.1   Neural Networks

Ten groups of neural networks were built corresponding to ten arrangements of the six sets of variables. All the NN's had three layers; the input layer ranged from 5 to 14 neurons, the only hidden layer with 25 neurons, and the output layer with two neurons, one each indicating one of two possible outputs: with MetS and without MetS. Table 3 shows the PPV averages of ten neural networks built with different initial weights, but with the same ten training sets. The PPV ranges from 32.8% when are include all sets of variables, to 45.4% when using as input layer to the anthropometrics and physical activity variable sets. When only anthropometrics variables are included in input layer (Table 3, row 1) a PPV of 38.8% is reached. Combined with anthropometric set variables, the variable Smoking is the second with high PPV percentage (41.6%) followed by Metabolic impairments (41.2%), then by Metabolic impairments+Mother family-Inherited background (40.6%), and then by Metabolic impairments+Mother+Father family-inherited background (39.8%). The standard deviation of the averages of ten NN's of the ten input layers ranged from 10.7 to 16.0, the first corresponding to the lower average of PPV, and second to the higher average of PPV.

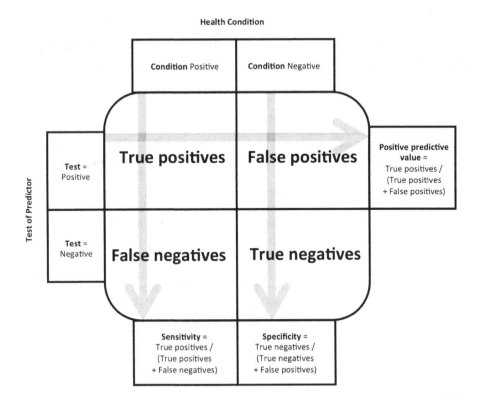

**Fig. 1.** Schematic representation of the concept of Positive Predictive Value (PPV) of a classifier

## 4.2   The Neural Networks as Predictors of MetS

As one of the objectives to build a neural network was to account with a classifier that helps to identify MetS in a population with the same characteristics of the training set, it is important to compare its efficiency vs. the one used previously. Up to day, the way to detect MetS is measuring directly the five parameters that formally define it (Table 1). With this procedure, the percentage of population with MetS detected in Mexican young population was equal to the prevalence of such syndrome, i.e.,14.6% [4,10]. Detecting MetS using NN's results, in average, a 45.4% if anthropometrics and physical activity variables are included at input layer (Table 3). Thus, it could be said that NN as predictor improves the MetS identification by three fold compared with the traditional method.

```
#
# R functions to generate the neural networks
#

my_sample<- c(sample(1:100,70),
        sample(101:200,70),
        sample(201:300,70),
        sample(301:400,70),
        sample(401:500,70),
        sample(501:600,70),
        sample(601:700,70),
        sample(701:826,78))

my_neural_network<- nnet(MetS_CLASS~SEX+WC+BMI+WIGHT+HEIGHT,
        data=my_data,
        subset=my_sample,
        size = 25,
        rang = 0.8,
        decay = 5e-2,
        maxit = 2000)

table(my_data$MetS_CLASS[-my_sample],
        predict(my_neural_network,
        my_data[-my_sample,],
        type = "class"))
```

**Fig. 2.** Functions and statements in R language used to generate the neural networks

## 5   Discussion

There are practically infinite ways of building a NN based on the noninvasive data, some of the decisions in the process include: the variables set as input layer; the way of categorize, both, qualitative and quantitative variables; the architecture of the NN, i.e., number of layers and neurons; the training algorithm; the initial weights of the connections; the proportions and list of cases of the training and validation sets; the structure of the output layer. All those conditions finally determine the efficiency of a NN as classifier, in the particular case of predicting MetS in young population, other conditions include the population where the prediction will be done, despite the population of the training set belongs to the same universe.

Anthropometrics variables combined with the physical activity seems to be the more important predictive factors, while the less important considered in the study are the reported ingest of vegetables or carbohydrates. To increase the PPV this finding suggests disaggregating the physical activity differentiating in separate neurons the kind of physical activity, because this study was summarized by the hours of exercise at week. Also, the vegetables and carbohydrates variables, were summarized to the numbers of meals were the students reported to include it, so, it could be an alternative to use the number of portions reported by the student.

Anthropometrics variables seem to be important, but this suggestion should have in mind that is true in the context of NN, as a figure it is illustrative to consider that a body mass index (BMI) in the range of 25 to 26 only captured 13.8% of the population with MetS [11].

Coinciding with other studies [6], the anthropometrics variables were the most important predictive factors. A study to predict MetS in patient with second generation antipsychotics treatment built a NN, included as input variables the anthropometrics, blood pressure and medications, and found a PPV 67.5% [12]. Other combinations of input variables need to be tested to search a higher PPV, and the results of this study could guide that process. Clearly a PPV reaching with the built NN is low if considering to predict MetS in an individual, i.e., in the clinic context, nevertheless in the context of public health, represents to reduce costs and the complexity of the logistics.

The PPV of NN including all the variables suggests that the factors involved in the study are non-linearly related to the outcome.

**Table 2.** Variables used to build the neural networks

| Variable set | Variable | Description |
|---|---|---|
| MetS Class (output variable) | MetS_CLASS | Metabolic syndrome present (yes/no) |
| Anthropometrics | WC | Waist circumference (cm) |
| Anthropometrics | SEX | Sex (female or male) |
| Anthropometrics | HEIGHT | Height |
| Anthropometrics | WEIGHT | Weight |
| Anthropometrics | BMI | Body mass index |
| Physical activity | PHYS_ACT | Hours a week of physical activity |
| Beverages | WATER | Water (ingest of liters a week) |
| Beverages | SODA | Non diet soda (ingest of liters a week) |
| Smoking | SMOKING | Whether the student smokes or not |
| Meals | VEGETABLES | Number of meals (out of 5) that the student reported to eat vegetables |
| Meals | CARBOHY | Number of meals (out of 5) that the student reported to eat carbohydrates |
| Metabolic impairments | MET_IMPAIR | Number of diseases reported by the student itself, including obesity, high blood pressure, and high blood glucose |
| Family-inherited background | FIB_MOTHER | Number of diseases related to MetS reported has the mother |
| Family-inherited background | FIB_FATHER | Number of diseases related to MetS reported has the father |

**Table 3.** Percentages of Positive Predictive Value of 10 neural networks to detect MetS in young

| Set of input variables | Avg.±SD | Max | Min | Neurons in input layer |
|---|---|---|---|---|
| 1 Anthropometrics | 38.8±12.8 | 50.2 | 28.7 | 5 |
| 2 Anthr. + Physical activity | 45.4±16.0 | 62.6 | 28.9 | 6 |
| 3 Anthr. + Beverages | 38.0±11.5 | 48.3 | 30.1 | 7 |
| 4 Anthr. + Smoking | 41.6±15.2 | 55.0 | 27.8 | 6 |
| 5 Anthr. + Meals: vegetables | 36.4±13.9 | 49.7 | 16.7 | 6 |
| 6 Anthr. + Meals: carbohydrates | 36.9±12.3 | 48.3 | 19.8 | 6 |
| 7 Anthr. + Met. impairments | 41.2±14.8 | 56.8 | 25.8 | 6 |
| 8 Anthr. + Met. impair. + FHB mother | 40.6±13.3 | 51.0 | 29.1 | 7 |
| 9 Anthr. + Met. impair. + FHB mother +father | 39.8±14.4 | 55.5 | 24.0 | 8 |
| 10 All variables | 32.8±10.7 | 48.3 | 24.6 | 14 |

Variables are grouped as in Table 2. Met. impairments = Metabolic impairments reported by the young, including obesity, high blood pressure, high blood glucose. FHB = family-inherited background from mother or father.

# 6    Conclusions

The maximum PPV reached with the noninvasive variables included in the study was 45.4%, i.e., the proportion of individuals that have MetS out of all identified by the NN. This percentage is three fold compared with the prevalence of the MetS in the population analyzed of 14.6%. This finding needs to be tested applying the NN to a population and performing clinical test that will confirm, or deny, the prediction of having MetS.

The anthropometrics variables, including sex, height, weight, waist circumference, and body mass index, combined with the physical activity reported by the student, are important variables to predict MetS in young; while the number of meals were the individual includes vegetables and carbohydrates seems to be of low importance as predictor of MetS.

Other combinations of variables and also other forms to summarize the variables as input neurons could be explored to improve the PPV reached by the NN's.

**Acknowledgments.** This study was supported by grant PAPIIT IN223113 DGAPA, U.N.A.M. We thank the staff of Grupo Diagnóstico Médico PROA S.A. de C.V. (Laboratorio CARPERMOR) that took and analyzed the blood samples. F.E.S. Iztacala, U.N.A.M., supported economically part of the work (P. Dávila-Aranda). RV-M is a visiting Professor at UACJ, supported by a fellowship from DGAPA, UNAM.

# References

1. Alberti, K., Eckel, R., Grundy, S., Zimmet, P., Cleeman, J., Donato, K., Fruchart, J., James, W., Loria, C., Smith, S.J.: International Diabetes Federation Task Force on Epidemiology and Prevention, National Heart, Lung, and Blood Institute, American Heart Association, World Heart Federation, International Atherosclerosis Society, International Association for the Study of Obesity: Harmonizing the metabolic syndrome: a joint interim statement of the International Diabetes Federation Task Force on Epidemiology and Prevention; National Heart, Lung, and Blood Institute; American Heart Association; World Heart Federation; International Atherosclerosis Society; and International Association for the Study of Obesity. Circulation 120, 1640–1645 (2009)
2. Grundy, S., Cleeman, J., Daniels, S.: Diagnosis and management of the metabolic syndrome. an american heart association/national heart, lung, and blood institute scientific statement. Circulation 112, 2735–2752 (2005)
3. SINAIS, Sistema Nacional de Información en Salud, México government, http://sinais.salud.gob.mx/descargas/xls/m_005.xls
4. Jiménez-Flores, J., Murguía-Romero, M., Mendoza-Ramos, Sigrist-Flores, S., Rodríguez-Soriano, N., Ramírez-García, L., Jesús-Sandoval, R., Álvarez-Gasca, M., Orozco, E., Villalobos-Molina, R., Méndez-Cruz, A.: Metabolic syndrome occurrence in university students from méxico city: the binomium low hdl/waist circumference is the major prevalence factor. Open Journal of Preventive Medicine 2, 177–182 (2012)
5. Murguía-Romero, M., Jiménez-Flores, R., Villalobos-Molina, R., Méndez-Cruz, A.: Estimating the geographic distribution of the metabolic syndrome prevalence in young mexicans. Geospatial Health 2, 43–50 (2010)
6. Hirose, H., Takayama, T., Hozawa, S., Hibi, T., Saito, I.: Prediction of metabolic syndrome using artificial neural network system based on clinical data including insulin resistance index and serum adiponectin. Comput. Biol. Med. 41, 1051–1056 (2011)
7. Ushida, Y., Kato, R., Niwa, K., Tanimura, D., Izawa, H., Yasui, K., Takase, T., Yoshida, Y., Kawase, M., Yoshida, T., Murohara, T., Honda, H.: Combinational risk factors of metabolic syndrome identified by fuzzy neural network analysis of health-check data. BMC Med. Inform. Decis. Mak. 12, 80 (2012)
8. Altman, D., Bland, J.: Diagnostic test 2: predictive values. BMJ 309, 102 (1994)
9. R Development Core Team: R: A language and environment for statistical computing. R Foundation for Statistical Computing, Vienna, Austria (2011), http://www.R-project.org ISBN 3-900051-07-0
10. Murguía-Romero, M., Villalobos-Molina, R., Méndez-Cruz, R., Jiménez-Flores, R.: Heuristic search of cut-off points for clinical parameters: Defining the limits of obesity. In: Batyrshin, I., Sidorov, G. (eds.) MICAI 2011, Part I. LNCS, vol. 7094, pp. 560–571. Springer, Heidelberg (2011)
11. Murguía-Romero, M., Jiménez-Flores, R., Villalobos-Molina, R., Mendoza-Ramos, M., Reyes-Reali, J., Sigrist-Flores, S., Méndez-Cruz, A.: The body mass index (bmi) as a public health tool to predict metabolic syndrome. Open Journal of Preventive Medicine 2, 59–66 (2012)
12. Bai, C.C.L., Chen, Y., Hwang, J., Chen, T., Chiu, T., Li, H., Easy, Y.: low-cost identification of metabolic syndrome in patients treated with second-generation antipsychotics: artificial neural network and logistic regression models. J. Clin. Psychiatry 71, 225–234 (2010)

# Homogeneous Population Solving the Minimal Perturbation Problem in Dynamic Scheduling of Surgeries

Adriana Pérez-López[1,*], Rosario Baltazar[1], Martín Carpio[1], Hugo Terashima-Marin[2], Dulce J. Magaña-Lozano[2], and Hector J. Puga[1]

[1] División de Estudios de Posgrado e Investigación, Instituto Tecnológico de León,
Av. Tecnológico S/N, 37290 Guanajuato, México
adriana_perez@ieee.com, r.baltazar@ieee.org,
jmcarpio61@hotmail.com
[2] Centro de Computación Inteligente y Robótica, Tecnológico de Monterrey,
Campus Monterrey, Av. Eugenio Garza Sada 2501, Monterrey, N.L. 64849 México
terashima@itesm.mx

**Abstract.** The Instituto Mexicano del Seguro Social (IMSS) is the federal government medical institution with many hospitals around the country. Usually, the surgical operating areas within hospitals are constantly requested for emergency surgeries which trigger continuous changes in the established schedule, and having an effect in other factors such as doctors, nurses and patients, as well. In this paper, we tackle this type of dynamic scheduling problem with minimal perturbation by using and comparing two types of approaches: A Segmentation-based heuristic and a Genetic-Algorithm-based schema. The GA-based model which includes homogenous population (GA-HPop) obtains the best performance when tested with a set of real instances. It gets the best characteristics of Genetic Algorithm and adding changes, ensuring a new solution as possible close to original solution.

**Keywords:** Dynamic Scheduling, Minimal Perturbation Problem, Genetic Algorithm, Segmentation Heuristic, Rescheduling.

## 1 Introduction

Scheduling resources in an institution is of great importance because available resources and unused represents lost money for the company if there is not a good schedule of activities. Then, each dynamic scheduling searches the resources optimization [1], however according to field of study the goal is solve the minimize perturbation problem, it consists of finding ways to change as little as possible the original scheduling when to try insert new task to schedule [2].

Actually the Instituto Mexicano del Seguro Social, (IMSS) is the federal government medical institution with many hospitals around the country, does first schedule of surgeries manually through a spreadsheet every week, interactive computer application program, however the surgical operating are constantly requested for emergency surgeries which trigger continuous changes in the established schedule, triggering a domino

---

* Corresponding author.

F. Castro, A. Gelbukh, and M. González (Eds.): MICAI 2013, Part I, LNAI 8265, pp. 473–484, 2013.

effect, where if a surgery is postponed the next surgeries will be postponed too, in the best case the affected surgeries will be scheduling next week regardless their emergency.

The Minimal Perturbation Problem within Dynamic Scheduling is a topic that has already been studied previously [3], It has been solved in the past with various techniques such as Multiagent Systems in the manufacture and transportation area [4], [5], heuristics such as BackTracking [2], Iterative Forward Search Algorithm in timetabling area among other [6], [7], [8] where each one of them with the goal reduce the disrupcions and different approach to medical area.

Genetic Algotithms (GA) have been used in many ways for solving optimization problems and other hybrid algorithms have been produced too, in the last forty years GA has been studied to solve different optimization problems of dynamic scheduling, in which the process of crossover and mutation is changed [9], [10], [1]. In the approach we present in the paper, we focus in the population, a similar population to original solution instead to population that search genetic diversification, thereby generating GA-HPop, which is a algorithm that gets the best desirable skills of GA to solve the Minimal Perturbations Problem in dynamic scheduling, gives priority the most urgent surgeries and postpones or disrupting the surgeries scheduled with state less emergency; getting a better performance than GA and a specific heuristic. GA-Hop is done to $n$ surgeries, $m$ surgery rooms, can be applied any hospital with business rules similar to IMSS.

The paper is organized as follows: Section 2 discusses about the approach in dynamic scheuduling of surgeries, where seek the minimize disruption of original schedule (section 3.1). The way to solve it, is use Genetic Algorithm, where even knowing good performance is possible improve, making some changes explain section 4.2, and subsequently show the results obtained in section 5, also the performance of GA and GA-HPop, finally concludes and shows future works will be produced by solution of minimal perturbations in scheduling dynamic of surgeries, GA-HPop.

## 2   Dynamic Scheduling

Heuristics are commonly used to solve many optimization problems, but they may get trapped in local optima [11]. Fuzzy logic, neural networks have great learning ability and quick evolution of system but do not keep guarantee to get the best decision [11].

The dynamic scheduling problem, called also rescheduling [12], is used in hospitals, when there are some complications or emergencies lead to cancel any surgery [13]. A process used to solve cancelation of surgeries is that each element must estimate a probability [13] but hardly to control the external enviroments or predict events, only possible make an approximate. The arrival of semi-urgent surgeries is unpredictable [14], so should have a compensation between surgeries cancelled and select surgeries, then Markov theory and Poisson distributed are established as tool to help the scheduling process, having approximated about what will happen, saving time for the events expected and there will be no disturbances.

The agents to diagnostic service scheduling is commonly used [4], but the agility, distribution, decentralization, reactivity and flexibility are advantages of combination of Artificial Intelligence with biological inspiration [15].

Besides the metaheuristics solve the dynamic scheduling with *predictive-reactive scheduling* approach [16], are a good tool to find a solution because the metaheuristics are constantly adapting according to change [17], as in the case UMDA and ACO [18], both metaheuristics have similar paradigm. The Genetic Algorithm is algorithm commonly used for a good performance and solution diversity that generate during the process [10]. GA has solved the JobShop scheduling problem in dynamic environment, observing the behavior of GA and managing its weakness so getting a better result.

# 3 Dynamic Scheduling of Surgeries

The dynamic scheduling implies updating a predefined schedule, in response to external changes that are not manageable, such as adding task, lack of resources [5].

The model studied in the scheduling of surgeries is named dynamic scheduling, where the activities, resources and process of time are predefined, and subsequently alter the schedule with new activities, this alteration is named re-scheduling. In this particular case the re-scheduling of surgeries into medical area is necessary to consider hours of service, duration of service, patient's importance criterion, and changes made on original schedule. Moreover, it is important to consider, every surgery has medical area, every medical area has surgery hours with itself surgery rooms; time for morning service is 360 min. According to data of IMSS.

The dynamic scheduling for surgeries problem is represented here as constraint satisfaction problem (CSP). A CSP is a 3-tuple $(X, D, C)$ where $X$ is a set of $n$ surgeries $\{x_1, ..., x_n\}$, $D$ is a set of $m$ surgeries rooms $\langle D_1, ..., D_m\}$, and the restrictions $C$ are hours of service of surgeries rooms is $360\ minutes$, days and surgeries rooms assigned to surgeries is according to medical area, and The surgeries with emergency *type 1* must be priority; where Emergency *type 1* The most emergency and Emergency *type 2* Less emergency.

## 3.1 Minimal Perturbation Problem

When introduced a variant to solution, it generates new solution based on original solution, the intention in the minimal perturbation problem is search a new solution closer possible to original solution [19] [6]. The objective in this investigation is generate a new schedule based on the original, searches the minimal alteration on the original schedule.

The minimal perturbation problem consists a $\Theta$ is the original solution, a $\Theta'$ is the new solution, and $\delta$ is the function which defines the distance between the two solution. The solution of scheduling of surgeries problem is given in 1, being a minimal distance $\Theta$ to $\Theta'$ i.e. $\delta(\Theta, \Theta')$. Where the distance is measured in days, because the goal is, the surgeries are scheduled as soon as possible, and fewest surgeries are postponed. i.e.

$$\delta(\Theta, \Theta') = \sum_{i=0}^{n} |diaSur_i - diaSur_i'| \cdot (3 - urgSur_i) \tag{1}$$

Where $diaSur_i$ is a day assigned of the surgery $c_i$ belonging to original solution ($\Theta$), $diaSur_i'$ is a day assigned of the surgery $c_i$ belonging to new solution($\Theta'$), and $urgSur_i$ is a emergency of surgery $x_i$.

The reason to subtract, is to give preference to surgeries *type 1* and it does not to move. The number three changes the value assigned to give more preference to *type1*, otherwise, the surgeries *type 1* would have preference to postponed. The results going to have two schedules, the first is the schedule before the arrival of new surgeries, i.e. the original schedule; the second is the reschedule proposed, which, the new surgeries have been added original schedule, so the new schedule should be so similar to original schedule.

## 4    Proposed Model

The algorithm proposed, GA-HPop, is compared with deterministic heuristic specified to solve the dynamic scheduling of surgeries, GA-HPop also is compared with original GA, and establishing a level of performance in dynamic scheduling of surgeries.

### 4.1    Segmentation Heuristics for Scheduling Surgeries (SH)

The segmentation heuristics are inspired in divide and conquer strategy, which break up a problem into several smaller instances of the same problem, solve these smaller instances, and then combine the solutions into a solution to the original problem [20]. Steps Segmentation Heuristics are shown below [21].

**Breaking :** Dividing it into subproblems i.e. instances smaller to same type of problem.
**Scheduling :** Recursively solving these subproblems.
**Update :** Appropriately combining their answers.

The Segmentation Heuristic for scheduled surgeries is a simply way to solve dynamic scheduling but it is not always the optimal, the algorithm used (see Algorithm 1) requires the original scheduler ($OrigSched$) and a vector with the news surgeries to scheduling ($nsurgery$) where a $nsurgery_i$ is an element $i$ of vector of new surgeries to schedule.

---

**Algorithm 1.** The Segmentation Heuristic for scheduling surgeries

---

**Require:** $(OrigSched, nsurgery)$
1: Do j=0
2: **repeat**
3:    $segment \leftarrow call$ segmentation($OrigSched$)
4:    $nsurgery_i \leftarrow$ select($nsurgery$)
5:    $segment' \leftarrow call$ insert ($segment, nsurgery_i$)
6:    $OrigSched \leftarrow llamar$ update($OrigSched, segment'$)
7:    $j \leftarrow j + 1$
8: **until** $j < totalnsurgery$

---

Segmenting a problem in this context, means dividing the original scheduler (*OrigSched*) by day, selecting the day with more time die and its adjoining. The days selected are called *segment*, this segment will be used to insert each $nsurgery_i$ according to the algorithm (see Algorithm 2).

---

**Algorithm 2.** Heuristic to insert the segment in order by emergency and time.

---

**Require:** (*segmento, nsurgery*)

1: Do $position = 0$
2: Do $stop$ = size of segment $+1$
3: $segment'$ ← *call* insert( *position, nsurgery* )
4: $segment$ ← *call* orderSizeEmergency(*segment*)
5: **repeat**
6:    $position$ ← $position + 1$
7:    $segment'$ ← insert( *position, segment$_{position}$* )
8: **until** $position < stop$

---

Finally, when a segment has been inserted the new surgery, $nsurgery_i$; the original scheduler, *OrigSched*, is updated, adding the segment with the new surgeries scheduled, this process is repeated while there are new surgeries to schedule.

## 4.2   Genetic Algorithm with Homogeneous Population (GA-HPop)

Genetic Algorithms are inspired by the evolutionary process in nature, where the evolutionary process of nature, consisting of individuals in a population that compete for survival, those individuals who succeed search to perpetuate the species through reproduction, i.e. the predominant population genes enhancing species will increase [22].

The classic Genetic Algorithm used a population of individuals, each individal is a possible solution, these individuals are binary chain that represent genetic material; each element of genetic chain is called *gen*. Generally the individuals selected are those with the best fitness, then, to do a transformation process helped to find a optimal solution.

The proposed GA-HPop keeps the same features as the classic GA, but with the peculiarity that its members tends to be homogeneous, meaning tends, to be clones of the initial solution, because the goal is get a solution as most similar possible to original scheduler. The Stopping criterion is measured by function call, each evaluation of the individual is a function call.

The steps to Genetic Algorithm with Homogeneours Population can see in Algorithm 3 and next lines explain the process.

---

**Algorithm 3.** Genetic Algorithm with Homogeneous Population

---
1:    $P$ = Initialize population
2:    EvaluatePopulation($P$)
3:    **repeat**
4:      $P' \leftarrow$ Elitism($P$)
5:      $P' \leftarrow$ Selection($P$)
6:      $P' \leftarrow$ CrossOver($P$)
7:      $P \leftarrow$ Mutation($P$)
8:      EvaluatePopulation($P$)
9:      $P \leftarrow P'$
10:      $P \leftarrow$ Intensifier($P$)
11:    **until** Stopping criterion is met
12:    **return** BestIndividual

---

**Initialize Population.** The GA-HPop starts a homogeneous population, i.e. a clon population of the original solution, putting the new surgeries in first position, ensuring each individual begin the same way. The individual has a chain of integer numbers (see Figure 1), which indicate id of surgerie. Beginning a similar population helps to do not generate individuals completely different for the solution, so not generate individuals that don't help to find a good solution.

**Elitism.** After initialize population with clones, the best individuals are selected, but on first generation as each individual will be similar itself, because the goal is keep the original solution for later generations, in next generations the goal is keep the best individuals, either homogeneous individual or a better individuals found which it is individuals closest to the original schedule.

**Selection.** Once the elitism process has done its job, the next step is the crossover, before the population will be crossover, the individuals selected are known as parents; the method for selection is called *tournament*. Through tournament selection where subgroups of individuals are chosen from larger population, the best individual of subgroup is chosen.

**Crossover.** The parents selected in step of selection will be reproduced; the method used is *annular cross* where the parents do interchange of information like as Figure 1. Whereas the chromosome is a ring, the annular cross $C1$ is defined indicating the place or point of crossing and establishing a $C4$ half ring length, so the genes are exchanged during the crossover.

**Mutation.** In the mutation, an individual is selected randomly, the chain's individual is mutated; a gen i.e. a *id* of surgery is selected and moved from its place, producing a new individual, with differents characteristics and different fitness. Has selected only a gene to mutate to not alter significantly the individual.

**Intensifier.** The intesifier revises how many individuals are differents to original solution, if the population exceeds a given percentage, part of population will be replaced by the homogeneous population, original solution. This ensures not to lose part of the population that is close to the origial solution.

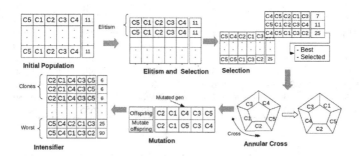

**Fig. 1.** Process of Genetic Algorithm with Homogeneours Population (GA-HPop)

## 5  Experiments and Results

The instances used to test the performance of the proposed algorithms were taken from real data in an IMSS hospital, and modified accordingly by using *Poisson Process*, tool used to simule the arrival patients, data from year 2011. The instances obtained, are formed for three types files, with different extensions, depending on the contents of the file:

***File.cld***  contains original schedule; it is obtained from previous studies, where the solution of static scheduling, are surgeries optimally scheduled [23]. its content is showing in Table 1, in the first column.

***File.txt***  is provided from real data of IMSS, the assigned days for each surgery in 2011, from monday to friday in morning duty. Nevertheless, the system is ready for add or reduce the number of operating rooms or change the assigned days.

***File.dat2***  was done from *Poisson Process*, simulating the arrival process of patients that need a emergency surgery, its content is showing in Table 1, in the second column.

Table 1 presents surgeries to scheduling, and the minutes with goal to show that would be possible schedule every surgery, if and only if all week were in a single block where assign tasks, however its wrong, because, there are five blocks according of the five days for week.

Moreover, Table 1 shows instances will not be possible schedule, even considering only block of *given time*, because the total time of scheduled surgeries and new surgeries is greater than *given time for week*, for exaple in instance *INST2, INST6, INST8, INST9*, view Table 1, which has *given time* smaller than sum *time of surgeries scheduling* and *time of new surgeries*. it is clear that the measure of time given is minutes.

Additionaly, four test collections were generated, each group has three kinds of file, which, 25 file with extension *dat2*, that contains the new surgeries to schedule, a file

**Table 1.** Contain surgeries and times of instances out of programme surgeries

| Instance | No. Surgeries Scheduled | No. New Surgeries to Schedule | Time of Surgeries Scheduling | Time of new surgeries | given time for week |
|---|---|---|---|---|---|
| INST1 | 9 | 1 | 1,815 | 150 | 2,160 |
| INST2 | 13 | 3 | 2,310 | 540 | 2,520 |
| INST3 | 22 | 3 | 4,665 | 450 | 5,400 |
| INST4 | 11 | 4 | 1,380 | 255 | 1,800 |
| INST5 | 39 | 8 | 4,769 | 870 | 7,200 |
| INST6 | 6 | 1 | 1,035 | 195 | 1,080 |
| INST7 | 26 | 3 | 3,285 | 285 | 3,600 |
| INST8 | 24 | 6 | 3,390 | 465 | 3,600 |
| INST9 | 10 | 2 | 2,490 | 420 | 2,880 |
| INST10 | 40 | 4 | 6,045 | 555 | 6,840 |

*txt* with restrictions of surgeries room and other file with extension *cld* that contain the original scheduler. Figure 2 shows the four groups, which, easy schedule has a original schedule with average of 50.62 free minutes for surgery room and some rooms free completely. Dificult schedule has an average 45.90 minutes of free time for room surgery in a week. Each group contains 25 files with extension *dat2*, easy *file.dat2* have an average of 180.60 minutes, its surgeries has a medical area where the *file.cld* contains more free time. Difficult *file.dat2* has a average of 601.00 minutes every file.

*Group A* has an average of 26.68 scheduled surgeries, the algorithm must schedule an average of 4 new surgeries. The *Group B* has average 23.96 surgeries in original schedule and 4 new surgeries to add. The *Group C* has an average of 18.52 surgeries in original schedule and 3 surgeries to add to schedule. the last group, *Group D* has a easy schedule with easy surgeries that has an average of 16.6 surgeries inside original schedule and 3 surgeries to insert in original schedule. The easiness of an instance is determined according to the number of surgeries and minutes that contains.

GA and GA-HPop solved the dynamic scheduling with a population of 50 individuals in GA and GA-HPop, a 20% of elitism with a mutation of 1% and 10% of scouts. This data has been selected because the last studies GA for case of static scheduling

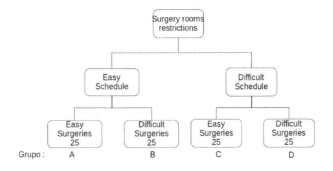

**Fig. 2.** Diagram of group of instances to GA-HPop

of surgeries [23] getting better results, the stopping method is called to function, given 10, 000 calls to function, both GA and GA-HPop are equals for number calls to function. In the case of SH don't is necessary the initial data or number of calls function.

The results obtained with the generated instances are shown in Table 2, where the results are presented according to the fitness funtion. Results of objective function do not only represent the moves of surgeries, represent also how many days was postponed the surgery. Thereby, SH shows as good performance as GA, comparing GA-HPop shows a better fitness than GA.

**Table 2.** Results according to the fitness function from Genetic Algorithm with Homogeneous Population (GA-HPob), Genetic Algorithm (GA) and Segmentation Heuristic (SH)

| Instance | | Median | | Desviation | | Best | |
|---|---|---|---|---|---|---|---|
| - | SH | GA | GA-HPob | GA | GA-HPop | GA | GA-HPop |
| INST1 | 6.00 | 8.00 | 6.00 | 7.20 | 3.41 | 5.00 | 5.00 |
| INST2 | 25.00 | 16.00 | 15.00 | 9.82 | 7.62 | 12.00 | 12.00 |
| INST3 | 12.00 | 19.00 | 12.50 | 7.69 | 6.56 | 13.00 | 12.00 |
| INST4 | 26.00 | 11.50 | 8.50 | 3.70 | 17.78 | 9.00 | 8.00 |
| INST5 | 58.00 | 71.50 | 39.50 | 18.32 | 19.51 | 41.00 | 37.00 |
| INST6 | 8.00 | 5.00 | 5.00 | 5.06 | 2.53 | 7.00 | 7.00 |
| INST7 | 15.00 | 15.00 | 12.50 | 19.04 | 13.10 | 13.00 | 12.00 |
| INST8 | 42.00 | 26.50 | 25.00 | 22.08 | 4.83 | 33.00 | 25.00 |
| INST9 | 10.00 | 16.50 | 9.00 | 13.59 | 5.57 | 13.00 | 13.00 |
| INST10 | 35.00 | 49.50 | 35.50 | 21.00 | 16.10 | 37.00 | 25.00 |

Besides, it is important to compare the fitness function versus standard deviation, which measures the uncertainty showing the dispersion of the data in relation with average, in case for SH it is zero because SH is deterministic algorithm, nevertheless, GA-HPop provides a standard deviation smaller over GA, except two of instances: *INST4* and *INST5*. This algoritm worked each instance ten times with ten thousand calls to function where the best fitness were obtained by GA-HPop.

Table 3 shows the number surgeries affected after scheduling, because its goal is present the impact from approach of number of patients that will be affected, independently of how long has postponed in the surgeries. In the case GA and GA-HPop the number of changes is given by median like the number of surgeries without schedule, it is because both the GA and the GAHPop are not deterministic algorithms such as the SH heuristic. According the number of changes is easly look that GA-HPop has getting better results than SH y GA. Nevertheless for instance *INST4* SH hold a best performance than GA and Ga-HPop, according the median of unschedule surgeries, this means that for some cases SH can have a good performance, but seek a continous good performance like Ga-HPop performance; although *INST4* does not show good performance.

**Table 3.** Number of changes to schedule the new surgeries with Segmentation Heuristics (SH), Genetic Algorithm (GA) and Genetic Algorithm with Homogeneous Population (GA-HPop)

| Instance | No. changes | | | Surgery unschedule | | |
|---|---|---|---|---|---|---|
| - | SH | GA | GA-HPop | SH | GA | GA-HPop |
| INST1 | 2.00 | 2.00 | 1.00 | 1.00 | 1.00 | 1.00 |
| INST2 | 6.00 | 3.50 | 2.00 | 4.00 | 2.00 | 2.00 |
| INST3 | 5.00 | 4.50 | 2.50 | 2.00 | 2.00 | 2.00 |
| INST4 | 7.00 | 2.50 | 2.00 | 0.00 | 2.00 | 2.00 |
| INST5 | 13.00 | 10.00 | 5.50 | 5.00 | 6.00 | 5.00 |
| INST6 | 2.00 | 1.00 | 1.00 | 2.00 | 1.00 | 1.00 |
| INST7 | 5.00 | 4.50 | 2.00 | 2.00 | 2.00 | 2.00 |
| INST8 | 8.00 | 8.00 | 3.00 | 6.00 | 3.50 | 3.00 |
| INST9 | 4.00 | 2.00 | 2.00 | 3.00 | 2.00 | 2.00 |
| INST10 | 15.00 | 9.50 | 4.00 | 3.00 | 4.00 | 4.00 |

The GA performed well with the parameters, so we considered the same information for the GAHPop. The used parameters are population of 25 individuals, elitism group of 30%, percentage of mutation of 8% and limit of 40% of cloned individuals to start exploration. Comparing the group instances with GA and GA-HPop, GA-HPop gets a better performance than GA, because the columns shown in Table 4, indicate that GA-HPop are has results more lower than GA, and the goal is minimize all these points, then GA-HPop has better performance that GA in rescheduling of surgeries.

**Table 4.** Comparing the average of results obtained of group of instances solved with GA and GA-HPop

| | Average | | | | | |
|---|---|---|---|---|---|---|
| | | | Median of surg affected | | Median of surg wihout scheduling | |
| Group | Median of Fitness | | | | | |
| | GA | GA-HPop | GA | GA-HPop | GA | GA-HPop |
| A | 28.76 | 18.32 | 8.16 | 4.42 | 3.12 | 2.58 |
| B | 24.50 | 11.96 | 7.58 | 2.74 | 3.08 | 1.86 |
| C | 12.88 | 7.16 | 4.48 | 1.56 | 1.28 | 1.06 |
| D | 5.86 | 3.76 | 1.92 | 0.84 | 0.70 | 0.64 |

# 6   Conclusion

Minimal Perturbations is a problem to scheduling of surgeries, because seek minimize the postponed surgeries to schedule the new surgeries. The mail goal is avoid the constant changes in schedule that it triggers dissatisfaction and waste of resources. However the problem is possible solve through algorithms as Segmentation Heuristics, and metaheuristics as Genetic Algorithm or an improve of GA to obtain better results.

GA according the steps explained has had better performance than a SH for scheduling surgeries, the Wilcoxon's signed-rank test affirms that GA has better performance than SH, into minimal perturbation problem in rescheduling of surgeries.

The changes of GA is the exploit its qualities and add peculiarities, geting to better performance, Wilcoxon's signed-rank test has showed that Genetic Algorithm with Homogeneous Population (GA-HPop) has a better performance than Genetic Algorithm

into minimal perturbation problem in rescheduling of surgeries. GA-HPop showed a better performance according the objetive function, the performance according the number of surgeries without schedule is the same as GA. However the role of the number of moves is better than GA into minimal perturbations problem of rescheduling surgeries.

GA-HPop according to analysis of results has been shown to have better performance against over GA and SH, it tries to approach the original schedule, while GA has genetic diversity and its individuals begin to move away from original schedule, GA-HPop generates similar individuals to original schedule and tries add new surgeries.

The behavior of GA-HPop to group of many instances has been desired, because the GA-HPop keep its stability in number surgeries affected and the dispersion the results according to the median. Moreover, even when in the tests of decrease of calls to function for GA-HPop, thought that GA could get advantage, but it was not, GA-HPop kept better performance than GA. GA-HPop has advantages of GA and additionally a better performance.

We have some ideas for future work, for example, to search for other algorithms that could further get better results, less perturbations in schedule, add other restriccions like lack of surgical equipment, changes of a surgical and others, the implementation of GA-HPop for a system led to IMSS's users, and thus may improve the institution service. And as desirable work, to generate a system with adaptive capabilities for rules of any medical institution.

**Acknowledgment.** Authors want to thank the Consejo Nacional de Ciencia y Tecnología (CONACyT), for their support to carry out this research through a scholarship to Adriana Rubí Pérez López, and thanks to the project 4310.11P of DGEST.

# References

1. Hao, X., Lin, L.: Job shop rescheduling by using multi-objective genetic algorithm. In: 2010 40th International Conference Computers and Industrial Engineering (CIE), pp. 1–6 (2010)
2. Barták, R., Müller, T., Rudová, H.: Minimal perturbation problem a formal view. Neural Network World 13, 501–511 (2003)
3. Hani El Sakkout, T.R., Wallace, M.: Minimal perturbation in dynamic scheduling. In: 13th European Conference on Artificial Intelligence, pp. 504–508 (1998)
4. Zhao, F., Wang, J., Jonrinaldi, J.: A dynamic rescheduling model with multi-agent system and its solution method. Journal of Mechanical Engineering 58, 81–92 (2012)
5. Montana, D., Vidaver, G., Hussain, T.: A reconfigurable multiagent society for transportation scheduling and dynamic rescheduling. In: Integration of Knowledge Intensive Multi-Agent Systems, pp. 79–84 (2007)
6. Zivan, R., Grubshtein, A., Meisels, A.: Hybrid search for minimal perturbation in dynamic csps. Constraints 16(3), 228–249 (2011)
7. Kuster, J., Jannach, D., Friedrich, G.: Applying local rescheduling in response to schedule disruptions. Annals of Operations Research 180, 265–282 (2010)
8. Elkhyari, A., Guéret, C., Jussien, N.: Constraint programming for dynamic scheduling problems. In: International Scheduling Symposium, pp. 84–89 (2004)
9. Davis, L.: Handbook of genetic algorithms. In: A Genetic Algorithms Tutorial (1991)

10. Dimitrov, T., Baumann, M.: Genetic algorithm with genetic engineering technology for multi-objective dynamic job shop scheduling problems. In: Proceedings of the 13th Annual Conference Companion on Genetic and Evolutionary Computation, GECCO 2011, pp. 833–834. ACM, New York (2011)
11. Ouelhadj, D., Petrovic, S.: A survey of dynamic scheduling in manufacturing systems. J. of Scheduling 12(4), 417–431 (2009)
12. Gly, L., Dessagne, G., Lrin, C.: Modelling train re-scheduling with optimization an operational research techniques: results and applications at sncf. In: World Congress on Railway Research (2006)
13. Pinedo, M.L.: Scheduling, Theory, Algorithms, and Systems. Springer (2008)
14. Zonderland, M., Boucherie, R., Litvak, N., Vleggeert-Lankamp, C.: Planning and scheduling of semi-urgent surgeries. Health Care Management Science 13(3), 256–267 (2010)
15. Godin, P., Wang, C.: Agent-based outpatient scheduling for diagnostic services. In: Systems Man and Cybernetics (SMC), pp. 1851–1856 (2010)
16. Moratori, P.B., Petrovic, S., Rodríguez, J.A.V.: Fuzzy approaches for robust job shop rescheduling. In: FUZZ-IEEE 2010, pp. 1–7 (2010)
17. de San Pedro, M., Eugenia, P.D., Marta, L., Villagra, A., Leguizamn, G.: Metaheurística ACO aplicada a problemas de planificación en entornos dinámicos. In: IX Workshop de Investigadores en Ciencias de la Computacion (2007)
18. Fernandes, C.M., Lima, C., Rosa, A.C.: Umdas for dynamic optimization problems. In: Proceedings of the 10th Annual Conference on Genetic and Evolutionary Computation, GECCO 2008, pp. 399–406. ACM, New York (2008)
19. Barták, R., Müller, T., Rudová, H.: A New Approach to Modeling and Solving Minimal Perturbation Problems. In: Apt, K.R., Fages, F., Rossi, F., Szeredi, P., Váncza, J. (eds.) CSCLP 2003. LNCS (LNAI), vol. 3010, pp. 233–249. Springer, Heidelberg (2004)
20. Exploring the Solution of Course Timetabling Problems through Heuristic Segmentation (2012)
21. Dasgupta, S., Papadimitriou, C.H., Vazirani, U.V.: Algorithms. Mc Graw Hill (May 2006)
22. Holland, J.: Algoritmos genéticos. Investigacion y Ciencia 192, 38–45 (1992)
23. Perez-Lopez, A., Baltazar, R., Carpio, M., Alanis, A.: Three metaheuristics solving a scheduling problem in a ria environment. In: VIII Encuentro Regional Académico III Encuentro Internacional Académico y de Investigación (2012)

# CUP Classification Based on a Tree Structure with MiRNA Feature Selection

Xiaoxue Zhang[1], Dunwei Wen[2], Ke Wang[1], and Yinan Yang[1]

[1] College of Communication Engineering, Jilin University, China
{xxzhang11,yangyn12}@mails.jlu.edu.cn, wangke@jlu.edu.cn
[2] School of Computing and Information Systems, Athabasca University, Canada
dunweiw@athabascau.ca

**Abstract.** Given the low sensitivity of identifying the origin of cancer tissues using miRNAs in previous research, we adopt a decision tree structure to build a new SVM based model for identifying a variety of Cancer of Unknown Primary Origin (CUP). We use an information gain based feature selection method provided by Weka to select miRNAs and combine them with previously recognized features to determine several most useful miRNAs. Next we design a layer-by-layer classification tree based on the expression levels of these selected miRNAs. Then we use a polynomial kernel SVM classifier, which is more effective in dealing with binary classification problem, for classification at each node of the decision tree structure. In our experiments, a final overall sensitivity of the test set reached 87%, and the sensitivity of identifying the metastatic samples in the test set significantly increased by 9%. The 10-fold cross-validation on this model shows that the sensitivity of the test set is not less than the sensitivity of the training set, indicating that the model has good generalization ability. Additionally, the use of general feature selection makes the approach of this paper more adaptable and suitable for other areas.

**Keywords:** miRNAs, SVM, CUP, feature selection, sensitivity.

## 1   Introduction

We can get abundant of protein-coding genes by regulating the expression levels of miRNAs (microRNA), and thus control the biological characteristics, so the expression levels of miRNAs can fully represent gene function level, which makes the use of miRNAs as biomarkers for cancer classification possible. There has been some research in this field in recent years. Kim and Cho [1] performed the feature extraction for miRNAs and compared the performance of multiple classifiers, dividing the samples into tumor tissues and normal tissues and obtained a recognition rate for the test data as high as 95%. Leidinger et al. [2] demonstrated that miRNAs in blood cells could be used as biomarkers to distinguish melanoma and achieved a classification accuracy of 97.4%. Although these studies proved the effectiveness of miRNAs in distinguishing tumors, they only used miRNA expression effectiveness for binary

F. Castro, A. Gelbukh, and M. González (Eds.): MICAI 2013, Part I, LNAI 8265, pp. 485–496, 2013.

classification problem, and they did not demonstrate the effectiveness of miRNAs for distinguishing a variety of tumors.

Cancer of Unknown Primary Origin (CUP) is the aggressive cancer with poor prognosis. The metastatic cancer cells of CUP may distribute in any part of the body. While diagnosing the CUP tissue origin is an important clinical application, they cannot be diagnosed by physical examination and pathological analysis. Thus it is very necessary to use gene expression profile to identify CUP tissue origin and this belongs to multiclass tumor classification problem. Shedden et al. [3] distinguished 14 types of cancer by an automatic pathology tree, but they have used 250 genes and the sensitivity only reached 83%, and if the number of gene has reduced to less than 100, the sensitivity of classification dropped to 80%. Later, a team of researchers [4] used nearly 600 genes to distinguish 13 types of cancer origins, the sensitivity achieved 90%, but the reduced number of genes caused a decline of sensitivity. These results show that we need to seek a better way which can be a good trade-off between sensitivity, the number of categories and the number of genes. Rosenfeld et al. [5] have proposed a decision-tree classifier (in Section 3) based on miRNAs to identify the metastatic carcinoma tissues. They used only 48 miRNAs to distinguish 22 types of cancer and reached an overall sensitivity of 86%. Compared with the work of Tothill et al. [4], this result used less cancer genes to classify more types of cancer and reached a high sensitivity, and it also focused on the metastatic samples in test set and made a detailed analysis, the sensitivity was 77%. It basically achieved a trade-off mentioned above, but the sensitivity of metastatic samples is low. Moreover, it used a logistic regression model to select features, which is domain specific and not very adaptable for other areas. Note that what we mentioned above are focused on some different situations of the research and may not be entirely comparable.

To address the deficiencies of the above studies, we perform a set of more suitable data processing, feature selection and training methods to enhance classification capability of the original decision-tree [5], which yields significant improvement in the sensitivity of metastatic samples in our experiments and also brings adaptability to our model.

The paper is organized as follows. Section 1 introduces the research background. Section 2 describes the main methods we proposed and Section 3 presents our experimental study. We make the comparison between our results and the previous results in Section 4, and finally a summary in Section 5.

## 2    Our Method

Feature selection and training SVM classifier at each node of Fig. 1 are our primary work (see Fig. 2). The idea is to use information gain associated method for the selection of miRNAs, then apply these selected features to train SVM classifier, and finally use test data to evaluate the classifier.

## 2.1  Feature Selection

Feature selection is an important way to improve the performance of a classification problem. The features we use for classification is the expression levels of miRNAs. There are some miRNA examples shown in Table 1. The first column is the name of miRNAs; their sequences are in the second column, the length of which ranges from 20 to 25; and the last column lists their expression levels, which are the features we used for our study. Basically, our feature selection method is based on the observation that, removing the miRNAs with weak distinguishing ability can improve accuracy, and removing the low importance miRNAs can accelerate the speed. Also, to improve the adaptability of the approach, we apply automatic feature selection techniques for selecting miRNAs before classification. More specifically, we use information gain of the attributes as our measure to select features, which, as Yu and Liu [6] have pointed out, is one of the most effective and fast methods, and the symmetry of which is a desired property for a measure of correlations between features.

**Table 1.** MiRNA samples

| miRNA name | Sequence(20-25) | Expression level |
|---|---|---|
| miR-124a | UUAAGGCACGCGGUGAAUGCCA | 7.4204 |
| miR-125b | UCCCUGAGACCCUAACUUGUGA | 10.8391 |
| miR-7 | UGGAAGACUAGUGAUUUUGUU | 6.64631 |

Let $X$ and $Y$ represent two attributes respectively, then the information gain of $X$ can be expressed as

$$IG(X \mid Y) = H(X) - H(X \mid Y) \tag{1}$$

where, $H(X)$ is the information entropy of $X$, $H(X \mid Y)$ is the information entropy of $X$ when observing attribute $Y$. When the information gain of $X$ is bigger than that of $Y$, we select attribute $X$ rather than attribute $Y$.

We choose three evaluation methods which are associated with information gain to select miRNAs, these methods are provided by Weka 3.6 [7]. They are the combination of Information Gain Ranking Filter and Attribute Ranking search strategy, the combination of Gain Ratio Feature Evaluator and Attribute Ranking search strategy, and the combination of CFS Subset Evaluator and Best first search strategy respectively.

**Information Gain Ranking Filter.** It evaluates an attribute according to the information gain *InfoGain* of the attribute related to the classes, which belongs to single attribute evaluation method.

$$InfoGain(Class, Attribute) = H(Class) - H(Class \mid Attribute) \tag{2}$$

Where *Class* represents class attribute, *Attribute* represents a single attribute. Now we can judge one miRNA according to the miRNA's *InfoGain*, which is related to the class attribute, and eventually find several miRNAs which have the most information gain constitute a feature set.

**Gain Ratio Feature Evaluator.** It evaluates an attribute based on the information gain ratio of a single attribute, which also belongs to single attribute evaluation method.

$$GainRatio(Class, Attribute) = \frac{H(Class) - H(Class \mid Attribute)}{H(Attribute)} \tag{3}$$

where, *Class* represents class attribute, *Attribute* represents a single attribute. It evaluates a miRNA according to the miRNA's information gain ratio, find several miRNAs whose information gain ratio are larger than others constitute a feature set.

**CFS Subset Evaluator.** It is a subset evaluation method. CFS [8] (Correlation-based Feature Selection) is an evaluation method that can be used to find a feature subset based on the feature correlation. The evaluation method can be given by

$$M_s = \frac{k \, \bar{r}_{cf}}{\sqrt{k + k(k-1)\bar{r}_{ff}}} \tag{4}$$

where, $M_s$ is the evaluation of a subset which has $k$ attributes, $\bar{r}_{cf}$ is the average correlations between attributes and classes and $\bar{r}_{ff}$ is the average correlations between attributes and other attributes. So the greater the correlation or the lower the redundancy between attributes and classes, the higher the evaluation value in the subset obtained by CFS algorithm. This algorithm is also related to the information gain, by which the correlations between attributes are given.

**Attribute Ranking.** It is a search strategy that used for sorting attributes based on the criterion values obtained by a given evaluation method. According to Weka 3.6, the Information Gain Ranking Filter and Gain Ratio feature evaluator are used together with Ranker. In the search process, Ranker calls the evaluation function to evaluate the miRNAs that are not at the attribute starting point, then sorting the criterion values of these miRNAs, and return miRNA sequence list to obtain a feature subset.

**Best First.** It is used together with CFS Subset Evaluator evaluation method. It is based on the best-first principle. The idea of this algorithm is applying a greedy hill-climbing method with traceback to search the attribute space with forward search (add one attribute every time) starting from an empty subset. Search will finish when the performance is not improved. Best First uses the given evaluation method to search a given data set and return the search result.

## 2.2   SVM Classification

The main purpose of SVM [9] is to deal with the binary classification problem based on max-margin principle. The idea is that the final decision of SVM is only determined by a fewer number of support vectors, which can ensure the lowest error rate with global optimum. These factors often make SVM a stronger candidate than other algorithms such as KNN and logistic regression, which were used by Rosenfeld et al. [5]. Similar to them, we first used a simple decision tree to perform the experiment, but the sensitivity for test samples was only 49%, consistent with their experiment, which is not acceptable. We thus adopted SVM classifiers in our study.

When using the SVM to do the classification, the primary form of the optimization problem [10] can be expressed as

$$
\begin{aligned}
\underset{w,b,\xi}{\text{minimize}} \quad & \frac{1}{2} w^T w + C \sum_{i=1}^{l} \xi_i \\
\text{subject to} \quad & y_i \left( w^T \phi(x_i) + b \right) \geq 1 - \xi_i \\
& \xi_i \geq 0.
\end{aligned}
\tag{5}
$$

In the formula, $y_i$ is the class label, $i = 1,...,l$, $x_i \in R^n$ and $y \in \{1,-1\}^l$, $C$ is the penalty parameter, and $C>0$. Now vector $x_i$ is mapped into a high dimensional space by function $\phi$.

In addition, $K(x_i, x_j) \equiv \phi(x_i)^T \phi(x_j)$ is called the kernel function. And the dual form of optimization problem (5) can be represented by

$$
\begin{aligned}
\text{maximise} \quad & W(\alpha) = \sum_{i=1}^{l} \alpha_i - \frac{1}{2} \sum_{i,j=1}^{l} y_i y_j \alpha_i \alpha_j K(x_i \cdot x_j) \\
\text{subject to} \quad & \sum_{i=1}^{l} y_i \alpha_i = 0, \quad \alpha_i \geq 0, i = 1,...,l
\end{aligned}
\tag{6}
$$

In the formula, $y_i$ is the class label, $i = 1,...,l$, $x_i \in R^n$ and $y \in \{1,-1\}^l$, $C$ is the penalty parameter, and $C>0$. $K(x_i, x_j) \equiv \phi(x_i)^T \phi(x_j)$ is kernel function. The use of the kernel function is to ensure that the optimization problem is convex, it can change the complexity of the data space, make the algorithm efficiency higher. So we use kernel-based SVM.

There are four commonly used kernel functions for SVM as follows

- linear: $K(x_i, x_j) = x_i^T x_j$
- polynomial: $K(x_i, x_j) = (\gamma x_i^T x_j + r)^d, \gamma > 0$
- radial basis function (RBF): $K(x_i, x_j) = \exp(-\gamma \|x_i - x_j\|^2), \gamma > 0$
- sigmoid: $K(x_i, x_j) = \tanh(\gamma x_i^T x_j + r)$

In above kernel functions, $\gamma$, $r$ and $d$ of them are all kernel parameters.

It has been proven that the performance of linear and sigmoid functions are similar to RBF ones in some cases [11, 12]. Because we have not found a detailed comparative analysis between RBF and polynomial kernel functions for similar classification problems, we test both kinds of kernel functions in our experiments individually.

## 3    Experiment Scheme Design

Our experiments used 336 cancer samples, the same as Rosenfeld et al. [5] used, containing 22 types of cancers (each cancer contains the primary cancer and its corresponding metastatic cancer), each sample contains 48 miRNA expression levels. Randomly select about 1/4 of each type of cancer sample as the test set, so that the final test set contains a total of 83 samples, and the remaining 253 samples constitute the training set. The whole classification process is performed on the basis of the decision tree structure (shown in Fig. 1) defined by Rosenfeld et al. [5]. There are 24 nodes in the structure. Binary classification is performed at each node and each leaf represents a type of cancer (a few exceptions are as follows: 'stomach*' includes both stomach cancers and gastroesophageal junction adenocarcinomas, 'head & neck*' includes cancers of head and neck and squamous carcinoma of esophagus, and 'GIST' is gastrointestinal stromal tumors). It should be noted that, at one node, the samples that have been classified before will no longer be input in the node for classification. This reduces the interference between the irrelevant samples. Data processing and training at each node are shown in Fig. 2. We use information gain associated method for feature selection of miRNAs and obtain the proper subset of miRNAs, and then use these selected miRNAs to train SVM classifier with a 10-fold cross-validation, which only uses the training partition, and in average, there are 71 samples in each node for training the SVM classifier, finally use test date to evaluate the classifier. We use Weka [13] as experiment platform, and use LibSVM [10] to perform SVM related tasks.

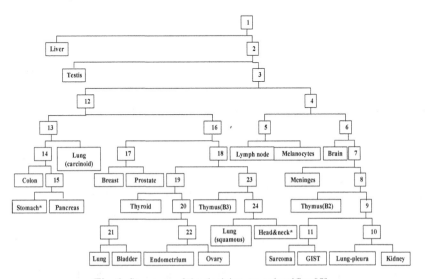

**Fig. 1.** Structure of the decision-tree classifier [5]

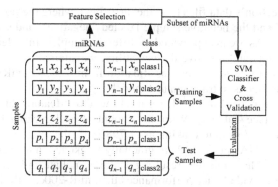

**Fig. 2.** Single node data processing

## 3.1    MiRNAs Feature Selection Process

This is the feature selection part of Fig. 2. Feature selection procedure [14] is shown in Fig. 3, the program selects features repeatedly, every time generate a new goodness value of the subset of miRNAs by an evaluation method, and compare with the old subset of miRNAs, if the performance of a new subset is better than the old one, then the new subset replaces the best subset. While performing feature selection, the stopping criterion is indispensable, as without it the program will never stop and we cannot get the result subset of miRNAs. In our experiment, we set the stopping criterion as a small number given by the program in Weka to make sure a complete iteration process, so that we can get the optimal feature subset. After getting the subset, we also perform a cross-validation on the training partition to evaluate it and make the final selection.

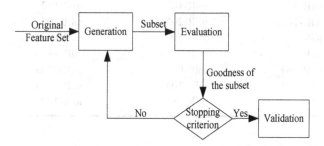

**Fig. 3.** Feature selection process with validation [14]

We used a built-in yet general attribute selecting option of Weka 3.6 for feature selection, which select miRNAs at each node as features for classification. This option requires the user to specify evaluation criteria and search strategy, and the evaluation criteria and search strategy need to be paired according to Weka. As mentioned above, we choose information gain based evaluation criteria, i.e., Information Gain Ranking Filter, Gain Ratio feature evaluator and CFS Subset Evaluator, in our experiments. More specifically, we use the first two evaluation methods together with the search strategy Attribute Ranking, and match the last evaluation method with the search strategy Best First.

In feature selection's data files (i.e., the .arff files), where the positive sample is labeled "positive" and the negative sample labeled "negative", and different expression levels 48 miRNAs are also provided in different samples. In order to achieve better classification results and improve the versatility, we attempt to find the certain miR-NAs which are most effective for classification from these 48 miRNAs, then use the subset of these miRNAs to train and test model.

For example, at node 3 in Fig. 1, we used the above feature selection method and got some results (see Table 2). With the amount of backtracking for Best First as 5 and the threshold of Attribute ranking as -1.798E308, the classification performances of the selected miRNAs in Table 2 are gradually weakened in the serial number order. We can see in Table 2 that the resulting features include miR-200c, miR-141 and miR-182, which provide better performances than miR-200c, miR-181a and miR-205 that are used in Rosenfeld et al. [5] instead. Considering their selection of miRNAs has guided by pathology theory, we incorporate it with our automatic selection, and finally choose miR-200c, miR-181a, miR-205, miR-141 and miR-182 as the miRNAs features for node 3 (in Fig. 4). These miRNAs can yield a local test sensitivity of 98% in our experiments, while the sensitivity of original features is 96%. This result shows that our improved feature selection is effective. Feature selection at other nodes is performed the same way as node 3.

**Table 2.** Feature selection results of different method

|    | Cfs + BestFirst | GainRatio + Ranker | InfoGain + Ranker |
|----|-----------------|--------------------|-------------------|
| 1  | miR-141         | miR-200c           | miR-200c          |
| 2  | miR-182         | miR-141            | miR-141           |
| 3  | miR-200c        | miR-375            | miR-375           |
| 4  | miR-31          | miR-182            | miR-182           |
| 5  | miR-181a        | miR-200a           | miR-205           |
| 6  | miR-9*          | miR-509            | miR-181a          |
| 7  | miR-152         | miR-146a           | miR-181b          |
| 8  | miR-509         | miR-9*             | miR-130a          |
| 9  | miR-205         | miR-205            | miR-146a          |
| 10 |                 | miR-181a           | miR-152           |

### 3.2    SVM Classification Processing

When training SVM classifier, we used Weka's interface for LibSVM for parameter setting, model training and validation. The same as feature selection part, there are 2 kinds of samples need to be input to SVM, one is the "positive" sample, and the other one is the "negative" sample. At first, we used RBF kernel SVM for classification while repeatedly adjusting the parameters, but the sensitivity still cannot exceed 86%, the result from Rosenfeld et al.'s experiment [5]. After using polynomial kernel, however, the performance had obvious improvement. So we decide to use polynomial kernel for our final experiments. We searched the suitable parameter values of polynomial kernel through repeated adjustments. For example, at node 3, the parameter setting of SVM is shown in Table 3, and the miRNAs we use to classify at node 3 shown in Fig. 4, and then a classification result on test set at node 3 shown in Fig. 5, where "a" represents the positive sample and "b" represents the negative sample. Fig. 5 shows that there are 79 samples correctly classified, and 2 samples incorrectly classified, so the sensitivity at node 3 is 97.5397%. Also, the area under ROC curve is 0.974 (close to 1), which is also part of the output results of our experiment program. We can see that our feature selection and SVM classification approach yield very good results.

**Table 3.** Parameter setting

| SVM type | Kernel type | gamma | degree | ceof0 |
|----------|-------------|-------|--------|-------|
| C-SVC | polynomial | 4.0 | 4 | 1.45 |

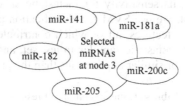

**Fig. 4.** MiRNAs used at node 3

```
a     b  ◄— classified as
47    1  | a=positive
 1   32  | b=negative
```

**Fig. 5.** Confusion matrix

# 4    Results and Analysis

Our experiment results and a comparison of them with the results of Rosenfeld et al. [5] are shown in Table 4. In Table 4, 'Union' is the method of Rosenfeld et al., 'SDTM' represents SVM Decision Tree Model, which is our method, and 'sens' represents sensitivity. The 1st column lists different types of cancer, 2 to 4 columns are the results of all 83 test samples, 5 to 7 columns are the results of metastatic samples included in test set, and the sample number of test set (TN) and metastatic sample number (MN) in test set is the same as Rosenfeld et al.'s [5]. We can see that our test sensitivity is 87%, only a slight improvement compared with Rosenfeld et al.'s 86%. For the part of metastatic samples included in test set, however, our sensitivity is 86%, a 9% increase compared to Rosenfeld et al.'s 77%. So in this more important part, we obtain a significant improvement. There are 13 types of cancer test sensitivity reach 100% in Rosenfeld et al.'s experiment, but ours can make 14 types achieve 100%, and specificities of most of the categories can achieve 100%. In addition, the experiment shares 131 metastatic samples, and we test on these samples with a sensitivity of 93.89%.

We applied a 10-fold cross-validation in searching the model parameters, and compared the cross-validation sensitivity of the training set to the final sensitivity of test set. It turns out that the sensitivities are similar in both cases. This means that the model we used is not over-fitting and has good generalization ability.

By re-selecting features on the basis of Rosenfeld et al.'s work as mentioned above, we added some useful features at each node, and thus provided more discriminative factors for classification, which greatly increases the information useful for classification and results in the higher accuracy. For the classification method, we choose polynomial kernel SVM, this is because generally it is better than other classifiers in handling binary classification problem, and free of local minimum. The method of Rosenfeld et al. is a combination of KNN and decision tree algorithm, the effect of any of which is not ideal, and the single decision tree algorithm in their work reached an average sensitivity of 78%, and specificity of 99%, with an even lower sensitivity of 71% by using single KNN algorithm (best situation when k=3). The authors thus used a "Union" method to combine both methods. Although it reached a higher sensitivity of 86%, its sensitivity for metastatic samples in test set was still low, only 77%. In contrast, we use SVM for classification and apply general feature selection methods to select features, all of which contribute to a significant 9% increase in the sensitivity of metastatic samples in test set, and at the same time, make our model more adaptable for similar applications than the previous work.

**Table 4.** Comparision of test results

| Cancer Type | Results of test set (%) | | | Results of metastases in test set (%) | | |
|---|---|---|---|---|---|---|
| | TN | Union sens | SDTM sens | MN | Union sens | SDTM sens |
| Bladder | 2 | 0 | 50 | 1 | 0 | 100 |
| Brain | 5 | 100 | 100 | 0 | | |
| Breast | 5 | 60 | 60 | 4 | 50 | 50 |
| Colon | 5 | 60 | 60 | 3 | 100 | 100 |
| Endometrium | 3 | 67 | 33 | 1 | 100 | 100 |
| Head&neck* | 8 | 100 | 100 | 0 | | |
| Kidney | 5 | 100 | 100 | 2 | 100 | 100 |
| Liver | 2 | 100 | 100 | 0 | | |
| Lung | 5 | 100 | 100 | 1 | 100 | 100 |
| Lung-pleura | 2 | 50 | 100 | 0 | | |
| Lymph-node | 5 | 80 | 100 | 0 | | |
| Melanocytes | 5 | 80 | 80 | 4 | 75 | 75 |
| Meninges | 3 | 100 | 100 | 0 | | |
| Ovary | 4 | 100 | 75 | 1 | 100 | 100 |
| Pancreas | 2 | 100 | 50 | 0 | | |
| Prostate | 2 | 100 | 100 | 0 | | |
| Sarcoma | 5 | 80 | 100 | 4 | 75 | 100 |
| Stomach* | 7 | 86 | 100 | 1 | 100 | 100 |
| Stromal | 2 | 100 | 100 | 0 | | |
| Testis | 1 | 100 | 100 | 0 | | |
| Thymus | 2 | 100 | 50 | 0 | | |
| Thyroid | 3 | 100 | 100 | 0 | | |
| Overall | 83 | 86 | 87 | 22 | 77 | 86 |

# 5    Conclusion

We have presented our work on improving the low sensitivity reported in the previous methods for identifying origins of metastatic cancer tissues through miRNAs. We enhanced the decision-tree based multiclass classification through general feature selection and stronger classifiers. Our proposed model achieved a sensitivity of 86% in identifying metastatic samples in test set, a significant improvement compared with 77% in the previous research. Also, the use of SVM classification, and general feature selection methods in our model, makes it more adaptable than the previous methods and more easily to be applied to other similar tasks. In the future, we will extend the model to more complex medical classification problems.

# References

1. Kim, K.J., Cho, S.B.: Exploring features and classifiers to classify microRNA expression profiles of human cancer. In: Wong, K.W., Mendis, B.S.U., Bouzerdoum, A. (eds.) ICONIP 2010, Part II. LNCS, vol. 6444, pp. 234–241. Springer, Heidelberg (2010)
2. Leidinger, P., Keller, A., Borries, A., Reichrath, J., Rass, K., Jager, S.U., Lenhof, H., Meese, E.: High-throughput miRNA profiling of human melanoma blood samples. BMC Cancer 10(1), 262 (2010)
3. Shedden, K.A., Taylor, J.M., Giordano, T.J., Kuick, R., Misek, D.E., Rennert, G., Schwartz, D.R., Gruber, S.B., Logsdon, C., Simeone, D., Kardia, S.L., Greenson, J.K., Cho, K.R., Beer, D.G., Fearon, E.R., Hanash, S.: Accurate molecular classification of human cancers based on gene expression using a simple classifier with a pathological tree-based framework. Am. J. Pathol. 163(5), 1985–1995 (2003)
4. Tothill, R.W., Kowalczyk, A., Rischin, D., Bousioutas, A., Haviv, I., Van Laar, R.K., Waring, P.M., Zalcberg, J., Ward, R., Biankin, A.V., Sutherland, R.L., Henshall, S.M., Fong, K., Pollack, J.R., Bowtell, D.D., Holloway, A.J.: An expression-based site of origin diagnostic method designed for clinical application to cancer of unknown origin. Cancer Research 65(10), 4031–4040 (2005)
5. Rosenfeld, N., Aharonov, R., Meiri, E., Rosenwald, S., Spector, Y., Zepeniuk, M., Benjamin, H., Shabes, N., Tabak, S., Levy, A., Lebanony, D., Goren, Y., Silberschein, E., Targan, N., Ben-Ari, A., Gilad, S., Ion-Vardy, N.S., Tobar, A., Feinmesse, M.R., Kharenko, O., Nativ, O., Nass, D., Perelman, M., Yosepovich, A., Shalmon, B., Polak-Charcon, S., Fridman, E., Avniel, A., Bentwich, I., Bentwich, Z., Cohen, D., Chajut, A., Barshack, I.: MicroRNAs accurately identify cancer tissue origin. Nature Biotechnology 26(4), 462–469 (2008)
6. Yu, L., Liu, H.: Feature selection for high-dimensional data: A fast correlation-based filter solution. In: Twentieth International Conference on Machine Learning, vol. 2(2), pp. 856–863 (2003)
7. Witten, I.H., Frank, E.: Data Mining: Practical machine learning tools and techniques. Morgan Kaufmann (2005)
8. Lu, X., Peng, X., Liu, P., Deng, Y., Feng, B., Liao, B.: A novel feature selection method based on CFS in cancer recognition. In: 2012 IEEE 6th International Conference on Systems Biology, pp. 226–231 (2012)
9. Cortes, C., Vapnik, V.: Support-vector networks. Machine Learning 20(3), 273–297 (1995)

10. Chang, C., Lin, C.: A library for support vector machines. ACM Transactions on Intelligent Systems and Technology 2(3), 1–27 (2011)
11. Keerthi, S.S., Lin, C.J.: Asymptotic behaviors of support vector machines with Gaussian kernel. Neural Computation 15(7), 1667–1689 (2003)
12. Lin, H.T., Lin, C.J.: A study on sigmoid kernels for SVM and the training of non-PSD kernels by SMO-type methods. Neural Computation, 1–32 (2003)
13. Hall, M., Frank, E., Holmes, G., Pfahringer, B., Reutemann, P., Witten, I.H.: The WEKA data mining software: an update. ACM SIGKDD Explorations Newsletter 11(3), 10–18 (2009)
14. Dash, M., Liu, H.: Feature selection for classification. Intelligent Data Analysis 1(3), 131–156 (1997)

# Machine Learning Techniques Applied to the Cleavage Site Prediction Problem*

Gloria Inés Alvarez[1], Enrique Bravo[2], Diego Linares[1], Jheyson Faride Vargas[1], and Jairo Andrés Velasco[1]

[1] Pontificia Universidad Javeriana Cali
{galvarez,dlinares,jheysonv,jairov}@javerianacali.edu.co
[2] Universidad del Valle
enrique.bravo@correounivalle.edu.co

**Abstract.** The Genome of the Potyviridae virus family is usually expressed as a polyprotein which can be divided into ten proteins through the action of enzymes or proteases which cut the chain in specific places called cleavage sites. Three different techniques were employed to model each cleavage site: Hidden Markov Models (HMM), grammatical inference OIL algorithm (OIL), and Artificial Neural Networks (ANN).

Based on experimentation, the Hidden Markov Model has the best classification performance as well as a high robustness in relation to class imbalance. However, the Order Independent Language (OIL) algorithm is found to exhibit the ability to improve when models are trained using a greater number of samples without regard to their huge imbalance.

## 1 Introduction

At present, good results have been obtained through the application of diverse machine learning techniques to many bioinformatics issues. In this paper, three machine learning techniques have been applied to the Potyvirus polyprotein cleavage site prediction problem. Two experiments were conducted to compare the performance of the grammatical Inference OIL alogrithm(OIL), Hidden Markov Models (HMM) and Artificial Neural Networks (ANN) on the prediction problem. Section I describes the Potyviridae family and its related cleavage site prediction problem. Section 2 briefly presents the three machine learning techniques applied. Section 3 describes the design of the experiments. Section 4 analyzes results of the experiments. And, Section 5 presents conclusions and proposals for future work.

---

* The translation for publication in English was done by John Field Palencia Roth, assistant professor in the Department of Communication and Language of the Faculty of Humanities and Social Sciences at the Pontificia Universidad Javeriana Cali. This work is funded by the Departamento Administrativo de Ciencia, Tecnología e Innovación de Colombia (COLCIENCIAS) under the grant project code 1251-521-28290.

F. Castro, A. Gelbukh, and M. González (Eds.): MICAI 2013, Part I, LNAI 8265, pp. 497–507, 2013.

## 2   The Cleavage Site Prediction Problem

Cleavage site prediction is a well-known problem in bioinformatics [1], [2], [3]; a problem which consists in finding the places where macromolecules are cut by specific peptidases and proteinases in the maturation process. This in turn leads to the securement of functional products. Cleavage sites in signal peptides, in viral coding segments, and in other biological patterns can be predicted, thus the problem is present in a great variety of species, from a virus to a human being. Additionally, cleavage sites may be viewed in either a primary, secondary or tertiary structure of a polyprotein; however, the prediction problem is based on the primary structure. The prediction of cleavage sites allows for the isolation of specific segments, the annotation of new sequences, and the comparison of all these findings with existing databases such as GenBank and PDB. Biologists have made predictions of various sites in biosequences, based on patterns which they have discovered. At times, these patterns show very little variability, for example: the termination codon for translation of proteins from messenger RNA is one of the following three: UAA, UAG, or UGA. However, cleavage sites are so variable that there exist tens or hundreds of different sequences marking each site. Therefore, due to the complexity of these cleavage site patterns, algorithms detect these patterns more easily. Potyviridae viruses, members of the largest plant virus family, are responsible for serious economic losses involving agricultural crops as well as grasses and ornamental plants. Thus, there is real interest in trying to understand and control these viruses effectively.

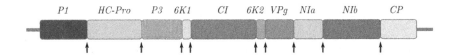

**Fig. 1.** Structure of a Potyvirus poliprotein. Arrows show cleavage sites.

Figure 1 shows segments and cleavage sites of the polyprotein obtained from the Potyvirus genome translation. This polyprotein is made up of amino acid sequences which encode the functional information of the virus typically in the following 10 segments: P1, HC-Pro, P3, 6k1, CI, 6K2, VPg-NIa, NIa and Nib-Pro.

From the computational point of view, the problem consists in learning nine models, one for each cleavage site. Each of these nine models must be able to distinguish the location of a given site based on fragments of a test sequence. Determining the most appropriate technique needed to train these binary classifier models for such a purpose is the express intention of this paper.

# 3   Description of Machine Learning Techniques

Grammatical Inference (GI) using OIL, Hidden Markov Models (HMM), and Artificial Neural Networks (ANN) are the three machine learning techniques used to predict the location of the nine cleavage sites. This prediction is based on the polyprotein obtained through the transcription of the genome of a Potyviridae family virus. In fact, due to the nondeterminism of the OIL algorithm, and the ability of HMM and ANN to produce different models depending on their initialization values, each technique generates a set of classifiers which participate in a voting system; thus, determining the prediction result.

## 3.1   Order Independent Language (OIL)

OIL is a non deterministic grammatical inference algorithm; it learns automata from positive and negative samples through a merging states technique. OIL was first proposed as an abstract theory [4], but later it proved to be useful in practical tasks of language learning [5]. OIL merges states in random order and yields different automata which, in turn, depend on the resultant order. Figure 2 presents a description of the algorithm: Lines 1 and 2 show how the positive and negative samples are ordered lexicographically; on line 3 $M$, a first empty automaton, is constructed; from lines 4 to 9, each positive sample is considered: if the current automaton $M$ accepts the sample, nothing happens; however if the sample is rejected, $M$ is redefined in order to accept the sample, thus being reduced by merging states as much as possible. It is important to note that the negative samples must be used during the reduction process in avoidance of merging states which cause the acceptance of any negative sample. In line 11, the algorithm returns $M$, the final model obtained.

## 3.2   Hidden Markov Model (HMM)

The states of the HMM statistical model are unobserved; but its outputs, which depend on hidden states, are visible [6]. The parameters of the model are the probabilities of transition among states as well as of emission of outputs from each state. The HMM is used in many fields of knowledge; here, its applications are used specifically to solve diverse problems of modeling and prediction in the field of bioinformatics.

## 3.3   Artificial Neural Network (ANN)

ANN is another well-evaluated machine learning technique for pattern recognition tasks [1], [2]; a technique which utilizes an adaptive massively parallel network of simple nonlinear computing elements for the acquisition of data based intelligence [7]. During the training phase, the ANN adaptive system changes its structure based on both external and internal information flows.

```
function OIL(D+, D−)
    posSamples ← lexicographical_sort(D₊)
    negSamples ← lexicographical_sort(D₋)
    M ← (Q, Σ, {0, 1, ?}, δ, q₀, Φ)
    for all pS ∈ posSamples do
        if M does not accept pS then
            M' ← (Q', Σ, {0, 1, ?}, δ', q'₀, Φ')
            M ← M ∪ M'
            M ← DoAllMergesPossible(M, negSample)
        end if
    end for
    return M
end function
```

**Fig. 2.** Order Independent Language (OIL) algorithm. OIL builds a Non-Deterministc Automaton from both positive and negative samples. D+ represents the positive training sample set. D- represents the negative training sample set.

### 3.4  Voting System

The three techniques described, OIL, HMM and ANN, are all characterized by their ability to produce several models from the same training data: OIL, due to its non deterministic behavior; and HMM and ANN, due to their dependance on initialization values. A mechanism used to exploit the advantages generated by this behavior is the voting system. This system allows for various models which can be coordinated to work together in the following way: first of all, an odd number of models are trained in order to predict the location of a cleavage site on a new sequence; then, all the models are fed the information sequence; finally, the subsequent answers are unified according to the majority.

## 4  Experiment Designs

Different procedures, both in the data preparation as well as in the tuning of the algorithms used, were employed in order to improve performance of the cleavage site prediction task on Potyvirus polyprotein sequences. This section presents the different procedures used.

### 4.1  Data Preparation

Based on the Potyvirus polyprotein sequences available in the public Swiss-Prot and TrEMBL databases, positive and negative samples were prepared. The totals of sequences prepared were: 86, manually annotated, which were found

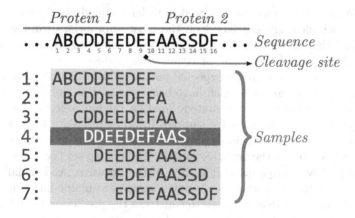

**Fig. 3.** Sampling process as made by a 6/4 sliding window

in the Swiss-Prot; and 9260, automatically annotated, which were found in the TrEMBL. Subsequently, the sequences which did not contain the 9 cleavage sites were eliminated, leaving 445; these constitute the data set used for this experiment.

A sliding window of a fixed size is used to move along the sequence in order to collect samples; each sequence contains many negative samples but only one positive sample for each determined site. Additionally, it is important to note that the cleavage site must be identified as a fixed spot within a window in order for the sample collected to be positive. Figure 3 illustrates a cleavage site and the possible samples which can be generated in its vicinity. This cleavage site is to be found between the ninth and the tenth amino acids of sequence fragment (between the E and the F), and all the samples are the same length of 10. However, the fourth sample is positive, because it contains the cleavage site in the expected position. A window of any given size could conceivably cause a collision if, within the corpus constructed by using that same window size, a given sample is detected as both positive and negative. Furthermore, collision counting guides the researcher towards determining the appropriate window size[1] by seeking to establish whether the complete pattern which pinpoints the cleavage site can be contained within a window of a given size. It is important to note that the window size which minimizes the number of collisions within the corpus in all probability contains the pattern marking the cleavage site completely.

In other words, the sliding window size was determined: based on the number of collisions per window size from 3 to 40 symbols each and taking into consideration all of the possible locations for the cleavage site while bearing in mind that in the event of a tie, the smallest window size is chosen.

---

[1] In the model, the window size represents that which biologically corresponds to the number of amino acids involved in the interaction between the polyprotein and the enzyme.

The following steps must be observed in order to build up the corpus which determines each cleavage site based on the most appropriate window selected as shown in Table 1. First of all, samples must be extracted from the sequence and then labeled as either positive or negative depending on whether or not the cleavage site is found to be in the expected position. Once all of the samples have been obtained, those samples which have been repeated as well as the negative sample in each collision are eliminated. Next, a random selection is made of both the positive and the negative samples in order to create both a training set and a testing set. The training set is created by using 80% of the positive sample as well as 80% of the negative sample. The testing set is created by using 20% of the positive sample as well as 20% of the negative. Additionally, Table 2 shows the quantity of training and testing samples available for each cleavage site. These training samples are used to construct the prediction models and the testing samples are used to compare model performance.

**Table 1.** Best window size as determined for each cleavage site prediction

| Cleavage Site | Window |
|---|---|
| 1 | 3/8 |
| 2 | 6/5 |
| 3 | 2/8 |
| 4 | 7/2 |
| 5 | 5/5 |
| 6 | 9/0 |
| 7 | 3/7 |
| 8 | 1/10 |
| 9 | 2/9 |

**Table 2.** Number of available samples per cleavage site

| Cleavage Site | Training | | Test | |
|---|---|---|---|---|
| | Positive | Negative | Positive | Negative |
| 1 | 72 | 143383 | 18 | 35846 |
| 2 | 39 | 143319 | 9 | 35830 |
| 3 | 56 | 138811 | 14 | 34703 |
| 4 | 80 | 210213 | 21 | 52554 |
| 5 | 84 | 220889 | 22 | 55223 |
| 6 | 101 | 210236 | 26 | 52559 |
| 7 | 68 | 193690 | 18 | 48423 |
| 8 | 84 | 230598 | 22 | 57650 |
| 9 | 100 | 230646 | 26 | 57662 |

## 4.2  Establishing Parameters for the Implementation of Machine Learning Algorithms

In order to establish parameters which take full advantage of the power of the implementation of Machine Learning Algorithms, careful thought was given to the way in which these techniques should be applied to the task of prediction.

First of all, and in order to predict the presence of a cleavage site in a test sample, the symbolic approach of OIL was applied. The OIL algorithm was implemented using the C++ language code. Since the OIL algorithm is non-deterministic, this allowed for the production of more than one solution based on a given training set. Fifteen models were generated in order to predict a determined cleavage site; a voting system being used in order to determine the sample label based on the fifteen models generated.

Secondly, and in order to predict the presence of a cleavage site in a test sample, the stochastic approach of HMM was applied. The HMM algorithm was implemented based on the Accord.net library; later customized. On the one hand, two models were constructed using the HMM algorithm for each cleavage site. One model was trained using only positive samples and the other model was trained using only negative samples. The maximum of the acceptance probabilities of the two models were used to determine the sample label; fifteen of these pairs were then trained for each cleavage site. On the other hand, in order to make use of the HMM algorithm, the number of states needed had to be established; values from two to fifteen states were evaluated experimentally and eight states were found to be the most appropriate.

Thirdly, the biologically inspired approach was applied using the ANN algorithm in order to predict the presence of a cleavage site in a test sample. The ANN algorithm was implemented as a multi-layer perceptron using the Matlab 2012 Neural Network Toolbox. The ANN algorithm was initiated using random values in the connections, allowing for different network configurations based on a given training set; once again, a voting system was used in order to determine the sample label based on the fifteen models generated just as was done in the OIL algorithm. Furthermore, the number of hidden layer neurons had to be established in order to make use of the ANN algorithm. Values between two and thirty-five were explored and fifteen was found to be the most appropriate number of hidden layer neurons. Moreover, the decision to use fifteen models to build the voting system resulted from previous experiments where a set from three to fifty-one models for the OIL algorithm was used; this in turn led to the discovery that beyond a set of fifteen there was no marked or significant improvement in the prediction outcome. To sum up, after having taken the decisions here presented, the three programs were ready to be used in the task of cleavage site prediction. In the following section, the results of the application will be shown and based on these it was possible to determine the technique which could best be used when solving the prediction problem.

### 4.3    Description of Experiments Performed

In order to compare the OIL, HMM and ANN algorithms when used to predict the polyprotein cleavage sites, two experiments were performed. The first experiment tested the three algorithms based on that corpus which contained ten negative samples for each positive one; the second experiment tested the three algorithms based on all of the available data which contained dozens of thousands of negative samples for each positive one. It should be noted that this second experiment created an adverse situation for most of the automatic learning methods because it favored over-training of the models; a situation which was evident in the ANN that could not be trained correctly under these adverse circumstances.

## 5    Result Analyses

In order to evaluate the performance of the techniques, the following well-known measurements in the field of Machine Learning were used: sensitivity, specificity, accuracy and the Matthews Correlation Coefficient. The calculation of these metrics was based on the values of the confusion matrix for binary classification, these are: 1) the true positives, which are the positive test samples labeled by the model as such; 2) the true negatives, which are the negative test samples labeled by the model as such; 3) the false positives, which are the test samples, that being negative are labeled positive by the model; and, 4) the false negatives, these are the test samples which, being positive, have been classified by the model as negative. The definition of these metrics was made in the following ways; 1) sensitivity as the ratio between the number of true positives and the total of the positive samples in the test conjunct; 2) specificity as the ratio between the number of true negatives and the total of negative samples in the test conjunct; 3) accuracy as the ratio between the number of well-classified samples and the total of samples in the test conjunct; and, 4) the Matthews Correlation Coefficient (MCC for short) [8] is considered a very complete measure, because it incorporates in its calculation all of the confusion matrix values for binary classification. Additionally the MCC value varies within the range [-1, 1] as well as measuring the grade of learning achieved: a value of zero corresponds to a random prediction, 1 reflects a perfect correspondence between the expected answer and that of the model, and -1 reflects a total discrepancy between the expected answer and the model.

Once the afore-mentioned metrics were applied to the results of experiments 1 and 2, the data presented in Tables 3 and 4 were obtained. Table 3 shows how some metrics weren't useful in the discrimination of the machine learning technique behavior while additionally allowing for the conclusion that HMM had the best performance in experiment 1. It should be noted that both the accuracy and the specificity metrics did not help discriminate between one technique and another since the values among all were similar. However, the metric which produced the most information was the MCC. In this metric, both OIL and ANN exhibited a low and similar performance while HMM showed a greater

**Table 3.** Results for experiment 1 using OIL, HMM and ANN for each of the 9 Cleavage Sites. These methods used the following metrics: Sensitivity (SE), Specificity (SP), Accuracy (AC), and the Matthews Correlation Coefficient (MCC).

| Cleavage | OIL | | | | HMM | | | | ANN | | | |
|---|---|---|---|---|---|---|---|---|---|---|---|---|
| Site | SE | SP | AC | CC | SE | SP | AC | CC | SE | SP | AC | CC |
| 1 | 0.84 | 0.97 | 0.97 | 0.11 | 0.93 | 0.99 | 0.99 | 0.27 | 0.40 | 0.99 | 0.99 | 0.10 |
| 2 | 0.62 | 0.97 | 0.97 | 0.07 | 0.87 | 0.99 | 0.99 | 0.31 | 0.79 | 0.99 | 0.99 | 0.20 |
| 3 | 0.63 | 0.96 | 0.96 | 0.05 | 0.77 | 0.99 | 0.99 | 0.17 | 0.04 | 0.99 | 0.99 | 0.01 |
| 4 | 0.84 | 0.97 | 0.97 | 0.09 | 0.76 | 0.99 | 0.99 | 0.18 | 0.53 | 0.98 | 0.98 | 0.09 |
| 5 | 0.85 | 0.96 | 0.96 | 0.08 | 0.92 | 0.99 | 0.99 | 0.41 | 0.46 | 0.98 | 0.98 | 0.07 |
| 6 | 0.78 | 0.96 | 0.96 | 0.09 | 0.78 | 0.98 | 0.98 | 0.13 | 0.03 | 0.99 | 0.98 | 0.00 |
| 7 | 0.79 | 0.97 | 0.97 | 0.09 | 0.66 | 0.99 | 0.99 | 0.21 | 0.29 | 0.98 | 0.98 | 0.04 |
| 8 | 0.53 | 0.97 | 0.97 | 0.06 | 0.60 | 0.99 | 0.99 | 0.19 | 0.21 | 0.98 | 0.98 | 0.03 |
| 9 | 0.79 | 0.94 | 0.94 | 0.11 | 0.82 | 0.98 | 0.98 | 0.21 | 0.21 | 0.99 | 0.99 | 0.10 |

level of prediction success. Table 4 shows the results for experiment 2, notice that the results for ANN were not reported given that it was no possible to train it correctly. Sensitivity of OIL was poor, it seemed to be over-trained. However, using MCC for comparison, in some cleavage sites, the performance of HMM was superior to that of OIL, but in other cases the opposite happened, thus neither one nor the other could be established as superior. Furthermore, while comparing Tables 3 and 4, it was noted that while allowing for the imbalance, OIL improved its MCC significantly in almost all the sites, given that HMM remained stable. In the sites 2 and 3 the MCC for OIL could not be calculated due to the fact that one of the confusion matrix values was zero, rendering as indeterminate the mathematical expression.

It is important to note that ROC curves are not reported because both OIL and HMM classifiers produce discrete answers and we have not a threshold value to be modified in order to produce such kind of graphics.

**Table 4.** Results for experiment 2 using OIL and HMM for each of the 9 Cleavage Sites

| Cleavage | OIL | | | | HMM | | | |
|---|---|---|---|---|---|---|---|---|
| Site | SE | SP | AC | CC | SE | SP | AC | CC |
| 1 | 0.28 | 0.99 | 0.99 | 0.47 | 0.93 | 0.99 | 0.99 | 0.26 |
| 2 | 0 | 1 | 0.99 | - | 0.85 | 0.99 | 0.99 | 0.47 |
| 3 | 0 | 1 | 0.99 | - | 0.77 | 0.99 | 0.99 | 0.18 |
| 4 | 0.26 | 1 | 0.99 | 0.51 | 0.76 | 0.99 | 0.99 | 0.19 |
| 5 | 0.39 | 0.99 | 0.99 | 0.60 | 0.92 | 0.99 | 0.99 | 0.38 |
| 6 | 0.09 | 1 | 0.99 | 0.30 | 0.81 | 0.97 | 0.97 | 0.11 |
| 7 | 0.33 | 0.99 | 0.99 | 0.54 | 0.66 | 0.99 | 0.99 | 0.21 |
| 8 | 0.03 | 1 | 0.99 | 0.18 | 0.60 | 0.99 | 0.99 | 0.22 |
| 9 | 0.33 | 0.99 | 0.99 | 0.48 | 0.78 | 0.98 | 0.98 | 0.21 |

# 6 Conclusions and Future Work

The following conclusions can be made based on analyses of the data collected during Experiment 1. First of all, the best performance results were obtained by HMM, for in spite of having few positive samples in the training corpus data, high levels of sensitivity were obtained. Additionally, the results for the MCC showed a clear level of learning, thus signifying that the results could not be attributed to chance. Secondly, although the OIL algorithm showed acceptable sensitivity values, its MCC showed a lesser level of learning while trained using the same data as HMM. Finally, ANN was clearly established as the least effective of the three techniques.

The following conclusions can be made based on analyses of the data collected during Experiment 2. First of all, the performance results obtained by HMM remained very much the same to those obtained during Experiment 1 in both sensitivity and in MCC. Additionally, the performance of OIL increased significantly, especially in its MCC. This is noteworthy because it shows that the method is capable of significantly increasing its learning in spite of a marked imbalance between the number of positive and negative samples. This significant increase is also unexpected because theoretically, inductive methods decrease in performance effectiveness when over-trained. However, it is necessary to note here that there were two cleavage sites for which it was impossible to calculate the MCC for OIL due to a zero in the confusion matrix.

These results clearly mark various possible lines to follow in future research. The first recommendation is to use HMM for cleavage site predictions; HMM showed tolerance to the imbalance of training samples while maintaining a high performance in sensitivity as did MCC in both experiments. Additionally, the results obtained using HMM allowed for the calculation of all of the metrics for all of the cleavage sites. The second recommendation is that a more detailed study be made regarding OIL's noted capacity for increased learning while using unbalanced data; achieving a confirmation of this capacity would create possibilities for the application of the algorithm in certain tasks where the imbalance is inevitable or even necessary.

In conclusion, this research showed that each technique has both its own strengths and weaknesses. It would be worthwhile to consider designing hybrid models which would use these various techniques in such a way that their strengths could be made advantageous and their weaknesses be limited.

# References

1. Bendtsen, J.D., Nielsen, H., von Heijne, G., Brunak, S.: Improved prediction of signal peptides: SignalP 3.0. Journal of Molecular Biology 340(4), 783–795 (2004)
2. Nielsen, H., Brunak, S., von Heijne, G.: Machine learning approaches for the prediction of signal peptides and other protein sorting signals. Protein Engineering 12(1), 3–9 (1999)

3. Leversen, N.A., de Souza, G.A., Målen, H., Prasad, S., Jonassen, I., Wiker, H.G.: Evaluation of signal peptide prediction algorithms for identification of mycobacterial signal peptides using sequence data from proteomic methods. Microbiology 155(7), 2375–2383 (2009)
4. Álvarez, G.I.: Estudio de la mezcla de estados determinista y no determinista en el diseño de algoritmos para inferencia gramatical de lenguajes regulares. PhD thesis, Universitad Politécnica de Valéncia, Departamento de Sistemas Informáticos y Computación (2008)
5. Garćia, P., de Parga, M.V., Álvarez, G.I., Ruiz, J.: Universal automata and NFA learning. Theoretical Computer Science 407(1-3), 192–202 (2008)
6. Rabiner, L.: A tutorial on hidden markov models and selected applications in speech recognition. Proceedings of the IEEE 77(2), 257–286 (1989)
7. Haykin, S.: Neural Networks: A Comprehensive Foundation, 2nd edn. Prentice Hall PTR, Upper Saddle River (1998)
8. Baldi, P., Brunak, S., Chauvin, Y., Andersen, C.A.F., Nielsen, H.: Assessing the accuracy of prediction algorithms for classification: an overview. Bioinformatics 16(5), 412–424 (2000)

# Human Heart Segmentation
# Based on Differential Evolution
# and Active Contours with Shape Prior

Ivan Cruz-Aceves, Juan Gabriel Avina-Cervantes,
Juan Manuel Lopez-Hernandez, Ma. De Guadalupe Garcia-Hernandez,
Sheila Esmeralda Gonzalez-Reyna, and Miguel Torres-Cisneros

Universidad de Guanajuato, División de Ingenierías Campus Irapuato-Salamanca,
Carretera Salamanca-Valle de Santiago Km 3.5+1.8 Km Comunidad de Palo Blanco,
C.P. 36885 Salamanca, Gto., México
{i.cruzaceves,avina,jmlopez,garciag,se.gonzalezreyna,mtorres}@ugto.mx

**Abstract.** Active contour model is an image segmentation technique
that uses the evaluation of internal and external forces to be attracted
towards the edge of a target object. In this paper a novel image segmentation method based on differential evolution and active contours with
shape prior is introduced. In the proposed method, the initial active
contours have been generated through an alignment process of reference
shape priors, and differential evolution is used to perform the segmentation task over a polar coordinate system. This method is applied in
the segmentation of the human heart from datasets of Computed Tomography images. To assess the segmentation results compared to those
outlined by experts and by different segmentation techniques, a set of
similarity measures has been adopted. The experimental results suggest
that by using differential evolution, the proposed method outperforms
the classical active contour model and the interactive Tseng method in
terms of efficiency and segmentation accuracy.

**Keywords:** Active Contour Model, Differential Evolution, Human
Heart, Image Segmentation, Shape prior.

## 1 Introduction

In clinical practice the Computed Tomography (CT) scanning is an effective
method for the monitoring and diagnosis of cardiac disease. The process carried
out by cardiologists can be subjective and time-consuming because it is based
on a visual examination followed by a manual delineation of the human organ.
Due to this, the application of automatic image segmentation methods plays an
important and challenging role.

In recent years, numerous approaches have been introduced for the automatic
medical image segmentation such as, region growing in pelvic injuries [1], templates for atlas in radiotherapy [2], watershed transform for tumors in mammograms [3], and active contour model in mammographic images [4] and human

F. Castro, A. Gelbukh, and M. González (Eds.): MICAI 2013, Part I, LNAI 8265, pp. 508–519, 2013.

prostate [5]. The active contour models (ACM) was introduced by [6] and it consists of an energy-minimizing spline composed of control points also called snaxels. This spline evolves through time according to the shape of a target object by evaluating internal and external forces. The traditional ACM implementation presents two shortcomings, firstly, the initialization of snaxels must be close to the target object, otherwise, failure of convergence will occur and, secondly, ACM is prone to be trapped into local minima because of the presence of noise. To solve these shortcomings some improvements have been suggested to adapt different methods working together with ACM including graph cut [7], statistical methods [8], population-based methods such as genetic algorithms [9,10] and particle swarm optimization (PSO) [11,12]. The performance of the ACM with population-based methods is suitable since the ACM becomes more robust, stable and efficient in the local minima problem.

Differential Evolution (DE) is a population-based method proposed by [13,14] similar to evolutionary algorithms. DE has become very popular to solve optimization problems with nonlinear functions with low computational time. In the classical implementation, the efficiency of the obtained results directly depends of three main parameters such as population size, differentiation factor and crossover rate. As DE is easy to implement, not computationally expensive and robust in the presence of noise, it has been used in many real-world applications including text summarization [15], job shop scheduling problem [16] and parameter estimation for a human immunodeficiency virus (HIV) [17].

In this paper, we introduce a novel image segmentation framework based on the theory of Active Contour Models with shape prior and Differential Evolution. The proposed framework is an adaptation of [18], here we use DE instead PSO to perform the optimization task increasing the exploitation capability regarding the classical Active Contour Model and the interactive Tseng method. Additionally, this framework uses the alignment process proposed in [19] to obtain an initial shape contour of the target object, which is scaled to different size to generate potential solutions. This proposed framework is applied in the segmentation of the human heart on Computed Tomography images from different patients, and the segmentation results are evaluated according to different similarity measures with respect to regions outlined by experts.

The paper is organized as follows. In Section 2, the fundamentals of the classical implementation of ACM and Differential Evolution are introduced. In Section 3 the proposed image segmentation framework is presented, along with a set of similarity measures. The experimental results are discussed in Section 4, and from the similarity analysis conclusions are given in Section 5.

## 2   Background

In this section, the fundamentals of the Active Contour Model and Differential Evolution optimization method are described in detail.

## 2.1  Active Contour Models

The traditional Active Contour Model (ACM) is a parametric curve that can move within a spatial image domain where it was assigned [6]. This curve is defined by $p(s,t) = (x(s,t), y(s,t)), s \in [0,1]$, where it evolves through time $t$ to minimize the total energy function given by the following:

$$E_{snake} = \int_0^1 [E_{int}(p(s,t)) + E_{ext}(p(s,t))]ds \tag{1}$$

This energy function consists of two energies, the internal energy $E_{int}$ to maintain the search within the spatial image domain and to control the shape modification of the curve, and the external energy $E_{ext}$, which is defined by the particular gradient features of the image. On the other hand, the computational implementation of the traditional ACM uses a set of $n$ discrete points $\{p_i | i = 1, 2, \ldots, n\}$, and the energy function is given by (2), which evaluates the actual control point to minimize the $k_i$ index in the $W_i$ searching window using (3).

$$E_{i,j} = E_{int} + E_{ext} \tag{2}$$

$$E_{snake} = \sum_{i=1}^n E_{i,k_i}, \quad k_i = \arg\min_j(E_{i,j}), j \in W_i \tag{3}$$

Because of the traditional ACM presents the drawbacks of initialization and local minima, Chan & Vese [20] proposed the integration of a shape prior constraint within the traditional ACM. This method is given by the following:

$$E_T = w_1 E_1 + w_2 E_2 + w_3 E_3 \tag{4}$$

where $E_T$ is the total energy function composed of the energies $E_1$, $E_2$, $E_3$ and their weighting factors $w_1$, $w_2$, $w_3$. $E_1$ represents the active contour, $E_2$ is the shape energy defined as the difference between the active contour and the shape template expressed as follows:

$$E_2 = \int_\Omega \left( H(\phi) - H(\varphi_T(B^T)) \right)^2 dxdy \tag{5}$$

where $\Omega$ represents the image domain, $H(\cdot)$ is the Heaviside function, $\phi$ is the signed distance function, $\varphi_T$ is the deformed template and $B^T$ is the transformation matrix consisting of translation $[t_x, t_y]^T$ in the horizontal and vertical axes, the scaling factor $[s]$ and the rotation angle parameter $[\theta]$, as follows:

$$B^T = \underbrace{\begin{bmatrix} 1 & 0 & t_x \\ 0 & 1 & t_y \\ 0 & 0 & 1 \end{bmatrix}}_{M(a,b)} \times \underbrace{\begin{bmatrix} s & 0 & 0 \\ 0 & s & 0 \\ 0 & 0 & 1 \end{bmatrix}}_{H(s)} \times \underbrace{\begin{bmatrix} \cos\theta & -\sin\theta & 0 \\ \sin\theta & \cos\theta & 0 \\ 0 & 0 & 1 \end{bmatrix}}_{R(\theta)} \tag{6}$$

Finally, the energy $E_3$ represents the image-based force with an image intensity $I$ and the gradient operator $\nabla$ calculated as follows:

$$E_3 = \int_\Omega (\nabla H(\phi) - \nabla I)^2 dxdy \tag{7}$$

The three energies are iteratively evaluated until the difference between the previous and actual segmented object becomes stable. Although the initialization drawback of the traditional ACM is solved through the Chan & Vese method, this method remains prone to be trapped into local minima. A suitable alternative to overcome this drawback is to use population-based methods such as Differential Evolution, which is described in the following Section.

## 2.2   Differential Evolution

Differential evolution is a stochastic real-parameter method proposed by [13,14] to solve numerical global optimization problems. DE consists of a set of potential solutions, called individuals $X = \{x_1, x_2, \ldots, x_{Np}\}$, where $Np$ is the population size. The individuals are iteratively improved by using different variation operators, and the solution is chosen to be the individual with the best fitness according to an objective function.

The main idea of the DE method consists of the mutation, crossover and selection operators based on the floating-point encoding. The mutation operator is used to create a mutant vector $V_{i,g+1}$ at each generation $g$ based on the distribution of the current population $\{X_{i,g} | i = 1, 2, \ldots, Np\}$ through the following strategy,

$$V_{i,g+1} = X_{r1,g} + F(X_{r2,g} - X_{r3,g}), \quad r1 \neq r2 \neq r3 \neq i \tag{8}$$

where $F$ is the differentiation factor, and $r1$, $r2$ and $r3$ represent the indexes of three different individuals and uniformly selected from the set $\{1,\ldots,Np\}$. The second operator is the crossover, which uses (9) to create the trial vector $U_{i,g+1}$ as follows:

$$U_{i,g+1} = \begin{cases} V_{i,g+1}, & \text{if } r \leq CR \\ X_{i,g}, & \text{if } r > CR \end{cases} \tag{9}$$

where $r$ represents a uniform random value on the interval $[0,1]$, which is compared with the $CR$ (crossover rate) parameter. If $r$ is bigger than $CR$, the current information of individual $X_{i,g}$ is preserved, otherwise the information from the mutant vector $V_{i,g+1}$ is copied to the trial vector $U_{i,g+1}$. Subsequently, the selection procedure is applied by using (10). This procedure selects according to a fitness function, the better one between the trial vector $U_{i,g+1}$ and the current individual $X_{i,g}$.

$$X_{i,g+1} = \begin{cases} U_{i,g+1}, & \text{if } f(U_{i,g+1}) < f(X_{i,g}) \\ X_{i,g}, & \text{otherwise} \end{cases} \tag{10}$$

According to the previous description, the traditional DE method is described below.

1. Initialize number of generations $G$, population size $Np$, value of differentiation factor $F$, and value of crossover rate $CR$.
2. Initialize each individual $X_i$.
3. For each individual $X_{i,g}$ , where $g = \{1, \ldots, G\}$:
   (a) Calculate $V_{i,g+1}$ by using the mutation step (8).
   (b) Assign $U_{i,g+1}$ according to the crossover operator (9).
   (c) Update $X_{i,g+1}$, if $U_{i,g+1}$ is better than $X_{i,g}$ by applying the selection step (10).
4. Stop if the convergence criterion is satisfied (e.g., stability or number of generations).

## 3   Proposed Image Segmentation Framework

The proposed framework based on the theory of Active Contour Models and Differential Evolution is described in Section 3.1. Moreover, to evaluate the performance of the segmentation results, the Jaccard and Dice indexes are introduced in Section 3.2.

### 3.1   Scaled Active Contours Driven by Differential Evolution

Because of the disadvantages of the classical active contour model discussed above, Differential Evolution and scaled templates have been adopted. These templates are acquired from an alignment process of reference images to overcome the initialization drawback and DE is used to solve the local minima problem. Since the methodology of the proposed framework allows directly apply the optimization method in the segmentation problem, the advantages of robustness, efficiency and low computational time are inherently preserved. In Figure 1 the segmentation process performed by the proposed framework is described below.

The proposed framework consists on three steps. Firstly, the construction of a shape template by using an alignment process of a set of reference images is required. This alignment process consists in the estimation of the parameters $[a, b, s, \theta]^T$ according to [19] as follows:

$$\begin{bmatrix} \tilde{x} \\ \tilde{y} \\ 1 \end{bmatrix} = M(a,b) \times H(s) \times R(\theta) \times \begin{bmatrix} x \\ y \\ 1 \end{bmatrix} \qquad (11)$$

where $M(a,b)$ represents the translation matrix on the horizontal $x$ and vertical $y$ axes, $H(s)$ is the scale matrix and $R(\theta)$ is the rotation matrix. The product of these matrices is used to apply the gradient descent method in order to minimize the following energy function:

$$E_{alig} = \sum_{i=1}^{n} \sum_{j=1, j \neq i}^{n} \left\{ \frac{\int \int_{\Omega} (\tilde{I}^i - \tilde{I}^j)^2 dA}{\int \int_{\Omega} (\tilde{I}^i + \tilde{I}^j)^2 dA} \right\} \qquad (12)$$

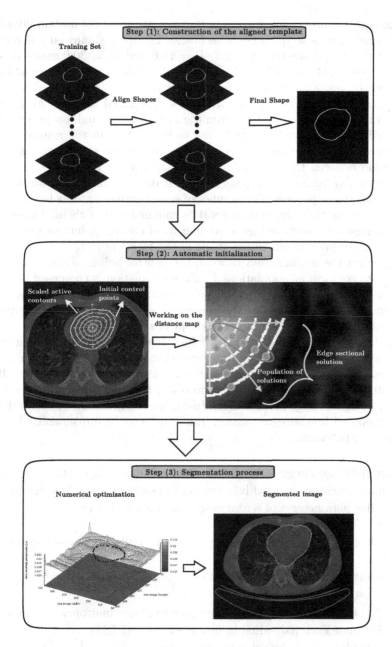

**Fig. 1.** Process of the proposed image segmentation method

where $\Omega$ represents the image domain and $\tilde{I}$ represents the transformed image. The final procedure in this step involves obtaining the final shape template, which is acquired through the maximum shape boundary from the whole set of superimposed transformed images.

Secondly, a preprocessing stage is performed. We use a 2D median filter ($3\times3$ window size) to remove the noise from image. Then, the Canny edge detector is applied with the parameters $\sigma = 1.3$, $T_l = 10.0$ and $T_h = 30.0$ experimentally tuned to preserve the real edges of the human heart from the background image. Subsequently, the Euclidean distance map (EDM) [21] is computed as potential surface to perform the optimization task. The EDM assigns high potential values to image pixels located far from the human heart, and low potential values (ideally zero) to pixels located close to the heart. On the resulting EDM, the automatic initialization process is performed through the maximum mutual information between the final template and the current test image. The $n$ initial scaled active contours are generated by scaling the final template from the previous alignment process. The number of scaled active contours has to be considered assuming that the human heart is confined within them. These scaled contours must be discretized by a number $m$ of control points to smooth and adapt the resulting contour to the shape of the target object.

To perform the optimization process, the control points are assigned as individuals to conform $m$ populations $P$. Each population is composed of control points of different contours with the same position label. The final step of the proposed framework consists on the numerical optimization followed by the image segmentation result. The numerical optimization is performed on the Euclidean distance map (range [0,255]), which represents the fitness function in the optimization process. Differential Evolution is applied for each population $P_i$ separately in order to minimize the nearest edge sectional solution. If the DE strategy for each population $P_i$ is finished, the final segmentation result is acquired by connecting the best individual of each population to each other.

The proposed image segmentation framework can be implemented by using the following procedure:

1. Align reference images according to [19] and obtain final template.
2. Perform maximum mutual information to positioning the final template.
3. Initialize parameter $n$ of scaled active contours and parameter $m$ of control points.
4. Initialize the DE parameters: generations, differentiation factor and crossover rate.
5. Generate $m$ populations assigning the control points as individuals.
6. For each population $P_i$:
   (a) Apply restriction of the search space to ignore improper solutions.
   (b) Evaluate each individual in fitness function (EDM).
   (c) Calculate $V_{i,g+1}$ by using the mutation step (8).
   (d) Assign $U_{i,g+1}$ according to the crossover operator (9).
   (e) Update $X_{i,g+1}$, if $U_{i,g+1}$ is better than $X_{i,g}$ by applying the selection step (10).
7. Stop if the convergence criterion is satisfied (e.g., stability or number of generations).

## 3.2   Validation Metrics

To assess the performance of the proposed framework on medical images, Jaccard and Dice indexes have been adopted to analyze the segmentation results between the regions outlined by experts and the regions obtained by computational methods.

The Jaccard $J(A, B)$ and Dice $D(A, B)$ indexes are similarity measures used for binary variables [3], which are defined in the range $[0, 1]$ and they are computed using (13) and (14), respectively. In our tests, $A$ represents the regions outlined by experts (ground truth) and $B$ represents the automatic segmented region by computational methods.

$$J(A, B) = \frac{A \cap B}{A \cup B} \qquad (13)$$

$$D(A, B) = \frac{2(A \cap B)}{A + B} \qquad (14)$$

In these indexes, if the regions $A$ and $B$ are completely superimposed the obtained result is 1.0, otherwise, if these two regions are completely different the obtained result is 0.

In Section 4, the segmentation results obtained from the proposed framework on computed tomography images are analyzed by the similarity metrics.

## 4   Experimental Results

In this section, the proposed image segmentation framework is applied for segmenting the human heart in Computed Tomography images. The computational simulations are performed with an Intel Core i3 with 4Gb of memory and 2.13Ghz using the GNU Compiler Collection (C++) version 4.4.5.

In Figure 2(a) a CT image of the human chest is illustrated, in order to have better understanding of the segmentation task. Figure 2(b) shows the resulting Euclidean distance map of the test image, in which the optimization process is applied. In Figures 2(c) and (d) the human heart outlined by expert 1 and expert 2 are presented to have reference ground truth for the experiments with the proposed methodology.

In Figure 3 the human heart segmentation results on a subset of Computed Tomography images are introduced. The whole dataset is composed of 144 CT images with size $512 \times 512$ pixels from different patients. In Figure 3(a) the manual delineations of the human heart made by cardiologists are presented. Figure 3(b) illustrates the segmentation results obtained via the traditional implementation of Active Contour Model, where the fitting problem and local minima problem are clearly shown. The ACM parameters were set according to [11] as 45 control points, $\alpha = 0.017$, $\beta = 0.86$ and $\gamma = 0.45$, obtaining an average execution time of 0.172s per image. Figure 3(c) presents the segmentation results obtained through the interactive Tseng method, in which, each control point is provided interactively by the user. The parameters of this implementation were

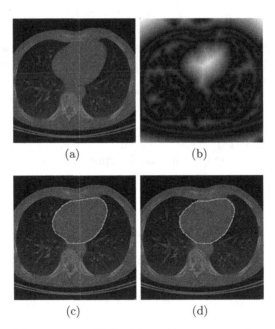

(a)                    (b)

(c)                    (d)

**Fig. 2.** CT image: (a) test image, (b) Euclidean distance map of test image, (c) human heart outlined by expert 1 and (d) human heart outlined by expert 2

set as 45 control points, window size 30×30 pixels, and for each control point 9 particles are created, given an average execution time of 0.214s per image. Even though the use of a square matrix in the Tseng method obtained suitable segmentation results, this method presents problems to fit the real human heart boundary accurately. Finally, in Figure 3(d) the segmentation results obtained by using the proposed segmentation framework presents an appropriate human heart segmentation. This method avoid the local minima and it fits the human heart accurately with parameters set as number of scaled contours = 9, number of control points = 45, iterations = 10, crossover rate = 0.9, and the differentiation factor = 0.5, obtaining an average execution time of 0.223s per image. The differentiation factor was experimentally tuned to perform local exploitation and reduce the number of improper solutions.

From the aforementioned dataset of CT images, in Table 1 the average of the segmentation results obtained by the classical ACM, interactive Tseng method and our proposed framework is compared to those regions delineated by cardiologists. The similarity results suggest that the proposed method can lead to more efficiency in human heart segmentation with respect to the comparative methods, which can significantly help cardiologists in clinical practice. The quality of the human heart segmentation results obtained with the proposed framework depends on parameter selection. We used a experimentally tuned value as differentiation factor to perform local exploitation, and the constant parameters in our experiments are suitable for other images, since the DE method is directly applied to minimize one edge sectional solution for each polar area.

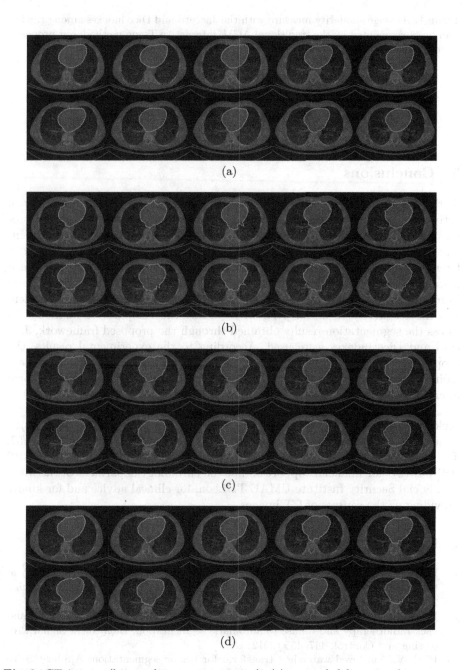

**Fig. 3.** CT images (human heart segmentation): (a) manual delineation by experts, (b) results of traditional ACM, (c) results of interactive Tseng method and (d) results of proposed implementation

**Table 1.** Average similarity measure with the Jaccard and Dice indexes among the human heart segmented by the traditional ACM, interactive Tseng method, our proposed method, and the regions outlined by experts of the CT dataset

| Comparative | Similarity Measure | |
|---|---|---|
| Studies | Jaccard index $(J)$ | Dice index $(D)$ |
| ACM vs Experts | 0.6666 | 0.8000 |
| Tseng vs Experts | 0.8000 | 0.8888 |
| Proposed method vs Experts | 0.8367 | 0.9111 |

## 5   Conclusions

In this paper, a novel image segmentation framework based on the theory of active contour models with shape prior and differential evolution has been introduced. The proposed framework uses an alignment process to generate different scaled contours according to the shape of the target object. Subsequently, differential evolution is used to perform the segmentation task within constrained polar sections. This novel framework was used to segment the human heart from Computed Tomography images allowing to overcome the local minima problem and the sensitivity to initial position regarding the comparative methods. To assess the segmentation results obtained through the proposed framework, Jaccard and Dice indexes were used. According to the experimental results, the proposed framework is suitable to the human heart segmentation, since the exploitation capability of differential evolution is efficient to overcome the local minima problem to fit the heart boundary accurately.

**Acknowledgments.** This research has been supported by the National Council of Science and Technology of México (CONACYT) under Grant 241224-218157. The authors thanks "Programa Integral de Fortalecimiento Institucional 2012 (PIFI-2012)" for financial support and at the cardiology deparment of the Mexican Social Security Institute UMAE T1 Leon, for clinical advice and for kindly providing us the sources of CT images.

## References

1. Davuluri, P., Wu, J., Tang, Y., et al.: Hemorrhage detection and segmentation in traumatic pelvic injuries. Computational and Mathematical Methods in Medicine 2012, 12 (2012)
2. Parraga, A., Macq, B., Craene, M.: Anatomical atlas in the context of head and neck radiotherapy and its use to automatic segmentation. Biomedical Signal Processing and Control, 447–455 (2012)
3. Hsu, W.: Improved watershed transform for tumor segmentation: Application to mammogram image compresion. Expert Systems with Applications 39, 3950–3955 (2012)
4. Jumaat, A., Rahman, W., Ibrahim, A., Mahmud, R.: Segmentation of masses from breast ultrasound images using parametric active contour algorithm. Procedia Social and Behavioral Sciences 8, 640–647 (2010)

5. Liu, X., Haider, M., Yetik, I.: Unsupervised 3d prostate segmentation based on diffusion-weighted imaging mri using active contour models with a shape prior. Journal of Electrical and Computer Engineering, 11 (2011)
6. Kass, M., Terzopoulos, A.W.D.: Snakes: Active contour models. International Journal of Computer Vision 1, 321–331 (1988)
7. Cheng, Y., Wang, Z., Hu, J., Zhao, W., Wu, Q.: The domain knowledge based graph-cut model for liver ct segmentation. Biomedical Signal Processing and Control 7, 591–598 (2012)
8. Wang, L., He, L., Mishra, A., Li, C.: Active contours driven by local gaussian distribution fitting energy. Signal Processing 89, 2435–2447 (2009)
9. Ballerini, L.: Genetic snakes for medical images segmentation. In: Poli, R., Voigt, H.-M., Cagnoni, S., Corne, D.W., Smith, G.D., Fogarty, T.C. (eds.) EvoIASP 1999 and EuroEcTel 1999. LNCS, vol. 1596, pp. 59–73. Springer, Heidelberg (1999)
10. Talebi, M., Ayatollahi, A., Kermani, A.: Medical ultrasound image segmentation using genetic active contour. Journal of Biomedical Science and Engineering 4, 105–109 (2011)
11. Tseng, C., Hiseh, J., Jeng, J.: Active contour model via multi-population particle swarm optimization. Expert Systems with Applications 36, 5348–5352 (2009)
12. Shahamatnia, E., Ebadzadeh, M.: Application of particle swarm optimization and snake model hybrid on medical imaging. In: Proceedings of the Third International Workshop on Computational Intelligence in Medical Imaging, pp. 1–8 (2011)
13. Storn, R., Price, K.: Differential evolution - a simple and efficient adaptive scheme for global optimization over continuous spaces. Technical Report TR-95-012, International Computer Sciences Institute, Berkeley, CA, USA (1995)
14. Storn, R., Price, K.: Differential evolution – a simple and efficient heuristic for global optimization over continuous spaces. Journal of Global Optimization 11, 341–359 (1997)
15. Alguliev, R., Aliguliyev, R., Mehdiyev, C.: psum-sade: A modified p-median problem and self-adaptive differential evolution algorithm for text summarization. Applied Computational Intelligence and Soft Computing 13 (2011)
16. Zhang, R., Wu, C.: A hybrid differential evolution and tree search algorithm for the job shop scheduling problem. Mathematical Problems in Engineering, 20 (2011)
17. Ho, W., Chan, A.: Hybrid taguchi-differential evolution algorithm for parameter estimation of differential equation models with application to hiv dynamics. Mathematical Problems in Engineering, 14 (2011)
18. Cruz-Aceves, I., Avina-Cervantes, J., Lopez-Hernandez, J., et al.: Unsupervised cardiac image segmentation via multi-swarm active contours with a shape prior. Computational and Mathematical Methods in Medicine, 15 (2013)
19. Tsai, A., Yezzi, A., Wells, W., Tempany, C., Tucker, D., Fan, A., Grimson, W., Willsky, A.: A shape-based approach to the segmentation of medical imagery using level sets. IEEE Transactions on Medical Imaging 22, 137–154 (2003)
20. Chan, T., Vese, L.: Active contours without edges. IEEE Transactions on Image Processing 10, 266–277 (2001)
21. Cohen, L., Cohen, I.: Finite-element methods for active contour models and balloons for 2-d and 3-d images. IEEE Transactions on Pattern Analysis and Machine Intelligence 15, 1131–1147 (1993)

# Detection of Human Retina Images Suspect of Glaucoma through the Vascular Bundle Displacement in the Optic Disc

José Abel de la Fuente-Arriaga[1], Edgardo Manuel Felipe-Riverón[2,*],
and Eduardo Garduño-Calderón[3]

[1] Tecnológico de Estudios Superiores de Jocotitlán,
Carretera Toluca-Atlacomulco Km. 44.8, C.P. 50700, Estado de México, Mexico
[2] Centro de Investigación en Computación, Instituto Politécnico Nacional,
Juan de Dios Bátiz s/n, C.P. 07738, D.F., Mexico
[3] Centro Oftalmológico de Atlacomulco,
Libramiento Jorge Jiménez Cantú 1208, C.P. 50450, Estado de México, Mexico
abeldlfa@gmail.com, edgardo@cic.ipn.mx, edugarcal@yahoo.com

**Abstract.** This work presents a methodology for detecting human retina images suspect of glaucoma based on the measurement of displacement of the vascular bundle caused by the growth of the excavation or cup. The results achieved are due to the relative increase in size of the cup or excavation that causes a displacement of the blood vessel bundle to the superior, inferior and nasal optic disc areas. The method consists of the segmentation of the optic disc contour and the vascular bundle located within it, and calculation of its displacement from its normal position using the chessboard metric. The method was successful in 62 images of a total of 67, achieving an accuracy of 93.02% of sensitivity and 91.66% of specificity in the pre-diagnosis.

**Keywords:** Glaucoma detection, vascular bundle displacement, excavation detection, optic papilla segmentation, chessboard metric.

## 1 Introduction

Application of noninvasive techniques in automatic retina analysis is an important area in medicine [1]. The information achieved from the analysis of these digital images permits to decide about the existence of ocular diseases as the glaucoma [2].

The optic disc or optic papilla is the clearest area in images of the rear pole of the retina. In a normal papilla, the vascular network coming out from the choroids travels through the center of the nervous fibers that constitutes the optic nerve, which goes through a tube-like structure toward the brain. Glaucoma, an ocular asymptomatic neuropathy, is caused by an excessive intraocular pressure that creates an excavation (or cup) in the papilla that damages the optic nerve. This excavation produces a thickening of the wall of the papilla, which moves the cluster of veins and arteries (called

---

* Corresponding author.

F. Castro, A. Gelbukh, and M. González (Eds.): MICAI 2013, Part I, LNAI 8265, pp. 520–531, 2013.

also vascular bundle), toward the nasal side of the affected eye. In time, the optic nerve is damaged, and if it is not medically treated in time, it causes first a progressive irreversible loss of peripheral vision and finally leads to blindness.

Between a 12% and a 15% of the total world population is affected by various degrees of blindness due to glaucoma [2, 3] and in Mexico glaucoma represents the second cause of blindness [4]. Consequently, it is important to work in the search of new methods for effective early detection of glaucoma.

The clinical procedures for the diagnosis of glaucoma are: (a) Analysis of the clinical history; (b) measurement of the intraocular pressure; (c) analysis of alterations in the optic disc; and (d) functional study of the visual field (Campimetry test).

We use the term pre-diagnosis, to emphasize that the (final) diagnosis is done exclusively by the physician specialized in glaucoma.

This work presents a new method for the pre-diagnosis of glaucoma based in morphological alterations detected within the optic disc (initial test for the disease identification). The approach is based on the close relationship found between the vascular bundle displacement and the excavation growth within the optic disc in the superior, inferior and nasal zones. It is possible using the proposed method to classify normal images (with a physiological excavation) and glaucoma suspect images, even when they are in its initial stages of development.

The method was tested using 67 retina images of 43 patients (20 healthy and 23 suspect patients), which 24 are retinal images from 20 normal patients, and the rest of 43 images are formed by 21 isolated images and 11 pairs of images from 23 suspect patients. Images of the database used in this research were supplied by a physician specialized in glaucoma and used without performing any pre-processing before use. This group of images is a part of the private collection of retinal images that belongs to the Center for Computing Research of the National Polytechnic Institute, Mexico.

## 2    Background

A medical procedure used in the detection of glaucoma consists of evaluating the morphological alterations in the optic disc, visible with the help of instruments such as a slit lamp; high-power convex lenses [7]; optical photographs of the retina [5]; retinal confocal tomography [8, 9]; laser polarimetry tomography [8, 9], and optical coherence tomography [8, 10]. The performance and reproducibility of papillary measurements in glaucomatous retinas have been successfully evaluated and compared in numerous investigations [11].

The analysis of glaucoma begins with the detection and evaluation of some parts of the retina, mainly the optic disc (or optic papilla), the excavation and the blood vessels located within it (vascular bundle), since in function of its characteristics is possible to reach to important and valuable clinical findings. The main characteristics more frequently analyzed are the measurement of the Cup/Disc ratio and the reviewing of the neuro-retinal rim thickness, which in normal eyes is thicker in the inferior zone. The images used in this research are all retina fundus images, namely those that are captured through the eye pupil.

Essentially, even with a large variety of methods for the detection of the optic disc and cup, based primarily on thresholding methods as Otsu [6] and in the use the standard deviation [12, 14]; dynamics border methods as the circular Hough transform [15, 24] and the active contours (Snakes) [20, 22, 23, 24]; interpolation methods of borders as spline [16, 22, 23], clustering methods [18, 19]; and the combination of some of them, such as the OOCE rule which uses the Otsu thresholding method, the Opening morphologic operator (defined as the erosion followed by an dilation), the Closing morphologic operator (defined as the dilation followed by an erosion) and the External border method [13], the success of the segmentation process had difficulties caused mainly by the natural coverage of the blood vessels coming from the choroid, since their leaving from and spreading on the retina cover parts of the optic disc. To solve this difficulty authors has attempted to reduce the effect of the blood vessel by the use of the Black-Top-Hat morphologic operator (defined as the difference between the original image and its morphological closing) for the detection of the blood vessels [17], and the Opening and Closing operators for remove them [12, 24], However, these problems sometimes even precludes the exact contour detection of the optic disc and the possible excavations. Despite this, many reported results on glaucoma detection are based only on the Cup/Disc ratio [13], where if the diameter of the cup (or its equivalent in area) exceeds to 0.4 of the diameter (or area) of the optic papilla, then the eye probably becomes glaucomatous and cause invariably blindness in the patient, such as [14, 15] and [16]; they show accuracy between 60% to 94% of sensitivity and 82% to 94.7% of specificity in pre-diagnosis. Other works measure this same characteristics using pairs of stereo retinal images to find the disparity of the corresponding points of both images [20] achieving accuracy of 87% of sensitivity and 82% of specificity. However, even achieving results within the reported international ranges, this remains a subject of much controversy.

Other authors, have reviewed other characteristics, combining the Cup/Disc ratio and the analysis of vessel bends or kinks, which are small vessels that when they come out from the excavation provide physiological validation for the boundary cup [22, 23], achieving accuracy between 18.6% to 81.3% of sensitivity and 45.5% to 81.8% of specificity, and the ISNT rule [12, 18] and [19], where, instead of measuring the neuroretinal rim thickness, they measure the proportion of the blood vessels in the inferior, superior, nasal and temporal disc zones, achieving accuracy between 97.6% to 100% of sensitivity and 80% to 99.2% of specificity in the pre-diagnosis.

# 3     Methodology

This work presents a new classification method of retina images with excavation suspect of glaucoma. The method relies only on the analysis of morphological alterations that can be detected within the optic disc, even when the excavation is in the initial stage of glaucoma.

The method proposes a different way for the detection of the excavation, where it is not necessary to detect the exact contours of the disc and the excavation, commonly required by current method. The method is based in the analysis of the vascular bundle displacement within the optic disc due to the excavation, since we have observed a near correlation between the excavation growth and the blood vessels displacement in the inferior, superior and nasal optic disc zones. The proposed method consists of the following steps: 1. RGB image acquisition; 2. Segmentation of the optic disc region; 3. Detection of a reference point in the excavation or cup; 4. Detection of centroids of three zones of the vascular bundle; 5. Measurement of the distance between the reference point of the cup to the three centroids. Now we will describe in detail each procedure.

1.    The proposed method was evaluated in 43 patients (20 healthy and 23 diseased), using 67 RGB retina images (24 normal and 43 suspect) of size 720 pixels of width and 576 pixels of height, in a JPG or BMP graphic format, which exhibit normal and suspect retinas with glaucoma at different stages of development. Images were acquired with a conventional eye fundus camera [5] and previously evaluated by an ophthalmologist specializing in glaucoma. Figure 1 shows an eye fundus image of our collection with the most important anatomic parts indicated: a. Optic disc; b. excavation or cup; c. vascular bundle; d. blood vessels; e. macula and fovea, whose excavation according to a specialist is classified in this case as suspect of glaucoma, due to the excessive size of the excavation with respect to the size of the optic disc.

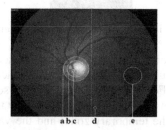

**Fig. 1.** Optical color eye fundus image classified as suspect of glaucoma showing the following anatomic parts: a. optic disc; b. excavation or cup; c. vascular bundle; d. blood vessels; e. macula and fovea

2.    The objective of the optic disc region segmentation is to obtain approximately the diameter of the disc to be used in the process of result normalization.

    We use the method developed in [24] for the optic disc segmentation. This method consists of six steps from which we occupy only the first five because we need only the segmentation of the optic disc area; we do not use the optic disc contour segmentation mentioned in the sixth step. The method in general find the region of interest (ROI), the elimination of the arterioles and venules and finally segments the optic disc with the use of morphological operators and the combination of the circular Hough transform and active contours. The method has an accuracy of 92.5% and is robust in images with low contrast, high levels of noise and edge discontinuities.

    The segmentation of the image shown in Fig.1 appears in Fig.2, where (a) shows the ROI containing the optic disc in RGB color model; (b) segmented optic disc area, and (c) the segmented area shown in (b) superimposed to the image shown in (a).

3.    The detection of a reference point in the excavation begins with the automatic segmentation of the excavation by the method developed in [13], which uses the OOCE (Otsu, Opening, Closing, External border) rule. There, an accuracy of 92.52% was achieved. Then, a reference point farther toward the temporal region is selected

as shown in Fig.3 marked with a cross enclosed by a rectangle, and denoted by the capital letter A. This zone was selected because it is where the excavation border is farther from the center of the optic disc. We assumed that the displacement of the vessel bundle to the left is a consequence of the growth of the excavation to the right.

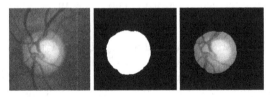

**Fig. 2.** Details of the optic disc contour which results from applying the algorithm detailed in [24]

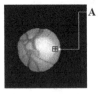

**Fig. 3.** Reference point in the excavation located at the temporal optic disc zone

4.    The detection of centroids of three zones of the vascular bundle (superior, inferior and nasal zones) is required for analyzing the displacement of blood vessels located within the optic disc. For this we take into account some reference points in the vascular bundle. These points approximately describe the tendency to grow in size of the excavation (located at the temporary zone) and the vascular bundle what is displaced to the nasal zone.

This step begins with the segmentation of blood vessels located within the optic disc (the vascular bundle). For this, the central point of the optic disc is obtained in figure 2(c), which serves as a reference point for coupling it individually with the three triangular masks shown in Fig. 4. The central point of each mask must match the central point of the optic disc, with the purpose of the right choice of the target zone, even when the masks protrude from the ROI (the point does not always coincide with the center of the ROI). Figure 4(a) shows the mask for the superior zone; 4(b) for the inferior zone, and 4(c) for the nasal zone, in the case that the image to be analyzed is from the left eye. If the image to be analyzed is from the right eye, then the mask should be the mirror image of that shown in Fig. 4(c).

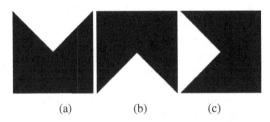

(a)              (b)              (c)

**Fig. 4.** Masks used for the segmentation of blood vessels located in different zones of the optic disc. (a) Mask for the superior zone; (b) for the inferior zone; (c) for the nasal zone (in case of the left eye).

The blood vessel segmentation is carried out in the red channel of the RGB images, since the best results were achieved with this channel probably due to the common orange-reddish color of the optic papilla. The segmentation uses the morphologic Black-top-hat operator and the Otsu for thresholding method [17]. The Black-top-hat is a morphologic transformation defined as the difference between the original image and its morphological closing. This highlights the elements deleted by the closing which, in this case, are the blood vessels located within the optic disc.

The result of the segmentation of blood vessels in the different zones is shown in Fig. 5, (a) superior zone; (b) inferior zone and (c) nasal zone.

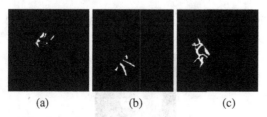

(a)                    (b)                    (c)

**Fig. 5.** Segmentation of blood vessels located in the different zones of the optic disc, (a) superior zone; (b) inferior zone; (c) nasal zone

To find the reference point that describes the trend in the position of vessels being analyzed, we calculate the centroid for each zone.

The centroid of a body coincides with the center of mass if the object density (area) is homogeneous or when the material distribution is symmetrical; however, if an area has irregular borders defined by relative complex mathematical expressions, the simplest method is to calculate the area of the objects (vessels) with help of the individual summations described in (1) [21].

$$A = \sum_{i=1}^{n} \Delta Ai \quad Qx = \sum_{i=1}^{n} \overline{yi} \Delta Ai \quad Qy = \sum_{i=1}^{n} \overline{xi} \Delta Ai \quad \overline{x} = \frac{Qy}{A} \quad \overline{y} = \frac{Qx}{A} \quad (1)$$

Where $\Delta Ai$ is the area of the $i^{th}$ element; $n$ is the number of elements; $\overline{yi}$ is the coordinate $y$ of the $i^{th}$ centroid of the element; $\overline{xi}$ is the coordinate $x$ of the $i^{th}$ centroid of the element; $\overline{x}$ is the coordinate $x$ of the centroid of the object; $\overline{y}$ is the coordinate $y$ of the centroid of the object.

The positions of centroids are shown in Fig. 6. They are marked by a cross enclosed by a rectangle, and denoted by capital letters. The letter B represents the centroid of vessels in the superior zone; the letter C the centroid of vessels in the nasal zone and the letter D represents the centroid of vessels in the inferior zone.

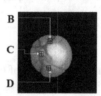

**Fig. 6.** Centroid of blood vessels located in the different zones of the optic disc, B: Superior zone; C: Nasal zone, and D: Inferior zone

5.    In this stage the blood vessels displacement is calculated with respect to the excavation growth, which is carried out by using the reference point of the cup (A in Fig. 3) and the vessel centroids (Fig. 6) in the zones defined by the masks (Fig. 5).

The measurement of the displacement consists of obtaining the distances $d_1$, $d_2$ and $d_3$ from the centroids B, C and D to the reference point A located in the temporal part of the excavation, as shown in Fig. 7. Since normally the vessel displacement is in the horizontal direction, distances are measured using the chessboard metric defined as:

$$d_c = \max(| x_2 - x_1 |, | y_2 - y_1 |) \tag{2}$$

Where $(x_1, y_1)$ are the coordinates of the first point and $(x_2, y_2)$ are those of the second.

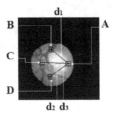

**Fig. 7.** Distance $d_1$, $d_2$ and $d_3$ between the centroids denoted by B, C and D and the reference point of the excavation A

The distances are normalized with respect to the horizontal diameter of the optic disc $D_h$. The normalized distance $d_n$ is:

$$d_n = \frac{100}{D_h} d \tag{3}$$

Where $D_h$ is the horizontal diameter of the optic disc and $d$ is the distance to normalize. The final result of the blood vessels displacement with respect to the proportional growth of the excavation is calculated using the average of the three normalized distances just measured.

For pre-diagnosing if an optic disc is suspect to suffer glaucoma or not, we need to use a cut point to decide the question. Tests were carried out with 67 images. The cut point was selected at a normalized distance of 45 pixels obtained empirically from our experiments. If the average of distances calculated was less than the cut point, then the retina was pre-diagnosed as normal. On the other hand, if the average of distances was equal or greater than 45, the retina is pre-diagnosed as suspect to have glaucoma.

# 4    Discussion of Results

Figure 8 shows some images from the collection of 67 images of human retinas which were analyzed using the proposed method.

The image population for the discussion of results was obtained in function of images with normal and suspect excavation.

The factors taken in account to select the test images population were: Images with suspect excavation; images with generalized thinning of the neuroretinal rim (a); having wide excavation and ostensible scleral holes (b); images with normal excavation. Rule ISNT preserved the excavation and the normal output of the papilla vessels (c), (d).

Figure 9 shows in detail the regions of interest (ROI) with the centroids and the reference points detected in different zones. The results achieved in these test images, were correct in all cases. The optic discs of the figures (a) and (b) have suspect excavations and the figures (c) and (d) have normal excavations.

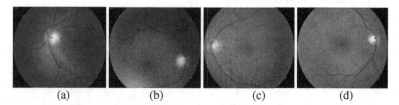

(a)              (b)              (c)              (d)

**Fig. 8.** Some images used for the test of the proposed method

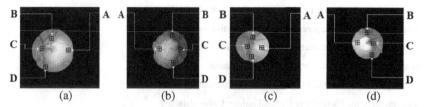

(a)              (b)              (c)              (d)

**Fig. 9.** Detail of the regions of interest (ROI) of the optic disc with the centroids and reference points detected in different zones: (a) and (b) images with suspect excavation; (c) and (d) images with normal excavation

The proposed method was tested with 67 retina images of real patients from which 24 were normal and 43 suspect to have glaucoma. From achieved results, 40 images had True Positives (*TP*), 22 images had True Negatives (*TN*), 2 images had False Positives (*FP*) and 3 images had False negatives (*FN*).

To calculate the Sensitivity and Specificity, we used the following expressions based on the results above:

$$Sensitivit\,y = \left(\frac{TP}{TP + FN}\right)100 = \left(\frac{40}{40 + 3}\right)100 = 93.02\%$$

$$Specificit\,y = \left(\frac{TN}{TN + FP}\right)100 = \left(\frac{22}{22 + 2}\right)100 = 91.66\% \qquad (4)$$

Then, it was achieved a Sensitivity of 93.02% and a Specificity of 91.66%, with an area under the curve of 0.923.

In Table 1 are shown our results and some related to other state of the art solutions. The number of samples and the origin of the retina image databases in each case are listed below the table. Conversely, these ranges allow appreciating a confidence interval of the diverse method accuracies, demonstrating that the results achieved by the proposed method are within the range of those achieved by other state of the art solutions.

**Table 1.** Comparison of our results with those achieved by other state of the art solutions

| # | Type of analysis | Sensitivity | Specificity |
|---|---|---|---|
| 1 | Cup/Disc ratio [13][1], [14][2], [15][3], [16][4] | 60% to 94% | 82% to 94.7% |
| 2 | Cup/Disc ratio used pairs of stereo retinal images [20][5] | 87% | 82% |
| 3 | Cup/Disc ratio and vessel bends [22][6], [23][7] | 18.6% to 81.3% | 45% to 81.8% |
| 4 | Cup/Disc ratio and ISNT rule [12][8], [18][9], [19][10] | 97.6% to 100% | 80% to 99.2% |
| **5** | **The proposed method[11]** | **93.02%** | **91.66%** |

[1] 107 images, from the Center for Computing Research of IPN database.

[2] 140 images, from the Singapore Eye Research Institute database.

[3] 90 images, from the Manchester Royal Eye Hospital database.

[4] 45 image, from the Gifu University Hospital database.

[5] 98 images pairs, from the Gifu University Hospital database.

[6] 138 images, from the Particularly Ophthalmology Clinic database.

[7] 27 images, from the Singapore Eye Research Institute database.

[8] 61 images, from the Kasturba Medical College database.

[9] 550 images, from an Aravind Eye Hospital database.

[10] 36 images, from an Aravind Eye Hospital database.

[11] 67 images, from the Center for Computing Research of IPN database.

Figure 10 shows two normal images that were classified as suspect of glaucoma. Fig. 10(a) has a Cup/Disc ratio less than 0.4 and meets the exigencies of the ISNT rule. Fig. 10(b) has a Cup/Disc ratio equal to 0.4 and also meets the exigencies of the ISNT rule. Then, both images have a pre-diagnosis of normal given by the specialist.

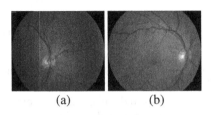

(a)                 (b)

**Fig. 10.** Normal images classified as suspect of glaucoma

Figure 11 shows two out of three retinal images that caused false negative results. They are suspect of glaucoma (diagnosis given by the specialist) and the system gave a result of healthy optic disc.

Fig. 11(a) has an excavation with inferior polar notch, and a lightly asymmetric Cup/Disc ratio 0.4H (horizontal) and 0.5V (vertical). Fig. 11(b) presents a loss of nervous fibers (it is observed the channel without fibers, below of the superior temporal vascular bundle) at XI (eleven o'clock) that coincides with the superior notch of the excavation, having a vertical predominance.

Figure 11(c) shows another situation, even when this appears as normal image belongs to a pair of image (in the work was used 11 pairs of images) of a patient with glaucoma; that is not a common situation. This occurs frequently when the glaucoma is caused by a traumatism, where only one optic disc is strongly affected and the other remains as normal. The fact of the high Cup/Disc ratio asymmetry is the reason by which the optic disc of that eye does not satisfy the ISNT rule to be considered as suspect of glaucoma.

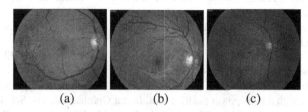

(a)               (b)               (c)

**Fig. 11.** Images that caused false negatives with the proposed method

As it is shown in Table 1, the sensitivity and the specificity in pre-diagnosis of our proposed method is within the results achieved in the state of the art related solutions. Analyzing the results in detail, images where our method failed, it was observed that the expert pre-diagnosis are suspect because apart of the growth characteristics of the excavation, there is also the presence of nicks and localized loss optical fiber. On this basis, we can say that the effectiveness of the method presented is high.

# 5    Conclusion

This paper presents a method for classifying color images of human retinas suspect of having glaucoma on the basis of the displacement of the vascular bundle produced caused by the excavation growth in the optic disc. A close relationship was found between the excavation growth and the vascular bundle displacement in the superior, inferior and nasal optic disc zones.

The proposed methodology achieved an accuracy of the 93.02% of sensitivity and 91.66% of specificity in the pre-diagnosis, even with excavations in early stages of development. This shows that the proposed approach is effective and can be used as a method for developing new ophthalmic medical systems suitable for computerized pre-diagnosis.

**Acknowledgments.** The authors of this paper wish to thank the Centro de Investigación en Computación (CIC), Mexico; Research and Postgraduate Secretary (SIP), Mexico, and Instituto Politécnico Nacional (IPN), Mexico, for their economic support.

# References

1. Gili-Manzanaro, G., Carrasco, F.C., Martín-Rodrigo, J.C., Yangüela-Rodilla, J., Arias-Puente, A.: Análisis digital de la papila con cámara de fondo de ojo convencional: estudio de variabilidad. Arch. Soc. Esp. Oftalmol. de Madrid 79(3) (2004)
2. Consejo de salubridad general: Aspectos Generales. Centro Nacional de Excelencia Tecnológica en Salud: Diagnóstico y Tratamiento del Paciente Adulto con Glaucoma de Ángulo Abierto, 10–26. Secretaría de Salud, México (2009)
3. Elolia, R., Stokes, J.: Monograph Series on Aging-related Diseases: XI. Glaucoma. Chronic Diseases in Canada 19(4) (1998)
4. Felipe-Riverón, E.M., Morales-Güitrón, S.L., Ortiz-Yánez, S.: Detección automática de la normalidad de las retinas humanas. Tesis de Maestría en Ciencias de la Computación CIC-IPN, México (2004)
5. Gili Manzanaro, G.: Fotografía de fondo de ojo con filtros. Boletín de a Soc Oftalmol de Madrid (44) (2004)
6. Otsu, N.: A threshold Selection Method from Gray-Level Histogram. IEEE Trans. Systems, Man and Cybernetics SMC-9(1), 62–66 (1976)
7. Ansari-Shahrezaei, S., Maar, N., Biowski, R., Stur, M.: Biomicroscopic measurement of the optic disc with a high-power positive lens. Invest Ophthalmol. Vis. Sci. 42(1) (2001)
8. Fernández-Argones, L., Piloto-Díaz, I., Coba-Peña, M., Pérez-Tamayo, B., Domínguez-Randulfe, M., Trujillo-Fonseca, K.: Sistemas de análisis digital de imágenes en el glaucoma. Rev. Cubana Invest. Biomédica 28(3) (2009)
9. Mendoza-Santiesteban, C.E., Santiesteban-Freixas, R., González-García, A., González-Hess, L., Mesa-Hernández, E., Perdomo-Trujillo, Y., Alemañy-Rubio, E., Eguia, F., Vidal-Casalís, S.: La tomografía de coherencia óptica en el diagnóstico de enfermedades de la retina y el nervio óptico. Rev. Cubana Oftalmol. 18(2) (2005)
10. Duch-Tuesta, S., Buchacra-Castellano, O.: Tomografía de coherencia óptica en glaucoma. Infothea 43 (2006)
11. De la Fuente-Arriaga, J.A., Garduño-Calderón, E., Cuevas-de la Rosa, F.J.: Estado actual de las técnicas computacionales para la valoración del disco óptico en glaucoma. Memorias del Congreso Mexiquense CTS+I 1(1), 155–161 (2011)
12. Nayak, J., Acharya, R.: Automated Diagnosis of Glaucoma Using Digital Fundus Images. J. Med. Syst. 33(5) (2009)
13. Felipe Riverón, E.M., del Toro Céspedes, M.: Measurement of Parameters of the Optic Disk in Ophthalmoscopic Color Images of Human Retina. In: Sanfeliu, A., Martínez Trinidad, J.F., Carrasco Ochoa, J.A. (eds.) CIARP 2004. LNCS, vol. 3287, pp. 661–668. Springer, Heidelberg (2004)
14. Liu, J., Wong, D.W.K., Lim, J.H., Li, H., Tan, N.M., Wong, T.Y.: ARGALI: an automatic cup-to-disc ratio measurement system for glaucoma detection and AnalysIs framework. In: Proc. of SPIE, Medical Imaging 2009: Computer-Aided Diagnosis, vol. 7260 (2009)
15. Abdel-Ghafar, A., Morris, A., Ritchings, B., Wood, C.: Detection and Characterization of the Optic Disk in Glaucoma and Diabetic Retinopathy. UMIST 88 (2004)

16. Hatanaka, Y., Noudo, A., Sawada, A., Hara, T., Yamamoto, T., Fujita, H.: Automated Measurement of Cup to Disc Ratio Based on Line Profile Analysis in Retinal Images. In: 33rd Annual International Conference of the IEEE EMBS, Boston (2011)
17. Muramatsu, C., Nakagawa, T., Sawada, A., Hatanaka, Y., Hara, T., Yamamoto, T., Fujita, H.: Automated segmentation of optic disc region on retinal fundus photographs: Comparison of contour modeling and pixel classification methods. Computer Methods and Programs in Biomedicine 101(1) (2010)
18. Kavitha, S., Duraiswamy, K.: An efficient decision support system for detection of glaucoma in fundus images using ANFIS. International Journal of Advances in Engineering & Technology 6(1), 226–240 (2012)
19. Narasimhan, K., Vijayarekha, K.: An efficient automated system for glaucoma detection using fundus image. Journal of Theoretical and Applied Information Technology 33(1) (2011)
20. Muramatsu, C., Nakagawa, T., Sawada, A., Hatanaka, Y., Yamamoto, T., Fujita, H.: Automated determination of cup-to-disc ratio for classification of glaucomatous and normal eyes on stereo retinal fundus images. Journal of Biomedical Optics 16(9) (2011)
21. Gere, J.M., Goodno, B.J.: Repaso de centroides y momentos de inercia. Cervantes-González, S.R: Mecánica de materiales. Cengage Learning, 901–927 (2009)
22. Joshi, G.D., Sivaswamy, J., Krishnadas, S.R.: Optic disk and cup segmentation from monocular color retinal images for glaucoma assessment. IEEE Transactions on Medical Imaging 30(6), 1192–1205 (2011)
23. Liu, J., Wong, D.W.K., Lim, J.H., Li, H., Tan, N.M., Wong, T.Y.: Automated detection of kinks from blood vessels for optic cup segmentation in retinal images. In: Proc. of SPIE, Medical Imaging 2009: Computer-Aided Diagnosis, vol. 7260, pp. 72601J-1–72601J-8 (2009)
24. De la Fuente-Arriaga, J.A., Felipe-Riverón, E.M., Garduño-Calderón, E.: Segmentación del disco óptico en imágenes de retina mediante la transformada de Hough y los contornos activos. Research in Computer Science 58, 117–131 (2012)

# Blood Vessel Segmentation in Retinal Images Using Lattice Neural Networks

Roberto Vega[1], Elizabeth Guevara[2], Luis Eduardo Falcon[1],
Gildardo Sanchez-Ante[1], and Humberto Sossa[2]

[1] Tecnológico de Monterrey, Campus Guadalajara
Computer Science Department
Av. Gral Ramon Corona 2514,
Zapopan, Jal, México
ri.vega@itesm.mx
[2] Instituto Politécnico Nacional-CIC
Av. Juan de Dios Batiz S/N, Gustavo A. Madero 07738
México, Distrito Federal, México

**Abstract.** Blood vessel segmentation is the first step in the process of automated diagnosis of cardiovascular diseases using retinal images. Unlike previous work described in literature, which uses rule-based methods or classical supervised learning algorithms, we applied Lattice Neural Networks with Dendritic Processing (LNNDP) to solve this problem. LNNDP differ from traditional neural networks in the computation performed by the individual neuron, showing more resemblance with biological neural networks, and offering high performance on the training phase (99.8% precision in our case). Our methodology requires four steps: 1)Preprocessing, 2)Feature computation, 3)Classification, 4)Postprocessing. We used the Hotelling $T^2$ control chart to reduce the dimensionality of the feature vector from 7 to 5 dimensions, and measured the effectiveness of the methodology with the $F_1 Score$ metric, obtaining a maximum of 0.81; compared to 0.79 of a traditional neural network.

## 1 Introduction

**Diabetic Retinopathy**, a complication of diabetes mellitus, affects up to 80% of diabetics and causes blindness even in developed countries like the US [1]. **Arteriosclerosis**, the hardening and thickening of the walls of the arteries, contributes to the development of cardiovascular diseases; the leading cause of death in people over age 45. It has an overall prevalence of circa 30% [2] and [3]. Finally, **hypertension**, or high blood pressure, is a factor for myocardial infarction, stroke, ischemia, and congestive heart failure. According to recent studies, the overall prevalence of hypertension is about 25 % of the population [4]. These three diseases share at least three facts: 1) They affect a significant portion of the population; 2) They have to be monitored once diagnosed, and 3) All three can be diagnosed and monitored through the observation of the retina [5].

The retina is a unique site where the blood vessels can be directly visualized non-invasively and *in vivo* [6]. Nowadays, digital ophthalmoscopes are able to

F. Castro, A. Gelbukh, and M. González (Eds.): MICAI 2013, Part I, LNAI 8265, pp. 532–544, 2013.
© Springer-Verlag Berlin Heidelberg 2013

take quite clear images of the retina, with the possibility of storing them in a digital format and offering the opportunity for automated image processing and analysis. Although this idea has attracted the attention of many research groups, the problem is still not completely solved. The images of the retina present important technical challenges, both in their capture as well as in the processing. These challenges are described by Abramoff et al. at [7].

The three most important areas of active research in retinal imaging include: development of cost-effective digital equipment to capture retinal images, development of techniques to study the function of the retina using oxymetry or near-infrared analysis, and development of image processing and analysis algorithms that allow the classification of retinal images for automated diagnosis. In many cases, a set of features of the vascular structure of the retina can establish a probable diagnosis. Parameters such as diameter, color, curvature and opacity of blood vessels may serve as a basis for diagnosis, treatment, and monitor of the aforementioned diseases [8] and [9].

In this work, we focus on the application of one machine learning algorithm to extract the vascular (blood vessel) structure from retinal images, so that in a further step, future parameters such as the ones described can be quantified. In particular, we report here the results of using a different configuration of neural network called Lattice Neural Network with Dendrite Processing (LNNDP).

The remainder of the paper is organized as follows: Section 2 describes current advances in retinal image processing, Section 3 introduces Lattice Neural Networks with Dendrite Processing, Section 4 presents our methodology, Section 5 describes experiments and results and finally, Section 6 presents the conclusions and future work.

## 2   Previous Work

In general, the correct interpretation of medical images is a complex task because of the steps that are needed: preprocessing, segmentation, classification and recognition. The two steps that are related with the work described in this paper are segmentation and classification. In a pioneering work, Goldbaum et al., [10] introduced an image management system called STARE (structured analysis of the retina). In such work the authors described, in theory, what things could be done for each step; however, they do not offer any results. Hoover et al. [11] presented a method to segment and extract blood vessels in retinal images by using local and global vessel features cooperatively. They first generated a new image that represents the strength of a matched filter response (MFR), and then a classification step done through threshold probing. Other authors have focused on the same problem: segmenting blood vessels. For instance, the work reported in [12] focuses only on the extraction of image ridges, which coincide approximately with vessel centerlines. Those centerlines classify neighboring pixels either as vessel or not. The authors in [13], tried to classify arteries and veins. They compared two feature extraction methods and two classification methods based on support vector machines and neural networks. As for feature extraction, one method is based on the vessel profile, while the other is based on a region of interest around the vessel pixel found on the center line. Given a hand-segmentation of vessels, their approach correctly classifies 95.32 % vessel pixels. There is no information on how much time this process takes. Other approaches have used color to perform the segmentation, such as in [14] and in [15]. Maruthusivarani et al. compared two different segmentation methods for blood vessel extraction: a local entropy based thresholding, and a morphological operation [16]. The authors of [17] also compared three methods (moment invariants [18], morphological image processing, and hybrid filtering). The work of Fraz et al. reports the application of linear discriminant analysis [5]. Probing methods have also been proposed, allowing the segmentation in pieces [11]. In [19] a graph-based approach was used to connect the pixels.

## 3    Lattice Neural Networks

The analysis of retinal images is a classification problem in which a given blood vessel is labeled as blood vessel or non blood vessel. One possible way of solving classification problems is through the use of artificial neural networks (ANN). This approach seems attractive because an ANN can be used to estimate only the behavior of a function from observations, rather than obtaining the model equation itself. Thus, if the ANN is fed with images in which blood vessels are hand labeled, then the network may discover the inherent properties of the images, allowing the proper classification of new images.

Some researchers have argued that traditional ANN models bear little resemblance with the biological neural networks [20] and [21]; thereby driving the design of new generations of neural networks: Lattice Neural Networks (LNN), Morphological Neural Networks [22] and Spiking Neural Networks, among others. New findings in neurocomputing propose that the primary autonomous computational unit in brain capable of realizing logical operations are the dendrtites. Therefore, Ritter et al. proposed a new paradigm of LNN that considers computation in the dendritic structure as well as in the body of the neuron. In a single layer feedforward neural network has been observed that there are no convergence problems and the speed of learning exceeds traditional back propagation methods [21]. Morphological neural networks (MNN) derive their name from the study of morphological transformations. Two such operations are dilation and erosion which are used to perform shape analysis [23] and [24].

In a traditional ANN the activation function is given by a linear combination of the weights and the input vector, adding also a term called "bias". In contrast, in a LNN the activation function is given by computing logical operations AND and OR, as well as the sum.

In order to train the LNNDP, we used a modified version the model proposed by Ritter and Schmalz [25]. This model proposes a set of $n$ input neurons $N_1, \ldots, N_n$, where $n$ is the number of features in the input vector, and $m$ output neurons $M_1, \ldots, M_m$, where $m$ is the number of classes in which the data is classified. Fig. 1 shows a representation of the LNNDP.

In this model, the weight of the axonal branch of neuron $N_i$ terminating on the $k-th$ dendrite $D_k$ of $M_j$ is denoted by $\omega_{ijk}^l$, where the superscript $l \in \{0,1\}$ distinguishes between excitatory ($l = 1$, marked as a black dot on Fig. 1), and inhibitory ($l = 0$, marked as an open dot on Fig. 1) input to the dendrite. The computation of the $k$-th dendrite $D_k$ of $M_j$ is given by:

$$\tau_k^j(x) = p_{jk} \bigwedge_{i \in I(k)} \bigwedge_{l \in L(i)} (-1)^{1-l}(x_i + \omega_{ijk}^l) \tag{1}$$

where $x = (x_1, \ldots, x_n)$ denotes the input value of the neurons $N_1, \ldots N_n, I(k) \subseteq \{1, \ldots, n\}$ corresponds to the set of all input neurons with terminal fibers that synapse on the $k$-th dendrite $D_k$ of $M_j$, $L(i) \subseteq \{0,1\}$ corresponds to the set of terminal fibers $N_i$ that synapse on the $k$-th dendrite $D_k$ of $M_j$, and $p_{jk} \in \{-1,1\}$ denotes inhibitory or excitatory response of the $k$-th dendrite $D_k$ of $M_j$ to the received input. The total output of the neuron $M_j$ is given by the equation:

$$\tau^j(x) = p_j \bigvee_{k=1}^{K_j} \tau_k^j(x) \tag{2}$$

where $K_j$ represents the total number of dendrites in the neuron $M_j$, $\tau_k^j(x)$ is the output of the dendrite $k$ of neuron $M_j$; $p_j = 1$ to denote that the particular input is accepted; and $p_j = 0$ to denote that the particular input is rejected. Finally, according to [25] the input vector $x$ is assigned to the class whose neuron results in the biggest value:

$$y = \bigvee_{j=1}^{m} \tau^j(x) \tag{3}$$

where $m$ is the number of classes, and $\tau^j(x)$ is the output of the neuron $M_j$.

## 4   Methodology

### 4.1   Image Acquisition

To evaluate the proposed methodology, we used the publicly available database STARE [11]. This database contains 400 retinal images with several pathologies, including various types of diabetic retinopathy, vein occlusion, and artery occlusion. In 20 of the 400 images, the blood vessels are hand labeled by two independent experts. These 20 images were used, selecting the labeling of the first expert as ground truth. The retinal fundus slides used were originally captured with a TopCon TRV-50 fundus camera at 35 field of view. The slides were digitalized to produce 605 x 700 color images, 24 bits per pixel. Half of the images are of patient retinas with no pathology, and the other half of the images are of retinas containing pathologies that obscure or confuse the blood vessel appearance, making the vessels harder to identify [11]. An example of each kind of image, as well as its hand labeled segmentation, is shown in Fig. 2.

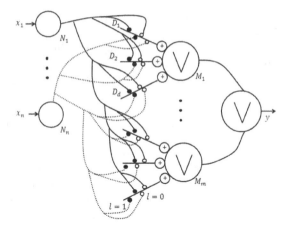

**Fig. 1.** Representation of a lattice neural network with dendritic computing

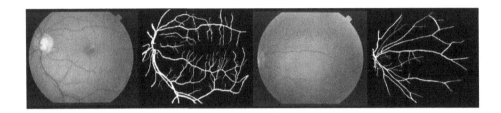

**Fig. 2.** Left: Normal fundus image and its segmentation, Right: Pathology fundus image and its segmentation

## 4.2 Preprocessing and Feature Extraction

In a dendritic model, a set of $n$ input neurons $N_1, \ldots, N_n$ accepts as an input a vector $x = (x_1, \ldots, x_n) \in R^n$ [24]. Marin, et al. proposed a neural network scheme for pixel classification and computed a 7-D vector composed of gray-levels and moment invariants for pixel representation [18]. In this work, we used a similar methodology to obtain a 7-D feature vector. The procedure is summarized as follows:

Since color fundus images often show important lighting variations, poor contrast and noise, a preprocessing step is needed. The steps involved in this stage are: 1) Vessel central light reflex removal, 2)Background homogenization, and 3)Vessel enhancement.

- *Vessel central light reflex removal*: The green layer of the image was isolated from the images because it shows the highest contrast between blood vessels and background [12]. Then, a morphological opening was implemented on the green layer in order to remove the light streak included in some vessels.

The structuring element used in the operation was an eight-connectivity, three-pixel diameter disc. The resultant image is labeled as $I_\gamma$.

- *Background homogenization*: In order to remove background lighting variations, a shade-corrected image is obtained from a background estimate. First, a $3 \times 3$ mean filter is applied over $I_\gamma$, followed by a convolution with a Gaussian kernel of $9 \times 9$, using a mean $\mu = 0$, and variance $\sigma^2 = 1.8$. Then, a background image ($I_b$) is obtained applying a $25 \times 25$ median filter. To obtain the shade corrected image, the background image is subtracted from the image after the morphological opening:

$$D(x,y) = I_\gamma(x,y) - I_b(x,y) \qquad (4)$$

Then the image was linearly transformed to cover all possible ranges of gray-levels $[0, 255]$. This new image is called $I_{SC}$. The transform implements the equation [26]:

$$N_{x,y} = \frac{N_{max} - N_{min}}{O_{max} - O_{min}} \times (O_{x,y} - O_{min}) + N_{min} \qquad (5)$$

where, $N_{max}, N_{min}, O_{max}$ and $O_{min}$ are the desired maximum and minimum gray level values of the new, and old histograms respectively; and $O_{x,y}$ is the value of the pixel to be changed. Finally, to reduce the influence of intensity variations along the image, a homogenized image $I_H$ is obtained displacing toward the middle of the histogram the pixel intensities of the images. This is accomplished by applying the transformation function:

$$g_{Output} = \begin{cases} 0 & \text{if } g < 0 \\ 255 & \text{if } g > 255 \\ g & \text{otherwise} \end{cases} \qquad (6)$$

where

$$g = g_{Input} + 128 - g_{InputMax} \qquad (7)$$

where $g_{Input}$ and $g_{Output}$ are the gray-level values of the input and output images. $g_{InputMax}$ represents the mode of the pixel-value intensities in $I_{SC}$.

- *Vessel Enhancement*: This step is performed by estimating the complement image of $I_H$, $I_H^c$, and then applying a morphological Top-Hat transformation using as a structuring element a disc of eight pixels in radius. The vessel enhanced image, $I_{VE}$ is then defined as:

$$I_{VE} = I_H^c - \gamma(I_H^c) \qquad (8)$$

where $\gamma$ is the morphological opening operation.

Once the preprocessing stage is finished, the resultant images $I_H, I_{VE}$ are used to extract a 7 feature vector for each pixel in the image. The effect of each step in the preprocessing stage is shown in Fig. 3.

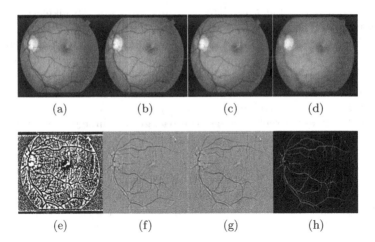

**Fig. 3.** (a) Green layer of the image. (b) Image after morphological opening. (c) Image after gaussian filter. (d)Image after applying a median filter. (e) Difference of (b) and (d). (f) Normalization of (e). (g) Homogenized image. (h) Image after top-hat transformation.

The features are divided in two groups:

- Gray level features: based on the gray-level intensity if the pixel of interest, and a statistical analysis of its surroundings. For these features, we use $I_H$.
- Moment invariants-based features: features based on moment invariants for small regions formed by a window centered at the pixel of interest. For these features, we use $I_{VE}$.

In the following equations, which define the features, $S^w_{(x,y)}$ represents the set of points in a window of $w \times w$, centered at the pixel $(x, y)$. The five gray level features can be expressed as:

$$f_1(x,y) = I_H(x,y) - min_{(s,t)\in S^9_{x,y}}\{I_H(s,t)\} \tag{9}$$

$$f_2(x,y) = max_{(s,t)\in S^9_{x,y}}\{I_H(s,t) - I_H(x,y)\} \tag{10}$$

$$f_3(x,y) = I_H(x,y) - mean_{(s,t)\in S^9_{x,y}}\{I_H(s,t)\} \tag{11}$$

$$f_4(x,y) = variance_{(s,t)\in S^9_{x,y}}\{I_H(s,t)\} \tag{12}$$

$$f_5(x,y) = I_H(x,y) \tag{13}$$

The moment invariant features proposed were the logarithm of the first and second moments of Hu in a window of $17 \times 17$ centered at the pixel of interest, which are defined as:

$$f_6(x,y) = \log(\eta_{20} + \eta_{02}) \tag{14}$$

$$f_7(x,y) = \log((\eta_{20} + \eta_{02})^2 + 4\eta_{11}^2) \tag{15}$$

where

$$\eta_{pq} = \frac{\mu_{pq}}{(\mu_{00})^{(\frac{p+q}{2}+1)}}; p+q \geq 2 \tag{16}$$

$$\mu_{pq} = \sum_x \sum_y (x - \overline{x})^p (y - \overline{y})^q f(x,y); x, y \in S_{x,y}^{17} \tag{17}$$

$$\overline{x} = \frac{m_{10}}{m_{00}}; \overline{y} = \frac{m_{01}}{m_{00}} \tag{18}$$

$$m_{ij} = \sum_x \sum_y x^i y^j f(x,y); x, y \in S_{x,y}^{17}. \tag{19}$$

## 4.3 Classification

The seven features were calculated for each pixel in the 20 images. Then, we took a reference image and extracted 30,000 random pixels (half hand-labeled as blood vessels, and half as non-blood vessels) to train the neural network.

According to Ritter and Schmalz in [21], there are two different approaches to learning in LNNDP: training based on elimination, and training based on merging. In this work, we used the training based on merging, which is based in the creation of small hyperboxes of $n$ dimensions around individual patterns, or small groups of patterns belonging to the same class.

Training is completed after merging all the hyperboxes for all patterns of the same class. Because this approach is used, the values of $p$ in equations 16, and 17 are set to 1. Sossa and Guevara proposed an efficient method for the training of LNNDP [25]. The process is summarized as follow:

Given $p$ classes of patterns $C^a$, $a = 1, 2, p$, each with $n$ attributes:

1. Create an hypercube $HC^n$, that includes all the patterns in the set.
2. Verify if all the hypercubes enclose patterns of just one class. If that is the case, label the hypercube with the name of the corresponding class and proceed to step 4, else proceed to step 3.
3. For all the hypercubes that have patterns of more than one class, divide the hypercube into $2^n$ smaller hypercubes. Check if the condition stated on step 2 is satisfied.
4. Based on the coordinates on each axis, calculate the weights for each hyper cube that encloses patterns belonging to $C^a$.

In this method, each hypercube is represented by a dendrite $D_k$, and each class of patterns is represented by an output neuron $M_j$. Since the number of hyperboxes for each class may vary, each class may have different number of dendrites. Each input neuron $N_i$ will connect to an output neuron $M_j$ through a dendrite $D_k$ at two different points: one excitatory ($l = 1$), and one inhibitory ($l = 0$). The weight $\omega_{ijk}^l$ associated with each connection will be the borders of the hypercube represented by $D_k$ over the axis $i$. The lowest value of the border will be assigned to $-\omega_{ijk}^1$, while the highest value will be assigned to $-\omega_{ijk}^0$. Figure 4 shows an example of how weights would be assigned to a hypercube $n = 2$.

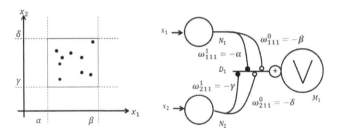

**Fig. 4.** Example of weight definition of an hypercube of $n = 2$

## 4.4 Postprocessing

In order to improve the results, we implemented a postprocessing stage. As it will be shown in the following section, the images predicted by the neural network contain "salt and pepper" noise, and small regions misclassified as blood vessels. The first step consists in applying a median filter using a mask of $5 \times 5$. This filter eliminates most of the isolated points labeled as blood vessels, although it can also add some points that were not in the original prediction. In order to eliminate these new points, we made the conjunction of the original and filtered images. Finally, we classified as non-vessel the regions whose area was below 25 pixels. In this case, the area of a region is the number of pixels connected.

## 5   Experiments and Results

In a first experiment, using the proposed methodology, we achieved an accuracy of 99.02% in the training phase. 4844 dendrites were in the neuron that classifies the pixels as blood vessels, and 4786 dendrites in the one that classifies them as non blood vessels. The weights obtained in the training phase were used to make the segmentation of the 20 images on the dataset.

In a second experiment, we made a control chart in order to eliminate outliers in the training set that could diminish the performance of the neural network. The most familiar multivariate control procedure is the Hotelling $T^2$ control chart for monitoring the mean vector of the process [27], so we used this procedure as a first choice. After implementing this control chart, we expected to label about 1% as outliers; however, about 6.6% of the samples fell in this category. A more profound analysis of this behavior made us realize that the features $f_4$ and $f_6$ were the cause of so many outliers. After removing these features, the percentage diminished to 2.4%. We removed the outliers from the new 5 dimensional feature set and we ran the experiment again. This experiment created 6966 dendrites for the first class and 6611 for the second class, and it achieved an accuracy of 99.8% in the training phase.

Finally, we ran a third experiment training the network with 3 images instead of just one. In this last experiment we used the 5 dimensional feature vector.

Although could be expected that a lattice neural network achieved 100% accuracy in the training set, this was not the case because some pixels with the same feature vector were classified sometimes as blood vessels, and some other times as non vessels. This behavior could have been caused by noise in the images, in the data, or human error in the hand labeling process. Usually, the stop criterion for a LNNDP is that all of the patterns must be correctly classified; if, however, the same pattern belongs to different classes, the stop will never occur. In order to avoid convergence problems caused by inconsistencies in the data, we had to re-label the pixels whose feature vector belonged to different classes. The re-classification criterion was to assign all the pixels with the same feature vector to the most frequent class present in this feature vector. For example, if nine identical pixels were labeled as class 0, and one pixel as class 1, then all the pixels were re-labeled as class 0.

In order to evaluate the predicted images, we used a metric called $F_1 Score$, which is defined as:

$$F_1 Score = \frac{(2 * truePositives)}{(2 * truePositives + falseNegatives + falsePositives)}$$

Table 1 lists the results of the different experiments implemented over the 20 images of the dataset before postprocessing (bp), and the results after post-processing (ap) in the experiment 2; the experiment which had the best results. Figure 5 shows an example of the prediction made by the neural network in each experiment. The proposed neural network with dendritic processing is also compared with a multilayer perceptron with 9 dendrites in the hidden layer (NN9), and our implementation of the methodology proposed by Martín et al. [18], which consists of a neural network with 3 hidden layers, each containing 15 hidden units. The results of our implementation of the methodology proposed by Marin et al. showed a lower performance than the results reported by them. This difference could be caused by the selection of the training set: they chose the training set manually, while we chose it randomly.

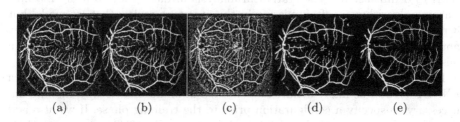

(a)          (b)          (c)          (d)          (e)

**Fig. 5.** (a) Exp. 1 bp. (b) Exp. 2 bp. (c) Exp. 3 bp. (d) Exp. 1 ap. (e) Hand-labeled image.

**Table 1.** Results of the experiments show a better performance applying a LNNDP using a 5 dimensional feature vector

|  | Exp. 1 bp | Exp. 2 bp | Exp. 3 bp | NN9 | Exp. 2 ap | Marín et. al |
|---|---|---|---|---|---|---|
| Average $F_1 Score$ | 0.5490 | 0.5539 | 0.4183 | 0.5587 | **0.6616** | 0.6565 |
| Min $F_1 Score$ | 0.4149 | 0.3805 | 0.2803 | 0.2579 | 0.4232 | **0.4287** |
| Max $F_1 Score$ | 0.6586 | 0.6722 | 0.5123 | 0.7351 | **0.8123** | 0.7916 |

## 6    Conclusions

The use of a LNNDP could solve the problem presented, showing a better performance (about 2% in the best case) when compared with the use of multilayer perceptron, and presenting a very high performance (99.8%) on the training set. Unfortunately, we could not compare our results against many other works available in literature because their algorithms used accuracy as metric, while we used $F_1 Score$. The problem with accuracy is that between 92% and 95% of the pixels in the images are non blood vessels, so an algorithm that always label a pixel as non blood vessel will have 92% - 95% of accuracy, giving a false idea of good performance. The metric $F_1 Score$ gives a more realistic evaluation by calculating the relationship between true positives, false negatives, and false positives. In this way, an algorithm that always label the pixels as non blood vessels will have a grade of 0, and an algorithm that labels all the pixels correctly will have a grade of 1.

We ran three experiments to evaluate the performance of three different training sets. The best result was obtained with the training set obtained by a single image, and characterized by a feature vector of 5 dimensions. Contrary to intuition, adding more images to the training set reduced the performance of the LNNDP. This was due to the high variety of the images in the database. Besides,we implemented six different methodologies to remove noise and false positives; however, most of them also removed fine details of the images. We presented the one that obtained better results. Finally, the Hotelling $T^2$ control chart allowed us to reduce the dimensionality of the training set from 7 dimensions to 5 dimensions. The statistical analysis of data prior to using machine learning algorithms is often missing in the literature review that we made, but it proved to be very usefull in our implementation. In this way, our methodology not only performed better that traditional neural networks, but also included a missing step in previous works.

Besides the aforementioned characteristics, we want to point out that a LNNDP creates as many dendrites as needed in an automatic way, making unnecessary to specify a configuration prior to the training phase. If we also add that the performance of the training phase is usually 100%, we can conclude that LNNDP is a powerful tool for solving classification problems.

**Acknowledgments.** The authors thank Tecnológico de Monterrey, Campus Guadalajara, IPN-CIC under project SIP 2013-1182, and CONACYT under project 155014 for the economical support to carry out this research. We also acknowledge professor Marco de Luna for his insight about statistical analysis, and all the reviewers for their valuable comments that helped us to improve this work.

# References

1. Agurto, C., Barriga, E., Murray, V., Nemeth, S., Crammer, R., Bauman, W., Zamora, G., Pattichis, M., Soliz, P.: Automatic detection of diabetic retinopathy and age-related macular degeneration in digital fundus images. Investigative Ophthalmology & Visual Science, 5862–5871 (2011)
2. Núñez Cortés, J., Alegria, E., Walther, L., Gimilio, J., Rallo, C., Morat, T., Prieto, J., Montoya, J.B., Sala, X.: Documento abordaje de la dislipidemia. sociedad española de arteriosclerosis (parte ii). Clínica e Investigación en Arteriosclerosis, 40–52 (2012)
3. Sy, R., Morales, D., Dans, A., Paz-Pacheco, E., Punzalan, F., Abelardo, N., Duante, C.: Prevalence of atherosclerosis-related risk factors and diseases in the philippines. Journal of Epidemiology, 440–447 (2012)
4. National Center for Health Statistics: Hypertension Among Adults in the United States 2009-2010 (2012)
5. Fraz, M., Remagnino, P., Hoppe, A., Barman, S.: Retinal image analysis aimed at extraction of vascular structure using linear discriminant classifier. In: International Conference on Computer Medical Applications (ICCMA), pp. 1–6 (2013)
6. Patton, N., Aslam, T., MacGillivray, T., Deary, I., Dhillon, B., Eikelboom, R., Yogesan, K., Constable, I.: Retinal image analysis: Concepts, applications and potential. Progress in Retinal and Eye Research 25, 99–127 (2006)
7. Abramoff, M., Garvin, M.K., Sonka, M.: Retinal imaging and image analysis. IEEE Reviews in Biomedical Engineering 3, 169–208 (2010)
8. Bernardes, R., Serranho, P., Lobo, C.: Digital ocular fundus imaging: A review. Ophthalmologica 226, 161–181 (2011)
9. Karthikeyan, R., Alli, P.: Retinal image analysis for abnormality detection-an overview. Journal of Computer Science 8, 436 (2012)
10. Goldbaum, M., Moezzi, S., Taylor, A., Chatterjee, S., Boyd, J., Hunter, E., Jain, R.: Automated diagnosis and image understanding with object extraction, object classification, and inferencing in retinal images. In: International Conference on Image Processing, pp. 695–698 (1996)
11. Hoover, A., Kouznetsova, V., Goldbaum, M.: Locating blood vessels in retinal images by piecewise threshold probing of a matched filter response. IEEE Transactions on Medical Imaging 19, 203–210 (2000)
12. Staal, J., Abramoff, M., Niemeijer, M., Viergever, M., Van Ginneken, B.: Ridge-based vessel segmentation in color images of the retina. IEEE Transactions on Medical Imaging 23, 501–509 (2004)
13. Kondermann, C., Kondermann, D., Yan, M.: Blood vessel classification into arteries and veins in retinal images. In: SPIE Medical Imaging, pp. 651247–651247 9 (2007)
14. Hijazi, M., Coenen, F., Zheng, Y.: Retinal image classification for the screening of age-related macular degeneration. In: Research and Development in Intelligent Systems XXVII, pp. 325–338 (2011)

15. Tariq, A., Akram, M.: An automated system for colored retinal image background and noise segmentation. In: IEEE Symposium on Industrial Electronics and Applications (ISIEA), Penang, Malaysia, pp. 423–427 (2010)
16. Maruthusivarani, M., Ramakrishnan, T., Santhi, D., Muthukkutti, K.: Comparison of automatic blood vessel segmentation methods in retinal images. In: International Conference on Emerging Trends in VLSI, Embedded System, Nano Electronics and Telecommunication System (ICEVENT), pp. 1–4 (2013)
17. Preethi, M., Vanithamani, R.: Review of retinal blood vessel detection methods for automated diagnosis of diabetic retinopathy. In: International Conference on Advances in Engineering, Science and Management (ICAESM), pp. 262–265 (2012)
18. Marin, D., Aquino, A., Gegundez-Arias, M., Bravo, J.: A new supervised method for blood vessel segmentation in retinal images by using gray-level and moment invariants-based features. IEEE Transactions on Medical Imaging 30, 146–158 (2011)
19. Lau, Q., Lee, M., Hsu, W., Wong, T.: Simultaneously identifying all true vessels from segmented retinal images. IEEE Transactions on Biomedical Engineering 60, 1851–1858 (2013)
20. Ritter, G., Iancu, L., Urcid, G.: Morphological perceptrons with dendritic structure. In: The 12th IEEE International Conference on Fuzzy Systems, FUZZ 2003, vol. 2, pp. 1296–1301 (2003)
21. Ritter, G., Schmalz, M.: Learning in lattice neural networks that employ dendritic computing. In: IEEE International Conference on Fuzzy Systems 2006, pp. 7–13 (2006)
22. Sussner, P.: Morphological perceptron learning. In: International Symposium on Intelligent Control (ISIC), held jointly with IEEE International Symposium on Computational Intelligence in Robotics and Automation (CIRA), Intelligent Systems and Semiotics (ISAS), pp. 477–482 (1998)
23. Ritter, G., Sussner, P.: An introduction to morphological neural networks. In: International Conference on Pattern Recognition, vol. 4, pp. 709–717 (1996)
24. Ritter, G., Beaver, T.: Morphological perceptrons. In: International Joint Conference on Neural Networks, IJCNN 1999, vol. 1, pp. 605–610 (1999)
25. Sossa, H., Guevara, E.: Efficient training for dendrite morphological neural networks (Submitted to Neurocomputing, 2013)
26. Nixon, M., Aguado, A.: Feature extraction & image processing. Newnes, Great Britain (2008)
27. Montgomery, D.: Introduction to Statistical Quality Control, 5th edn. Wiley, USA (2005)

# A Bayesian and Minimum Variance Technique for Arterial Lumen Segmentation in Ultrasound Imaging

Sergio Rogelio Tinoco-Martínez, Felix Calderon,
Carlos Lara-Alvarez, and Jaime Carranza-Madrigal

División de Estudios de Posgrado, Facultad de Ingeniería Eléctrica,
Universidad Michoacana de San Nicolás de Hidalgo,
Santiago Tapia 403, Centro, 58000 Morelia, Michoacán, México
http://www.umich.mx/

**Abstract.** Cardiovascular diseases (CVDs) are the worldwide leading cause of deaths. Based on ultrasound, primary assessment of CVDs is measurement of carotid intima-media thickness and brachial endothelial function. In this work we propose improvements to a state of the art automatic methodology for arterial lumen detection, based on graphs and edge detection, fundamental for cited tests. We propose a bayesian approach for segmenting the graph minimum spanning tree created with points between edges. Lumen is located applying three criteria on segmented trajectories: length, darkness, and our proposal, minimum variance. In 294 sonograms having manually established measurements, from a 1,104–sonogram set, mean and standard deviation error in brachial near wall detection was $14.6\,\mu m$ and $17.0\,\mu m$, respectively. For far wall they were $15.1\,\mu m$ and $14.5\,\mu m$, respectively. Our methodology maintains superior performance to results in recent literature that the original methodology presents, but surpasses it in overall accuracy.

**Keywords:** automatic detection, ultrasonography, carotid, brachial, lumen, bayesian, variance, graphs, polynomial fitting.

## 1 Introduction

Cardiovascular diseases (CVDs) are the worldwide leading cause of deaths [26]. The most disturbing pathology associated with CVDs is atherosclerosis, a progressive degeneration that reduces the *arterial lumen* (AL) and causes arterial wall thickening. Progressive development of this disease has been correlated with increased risk of CVDs [16].

Based on ultrasound, primary markers for CVDs and atherosclerosis assessment are measurement of the carotid intima-media thickness (IMT) [1], and measurement of the brachial artery endothelial function (BAEF) [4].

The IMT and BAEF tests require the detection of carotid and brachial lumen, respectively, in order to run properly. Calderon et al. [2] proposed in 2013 a graph-based algorithm for automatic AL detection in *ultrasound images* (USIs).

F. Castro, A. Gelbukh, and M. González (Eds.): MICAI 2013, Part I, LNAI 8265, pp. 545–557, 2013.

The algorithm first determines edges of the *ultrasound image* (USI), and then creates a graph with intermediate points between consecutive detected edge points (in a column basis). Later, it calculates the graph *minimum spanning tree* (MST), and does a segmentation process of those trajectories likely to be the true AL, using only a criterion based on distance between connected nodes.

Trajectory representing the true AL is selected from those segmented ones, based on a linear combination of a length and a darkness criteria.

Calderon et al. pointed out that their algorithm has superior performance to results reported in recent literature in this area. Nevertheless, in this paper we propose solution to two deficiencies their algorithm has.

Remainder of this paper is organized as follows: Section 2 presents a brief review of recent work in the area; Section 3, poses problems whose solution we propose in this article; Section 4, details the bayesian hypothesis test used for validating the trajectories segmentation process referred to in Section 3; Section 5 describes the *minimum variance criterion* (MVC) that is used to discriminate the true AL in those cases where the length criterion presents the inconsistencies explained in Section 3; Section 6, summarizes the methodology presented in this research for automatic AL detection in USIs; Section 7, describes tests performed and results obtained when methodology presented in Section 6 is applied on an USI set; and, Section 8, summarizes conclusions reached with work carried out.

## 2   Previous Work

In the absence of atherosclerotic plaque, B–mode ultrasound shows the wall of an artery as a regular pattern that correlates with anatomical layers. In the USI, the AL may be observed as a dark region flanked on its top and bottom by bright light stripes, which will turn out as edges considering the intensity profile of the pixels. Under this assumption, works presented in literature for arterial vessel segmentation apply different methods to locate these contrasting zones, and thus, determining both the lumen and different arterial measurements.

Early work is based on edge detection [17,22] and, later, on image gradient [12,20,8]. Methods included in these categories are fast in their calculation but sensitive to noise, artery morphology, and require manual intervention to get good results.

Other approaches apply linear programming [18,23] in order to establish a cost function based on a linear combination of several weighted measurements calculated from the USI, to segment the artery and the layers that it is made of. It has also been proposed [11] to apply this method at different USI scales to reduce computational cost. Techniques in this category can be fully automated, which limits variability in final results [24,9] due to skills and operator fatigue. However, they require system training and are sensitive to image noise, which directly affects the cost function.

The most used technique for arterial segmentation is the active parametric contours [25] or *snakes*, which adapts a deformable linear model to the border between the AL and the intima layer. Most of the published works [13,16,5] adopt the snakes formulation presented in [25]. Application of this method has not been fully automated; besides, is very sensitive to noise, requires tuning of those parameters that define the snakes, and results depend on chosen starting points as well as their number.

Other proposals consists in calculating local statistics on intensity of the USI pixels, coupled with the establishment of an acceptance/rejection threshold on membership of these pixels to the AL area [5]. It has also been proposed to improve this technique [14,6] using a fuzzy k-means classifier as an initialization stage for a snakes-based method to refine the detection process.

Hough transform has also been proposed for the arterial segmentation [10,21]. In longitudinal USIs the goal is to delineate dominant lines of the boundary between lumen and arterial walls, and in transversal USIs, the goal is to delineate the same boundary, but outlined as a circumference. Although Hough transform calculation is fast, it is effective only when processing images in which the artery appears in a straight and horizontal way.

Finally, a recent work has proposed a fully automated technique for arterial detection [16] based on local maxima in pixels intensity of the USI, applying a linear discriminant to these *seed points*, with a fuzzy k-means classifier as a refinement stage.

Next section outlines deficiencies of the methodology proposed by Calderon et al. for AL detection in USIs, and whose solution we propose in this article.

## 3  Problem Statement

Work presented by Calderon et al. in [2] faces difficulties in recognizing an AL in an USI that has noticeable discontinuities or cuts at the edges. To illustrate this, Fig. 1(a) shows trajectories likely to be selected as the true AL in a test USI, applying this algorithm.

When the graph MST is segmented, based on distance-between-connected-nodes criterion, trajectory that belongs to the true AL is broken into several ones (2 and 3 in Fig. 1(a)). In consequence, trajectory 1 is mistakenly chosen as the true AL. The solution proposed for this problem is to validate segmentation process by the hypothesis testing detailed in Section 4.

Equally important, when length criterion value $l_i$ for two or more trajectories that represent options likely to be selected as the real AL are above a certain threshold $u_{cl}$, algorithm of Calderon et al. is unable to select the correct choice.

To illustrate this, we take the USI in Figure 1(b) as an example. Trajectory 0 in this figure has 0.98661, 0.95766, and 1.94427 as values for the length, darkness, and their linear combination criteria, respectively. Trajectory 4 has 1.0, 0.87787, and 1.87787 as values for the same criteria. If we select the true AL based on length criterion, trajectory 4 would be correctly selected as the AL. If we select the true AL based on darkness criterion, trajectory 0 would be incorrectly selected as the AL. Finally, selection of Calderon et al. is based on the maximum linear combination of both criteria, i.e., trajectory 0 is selected as the AL, which is incorrect for this specific USI. To solve the problem above, without affecting overall performance of methodology, the MVC, explained in Section 5, is proposed.

Calderon et al. indicate that, for the whole set of test USIs, combination of length and darkness criteria produces the best results to select the real AL.

The following section describes in detail the procedure for validating the segmentation process that is used as part of the methodology for automatic AL detection presented in this paper.

## 4   Hypothesis Testing

To reduce over-segmentation produced by the methodology of Calderon et al., we propose to validate this segmentation process using a hypothesis testing [19].

Given point sets $D_1 = \{p_i\}$, $p_i = [x_i, y_i]^T$ and $D_2 = \{p_j\}$, $p_j = [x_j, y_j]^T$; such that $D_1 \cap D_2 = \emptyset$, of size $N_1$ and $N_2$, respectively; which have associated corresponding polynomial approximations $f(x_i; a_1)$ and $f(x_j; a_2)$ given by:

$$f(x; a) = a_0 + a_1 x + a_2 x^2 + a_3 x^3 + \cdots + a_m x^m \ . \tag{1}$$

One of the following hypotheses has to be demonstrated:

$H_0$: Sets $D_1$ and $D_2$ are partitions of the same set $D$ ($D = D_1 \cup D_2$), therefore, they can be characterized by a unique polynomial approximation $f(x, a)$.
$H_1$: Sets $D_1$ and $D_2$ are not partitions of the same set, therefore, they are characterized by polynomial approximations $f(x_1, a_1)$ and $f(x_2, a_2)$, respectively.

Decision criterion will be probabilistic, so that hypothesis $H_0$ will be valid if and only if (2) holds. Otherwise, the fulfilled hypothesis will be $H_1$.

$$P(H_0 \mid D_1, D_2) > P(H_1 \mid D_1, D_2) \ . \tag{2}$$

Applying Bayes' theorem and assuming that probability of both hypotheses is the same, $P(H_0) = P(H_1)$, the final decision criterion can be expressed as (3).

$$P(D_1, D_2 \mid H_0) > P(D_1, D_2 \mid H_1) \ . \tag{3}$$

In order to use decision criterion (3), probabilities $P(D_1, D_2 \mid H_0)$ and $P(D_1, D_2 \mid H_1)$ need to be estimated. We begin by estimating $P(D \mid H_0)$, given that $D$ is a single data set; for this, we assume that any polynomial with parameters $a$ has the same probability of being selected, therefore, it follows a uniform distribution, $P(a \mid H_0) = k_1$; and that errors between approximation $f(x_i, a)$ and the actual measurements $y_i$, follow a Gaussian model given by (4).

$$P(D \mid a, H_0) = k_1 \exp\left(-\frac{E(a)}{2\sigma^2}\right) = k_1 \exp\left(-\frac{\sum_{i=1}^{N}(f(x_i; a) - y_i)^2}{2\sigma^2}\right) \ . \tag{4}$$

Then, $P(D \mid H_0)$ can be written, considering the total probability law, as:

$$P(D \mid H_0) = k_1 k_2 \int_{\Omega} \exp\left(-\frac{E(a)}{2\sigma^2}\right) d^m a \ . \tag{5}$$

where $\Omega$ is the function domain, which is integrated in $m$ dimensions.

In order to solve (5), we determine the Taylor series expansion at point $a^*$, which is the least squares solution for $E(a)$, and integrate the exponential function in $m$ dimensions [19], which give us:

$$P(D \mid H_0) = k_1 k_2 \sqrt{\frac{(4\pi\sigma^2)^m}{|\nabla^2 E(a^*)|}} \exp\left(-\frac{E(a^*)}{2\sigma^2}\right) . \tag{6}$$

For calculation of probability $P(D_1, D_2 \mid H_1)$, assume that data sets $D_1$ and $D_2$ were generated by independent models, so that it can be written as:

$$P(D_1, D_2 \mid H_1) = P(D_1 \mid H_0)P(D_2 \mid H_0) . \tag{7}$$

Probabilities $P(D_1 \mid H_0)$ and $P(D_2 \mid H_0)$ are calculated using (6), and the obtained result for (7) is given by (8):

$$P(D_1, D_2 \mid H_1) = \frac{k_1^2 k_2^2 (4\pi\sigma^2)^m}{\sqrt{|\nabla^2 E(a_1^*)||\nabla^2 E(a_2^*)|}} \exp\left(-\frac{E(a_1^*) + E(a_2^*)}{2\sigma^2}\right) . \tag{8}$$

Sets $D_1$ and $D_2$ will be join if $P(D \mid H_0) > P(D_1, D_2 \mid H_1)$.

Next section describes the MVC, referred to in Section 3, for selecting the AL in those cases where the length criterion is inconsistent.

## 5   Minimum Variance Criterion

For AL selection cases where length criterion value exceeds a threshold $u_{cl}$ for two or more trajectories, we propose to use a MVC as a third discrimination criterion for selecting the true AL.

According to a radiologist observations and criteria, it can be considered that an AL has a smooth curvature in an USI, thus, when image edges are detected, the number of outlier edge points will be fewer as compared to the number in detected edges of channels or anatomical structures that resemble it. One way to calculate this is using the sample variance of the edge points.

We will do the variance calculation over the elements of a set $S_u$, comprised of the trajectories set whose number of edge points is greater than 95% of the number of points corresponding to the anatomical structure in the USI with the greatest number of them.

For our noise model given by (4), sample variance for the $j$-th anatomical structure in the USI can be calculated as:

$$\sigma_j^2 = \frac{1}{N_j - 1} \sum_{i=1}^{N_j} \left(f(x_i; a_j^*) - y_i\right)^2 . \tag{9}$$

MVC points out that the true AL is the one trajectory, given by (10), having the minimum value of the sample variance:

$$\min_j j^* = \sigma_j^2, \ j \in \{1, 2, \dots, |S_u|\} . \tag{10}$$

Note that the MVC is used only in those cases where more than one trajectory exists, i.e., that $|S_u| > 1$. Otherwise, linear combination of length and darkness criteria is used, as proposed by Calderon et al.

For USI in Fig. 1(b), we have that trajectories 0 and 4 have similar values of length criterion, but sample variance calculated with (9) gives us $\sigma_0 = 2.2321$ and $\sigma_4 = 0.3649$. It follows from the aforementioned that the selected true AL is given by trajectory 4.

Figure 1(c) shows the USI in Fig. 1(b), with the superimposing of the edges of the detected AL, based on the MVC.

The following section describes the methodology of Calderon et al. with changes we propose, for the AL segmentation in USIs.


## 6   Methodology

Detection procedure begins with an automatic histogram-based clipping of the USI, which removes information not necessary for the AL segmentation process. Resulting image is referred to as the original image $I$.

An USI $I$ is defined as a set of pixels $I(p_i)$, which represents a gray tone in a point having coordinates $p_i = [x_i, y_i]^T$, over image grid $R$ of size $N_{\text{Cols}} \times N_{\text{Rows}}$.

Next, and under the assumption that the AL in an USI is presented as a dark region flanked on its top and bottom by much clearer areas, edges of image $I$ are detected using Canny's algorithm [3]. These detected edges are represented as a set $B$, containing $N_B$ coordinate points $b_i = [x_i, y_i]^T$ such that:

$$B = \{b_i \in R \mid g(b_i) = 1, \forall b_i \in R\} \tag{11}$$

where $g$ is a binary image of same size as $I$, defined in (12).

$$g(b_i) \equiv g(x_i, y_i) = \begin{cases} 1 & \text{if } b_i \text{ is an edge,} \\ 0 & \text{otherwise.} \end{cases} \tag{12}$$

Later, a column $c$ of image $g$, a vector of 0s and 1s like (13), is built.

$$g(c, \ldots) = [0, 0, 1, 0, 1, 0, 0, 0, 1, 0, 0, 0, 1, 0, 0, 1, 0, 0 \ldots]^T . \tag{13}$$

Representation of these edges is done by storing their coordinates in an ordered array. For edge column in (13), its representation is given by (14):

$$\hat{B}_c = \{[c, 3]^T, [c, 5]^T, [c, 9]^T, [c, 13]^T, [c, 16]^T, \ldots\} = \{\hat{b}_k, \hat{b}_{k+1}, \hat{b}_{k+2}, \ldots\} \tag{14}$$

and the ordered representation of all edges of image $I$, equivalent to (11), is (15):

$$\hat{B} = \{\hat{B}_1, \hat{B}_2, \ldots, \hat{B}_c \ldots, \hat{B}_{N_{\text{Cols}}}\} = \{\hat{b}_1, \hat{b}_2, \hat{b}_3, \ldots, \hat{b}_k, \hat{b}_{k+1}, \hat{b}_{k+2} \ldots\} . \tag{15}$$

With this, there will be a couple of points $<\hat{b}_i, \hat{b}_{i+1}>$ in each column of the image with all edges, candidates to be the AL limits.

Methodology continues discarding pairs of consecutive edge points whose separation distances are below a preset threshold $A_{\text{Min}}$. Thus, set of points $B_{\text{L}}$ is defined, based on the ordered set of points $\hat{B} \equiv B$, as follows:

$$B_{\text{L}} = \{\hat{b}_1, \hat{b}_2, \ldots, \hat{b}_i, \hat{b}_{i+1} \ldots \mid (\hat{y}_{i+1} - \hat{y}_i) \geq A_{\text{Min}}, \, \hat{x}_i = \hat{x}_{i+1}\} \, . \qquad (16)$$

$B_{\text{L}}$ set is a subset of edge set $B$, therefore, lumen search universe is reduced.

It is also defined $V$, the set of points half of the way between the likely lumen limits given by the set $B_{\text{L}}$, as:

$$V = \{v_i \mid v_i = \frac{\hat{b}_i + \hat{b}_{i+1}}{2}, \, \hat{x}_i = \hat{x}_{i+1}, \forall \hat{b}_i \in B_{\text{L}}\} \, . \qquad (17)$$

In this way, for a point $v_i$ exists an associated pair $< \hat{b}_i, \hat{b}_{i+1} >$ such that $\hat{b}_i < v_i < \hat{b}_{i+1}$, and the three of them are in the same column of image $g$.

Figure 1(d) shows points of sets $B_{\text{L}}$ and $V$, superimposed on image $I$. Points of set $V$ are the options likely to be selected as the center of the real lumen.

Subsequently, an undirected graph $G = \{V, A\}$ is built from point set $V$, defined in (17). $V$ represents the graph nodes set, and $A$ the set of graph edges. Initially all nodes are connected, and the weight of each graph edge, $A_{ij}$, is the Euclidean distance $d(v_i, v_j)$ between points of set $V$ the edge connects.

Afterwards, the undirected graph is segmented and classified using weights $d(v_i, v_j)$, supporting these cutting process by the bayesian hypothesis test from Section 4. The minimum spanning tree (MST) $G^+$ for graph $G$, is calculated using Kruskal's algorithm. Figure 1(g) shows an example of created $G^+$.

In order to take the true AL trajectory out from the graph, a set $S$ of $N_{\text{G}}$ subgraphs is defined in (18). This set is the result of segmenting $G^+$, when cutting graph edges whose distances $d(v_i, v_j) > p_{\text{Max}}$ (a cutoff threshold), and that meet hypothesis $H_1$ (from Section 4) for nodes corresponding to subgraphs $G_i^+$ and $G_j^+$ that are connected by graph edge $A_{ij}$. Otherwise, when fulfilled hypothesis is $H_0$, graph edge $A_{ij}$ is kept intact, even when distance $d(v_i, v_j)$ exceeds $p_{\text{Max}}$. Cuts are carried out using a depth-first traversal on $G^+$.

$$S = \{G_1^+, G_2^+, \ldots, G_{N_{\text{G}}}^+\} \, . \qquad (18)$$

Figure 1(g) shows the graph MST, created with points indicating options likely to be selected as the center of the true AL for a test USI. Double-headed arrow marked as $H_1$ is an example of graph edge that exceeds distance threshold $p_{\text{Max}}$, and that meets hypothesis $H_1$; so to be cut. Single-headed arrow $H_0$ is an example of a graph edge that exceeds distance threshold $p_{\text{Max}}$, but that meets hypothesis $H_0$; so that should remain intact.

Process continues removing short trajectories that exist due to noise or muscle tissue layers in the USI. Hence, subgraphs $G_i^+$ which have a total node number below a threshold $N_{\text{Min}}$ are eliminated from set $S$, defining subgraph set $S^+$ as:

$$S^+ = S - \{G_i^+ \in S \mid N_{S_i} < N_{\text{Min}}\}, \quad i \in \{1, 2, \ldots, N_{\text{G}}\} \qquad (19)$$

being $N_{S_i}$ the node number of subgraph $G_i^+$.

Options likely to be the true AL has been decreased considerably up to this point, but there are still more than one option, so that the real AL is selected using the length, minimum variance, and darkness criteria.

Length criterion calculates total node number on each subgraph $G_i^+ \in S_i^+$, normalized between $[0, 1]$, according to the following equation:

$$l_i = \frac{N_{S_i}}{\max(N_{S_1}, N_{S_2}, \ldots, N_{S_{|S^+|}})}, \quad i \in \{1, 2, \ldots, |S^+|\}. \tag{20}$$

Now, if at the time of calculating length criterion $l_i$ for each subgraph $G_i^+$, it happens that more than one $l_i > u_{cl}$, the MVC (Section 5) will be used to determine the correct AL of the USI. Otherwise, the AL selection will be based on a linear combination of both length and darkness criteria.

For the darkness criterion the average value $\mu_j$ of gray tones of the corresponding area for each subgraph $G_j^+ \in S^+$ is calculated. To this end, each subgraph is traversed in each of its points $v_i$, sweeping in a column basis at intervals $[\hat{b}_i, \hat{b}_{i+1}]$ (according to (17)) of the original image $I$, as formulated next:

$$\mu_j = \frac{1}{N_{S_j^+}} \sum_{\forall v_i \in G_j^+} \left[ \frac{1}{\hat{y}_{i+1} - \hat{y}_i + 1} \sum_{\forall p \in [\hat{b}_i, \hat{b}_{i+1}]} I(p) \right], \quad \forall j \in \{1, 2, \ldots, |S^+|\} \tag{21}$$

being $N_{S_j^+}$ the node number in subgraph $S_j^+$.

Once the average is calculated, the darkness criterion is:

$$o_i = 1 - \frac{\mu_i}{\max(\mu_1, \mu_2, \ldots, \mu_{|S^+|})}, \quad \forall i \in \{1, 2, \ldots, |S^+|\}. \tag{22}$$

Darkness criterion, just as the length one, is normalized to range $[0, 1]$ so they can be combined. That is, the subgraph corresponding to the center of the true AL is the one with the maximum value of the sum of both criteria:

$$\max_i i^* = (l_i + o_i), \quad \forall i \in \{1, 2, \ldots, |S^+|\}. \tag{23}$$

Figures 1(e) and 1(h) show two examples of arterial USIs with superimposed edges corresponding to detected lumen in each case. In Fig. 1(e), corresponding to Fig. 1(a), an example of detection based on length and darkness criteria is shown. In Fig. 1(h), corresponding to Fig. 1(b), an example of detection based on MVC is shown.

Last step of proposed technique for AL detection fits a polynomial $f(x, a)$ of degree $m$, by means of the least squares method, to each of the point sets belonging to the edges of the detected AL. That is, to the sets of edge points $<\hat{b}_{i^*}, \hat{b}_{i^*+1}>$, related to the points $v_{i^*} \in G_{i^*}^+$.

Polynomial fitting is performed to the set of edge points $\hat{b}_{i^*}$ first, belonging to the edge $f_N(\hat{x})$ between the lumen and the near wall of the artery; and, later, to the set of edge points $\hat{b}_{i+1}^*$, belonging to the edge $f_F(\hat{x})$ between the lumen and the far wall of the artery.

In order to strengthen the polynomial fitting against noise in the USI, estimation of the polynomial model parameters is directed by means of the *RANdom SAmple Consensus* (RANSAC) algorithm.

Figure 1(f) shows the image with the fitted polynomial approximations by the least squares method and the RANSAC algorithm, on points of the AL edges shown in Fig. 1(e). Robust polynomial approximations, corresponding to Fig. 1(h), are shown in Fig. 1(c).

Once described the proposed AL detection methodology, the section below details tests and results obtained from its application.

# 7   Tests and Results

Tests were carried out on same database of USIs provided to Calderon et al. by the laboratory *Centro Unión* of Morelia, Michoacán, México. This database consists of 1,104 longitudinal B–mode ultrasound two-dimensional images of carotid and brachial arteries. All images were transferred to the computer through a DICOM communication port and logarithmically compressed to an 8-bit grayscale (256 gray shades). Axial resolution of the USIs is $76.9\,\mu m$ per pixel.

Parameters of the methodology were adjusted as follows: $A_{Min} = 20$ pixels, $p_{Max} = 10$ pixels, $N_{Min} = 100$ nodes, fitting polymonials degree $m = 3$, $\sigma = 32.0$ for bayesian hypothesis testing, and threshold $u_{cl} = 0.95$.

Initial test was to apply our methodology on each of the 1,104 USIs in the database then verify, qualitatively, the percentage of them in which correct pattern of a dark area flanked up and down by clearer areas was selected. In this test, 51 failures in the 1,104 USIs were found. Meanwhile, the algorithm of Calderon et al. failed in 85 of the same 1,104-USI set. This is, with proposed solutions to problems detailed in Section 3, our method accurately detected the AL in 34 pictures more than the original algorithm.

Later tests were carried out on the 294 USIs from general set which have measurements manually established by a radiologist. Process consisted in applying our technique to each image to get polynomial aproximations $f_N(\hat{x})$ and $f_F(\hat{x})$, for near and far arterial walls, respectively. Finally, error between manually established points $[x_N, y_N]^T$, $[x_F, y_F]^T$; and the estimated ones $f_N(x_N)$, $f_F(x_F)$; were calculated. Results for these tests are presented in Table 1.

**Table 1.** Error in measurements of the lumen-intima interface

|  | Near Wall | Far Wall |
|---|---|---|
| Average | $14.6\,\mu m$ (1.8 pixels) | $15.1\,\mu m$ (1.9 pixels) |
| Standard Deviation | $17.0\,\mu m$ (2.2 pixels) | $14.5\,\mu m$ (1.9 pixels) |

Calderon et al. pointed out that based on results reported in recent literature on the AL detection area, the automatic technique that achieves best performance [15] has an average error on the far wall of $35.0\,\mu m \pm 32.0\,\mu m$. Besides,

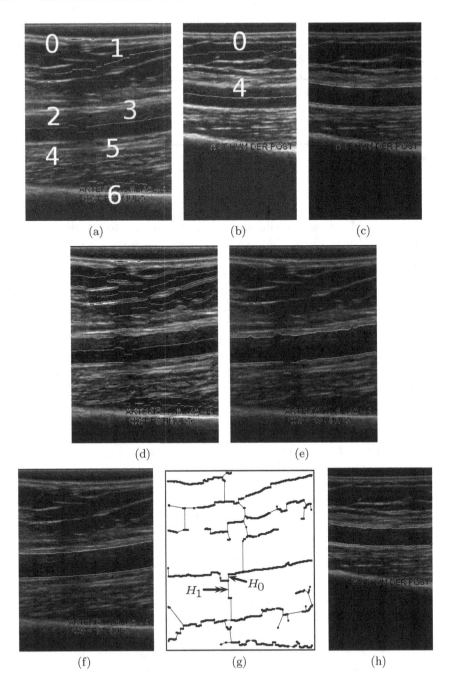

**Fig. 1.** (a) Options likely to be selected as the AL. (b) Inconsistency example. (c) Edges detected based on MVC (with polynomial fitting). (d) Points belonging to sets $B_L$ and $V$. (e) Edges detected based on length and darkness criteria. (f) Polynomial fitting. (g) MST. (h) Edges detected based on MVC.

the semiautomatic technique best performed [7] has an average error on the same wall of $21.0\,\mu m \pm 13.0\,\mu m$. In relation to the arterial near wall, they pointed out that only in work presented in [14] the obtained average error is given, which is of $75.0\,\mu m \pm 56.3\,\mu m$.

Based on results shown in Table 1, methodology presented in this paper maintains superiority of proposed technique by Calderon et al. over reported performance in recent studies for automatic [15] and semi-automatic [7] detection of the arterial far wall, as well as detection of the arterial near wall [14]. Moreover, our methodology produces an average improvement of $0.3\,\mu m$ in locating of the arterial far wall, over results of Calderon et al. On the other hand, in the near wall, our approach produces an average reduction of $0.7\,\mu m$. However, this result is generated at the expense of correctly detecting the AL in 34 USIs beyond those from the original methodology. Besides, additional number of images consists of USIs with features that generate greater difficulty in the discrimination process of the AL; which is markedly accounted for in results reported for our algorithm, and detection failures for the algorithm of Calderon et al.

It is worth mentioning that the algorithmic complexity of the hypothesis testing in (6) and (8) comes from the least squares solutions, which are of $\mathcal{O}(m^2(N_1+N_2))$. Calculation of Hessian determinants in (6) and (8) are of $\mathcal{O}(m^3)$ but, given that in our tests $m = 3$, we consider only the former. Also, calculating the MVC in (9) is of $\mathcal{O}(m^2 N_j)$, coming from the least squares fitting, as well. Meanwhile, the stages of the methodology with bigger complexity order, the edge detection and the MST calculation, have corresponding $\mathcal{O}(k_s^2 N_{Cols} N_{Rows})$ (being $k_s^2$ the size of the convolutional kernel) and $\mathcal{O}(N^2 \log(N))$, respectively.

Considering the above and that the edge detector is applied to the whole USI, that the MST is calculated from all the USI borders, and that the hypothesis testing and the MVC are calculated for only a few trajectories, it follows that the complexity we added to the methodology of Calderon et al. is not significant because $\mathcal{O}(k_s^2 N_{Cols} N_{Rows}) > \mathcal{O}(N^2 \log(N)) >> \mathcal{O}(m^2(N_1 + N_2)) + \mathcal{O}(m^2 N_j)$ due to $N_{Cols} N_{Rows} >> N_1, N_2, N_j$.

## 8    Conclusions

We presented a technique for automatic arterial lumen detection in carotid and brachial ultrasound images, which proposes a bayesian and a minimum variance criteria to address some flaws in methodology by Calderon et al. in [2].

Methodology in this work, as well as the original one, is robust to arterial morphology and orientation in an ultrasound image but, unlike the original, is robust with relation to discontinuities or cuts in the arterial edges. However, it is vulnerable to arterial pathologies or abnormal echogenic characteristics.

It should be noted that both our proposal and the original one, find the limit of their application in the edge detection algorithm. If this algorithm is unable to detect the arterial edges, for instance due to noise, the arterial lumen detection methodology will also be unable to select the correct arterial lumen.

Finally, in a laptop with an Intel® Core™ i5 at 2.30GHz processor, 4GB of memory, and software developed (but not yet speed-optimized) with the Open

Java Development Kit 7, on a Debian GNU/Linux system with a 64-bit kernel version 3.2.0, our technique processes each ultrasound image in a variable time up to 30 seconds. Nevertheless, we believe that real-time execution is possible, by means of process optimization and parallel processing use.

# References

1. Amato, M., Montorsi, P., Ravani, A., Oldani, E., Galli, S., Ravagnani, P.M., Tremoli, E., Baldassarre, D.: Carotid intima-media thickness by B-mode ultrasound as surrogate of coronary atherosclerosis: Correlation with quantitative coronary angiography and coronary intravascular ultrasound findings. European Heart Journal 28(17), 2094–2101 (2007)
2. Calderon, F., Tinoco-Martínez, S.R., Carranza-Madrigal, J.: Un algoritmo basado en grafos para la detección automática de la luz arterial en imágenes ultrasonográficas. Revista Iberoamericana de Automática e Informática Industrial (to appear, 2013)
3. Canny, J.: A computational approach to edge detection. IEEE Transactions on Pattern Analysis and Machine Intelligence PAMI-8(6), 679–698 (1986)
4. Celermajer, D.S., Sorensen, K.E., Bull, C., Robinson, J., Deanfield, J.E.: Endothelium-dependent dilation in the systemic arteries of asymptomatic subjects relates to coronary risk factors and their interaction. Journal of the American College of Cardiology 24(6), 1468–1474 (1994)
5. Delsanto, S., Molinari, F., Giustetto, P., Liboni, W., Badalamenti, S., Suri, J.S.: Characterization of a completely user-independent algorithm for carotid artery segmentation in 2-D ultrasound images. IEEE Transactions on Instrumentation and Measurement 56(4), 1265–1274 (2007)
6. Delsanto, S., Molinari, F., Liboni, W., Giustetto, P., Badalamenti, S., Suri, J.S.: User-independent plaque characterization and accurate IMT measurement of carotid artery wall using ultrasound. In: Proceedings of the 2006 IEEE Engineering in Medicine and Biology Society 28th Annual International Conference, vol. 1, pp. 2404–2407 (2006)
7. Destrempes, F., Meunier, J., Giroux, M.F., Soulez, G., Cloutier, G.: Segmentation in ultrasonic B-mode images of healthy carotid arteries using mixtures of Nakagami distributions and stochastic optimization. IEEE Transactions on Medical Imaging 28(2), 215–229 (2009)
8. Faita, F., Gemignani, V., Bianchini, E., Giannarelli, C., Ghiadoni, L., Demi, M.: Real-time measurement system for evaluation of the carotid intima-media thickness with a robust edge operator. Journal of Ultrasound in Medicine 27(9), 1353–1361 (2008)
9. Furberg, C.D., Byington, R.P., Craven, T.E.: Lessons learned from clinical trials with ultrasound end-points. Journal of Internal Medicine 236(5), 575–580 (1994)
10. Golemati, S., Stoitsis, J., Sifakis, E.G., Balkizas, T., Nikita, K.S.: Using the Hough transform to segment ultrasound images of longitudinal and transverse sections of the carotid artery. Ultrasound in Medicine and Biology 33(12), 1918–1932 (2007)
11. Liang, Q., Wendelhag, I., Wikstrand, J., Gustavsson, T.: A multiscale dynamic programming procedure for boundary detection in ultrasonic artery images. IEEE Transactions on Medical Imaging 19(2), 127–142 (2000)
12. Liguori, C., Paolillo, A., Pietrosanto, A.: An automatic measurement system for the evaluation of carotid intima-media thickness. IEEE Transactions on Instumentation and Measurement 50(6), 1684–1691 (2001)

13. Loizou, C.P., Pattichis, C.S., Pantziaris, M., Tyllis, T., Nicolaides, A.: Snakes based segmentation of the common carotid artery intima media. Medical and Biological Engineering and Computing 45(1), 35–49 (2007)
14. Molinari, F., Delsanto, S., Giustetto, P., Liboni, W., Badalamenti, S., Suri, J.S.: User-independent plaque segmentation and accurate intima-media thickness measurement of carotid artery wall using ultrasound. In: Advances in Diagnostic and Therapeutic Ultrasound Imaging, pp. 111–140. Artech House, Norwood (2008)
15. Molinari, F., Liboni, W., Giustetto, P., Badalamenti, S., Suri, J.S.: Automatic Computer-based Tracings (ACT) in longitudinal 2-D ultrasound images using different scanners. Journal of Mechanics in Medicine and Biology 9(4), 481–505 (2009)
16. Molinari, F., Zeng, G., Suri, J.S.: An Integrated Approach to Computer-Based Automated Tracing and IMT Measurement for Carotid Artery Longitudinal Ultrasound Images. In: Atherosclerosis Disease Management, pp. 221–251. Springer (2010)
17. Pignoli, P., Longo, T.: Evaluation of atherosclerosis with b-mode ultrasound imaging. The Journal of Nuclear Medicine and Allied Sciences 32(3), 166–173 (1988)
18. Schmidt, C., Wendelhag, I.: How can the variability in ultrasound measurement of intima-media thickness be reduced? studies of interobserver variability in carotid and femoral arteries. Clinical Physiology 19(1), 45–55 (1999)
19. Sivia, D.S., Skilling, J.: Data Analysis: A Bayesian Tutorial. Oxford University Press, USA (2006)
20. Stein, J.H., Korcarz, C.E., Mays, M.E., Douglas, P.S., Palta, M., Zhang, H., LeCaire, T., Paine, D., Gustafson, D., Fan, L.: A semiautomated ultrasound border detection program that facilitates clinical measurement of ultrasound carotid intima-media thickness. Journal of the American Society of Echocardiography 18(3), 244–251 (2005)
21. Stoitsis, J., Golemati, S., Kendros, S., Nikita, K.S.: Automated detection of the carotid artery wall in B-mode ultrasound images using active contours initialized by the Hough transform. In: Proceedings of the 2008 IEEE Engineering in Medicine and Biology Society 30th Annual International Conference 2008, pp. 3146–3149 (2008)
22. Touboul, P.J., Prati, P., Yves Scarabin, P., Adrai, V., Thibout, E., Ducimetiere, P.: Use of monitoring software to improve the measurement of carotid wall thickness by b-mode imaging. Journal of Hypertension 10(suppl. 5), S37–S42 (1992)
23. Wendelhag, I., Liang, Q., Gustavsson, T., Wikstrand, J.: A new automated computerized analyzing system simplifies readings and reduces the variability in ultrasound measurement of intima-media thickness. Stroke 28(11), 2195–2200 (1997)
24. Wendelhag, I., Wiklund, O., Wikstrand, J.: On quantifying plaque size and intima-media thickness in carotid and femoral arteries. comments on results from a prospective ultrasound study in patients with familial hypercholesterolemia. Arteriosclererosis, Thrombosis, and Vascular Biology 16(7), 843–850 (1996)
25. Williams, D.J., Shah, M.: A fast algorithm for active contours and curvature estimation. Computer Vision Graphics and Image Processing: Image Understanding 55(1), 14–26 (1992)
26. World Health Organization: Cardiovascular diseases. (March 2013), http://www.who.int/mediacentre/factsheets/fs317/en/index.html

# Detection of Masses in Mammogram Images Using Morphological Operators and Markov Random Fields

Verónica Rodríguez-López, Rosebet Miranda-Luna,
and José Anibal Arias-Aguilar

Universidad Tecnológica de la Mixteca, Km 2.5 Carretera a Acatlima
CP 69000 Huajuapan de León, Oaxaca, México
{veromix,rmiranda,anibal}@mixteco.utm.mx

**Abstract.** In this work we present a two stages method for detection of masses in mammogram images. In a first step, a mass contrast enhancement algorithm based on morphological operators is proposed. Afterwards, a Gaussian Markov Random Field (MRF) model is used for mass segmentation. In the MRF model, the image pixels are described by three statistical texture features of first order. Our approach was tested on 58 mammographic images of masses from MIAS database achieving a performance of 84.4%.

**Keywords:** Breast masses, Image Analysis, Mass detection, Mammogram, MRF segmentation.

## 1 Introduction

Breast cancer is considered a public health problem in the world. Recent evidence shows that breast cancer is a leading cause of death and disability among women in developing countries. For instance, in Mexico, it is the primary cause of death from malignant tumors among women [5]. Mammograms is currently the most effective tool for early detection of breast cancer. It is an X-ray picture of the breast which usually involve two views: craniocaudal (CC) and medio-lateral oblique (MLO).

Masses are the most important sign of breast cancer that radiologists seek in mammograms. The American College of Radiology (ACR) defines a mass as three-dimensional structure demonstrating convex outward borders, usually evident on two orthogonal views [1]. Radiologists describe masses by their location, size, shape, margin, and density characteristics. However, due to density of breast tissue and wide range of the mass characteristics, detection and description of this type of lesion are complex, tedious and time-consuming. Moreover, the success of these tasks depends on training, experience and judgment of radiologists.

Computer Aided Diagnosis systems (CADx) help experts in detection and diagnosis of mammographic lesions. The detection sensitivity without CADx is around 80% and with it is up to 90% [2]. The CADx systems involve the pre-processing, segmentation, and classification stages. In the pre-processing stage,

F. Castro, A. Gelbukh, and M. González (Eds.): MICAI 2013, Part I, LNAI 8265, pp. 558–569, 2013.

noise reduction, extraction of breast region and enhancement of images are performed. Suspicious regions are detected and outlined in the segmentation stage, and in the classification stage, they are classed as normal breast tissue, benign mass or malignant mass.

Due to the huge workload that specialists in mammograms analysis have, is important to provide them computational tools that aid in the early detection of masses. There are a number of Computer Aided Detection systems (CAD) available to specialists; however, they are not CADx [12]. The CADx systems help experts in detecting and diagnosis mammographic lesions. With this research we start the development of a CADx system. We intend to develop it for detection and diagnosis of masses (in a first version, identifying other abnormalities later) and make it available to public health institutions. In this work we investigate the identification of potential masses in breast area. The detection is performed with a special filter based on morphological operators and Markov Random Fields segmentation.

The paper is organized as follows. In Section 2, we describe some approaches for automated detection of masses in mammograms related with this work. The description of our approach for detection masses is presented in Section 3. The experimental results are presented in Section 4. Finally, conclusions and future work are given in Section 5.

## 2   Related Work

Several methods have been proposed for mammography mass detection. Excellent state of art reviews for this task are given in [9] and [2]. In [9], a quantitative evaluation of the seven most representative masses detection approaches is presented. All methods were evaluated using the MIAS database [13] and a private full-field digital mammograms database. In the case of MIAS database, they showed that a based region technique which uses Density-Weighted Contrast Enhancement and Gaussian filters (with a sensivity of 79%) was one of the best. A clustering method based on Iris filter got the best performance in both databases, with a sensitivity of 75.3% in the private database and sensitivity of 80.6% in the MIAS database.

Clustering methods are used for mass detection. Some of them are proposed by Rojas & Nandi [11], and Suliga et al. [14]. Rojas & Nandi [11] proposed a three stages method to perform mass detection. The first one is a multilevel adaptative process based on local statistical measure of the pixel intensities and morphological operators to enhance breast structures. In the next stage, the images are segmentated by applying thresholding and Gaussian filtering. Finally, the selection of suspicious regions is performed by means of a ranking system that uses 18 shape and intensity features. The method was tested on 57 mammographic images of masses from the MIAS database, and achieved a sensitivity of 80% at 2.3 false-positives per image. Suliga et al. [14] used a Markov Random Field (MRF) Model to group pixels with similar gray level intensity. Their algorithm was evaluated with a private database of 44 images and achieved a sensitivity of 82%. Other clustering technique that uses a MRF model is proposed in [6] with a 94% of sensitivity at 1.5 false positives per image.

## 3    Methods

Our approach for detecting masses consists of two main stages: mass contrast enhancement and mass segmentation.

### 3.1    Mass Contrast Enhancement

Masses are small regions most of the time hidden in dense breast tissue. With the aim to enhance the contrast of the possible mass regions, a special filter based on morphological operators is applied. The process is as follows.

1. The maximum diameter that a potential mass could have in the image is determined. To do that, the size of the breast area ($breast\_diam$) and the maximum size for the masses ($max\_size$) reported in the MIAS database are considered. The size of masses can not be larger than these two values. With these conditions, the maximum diameter is,

$$dmax\_mass = minimum(max\_size, breast\_diam) \qquad (1)$$

where $breast\_diam$ is the maximum width of the breast border.

2. The Top-Hat transform with a round structure of two-pixels diameter is applied to the image. With this operation, an image ($TH_1$) containing elements that are smaller than two pixels is obtained.

3. The original image is filtered again with the Top-Hat transform. In this case a round structure of $dmax\_mass$ diameter is used. The resulting image is denominated $TH_2$.

4. In order to extract all possible masses with size of $2 - dmax\_mass$ diameter, the image $TH_1$ is subtracted from the image $TH_2$. Then, to reduce the noise generated by subtraction, the morphological opening operation is applied. The final image is called $TH\_dif$.

5. Due to big size of the structural element in the second Top-Hat transformation, in the image $TH_2$ some bright elements appear on breast border that reduces contrast of the image. To resolve this problem, the open image used in the second Top-Hat transformation is thresholded and normalized. Finally, this normalized image $imOpenU$ is multiplied with the image $TH\_dif$. This last operation generates the output image of the mass contrast enhancement process.

An example of this process is shown in Fig. 1.

### 3.2    Mass Segmentation

The mass segmentation process is based on Markov Random Fields and texture features. The steps of the process are as follows:

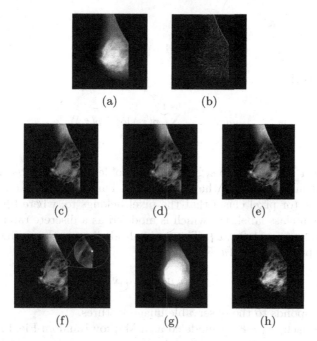

**Fig. 1.** Example of mass contrast enhancement process. (1a) Input image. (1b) First Top-Hat transformation of input image. (1c) Second Top-Hat transformation of input image. (1d) The result of subtracting (1b) from (1c). (1e) Noise removal of (1d). (1f) The element in image (1e) that reduces contrast. (1g) Normalization for the open image of second Top-Hat transformation. (1h) The result of multiplication between (1g) and (1f).

- The gray level values of the image are transformed to the range $[0, 1]$.
- For each pixel of the image, three textures features in a $3 \times 3$ window are obtained. This step computes the image features, **F**, which is the input to the segmentation step.
- Finally, regions with possible masses are obtained by Markov Random Field segmentation.

**Texture Features.** Due to the fact that masses appear in mammograms as bright regions surrounded by a dark inhomogeneous background [14], the following first-order statistics (considered as texture features) [3] are calculated:

- Mean

$$\mu = \sum_{i=0}^{L-1} z_i p(z_i) \tag{2}$$

where $p(z_i)$ is the fraction of pixels with gray level $z_i$, and $L$ is the number of possible gray levels.

– $R$

$$R = 1 - \frac{1}{1 + \sigma^2} \tag{3}$$

where $\sigma^2$ is the variance.

– Entropy:

$$e(z) = -\sum_{i=0}^{L-1} p(z_i) \log_2(p(z_i)) \tag{4}$$

**Segmentation Model.** The segmentation problem is formulated basically as finding an optimal labeling of the input image. That is, for each pixel $s$, to find the region-type (or pixel class) that the pixel belongs to, where the pixel class is specified by a class label, $w_s$, which is modeled as a discrete random variable taking values in $\Lambda = \{1, 2, ., L\}$. The optimal labeling, is the $\hat{w}$ that maximice the posterior probability, $P(w|\mathbf{F})$ [4],

$$\hat{w} = \arg\max_{w \in \Omega} P(w|\mathbf{F}) \tag{5}$$

where $\mathbf{F}$ corresponds to the observable image features.

In our approach, $P(w|\mathbf{F})$ is modeled as a Markov Random Field in the form,

$$P(w|\mathbf{F}) = \frac{1}{Z} \exp(-U(w, \mathbf{F})) \tag{6}$$

$$U(w, \mathbf{F}) = \sum_{s \in S} V_S(w_s, \vec{\mathbf{f_s}}) + \sum_{C \in \zeta} V_C(w_s, w_r) \tag{7}$$

where $Z$ is the normalizing constant, $U(w, y)$ is the posterior energy function, $V_S(w_s, \vec{\mathbf{f_s}})$ and $V_C(w_s, w_r)$ denote clique potentials of first and second order, respectively. $\zeta$ is the set of pair of neighboring pixels for the first order neighborhood system.

Information about the observations (image features) is represented in the first order potentials. Assuming that the image features are corrupted by Gaussian Noise, $n \sim N(0, \Sigma)$, these potentials have the form [4]:

$$V_S(w_s, \vec{\mathbf{f_s}}) = \ln(\sqrt{(2\pi)^3 |\Sigma_{w_s}|}) + \frac{1}{2}(\vec{\mathbf{f_s}} - \vec{\mu}_{w_s})\Sigma_{w_s}^{-1}(\vec{\mathbf{f_s}} - \vec{\mu}_{w_s})^T \tag{8}$$

where $\vec{\mu}_\lambda$ and $\Sigma_\lambda$ correspond to mean vector and covariance matrix of each label class $\lambda \in \Lambda$.

The second order clique potentials express relationship between neighboring pixel labels and controls the homogeneity in the regions. The Ising model [8] was used to define these potentials,

$$V_C(w_s, w_r) = \begin{cases} +\beta \text{ if } w_s \neq w_r \\ -\beta \text{ otherwise} \end{cases} \tag{9}$$

$\beta$ is the parameter which controls the homogeneity of the regions.

# 4   Experimental Results

In order to evaluate our mass detection method, two experiments were performed. In the first one, we analyzed the efficiency of our method for finding regions with masses. While, in the second experiment, we check their efficiency for detecting coherent mass regions. Results are presented with two measures: sensitivity and false positives per image. Sensitivity is the counting of the number of correctly regions identified as masses relative to all masses. Counting of the number of regions incorrectly identified as masses relative to all images is the false positives per image measure.

## 4.1   Data

Our method was tested on a subset of 58 images extracted from the Mammographic Image Analysis Society (MIAS) database [13]. There are few public mammogram databases, MIAS database is the most widely used, hence the interest for use it and compare our results. This database contains left and right breast images in MLO view that represent the mammograms of 161 patients with ages between 50 and 65. All images were digitized at a resolution of 1024×1024 pixels and at 8-bit grey scale level.

The test set of images contained masses annotated as circumscribed, miscellaneous (ill-defined masses) and spiculated. The circumscribed masses are characterized by well defined and sharply margins with an abrupt transition between lesion and surrounding tissue. Ill-defined masses have poorly defined and scattered margins, while in spiculated masses, margins are marked by radiating lines [7]. The summary of this dataset is shown in Table 1.

**Table 1.** Summary of MIAS images used

|  | Fatty | Fatty-Glandular | Dense-Glandular | Total |
|---|---|---|---|---|
| circumscribed | 13 | 8 | 3 | 24 |
| miscellaneous | 8 | 5 | 2 | 15 |
| spiculated | 5 | 7 | 7 | 19 |
| Total |  |  |  | 58 |

The ground-truth for the masses is their location and radius, provided in the MIAS annotations.

For decreasing the computational cost, all images were reduced by a factor of two. Moreover, the $3 \times 3$ median filter was applied to reduce speckle noise, and labels, tape artifacts, and pectoral muscle were manually extracted from the images with the help of the ImageJ program [10].

## 4.2   Parameters

The following parameters were used for the experiments:

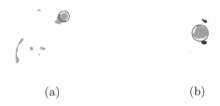

(a)                         (b)

**Fig. 2.** Some examples of results for detection of regions with masses. The detected regions with masses appear in grey and the black circle is the corresponding ground truth.

- **Number $L$ of label classes:** Three texture classes were considered in the segmentation model: mass, breast tissue, and background.
- **Initial labeling:** An initial segmentation of the image is obtained by using two thresholds $\{T1, T2\}$. These thresholds were heuristically chosen, considering that the background of the image is the darkest area, and the masses, the brightest ones. $T1 = 0.4$ and $T2 = 0.85$ were chosen values that had a good perfomance in the process.
- **Mean vector and covariance matrix of each class:** For the estimation of covariance matrices, independence between texture features were assumed. The parameters for mass and breast tissue classes were determined from to corresponding regions of the initial segmentation. For background class, taken into account that it represents a black uniform region, a zero mean vector and a diagonal covariance matrix with $\sigma^2 = 0.0001$ were considered.
- $\beta$ **parameter:** A value of $\beta = 1.9$ was experimentally determined.
- **Number of iterations:** Simulated annealing with Gibbs Sampler [8] was used to find the optimus labeling for segmentation. 50 iterations of this algorithm were enough to obtain satisfactory results.

### 4.3   Experimental Results for Detecting Regions with Masses

The performance of our method for detecting regions with masses was evaluated by verifing whether the region in the mammogram associated with the mass had any intersection with one of the suspect regions detected by the algorithm [9,14]. In the Fig. 2 are presented some examples of satisfactory results for this experiment.

In general, in this aspect, our method had a satisfactory sensitivity of 93% at 5.2 false positives per image. Due that a disk was used as structural element in the mass contrast enhancement stage, the linear pattern that characterizes a spiculated mass is blurred, so that some of these masses were missed by our method.

### 4.4   Experimental Results for Detection of Coherent Mass Regions

Another aspect evaluated of our method was their performance for detecting coherent mass regions [14]. In this case, a result was considered satisfactory if

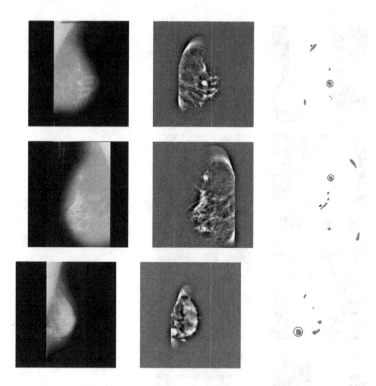

**Fig. 3.** Examples of results for detection of circumscribed masses. From left to right: original, mass contrast enhancement and segmentation images. From top to bottom: fatty, fatty-glandular and dense-glandular breast tissue.

the region detected by the algorithm falls completly inside of mass region. That is, if pixels of the detected regions correspond only to masses.

The general perfomance in this aspect was of 84.4% in sensitivity with 5.3 false positives per image. Some results for this experiment are presented in figures 3 and 4. As shown in these figures, the mass contrast enhancement process got an acceptable performance, hence almost all types of masses were properly detect in the segmentation stage. It can be seen from the results in Table 2 that masses with ambiguous margins (miscelloneous and spiculated) were the most difficult types to be properly detected.

**Table 2.** Coherent region detection results according to type of mass

| | |
|---|---|
| circumscribed | 96% |
| miscellaneous | 80% |
| spiculated | 73% |

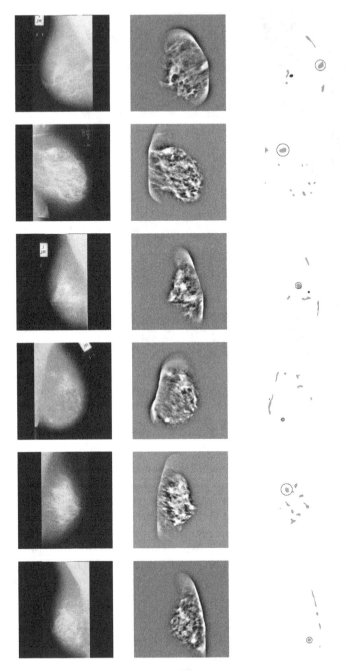

**Fig. 4.** Examples of results for detection of ill-defined (in the first three rows) and spiculated (in the last three rows) masses. From left to right: original, mass contrast enhancement and segmentation images. From top to bottom: fatty, fatty-glandular and dense-glandular breast tissue.

Table 3 compares the results obtained according to mass type and breast tissue. The easiest breast tissue to segment is the fatty, that produces black background in mammograms. In contrast, dense glandular is the most complex because appear as white regions and usually hide masses [7]. It is shown in Table 3 that the method got an acceptable efficiency for all type of breast tissue, even for the most difficult, the dense-glandular tissue. Also, it can be seen from this table that some masses that appear in mamograms with fatty breast tissue, were inappropriately detected by our method. This result may be explained by the fact that these masses are small (20-30 pixels in diameter), and some of them are located in the muscle pectoral border or surrounded by breast tissue with similar density.

**Table 3.** Coherent region detection results according to type of mass and breast tissue. The breast tissues are ordered from least to most complex.

|  | Fatty | Fatty-Glandular | Dense-Glandular |
|---|---|---|---|
| circumscribed | 92% | 100% | 100% |
| miscellaneous | 75% | 80% | 100% |
| spiculated | 80% | 71% | 71% |

We found that our average result for this experiment is comparable with the obtained by some detection works that used the MIAS database for testing. In Table 4 we compare our result with the obtained by Rojas & Nandi [11] and the two best methods (labelled as b1 and c2) evaluated by Oliver et al. [9]. From this table it can be seen that our sensitivity result outperformed all others. Although the false positives per image performance of our method was lower, it is acceptable.

On the other hand, when comparing our results for each type of mass with the two best methods evaluated by Oliver et al. [9], we noted that our method was the best in detection of circumscribe and ill-defined masses. Due to that b1 and c2 methods are based on gradient filter, they could detect the linear pattern

**Table 4.** Comparision of sensitivity at false positives per image of our approach with the obtained by other methods

| Our approach | 84.4% at 5.3 false positives per image |
|---|---|
| Method of Rojas & Nandi [11] | 80.0% at 2.3 false positives per image |
| b1 [9] | 79.0% at 4.1 false positives per image |
| c2 [9] | 80.6% at 3.8 false positives per image |

**Table 5.** Comparison of results for type of mass detection. The results show the sensivity of each method.

|  | circumscribed | ill-defined | spiculated |
|---|---|---|---|
| Our approach | 96.0% | 80.0% | 73.0% |
| b1 [9] | 86.5% | 65.4% | 76.2% |
| c2 [9] | 76.8% | 77.9% | 80.9% |

of spiculated masses, and it justify their superior performance with this kind of masses. This comparison is presented in Table 5.

## 5   Conclusions

A method for detection of masses in mammograms with a average performance of 84.4% has been presented. The preliminary results on circumscribed and ill-defined mass detection were presented. Although results for spiculated ones are shown, due to their characteristics, a special processing is required for them and is considered as future work. Our results are comparable with those obtained by other methods in the literature. It is important to note that this study focuses only in the part of segmentation, specifically in the identification of possible mass regions within all breast, determining if a region is a mass or normal tissue is also part of future work. In the segmentation, usually a lot of false positive regions are detected but they are discarded in a classification stage.

Refining the method for outlined mass margins, including automatic breast extraction process, are also being considered for future work.

**Acknowledgments.** Authors gratefully acknowledge funding from Mexican SEP (PROMEP program) research project PROMEP/103.5/12/4621.

## References

1. American College of Radiology, ACR: Breast Imaging Reporting and Data System BI-RADS, 4th edn. (2003)
2. Cheng, H., Shi, R.M., Hu, L., Cai, X., Du, H.: Approaches for automated detection and classification of masses in mammograms. Pattern Recognition 39(4), 646–668 (2006)
3. Gonzalez, R.C., Woods, R.E.: Digital Image Processing, 3rd edn. Prentice-Hall, Inc., Upper Saddle River (2006)
4. Kato, Z., Pong, T.C.: A Markov random field image segmentation model for color textured images. Image and Vision Computing (2006)
5. Knaul, F.M., Arreola-Ornelas, H., Lozano, R., Héctor, G.: México: Numeralia de cáncer de mama. Fundación Mexicana para la Salud (2011)
6. Li, H., Kallergi, M., Clarke, L., Jain, V., Clark, R.: Markov random field for tumor detection in digital mammography. IEEE Transactions on Medical Imaging 14(3), 565–576 (1995)
7. Malagelada, O.A.: Automatic mass segmentation in mammographic images. Ph.D. thesis, Universitat de Girona (2007)
8. Murphy, K.P.: Machine Learning: a Probabilistic Perspective. The MIT Press (2012)
9. Oliver, A., Freixenet, J., Martí, J., Pérez, E., Pont, J., Denton, R.E., Zwiggelaar, R.: A review of automatic mass detection and segmentation in mammographic images. Medical Image Analysis 14(2), 87–110 (2010)
10. Rasband, W.: J. National Intitutes of Health, USA, http://imagej.nih.gov/ij
11. Rojas, D.A., Nandi, K.A.: Detection of masses in mammograms via statistically based enhancement, multilevel-thresholding segmentation, and region selection. Computerized Medical Imaging and Graphics 32(4), 304–315 (2008)

12. Sampat, M., Markey, M., Bovik, A.: Computer-aided detection and diagnosis in mammography. In: Handbook of Image and Video Processing, ch.10.4, pp. 1195–1217. Elsevier Academic Press (2005)
13. Suckling, J.: The mammographic image analysis society digital mammogram database, http://peipa.essex.ac.uk/info/mias.html
14. Suliga, M., Deklerck, R., Nyssen, E.: Markov random field-based clustering applied to the segmentation of masses in digital mammograms. Computerized Medical Imaging and Graphics 32(6), 502–512 (2008),
    http://www.sciencedirect.com/science/article/pii/S0895611108000542

# A New Collection of Preprocessed Digital Mammograms

Juana Canul-Reich and Omar Trinidad Gutiérrez Méndez

División Académica de Informática y Sistemas (DAIS),
Universidad Juárez Autónoma de Tabasco (UJAT),
Cunduacán, Tabasco, Mexico
juana.canul@ujat.mx, omar.vpa@gmail.com

**Abstract.** We contribute with a publicly available repository of digital mammograms including both raw and preprocessed images. The study of mammographies is the most used and effective method to diagnose breast cancer. It is possible to improve quality of images for more accurate predictions of radiologists, by applying some preprocessing techniques. In this work we introduce a method for mammogram preprocessing. Our method includes the following processes: reduction of the work area, bit conversion, denoising using the adaptive median filter, contrast enhancement using histogram equalization, and image compression using histogram shrinking. Practical experiments were conducted on raw images in DICOM format from the Mammography Clinic at Hospital de Alta Especialidad Juan Graham Casasús located in Tabasco, Mexico. Results were evaluated by medical doctors.

**Keywords:** DICOM, mammogram database, reduction, bit conversion, denoising, contrast enhancement, preprocessing.

## 1 Introduction

Breast cancer is a serious health problem worldwide. It is the second most common type of cancer according to the World Health Organization [1]. Study of mammograms is the most effective and cheapest way to identify it in early stages. In Mexico, at least one in ten women could develop breast cancer [2]. There are similar numbers in Latin America. In these countries it is common to find radiologists using equipment of non-standard quality, which might lead to a number of false positives or false negatives in resultant diagnosis.

In order to improve diagnosis it is possible to modify the appearance of the image with image processing algorithms, however, before any of these algorithms could be applied it is highly recommendable to perform some preprocessing steps [3]. Preprocessing of mammograms is a classical problem in Computer Science, and yet an open field of research.

In this work we contribute with a new collection named Collection of Preprocessed Digital Mammograms (CPDM). All mammograms were collected from the Mammography Clinic at Hospital de Alta Especialidad Juan Graham Casasús located in Tabasco, Mexico. Each image underwent a hybrid preprocessing method

F. Castro, A. Gelbukh, and M. González (Eds.): MICAI 2013, Part I, LNAI 8265, pp. 570–581, 2013.

which is introduced here as well. The hybrid method is composed of five stages. Stage 1 focuses on the reduction of the work area. Stage 2 is an optional bit conversion. Stage 3 consists in image denoising. Stage 4 aims at contrast enhancement. Stage 5 looks for image compression. We used Matlab and the Image Processing Toolbox.

Original mammograms were all in DICOM format. DICOM stands for Digital Imaging and Communication in Medicine. It is a standard format for medical images created by American College of Radiology (ACR) in conjunction with National Electrical Manufacturers Association (NEMA) [4]. Each mammography study constitutes a case with four images minimum each, two for each breast.

The paper is organized as follows: a brief revision of related work is given in Section 2, description of CPDM is given in Section 3. Preprocessing method of each mammogram is described in Section 4. Section 5 exposes a discussion derived from our work, and Section 6 draws conclusions.

## 2    Related Work

Table 1 lists in order of release date some of the public mammographic databases. Information provided include name of the database, number of registered cases, number of images, view of the images either mediolateral oblique (MLO) or craniocaudal (CC), file format of images, and column named BIRADS indicates whether images in the database are classified under this standard.

Two well-known databases are the Mammographic Image Analysis Society Digital Mammogram Database (miniMIAS) [5] and the Digital Database for Screening Mammography (DDSM) [6]. Both databases contain screen-film mammographies, that is, images that were non-digital originally. All mammograms contained in miniMIAS are 8-bit images, all of them shown in MLO view only. DDSM is the biggest public database and the most highly cited in the literature. It contains images of 12 and 16 bits.

GPCalma [7] stands for Grid Platform for Computer Assisted Library for Mammography. It is a distributed database. It contains digitized images just as miniMIAS and DDSM do.

IRMA [8] stands for Image Retrieval in Medical Applications. It is an integration of some mammograms from four databases. One goal is to standardize the criteria for image classification based on tissue type and lesion description.

MIRaCLe [9] DB stands for Mammography Image reading for Radiologists' and Computers' Learning Database. It is a dynamic repository featuring an interface for querying the database. It is mainly used for radiologist training.

BancoWeb is a database created by Laboratório de Análise e Processamento de Imagens Médicas e Odontológicas (LAPIMO) [10]. The purpose of this work is to constitute itself as a resource for all interested in developing CAD systems.

MIDAS [11] stands for Mammographic Image Database for Automated Analysis. In addition to images, MIDAS provides genome sequence data. It allows users and developers to contribute in their research process.

Table 1. Some Public Mammographic Databases

| Name | No. cases | No. images | Views | File format | BIRADS |
|---|---|---|---|---|---|
| miniMIAS [5] | 161 | 322 | MLO | PGM | no |
| DDSM [6] | 2'620 | 10'480 | MLO & CC | LJPEG | yes |
| GPCalma [7] | 967 | 3'369 | MLO & CC | DICOM | no |
| IRMA [8] | Unknown | 10'509 | MLO & CC | Several | yes |
| MIRaCLe [9] | 196 | 204 | Unknown | Unknown | yes |
| BancoWeb [10] | 320 | 1'400 | MLO & CC | TIFF | yes |
| MIDAS [11] | 100 | 600 | MLO & CC | DICOM | yes |
| INbreast [12] | 115 | 410 | MLO & CC | DICOM | yes |

Recently, INbreast [12] was introduced. It contains full-field digital mammograms only. All images feature lesion location information. They provide a guideline to be considered for mammographic database construction.

# 3   Description of the Collection

## 3.1   Image Gathering

All mammograms were collected from the mammography clinic at Hospital Juan Graham Casasús located in Villahermosa, Tabasco, Mexico. We were granted access to each individual CD containing the mammogram study with the patient consent. All original mammograms were digital in DICOM format, which includes a file named DICOMDIR containing descriptive data on the location of files of the mammogram study. Thus, it allows for individual access to each image.

DICOM images were extracted from the CD. Private data such as patient identification was removed. Finally each image was made part of the collection in its original format.

## 3.2   Description of CPDM

CPDM holds a number of mammograms. CPDM constitutes itself as a source of medical images for use by the scientific community. It is publicly available. The collection includes both original and preprocessed images.

There is a card description associated to each mammogram which provides data of the patient such as birthday, date of study, sex, view of the image (CC - left and right, MLO - left and right) and BIRADS (Breast Imaging Report and Database System) classification. Patient identification information is omitted.

In the collection, each patient case is stored in a folder. A view for a mammogram is identified by the filename. For instance, the mediolateral oblique view for patient case 0001 is named 0001mlol.dcm. Table 2 shows an example of an image card information for this case.

**Table 2.** Example of an image card information

| # | Birthday | Date of study | BIRADS | View |
|---|----------|---------------|--------|------|
| 0001 | 1980-10-10 | 2011-07-21 | 4 | L-CC<br>R-CC<br>L-MLO<br>R-MLO |

The collection and source code used in this work can be found online at casi.ujat.mx/cpdm/index.html. Our goal is to increase the number of images and applications.

The total number of cases are 60, most of the cases have four images minimum corresponding to the four typical views of the breast. Some cases have more than four images.

## 4    Method for Preprocessing of Mammograms

Each mammogram in the collection was preprocessed using a hybrid method consisting of five stages as illustrated in Fig. 1.

### 4.1    Reduction of the Work Area

Original mammograms came with a wide dark empty area, which does not provide meaningful information to algorithms used in this work. The aim of reducing the work area is to get rid of this empty area as much as possible. The region of interest, in our case, the breast will be the main object contained in final images. Acceleration of processing time of algorithms as well as improvement of effectiveness in further stages are benefits derived from working on smaller areas. It is usual to perform this process as suggested in [13] and [14].

We applied a three-phase method based on [14] to accomplish this reduction: thresholding, object deletion, and automatic cutting. Fig. 2 shows each of these phases applied to a mammogram.

The first phase is thresholding whose aim is to separate the region of interest from the background. To achieve this, initially, the image is converted from *single precision* into *double precision*. The latter delivers more solid image border in the binarization process. Secondly, the value of thresholding for the image is calculated using a Matlab function called **graythresh** which implements method of Otsu [15]. Threshold value just calculated is used for pixel classification as

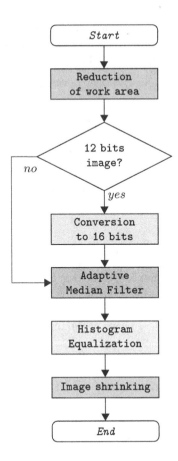

**Fig. 1.** Preprocessing method applied to each image in the collection

either 1 or 0. Third step is image binarization which is performed using a Matlab function called im2bw. Result of thresholding is shown in Fig. 2b.

Second phase is object deletion which consists of removing all small objects but the one of interest. For instance, Fig. 2b has a small label by the upper left corner which has been removed in Fig. 2c. What we actually do is to remove all objects with less than 10,000 pixels. We consider that a breast will never be of less than 10,000 pixels, and thus it will never accidentally be removed through this step. This process is performed using a Matlab function called bwareaopen.

Finally, automatic cutting phase consists of two steps. First step is to determine the location of the image border, which is accomplished with a Matlab function called bwboundaries. This function finds the boundaries of an object using the Moore-Neighbor tracing algorithm modified by Jacob's stopping criteria [16]. Borders are used to determine the extreme points of the breast, see Fig. 2d. Second step consists of cutting out the breast image using these extreme points, see Fig. 2e.

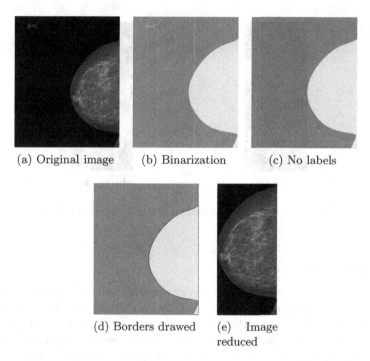

(a) Original image     (b) Binarization     (c) No labels

(d) Borders drawn     (e)  Image reduced

**Fig. 2.** Method for reduction of work area in a mammogram

## 4.2  Bit Conversion

All collected mammogram studies were obtained in the standard format DICOM. Mammograms in DICOM format are represented with 4096 gray scales, that is, these are 12-bit grayscale images [17]. Matlab represents these image matrices using 16 bits (65536 gray levels) [18]. When an image of 12-bits is displayed using a viewer of 16-bits, this just look like a dark squared area, see example in Fig. 3a. In order to correctly show the image it needs to be converted into a 16-bit image. We applied Eq. 1 to each value in the original image to get such conversion done.

$$\ell = \frac{2^n}{2^m}$$
$$c_{x,y} = i_{x,y} \times \ell,$$

(1)

where $\ell$ is a scalar value, $n$ is the number of bits in the target image, $m$ is the number of bits in the original image. The old matrix is represented with $i$ and the new one with $c$. $x$ and $y$ values refer to location of pixels in the matrices.

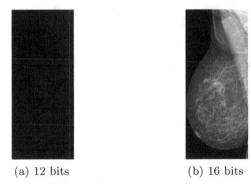

(a) 12 bits                    (b) 16 bits

**Fig. 3.** (a) original 12-bit image visualized in Matlab. (b) 16-bit image visualized in Matlab

### 4.3  Image Denoising

Noise is a kind of contamination images can acquire through the imaging process. It may be due to transmission errors, malfunctioning sensors, faulty memory locations, among other factors [19]. There are two types of noise usually present in mammograms, quantum and impulsive noise. In this work we focus our attention on removing impulsive noise from our mammograms as it is simpler.

The process for noise reduction is called denoising. It aims at preserving original image information after the process completes. We used the algorithm of Adaptive Median Filter (AMF) as implemented in [16].

The main idea of AMF is to remove noisy pixels, which are those surrounded by largely different pixel values in its neighborhood. As soon as AMF finds a noisy pixel it replaces it with the median value of its neighborhood, just as the Standard Median Filter (SMF) does. The difference between AMF and SMF is that in AMF no pixel replacement occurs if no noise is found.

The algorithm uses a window $w$ of $3 \times 3$ size that traverses the image. At each location, values for the minimum intensity $Zmin$, maximum intensity $Zmax$, and median intensity $Zmed$ are obtained. $Zxy$ is the center of $w$. $Smax$ is the maximum size $w$ can reach.

Algorithm AMF works in two levels, level A and level B. In *Level A* line 2 identifies an impulse $Zmed$ when condition evaluates to false. In this case, the size of $w$ increases (line 5) and level A is repeated while $w$ is less than or equal to its maximum size $Smax$ (line 6); otherwise, the central pixel $Zxy$ is changed to $Zmed$ which is the median of the pixels in the window $w$ (line 9).

True evaluation of condition in line 2 discards $Zmed$ as being an impulse; and the algorithm will continue with *Level B* (line 3).

In *Level B*, when the condition in line 11 evaluates to true, $Zxy$ is not an impulse, for which case the image remains the same (line 12); otherwise, the central pixel $Zxy$ is changed to $Zmed$ which is the median of the pixels in the window $w$ (line 14).

**Algorithm 1.** Adaptive median filtering algorithm as implemented in [16]

```
 1 Level A:
 2 if Zmin < Zmed < Zmax then
 3     go to Level B
 4 else
 5     increase the window size
 6     if w ≤ Smax then
 7         repeat Level A
 8     else
 9         output is Zmed
10 Level B:
11 if Zmin < Zxy < Zmax then
12     output is Zxy
13 else
14     output is Zmed
```

### 4.4 Contrast Enhancement via Histogram Equalization

The Global Histogram Equalization (GHE) is a technique used to redistribute the gray levels in an image. As a result, a contrast adjustment occurs, that is, low-contrast regions get more contrast and those with high contrast will experience a contrast decrease. A histogram equalization process applies a distribution function to make an adjustment in the data. GHE works on the entire image.

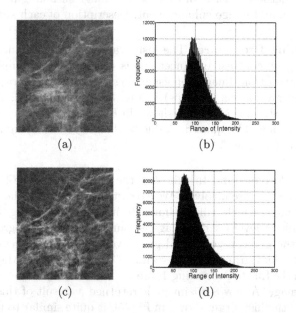

(a)          (b)

(c)          (d)

**Fig. 4.** Close-up of a mammogram. (a) Original lesion area, (b) histogram of (a), (c) same lesion area after CLAHE has been applied to it, (d) histogram of (c).

Pixel value distribution is not even throughout medical images. This is the reason why approaches based on Local Histogram Equalization (LHE) are more suitable for medical imaging. Local contrast enhancement is more important than global contrast enhancement in medical images [20].

The Adaptive Histogram Equalization (AHE) is an improved technique based on GHE. It consists in computing the histogram equalization for several regions in the image.

Contrast Limited Adaptive Histogram Equalization (CLAHE) is a special class of AHE. CLAHE limits the maximum contrast adjustment that can be made to any local histogram. This limitation is useful as the resultant image will not be too noisy [21].

In this work we used a function named `adapthisteq` [22] which is part of the Matlab Image Processing Toolbox. This function implements the CLAHE algorithm. Parameters of function `adapthisteq` can be setup with aid of radiologists. Final configuration would be applied to a specified area of the image. Fig. 4 shows an example of contrast enhancement using CLAHE.

### 4.5   Compression by Shrinking Histogram

This is the final phase in our method. It deals with image compression. A compressed image takes less time for transmission, processing, and less storage capacity. We applied a technique introduced by AbuBaker in [23] and [24]. It aims at compressing an image with minimal loss of quality.

The applied method consists of three steps: image shrinking procedure, pixel depth conversion, and image enhancement. Description of each step follows.

**Image Shrinking Procedure.** The histogram of image obtained either from image denoising or contrast enhancement is created. For example, Fig. 5a is the image obtained from image denoising. Fig. 5b is the histogram of image in Fig. 5a. Unused grey levels (or gaps) in Fig. 5b are eliminated. As a result, a right-skewed histogram is obtained, shown in Fig. 5c. A new image is generated from Fig. 5c, which will be quite dark due to the gray levels being located in the dark side section (see Fig. 5d).

**Pixel Depth Conversion.** In this step the goal is to reduce the size of the image. Three substeps are involved. We extract the histogram (shown in Fig. 6a) of the shrunk image, which will be similar to image shown in Fig. 5c. Then, the maximum shrinking level for the image is found based on histogram in Fig. 6a by computing the percentage of used gray levels (non-zero values) in the array representing the histogram. This percentage is input to the Matlab function `imadjust` from the Image Processing Toolbox. This function adjusts the intensity values in the image. A new 8-bit image is returned as result of this function.

The shape of the histogram shown in Fig. 5b is quite similar to the histogram of the resultant image shown in Fig. 6c. Peaks look the same, which indicates that the concentration of gray levels remains unchanged.

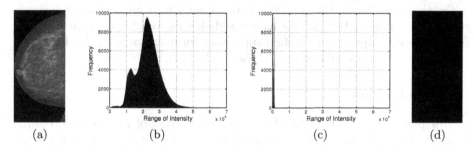

**Fig. 5.** Shrinking procedure. (a) original mammogram, (b) histogram of (a), (c) histogram shown in (b) after being shrunk, and (d) is the dark image generated from the shrunk histogram.

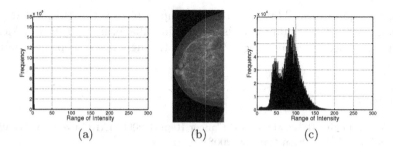

**Fig. 6.** (a) histogram generated from the dark mammogram shown in Fig. 5d, (b) 8-bit mammogram obtained from (a), (c) histogram of image (b), which is similar to histogram shown in Fig. 5b

**Enhancing Pixel Depth Conversion.** This step aims at improving brightness of the image obtained from pixel depth conversion. Afterwards, image conversion from 16 to 8 bits using an efficient coefficient takes place. Medical information carried by the image should be maintained. This final step is useful like a normalization process.

## 5   Discussion

Our repository includes preprocessed mammograms collected at Hospital de Alta Especialidad Juan Graham Casasús. We described each algorithm applied at each step of the preprocessing method. Regarding contrast enhancement where we applied CLAHE algorithm, we received help from a medical doctor who used a graphical user interface (GUI) we developed to setup input parameters of CLAHE for the image under experiment. The GUI enables us to observe the effect of diverse parameter values directly on the image. We used the set of parameter values for the image at its best look under the doctor's opinion. This is the step that needs to be completed for each image in the repository.

On the other hand, the location of the wound area on each mammogram remains incomplete. We plan on having radiologists working on it in the near future. The development of a system application for image consultation including search optimization would be part of the future work as well.

## 6    Conclusions

In this paper we have introduced CPDM, a collection of preprocessed digital mammograms. We described the method used for mammogram preprocessing, which is a combination of a number of algorithms. Obtaining medical resources to be offered as online material for research is always complicated. Main issue has to do with assuring to keep private information private, such as patient identification. Although the results obtained are good, further work can be done.

**Acknowledgements.** This research was supported by the Hospital de Alta Especialidad Juan Graham Casasús located in Villahermosa, Tabasco, Mexico. Funding was also obtained from PROMEP through research project number UJAT-CA-198.

## References

1. Boyle, P., Levin, B., et al.: World Cancer Report 2008. IARC Press, International Agency for Research on Cancer (2008)
2. Nacional de Estadística y Geografía (2008), http://www.inegi.org.mx
3. Ponraj, D.N., Jenifer, M.E., Poongodi, D.P., Manoharan, J.S.: A survey on the preprocessing techniques of mammogram for the detection of breast cancer. Journal of Emerging Trends in Computing and Information Sciences 2(12) (2011)
4. American College of Radiology, National Electrical Manufacturers Association, Digital Imaging and Communications in Medicine, http://medical.nema.org/standard.html (visited in August 2013)
5. Suckling: The mini-mias database of mammograms. In: Excerpta Medica. International Congress Series, vol. 1069, pp. 375–378 (1994)
6. Heath, M., Bowyer, K., Kopans, D., Moore, R., Kegelmeyer, P.: The digital database for screening mammography. In: Proceedings of the 5th International Workshop on Digital Mammography, pp. 212–218 (2000)
7. Lauria, A., Massafra, R., Tangaro, S.S., Bellotti, R., Fantacci, M., Delogu, P., Torres, E.L., Cerello, P., Fauci, F., Magro, R., Bottigli, U.: GPCALMA: an Italian mammographic database of digitized images for research. In: Astley, S.M., Brady, M., Rose, C., Zwiggelaar, R. (eds.) IWDM 2006. LNCS, vol. 4046, pp. 384–391. Springer, Heidelberg (2006)
8. Oliveira, J.E.E., Gueld, M.O., de A. Araúio, A., Ott, B., Deserno, T.M.: Toward a standard reference database for computer-aided mammography. In: vol. 6915, pp. 69151Y–69151Y-9 (2008)
9. Antoniou, Z.C., Giannakopoulou, G.P., Andreadis, I.I., Nikita, K.S., Ligomenides, P.A., Spyrou, G.M.: A web-accessible mammographic image database dedicated to combined training and evaluation of radiologists and machines. In: 9th International Conference on Information Technology and Applications in Biomedicine, ITAB 2009, pp. 1–4. IEEE (2009)

10. Matheus, B.R.N., Schiabel, H.: Online mammographic images database for development and comparison of CAD schemes. Journal of Digital Imaging 24(3), 500–506 (2011)
11. Fernandes, F., Bonifácio, R., Brasil, L., Guadagnin, R., Lamas, J.: Midas–mammographic image database for automated analysis. In: Mammography-Recent Advances, pp. 243–260. InTechOpen (2012)
12. Moreira, I.C., Amaral, I., Domingues, I., Cardoso, A., Cardoso, M.J., Cardoso, J.S.: Inbreast: toward a full-field digital mammographic database. Academic Radiology 19(2), 236–248 (2012)
13. Dehghani, S., Dezfooli, M.A.: A method for improve preprocessing images mammography. International Journal of Information and Education Technology 1(1) (2011)
14. Holguín, L.G.A., Álvarez, D., Guevara, M.L.: Pre-procesamiento de imágenes aplicadas a mamografías digitales. Scientia Et Technica (2006)
15. Otsu, N.: A threshold selection method from gray-level histograms. Automatica 11(285-296), 23–27 (1975)
16. Gonzalez, R.C.: Digital image processing using MATLAB, vol. 2. Pearson (2009)
17. Pianykh, O.S.: Digital Imaging and Communications in Medicine (DICOM): A practical introduction and survival guide. Springer (2011)
18. Mustra, M., Grgic, M., Delac, K.: Efficient presentation of DICOM mammography images using Matlab. In: 15th International Conference on Systems, Signals and Image Processing, IWSSIP 2008, pp. 13–16. IEEE (2008)
19. Motwani, M.C., Gadiya, M.C., Motwani, R.C., Harris Jr, F.C.: Survey of image denoising techniques. In: Proceedings of GSPX, Citeseer, pp. 27–30 (2004)
20. Mohan, S., Ravishankar, M.: Modified contrast limited adaptive histogram equalization based on local contrast enhancement for mammogram images. In: Das, V.V., Chaba, Y. (eds.) AIM/CCPE 2012. CCIS, vol. 296, pp. 397–403. Springer, Heidelberg (2013)
21. Pisano, E.D., Cole, E.B., Hemminger, B.M., Yaffe, M.J., Aylward, S.R., Maidment, A.D., Johnston, R.E., Williams, M.B., Niklason, L.T., Conant, E.F., et al.: Image processing algorithms for digital mammography: A pictorial essay. Radiographics 20(5), 1479–1491 (2000)
22. Zuiderveld, K.: Contrast limited adaptive histogram equalization. In: Graphics gems IV, pp. 474–485. Academic Press Professional, Inc. (1994)
23. AbuBaker, A.A., Qahwaji, R.S., Aqel, M.J., Saleh, M.H.: Mammogram image size reduction using 16-8 bit conversion technique. International Journal of Biological and Medical Sciences 2, 103–110 (2006)
24. AbuBaker, A.A., Qahwaji, R., Aqel, M.J., Al-Osta, H., Saleh, M.H.: Efficient pre-processing of USF and MIAS mammogram images. Journal of Computer Science 3(2), 67–75 (2007)

# Author Index